Vascular Surgery
Issues in Current Practice

Vascular Surgery
Issues in Current Practice

Edited by

Roger M. Greenhalgh, MA, MD, MChir, FRCS

Professor of Surgery
Charing Cross & Westminster Medical School
Department of Surgery
Charing Cross Hospital
London, England

Crawford W. Jamieson, MS, FRCS

Consultant Surgeon
St. Thomas' Hospital
Honorary Consultant Surgeon
St. Mary's and Hammersmith Hospitals
London, England

Andrew N. Nicolaides, MS, FRCS, FRCSE

Professor of Vascular Surgery, Honary Consultant Cardiovascular Surgeon,
Director, Irvine Laboratory
Irvine Laboratory for Cardiovascular Investigation and Research
St. Mary's Hospital Medical School
London, England

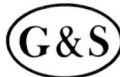

Grune & Stratton
Harcourt Brace Jovanovich, Publishers
London   Orlando   New York   San Diego   Boston
San Francisco   Tokyo   Sydney   Toronto

British Library Cataloguing in Publication Data

Vascular surgery: issues in current practice.
  1. Blood-vessels—Surgery
  I. Greenhalgh, Roger M. (Roger Malcolm)
  II. Jamieson, C. W.   III. Nicholaides, Andrew N.
  617′.413   RD598.5

  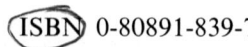 0-80891-839-7

Grune & Stratton, Ltd.
24/28 Oval Road
London   NW1 7DX

United States edition published by
Grune & Stratton, Inc.
Orlando, Florida   32887

Library of Congress Catalog Number 86-18353
International Standard Book Number 0-8089-1839-7
Printed in the United States of America
86 87 88 89   10 9 8 7 6 5 4 3 2 1

Contents

Contributors

BERNARD ALBAT
Aiguelongue Hospital
Montpellier, France

WILEY F. BARKER, MD, FACS
Professor of Surgery
University of California
Los Angeles, California, USA

KAREN BAXTER, SRN
Medical Lab Scientific Officer
Charing Cross Hospital
London, England

PETER R.F. BELL, MD, FRCS
Professor of Surgery
University of Leicester
Leicester, England

JOHN J. BERGAN, MD
Magerstadt Professor of Surgery
Chief, Division of Vascular Surgery
Northwestern University Medical
    School
Chicago, Illinois, USA

EUGENE F. BERNSTEIN, MD, PhD
Division of Vascular and Thoracic
    Surgery
Scripps Clinic and Research
    Foundation
La Jolla, California, USA

ALFRED BOLLINGER, MD
Professor and Head
Angiology Division
Department of Internal Medicine
Medical Policlinic
University Hospital
Zurich, Switzerland

ALLAN D. CALLOW, MD, PhD
Vascular Surgeon
Tufts University School of Medicine
New England Medical Center
Boston, Massachusetts, USA

T. CODDINGTON,
Senior Medical Officer
Department of Health and Social
    Security, Artificial Limb and Appli-
    ance Services

C. WILLIAM COLE, MD
Fellow in Vascular Surgery
University of California
School of Medicine
Los Angeles, California, USA

MARY PAULA COLGAN, MB
Vascular Research Fellow
Southern Illinois University
School of Medicine
Springfield, Illinois, USA

NATHAN P. COUCH, MD
Associate Professor of Surgery
Harvard Medical School
Brigham and Women's Hospital
Boston, Massachusetts, USA

SIMON G. DARKE, MD, FRCS
Consultant Surgeon
Royal Victoria Hospital
Bournemouth, Dorset, England

RICHARD H. DEAN, MD
Professor of Surgery
Head, Division of Vascular Surgery
Vanderbilt University School of
    Medicine
Nashville, Tennessee, USA

RALPH G. DePALMA, MD
Professor and Chairman
Department of Surgery
George Washington University
    Medical Center
Washington, D.C., USA

JOHN A. DORMANDY, FRCS
Consultant Vascular Surgeon
Department of Vascular Surgery
St. James' and St. George's Hospitals
London, England

A. DREW
Orthotist
Vascular Surgical Service
Charing Cross Hospital
London, England

H.J. DUNCAN, MB, BS
Department of Surgery
University of Adelaide
Adelaide, South Australia

WILLIAM K. EHRENFELD, MD
Professor of Surgery
Co-Chief, Vascular Surgery
University of California
San Francisco, California, USA

MARY ELLIS, BSc
Senior Medical Laboratory Scientific
    Officer
Charing Cross Hospital
London, England

I.B. FARIS, MD, FRACS
Department of Surgery
University of Adelaide
Adelaide, South Australia

MADELEINE R. FISHER, MD
Assistant Professor of Radiology
Northwestern University Medical
    School
Chicago, Illinois, USA

WILLIAM R. FLINN, MD
Assistant Professor of Surgery
Northwestern University Medical
    School
Chicago, Illinois, USA

PETER GLOVICZKI, MD
Fellow, Section of Vascular Surgery
Mayo Clinic
Department of Surgery
Mayo Graduate School of Medicine
Rochester, Minnesota, USA

ROGER M. GREENHALGH, MA,
MD, MChir, FRCS
Professor of Surgery
Charing Cross and Westminster
    Medical School
Department of Surgery
Charing Cross Hospital
London, England

JOERG DIETER GRUSS, MD
Head, Department of Vascular Surgery
Kurhessisches Diakonissenhaus
Kassel, Germany

J.T. HOBBS, MD, FRCS
Consultant Surgeon and Senior
    Lecturer
St. Mary's Hospital
London, England

LARRY H. HOLLIER, MD
Head, Section of Vascular Surgery
Mayo Clinic
Assistant Professor
Department of Surgery
Mayo Medical School and Mayo
    Graduate School
Rochester, Minnesota, USA

RUSSEL D. HULL, MBBS, Msc,
FRACP, FRCP(C), FACP, FCCP
Associate Professor
Department of Medicine
McMaster University
Chief of Medicine
Chedoke Division
Chedoke–McMaster Hospitals
Hamilton, Ontario, Canada

ANTHONY M. IMPARATO, MD
Professor of Surgery
Director, Division of Vascular Surgery
New York University Medical Center
New York, USA

CRAWFORD JAMIESON, MS,
    FRCS
Consultant Surgeon
St. Thomas' Hospital
Honorary Consultant Surgeon
St. Mary's and Hammersmith
    Hospitals
London, England

V.V. KAKKAR, FRCS, FRCSE
Professor of Surgical Science
Director of Thrombosis Unit
King's College School of Medicine and
    Dentistry
London, England

WALTER KOLTUN, MD
Research Fellow
Department of Surgery
Harvard Medical School
Brigham and Women's Hospital
Boston, Massachusetts, USA

DAVID A. KUMPE, MD
Associate Professor of Radiology
University of Colorado Health
    Sciences Center
Department of Surgery
Vascular Surgery Section
Denver, Colorado, USA

SUSAN LAING, MA, PhD
Research Fellow
Department of Surgery
Charing Cross Hospital
London, England

MAHIR S. MAHIR, FRCS(Ed)
Senior Surgical Research Fellow
Department of Vascular Surgery
St. James' Hospital
London, England

JOHN A. MANNICK, MD
Moseley Professor of Surgery
Harvard Medical School
Surgeon-in-Chief
Brigham and Women's Hospital
Boston, Massachusetts, USA

CLAIRE MARTIN,
Physiotherapist
Vascular Surgical Section
Charing Cross Hospital
London, England

WALTER J. McCARTHY III, MD
Associate in Surgery
Northwestern University Medical
    School
Chicago, Illinois, USA

C.N. McCOLLUM,
Senior Lecturer
Charing Cross and Westminster
Medical School
London, England

WESLEY S. MOORE, MD
Professor of Surgery
Chief, Section of Vascular Surgery
University of California
School of Medicine
Los Angeles, California, USA

PETER J. MORRIS, MA, PhD,
FRCS, FRCAS, FACS
Nuffield Professor of Surgery
Nuffield Department of Surgery
University of Oxford
John Radcliffe Hospital
Oxford, England

JOHN A. MURIE, MA, BSc, MD,
FRCS
Clinical Reader in Surgery
Nuffield Department of Surgery
University of Oxford
John Radcliffe Hospital
Oxford, England

ANDREW N. NICOLAIDES, MS,
FRCS, FRCSE
Professor of Vascular Surgery
Honary Consultant Cardiovascular
Surgeon
Director, Irvine Laboratory for
Cardiovascular Investigation and
Research
St. Mary's Hospital Medical School
London, England

STEVEN P. OKUHN, MD
Research Fellow in Vascular Surgery
University of California
San Francisco, California, USA

ANITA PATT, MD
Research Fellow
University of Colorado Health
    Sciences Center
Department of Surgery
Vascular Surgery Section
Denver, Colorado, USA

CHRISTINE A. PERSSON, MD
Resident-in-Training
University of Massachusetts Medical
    Center
Worcester, Massachusetts, USA

ALFRED V. PERSSON, MD
Chairman, Section of Peripheral
    Vascular Surgery
Director, Noninvasive Vascular
    Laboratory
Lahey Clinic Medical Center
Burlington, Massachusetts, USA

J.T. POWELL, MD, PhD
Lecturer
Department of Surgery and
Biochemistry
London, England

GARY E. RASKOB, BSc(Hons.),
MSc
Clinical Trial Specialist
Department of Medicine
McMaster University
Chedoke–McMaster Hospitals
Hamilton, Ontario, Canada

LINDA M. REILLY, MD
Assistant Professor of Surgery
Department of Surgery
Division of Vascular Surgery
University of California
San Francisco, California, USA

C. VAUGHAN RUCKLEY, MB, ChM,
FRCSE
Consultant Surgeon
Senior Lecturer in Clinical Surgery
Vascular Surgery Unit
The Royal Infirmary
Edinburgh, Scotland

ROBERT B. RUTHERFORD, MD
Professor of Surgery
University of Colorado Health
    Sciences Center
Department of Surgery
Vascular Surgery Section
Denver, Colorado, USA

A–MAJEED SALMASI, MD, PhD
Senior Research Fellow
Irvine Laboratory for Cardiovascular
    Investigation and Research
St. Mary's Hospital Medical School
London, England

TANSUKH N. SONECHA, MRCP, DTM&H
Senior Research Fellow
Irvine Laboratory for Cardiovascular
    Investigation and Research
St. Mary's Hospital Medical School
London, England

RONALD J. STONEY, MD, FACS
Professor of Surgery
Department of Surgery
Division of Vascular Surgery
University of California
San Francisco, California, USA

E. EUGENE STRANDNESS, Jr. MD
Head, Vascular Surgery Section
Seattle Veterans Administration
    Center
Professor of Surgery
University of Washington School of
    Medicine
Seattle, Washington, USA

DAVID S. SUMNER, MD
Professor of Surgery
Chief, Peripheral Vascular Service
Southern Illinois University
School of Medicine
Springfield, Illinois, USA

D.E.M. TAYLOR, MB, ChB, FRCS
Professor of Surgery
Royal College of Surgeons of England
London, England

JOHN TERBLANCHE, ChM, FRCS, FCS(SA)
Professor and Head
Department of Surgery
University of Cape Town and Groote
    Schuur Hospital
Cape Town, South Africa
Visiting Professor and Honorary
    Consultant Surgeon
Royal Free Hospital
London, England

ANDRÉ THEVENET, MD
Professor of Surgery
Aiguelongue Hospital
Montpellier, France

ROBERT L. VOGELZANG, MD
Assistant Professor of Radiology
Northwestern University Medical
    School
Chicago, Illinois, USA

J. WALLER
Prosthetist
Vascular Surgical Section
Charing Cross Hospital
London, England

JACQUELINE WALTON, BSc
Medical Laboratory Scientific Officer
Charing Cross Hospital
London, England

ANTHONY D. WHITTEMORE, MD
Assistant Professor of Surgery
Harvard Medical School
Brigham and Women's Hospital
Boston, Massachusetts, USA

JAMES S.T. YAO, MD, PhD
Professor of Surgery
Director, Blood Flow Laboratory
Northwestern University Medical
    School
Chicago, Illinois, USA

R. EUGENE ZIERLER, MD
Chief, Vascular Surgery Section
Seattle Veterans Administration
    Medical Center
Assistant Professor of Surgery
University of Washington School of
    Medicine
Seattle, Washington, USA

Introduction

This book has been published to coincide with the Second International Symposium in London in September 1986. As in the first International Vascular Symposium in 1981, a number of questions were raised and papers were submitted addressing these themes. On this occasion, speakers have been chosen to chair the appropriate session and who may give an invited commentary. Some of these speakers have been asked to produce a chapter so that it will be available to read at the Symposium. The authors had no opportunity to see the abstracts of the papers, and no attempt has been made to include material that will be delivered at the Symposium.

The book falls into five sections. In the first section, on risk factors and medical treatment, questions are posed which we feel should be considered, even though frequently our knowledge on these matters is much less than on technical and procedural matters. We recognise that the subject will advance yet further in a technical sense but that we must strive to understand the natural history of arterial disease in particular and constantly to ask ourselves what can be done by medical means of prevention in the community to limit the amount of surgery performed either now or in the future.

The second section, on investigation, represents an area in which perhaps the greatest advance has been made in the last five years. Non-invasive tests have been with us for some time, but the application of these tests to clinical practice lags behind the detailed knowledge of the test itself. Imaging techniques with Doppler B-mode Ultrasound and Duplex scanning have developed greatly since the First International Symposium. Digital subtraction angiography and CT scanning are now very much more widely available. We now recognise that coexistent lesions can be detected and that these are frequently asymptomatic and pose new questions of management. This area remains controversial. The detection of early subclinical disease is potentially important in the future and may herald a new wave of screening for arterial disease long before symptoms develop.

Section III addresses new trends in arterial reconstruction, asking questions concerning improvements in graft materials and, equally as important, reviewing the situations in which these graft materials are used to bypass arterial lesions. The test tube–built bioprosthesis of the future will certainly represent a major advance if the developmental problems can be overcome. Questions are asked addressing whether this is potentially the ideal graft for the future. The chapter questioning the influence of surgery on the risk of stroke is perhaps even more important now than five years ago. Presently, vascular surgeons are accustomed to neurologists organising multi-centre trials to test their arterial reconstructive procedures. The time has come when it may be inadequate merely to state how well our patients do after arterial recon-struction when controlled trials against medical treatment have not been performed.

Section IV is an array of special problems that confront the vascular surgeon and that have been identified by us to be ripe for discussion in 1986. Concerning the management of the amputee, for example, problems may be different in different parts of the world. Amputation services and rehabilitation programmes vary. It is perhaps timely to recognise that 80 percent of major amputations in the western world are caused by vascular disease; surely referring physicians should send their patients with ischaemic limbs to a vascular surgeon in the first instance. Not to do this will inevitably lead to a higher amputation rate in the community. If this approach requires that vascular surgical services be set up strategically across a country, then we vascular surgeons must state this quite clearly.

The final section concerns venous and pulmonary embolism problems, covering varicose veins, venous thrombosis, the post phlebitic limb, and venous reconstruc-tion. What becomes clear while reading these chapters is that fashions in the man-agement of venous thrombosis vary in different parts of the world and even in different parts of Europe. In Britain at the present time, acute deep vein thrombosis is seldom managed by surgical thrombectomy, but evidently this is not the case in Germany, Austria and central Europe. Such differences of fashion will make for admirable discussion in the Second International Vascular Symposium and it is hoped that this book, which will be available to all of the delegates, will be a useful companion at the time of the meeting and a record of current issues in vascular surgical practice.

R.M. Greenhalgh
C.W. Jamieson
A.N. Nicolaides

PART I

Risk Factors and Medical Treatment

John A. Dormandy
and Mahir S. Mahir

1

The Natural History of Peripheral Atheromatous Disease of Legs

INTRODUCTION

There are countless reports in the literature on the outcome of particular operations for the treatment of leg ischaemia. By contrast, relatively little has been published about the disease in terms of its prevalence in the population and its natural history in the vast majority of patients who never come to surgery. This neglect is undoubtedly due to the fact that atheromatous disease affecting the legs rarely, if ever, causes death directly. It is, however, an important cause of morbidity and identifies a group of patients who are at a very significant risk of death from the same disease affecting the vital circulations, although this may initially be asymptomatic.

PREVALENCE OF LEG ISCHAEMIA IN THE GENERAL POPULATION

There is very little information on the prevalence of asymptomatic arterial disease of the legs, although new data are available in Chapter 6. Widmer, Greensher, and Kannel showed that two-thirds of patients with proven arterial stenosis or occlusion reported no complaint on a questionnaire, and even after a detailed interview, one-third were symptom free.[1] This frequency of asymptomatic occlusion of peripheral arteries is quite comparable to autopsy studies of coronary arteries in which 30% of subjects with demonstrated occlusions had no symptoms prior to death.[2]

Table 1-1 summarises 11 published studies which looked at a random general population and observed the prevalence of symptoms of intermittent claudication. Some relied totally on questionnaires[3–7] while in others the presence of arterial disease was confirmed by an interview and examination,[1, 8–11] which in some

Table 1-1
Incidence and Prevalence of Intermittent Claudication in the General Population

First Author (Year of Publication)	Number of Subjects	Geographical Area	Total (%)		Age of Men At Observation	Men (%)		
			Men	Women		40–49 years	50–59 years	60–69 years
Widmer[1] (1964)	6400	Basle	0.8		15–64	0.6	4	3.8
Kannel[3] (1970)	4030	Framingham	1.8	1.2	30–74	0.3	0.5 (Age 55–64 years)	
Isacsson[11] (1972)	703	Malmo	1.1		55			
Richard[7] (1972)	3733	Paris	0.9		50–59	0.8	1.1	
Reid[4] (1974)	18,403	London	0.9		40–64	0.6	0.8	1.3
Bothing[5] (1976)	860	Moscow	6.9		50–54			
Bothing[5] (1976)	552	Berlin	3.4		50–54			
DeBacker[6] (1977)	8252	Belgium	1.4		40–59	0.8	2.3	
Hughson[9] (1978)	2925	Oxfordshire	2.2	1.2	40–69			
Reunanen[8] (1982)	10,962	Finland	2.1	1.8	30–59	1.9	4.6	
Widmer[10] (1985)	2630	Basle			>35	1.3 (Age 35–44 years)		6 (Age >65 years)

included noninvasive and invasive vascular tests.[1,10,11] In relation to the reliability of questionnaires, it is interesting that in the study by Isacsson[11] only one-third of the patients diagnosed as claudicants on the basis of the questionnaires proved to have true intermittent claudication and abnormal arterial flow when interviewed, carefully examined, and investigated. Widmer, Greensher, and Kannel[1] and Hughson, Mann, and Garrod[9] found a 30% false positive response to questionnaires. Kallero, investigating patients referred for symptoms suggestive of claudication, found that 38% had normal vascular tests.[12] Reunanen, Takkunen, and Aromaa, using clinical examination only, were able to confirm significant arterial insufficiency in only a third of men and a fifth of women with typical symptoms at interview.[8] Therefore, questionnaires, as the sole method of screening, tend to be unreliable. On balance, it would seem that false positive responses exceed the number of false negatives and therefore the prevalence of true intermittent claudication tends to be overestimated in studies which rely only on questionnaires for screening. This may account for the exceptionally high prevalence in the studies by Bothing and coworkers.[5] The reported prevalence will also depend on the population studied. For instance, the very low prevalence reported by Reid and coworkers[4] is probably related to the fact that their study population consisted of sedentary civil servants. Reunanen reported a higher prevalence among agricultural workers.[8] Taking these various factors into account when interpreting the figures in Table 1-1, it would seem that the prevalence of the symptomatic true claudication in men below the age of 50 is approximately 1–1.5%, rising rapidly with age with a 4–6% prevalence in the older age groups. The actual prevalence of atheromatous disease, much of it asymptomatic, is much higher.

INCIDENCE OF INTERMITTENT CLAUDICATION

Only in the Framingham[3] and Basle[10] studies were normal subjects followed over a period of years to determine the incidence of claudication. The 14 years' follow-up in the Framingham study probably gives the best indication of the risk of previously asymptomatic subjects developing claudication, although it is a questionnaire study. The incidence suddenly increases from 0.5% in men aged 50–59 to 3.8% in men aged 60–69 years. In the same population, the incidence of ischaemic strokes was about half and the incidence of ischaemic heart disease about four times that of claudication. In the Basle study[10] the diagnosis was based on careful examination as well as symptoms and the five-year incidence of occlusive peripheral arterial disease was 4% for the youngest (35–44 years) and 18% for the eldest group (over 65 years). However, only one-third of those with detectable disease had symptoms of intermittent claudication.

Apart from four studies,[1,3,8,9] only male populations were studied. However, in these four studies, there is surprisingly little difference in the prevalence and incidence between men and women, and the ratio of men to women is less than 2. In the Basle study,[10] there is no prevalence between men and women under the age of 40 years; above 40 the ratio becomes 1.6. In most of the studies looking at the disease at a later stage, the ratio of men to women is much higher, ranging from 3 to 13.[13–19] This would suggest that the prognosis of the local disease in women is much milder than in men. In the incidence of the disease, women lag behind men by about 10 years.[3] In both studies of the incidence of claudication, the incidence is found to increase in the presence of certain risk factors at entry. Widmer, Biland, and DaSilva showed that the incidence over a five-year follow-up was 2% in subjects free from risk factors against 11.4% in those with three risk factors present.[10] In the Framingham study, the presence of coronary artery disease increased the incidence of claudication 4.5 times.[3] As regards prevalence, the relative risk of having the disease in the presence of one risk factor is 3.1 and this increases to 22 in the presence of three risk factors.[9] The relative risk is 4–7 in the presence of coronary artery disease and 3–5.7 in the presence of diabetes mellitus.[8,9] The most important of all risk factors is smoking, where the risk of having the disease is increased nine times in patients who smoke more than 15 cigarettes a day.[9] There is controversy as to whether the prevalence of claudication is related to hypertension.[5,8,9] Other risk factors are thought to include high serum urate, cholesterol, triglyceride, and plasma fibrinogen.[8,9]

In summary, the available data suggest that the incidence and prevalence of intermittent claudication is much higher than generally suspected. In men over the age of 60 symptomatic claudication is about two to three times as common as diabetes mellitus, which is thought to be a common disease. The prevalence of asymptomatic atheromatous disease of the legs is even higher.

PROGRESS OF THE LOCAL DISEASE IN PATIENTS PRESENTING WITH INTERMITTENT CLAUDICATION

Traditionally, atheromatous disease of the legs has been regarded as falling in the specialist province of the vascular surgeon. Most reported series have therefore been concerned with the small proportion of claudicants referred to surgical departments. From the study by Hughson, Mann, and Garrod in Oxford[9] only 50% of the patients with claudication had consulted a doctor while in the study by Reid and coworkers[4] of over 18,000 subjects in London the comparable figure was only 10%. The vast majority of claudicants are never referred to a specialist centre. This must be partly due to the small number of angiologists, i.e., specialists concerned with the non-surgical treatment of leg ischaemia. Angiologists should be leading the investigation and management of the many patients complaining of intermittent claudication who are never referred to a vascular surgeon.

The classic study of the natural history of the claudicant was presented in the Hunterian lecture delivered by Bloor to the Royal College of Surgeons of England in 1960.[14] His account of approximately one and a half thousand patients presenting with claudication between 1947 and 1953 has probably not been bettered. He showed that during the first year after the onset of symptoms of claudication, only 10% became significantly worse.

Table 1-2 summarizes the data from eight studies which are not primarily surgical and therefore give the best approximation to what is likely to happen to the intermittent claudication of the average patient. Patients were followed for a maximum of 5–13 years from the time of presentation to a doctor. None of the subjects in the earlier series[14–16,18,20] had undergone arterial reconstruction, although lumbar sympathectomy was occasionally performed. There have been only

Table 1-2
Intermittent Claudication: Clinical Progress from
Presentation to a Doctor

First Author (Year of Publication)	Number of Patients	Follow-up (years)	Stable or Improved	Worse
LeFevre[16] (1959)	185	5	74.6	25.4
Bloor[14] (1961)	1476	4–10	71	29
Schadt[18] (1961)	362	9	93.3*	6.7*
Begg[20] (1962)	198	5–13	68.8	31.2
Taylor[15] (1962)	412	3–12	82.7	17.3
Ulrich[22] (1973)	304	0.6–6.4	75	25
Imparto[21] (1975)	104	0.5–8	79	21
Kallero[12] (1981)	193	8.5–11.5	78.8	21.1

* Survivors only.

three, relatively small, studies published in the last 20 years.[12,21,22] All the studies in Table 1-2 look at the outcome in all the patients who presented with intermittent claudication, except for the study by Schadt and coworkers[18] who looked at the progress in the survivors only and about 10% of the patients in their series had rest pain or severe symptoms at entry. Ulrich, Engell, and Siggaard-Andersen determined progress plethysmographically, and in claudicants more than half the extremities found to be normal at first examination had evidence of arterial obliterative changes at follow-up; thus unilateral disease soon becomes bilateral.[22] There is a remarkable general agreement that in approximately three-quarters of the patients the disease will symptomatically stabilise soon after its onset and only about a quarter will significantly deteriorate. Although symptomatically the prognosis is good, the underlying atheromatous disease almost certainly progresses with time.

Kallero followed nondiabetic claudicants over a period of 8.5–11.5 years and found that only 16% required arterial surgery.[12] The overall rate of reconstructive surgery in the Imparto and coworkers series was 21%, the proportion being more or less the same in the 79% who were stable or improved and the 21% who ultimately got worse.[21] In his review of reconstructive surgery in the Danish National Health Service, Eickhoff has found that only 9.6% of patients admitted to hospital for atherosclerotic disease of the lower limbs had reconstructive surgery.[23] Of over 2000 patients with chronic leg ischaemia referred to a vascular surgical unit in Sydney, only 22.6% required reconstructive arterial surgery.[24] The inappropriativeness of the surgical bias of most specialists dealing with this problem is emphasized by the fact that only between 10 and 22% of all claudicants presenting to a doctor came to any form of surgery. If on the basis of the studies by Hughson, Mann, and Garrod[9] and Reid and coworkers[4] it is assumed that only 10–50% of all claudicants consult a doctor then reconstructive surgery is only performed in 1–10% of all claudicants.

The incidence of amputation depends on the population studied and whether reconstructive operations were available at the time of the study (Table 1-3). In the two large general population epidemiological studies (group A), only 1.6[3] and 1.8%[10] of patients who had developed claudication came to amputation. In follow-up studies of patients referred to hospital before reconstructive arterial surgery was

Table 1-3
Chronic Leg Ischaemia: Incidence of Major Amputation

First Author (Year of Publication)	Number of Subjects	Follow-up (years)	Incidence of Amputation (%)
Group A. *General population screening*			
Kannel[3] (1970)	79	>14	1.6
Widmer[10] (1985)	239	7–15	1.8
Group B. *Early and nonoperative series*			
LeFevre[16] (1959)	185	5	11.9
Bloor[14] (1961)	1320	4–10	9.2
Schadt[18] (1961)	362	9	8.6
Begg[20] (1962)	198	5–13	5
Taylor[15] (1962)	412	3–12	10
Ulrich[22] (1973)	251	0.6–6.4	4
Imparto[21] (1975)	104	0.5–8	5.8
Kallero[12] (1981)	193	8.5–11.5	5.2
Group C. *Reconstructive surgery series (selected studies)*			
Hansteen[13] (1975)	307	8–16	3
Szilagyi[19] (1979)	531	0–15	24
Martinez[25] (1980)	376	3–13	4
Crawford[26] (1981)	949	0–25	6

widely established or in the early stage of the disease when arterial surgery was not indicated (group B) between 4 and 12% came to amputation.[12, 14–16, 18, 20–22] In all these studies the large majority of the patients only had claudication in the early stages of the disease. In the three later studies the amputation rate was near 5%, presumably because limb salvage surgery was more widely available. Group C compares a selection of more recent large surgical series and in three of these only 3–6% of patients ever came to amputation during the follow-up period.[13, 25, 26] In these surgical series only 75% of the patients at entry had intermittent claudication only; the rest had more severe manifestation of ischaemia.[13, 25, 26] The high amputation rate of 24% in the study by Szilagyi and coworkers can be explained at least partly by the fact that 75% of their patients had severe rest pain or more severe manifestation of the disease.[19]

Bad prognosis factors for limb survival include advanced age (above 65 years)[15] and distal vessel disease.[13, 25, 26] The amputation rate is about 2% in the absence of distal disease and 7% in its presence. The more severe the symptoms, the worse is the prognosis for the limb. An amputation rate of 3% in claudicants increases to 9% in those with rest pain,[25] while patients with severe claudication have an amputation rate more than three times that of mild claudication.[21] However, probably the most important risk factors are continuing smoking[17] and diabetes.[18] Jeurgens, Barker, and Hines showed, over a five-year follow-up, that none of the patients who stopped smoking at entry ever required an amputation, while 11.4% of those who continued smoking had a major amputation.[17] Diabetes increases the rate of major amputation almost five times,[18] and this again would explain the high incidence of amputation in the Szilagyi and coworkers series, where 55.4% of the patients were diabetic.

In summary the patient who newly develops intermittent claudication can therefore be cheered up by the knowledge that he has only a 25% chance of his symptoms continuing to deteriorate and only a 3–6% chance of ever requiring a major amputation. Unfortunately, part of the reason for this relatively optimistic outlook for the claudication itself is that most claudicants will die prematurely of atheromatous disease in a vital circulation.

NONFATAL CARDIAC AND CEREBROVASCULAR EVENTS

The apparent prevalence of coronary artery and cerebrovascular disease in patients presenting with atherosclerotic arterial disease of the lower limbs varies with the nature of the patients studied and the method of screening. In the Widmer, Biland, and DaSilva study of the incidence of claudicants in the general population, the total prevalence of coronary artery and cerebrovascular disease was 37% compared to 10% in an age-matched control group.[10] Table 1-4 summarises some of the other published studies on the prevalance of coronary artery disease in patients presenting with claudication. All but two[20,27] are surgical series.

The incidence of coronary artery disease depended on the method of screening. Most studies using clinical history and resting ECG for diagnosis showed a prevalence of 40–60% while in the Hertzer and coworker study,[28] using routine preoperative coronary angiography, coronary artery disease was detected in 90% of patients. It is interesting that in an earlier study by Hertzer, using clinical history and resting ECG alone, coronary artery disease was detected in only 47% of the patients.[29] In the remaining 53%, with negative clinical history and normal ECG, the 10-year survival was not significantly different from that in the general population and at five years the survival rates were almost identical. These results raise the question of whether we really need more sensitive tests than a resting ECG to detect significant coronary artery disease.

Table 1-4
Prevalence of Coronary Artery Disease at Presentation to a Doctor (Selected Studies)

First Author (Year of Publication)	Number of Patients	Method of Screening	Coronary Artery Disease (%)
Begg[20] (1962)	198	Clinical history + ECG	19
DeWeese[31] (1977)	103	Clinical history + ECG	34
Malone[30] (1977)	180	Clinical history + ECG	58
Hughson[27] (1978)	160	Clinical history + ECG	36
Szilagyi[19] (1979)	531	Clinical history + ECG	38.5
Crawford[26] (1981)	949	Clinical history + ECG	38
Hertzer[29] (1981)	256	Clinical history + ECG	47
Vecht[32] (1982)	100	Modified treadmill stress ECG	62
Hertzer[28] (1984)	381	Angiography	90
Brewster[33] (1985)	54	Dipyridamole stress–thallium imaging	63

Table 1-5 lists some selected studies of claudicants looking at the prevalence of concomitant cerebrovascular disease. Here again, the prevalence varies depending on the nature of the patient group and the method of screening. In the Begg and Richards study, which represents earlier nonoperative series relying on clinical history alone for the diagnosis of cerebrovascular disease, the prevalence is only 0.5%,[20] while in the Turnipseed, Berkoff, and Belzer series,[34] looking at a surgical group of patients using Doppler imaging, the prevalence of arterial disease is 52%. In the latter study, non-invasive testing showed that about half of the patients with cervical bruits had no significant carotid stenosis. Conversely, in the absence of clinical manifestation severe occlusive disease was shown to exist in 9% of the patients. More detailed review and discussion of the screening methods for the prevalence of concomitant coronary and cerebrovascular disease is discussed elsewhere, but it would seem that about half of all patients presenting with claudication have coronary artery disease detectable by simple clinical techniques, and a much lower proportion have cerebrovascular disease. It would therefore be interesting to quantify the chances of these patients developing symptomatic clinical evidence of myocardial or cerebral ischaemia.

Unfortunately, there are few data on the incidence of nonfatal myocardial infarction or cerebrovascular accidents in patients presenting with claudication. Bloor's study makes a general statement that nonfatal coronary and cerebral disease may have developed in at least 20% of claudicants still alive at five years.[14]

Table 1-6 lists the four studies with more detailed information on nonfatal myocardial and cerebrovascular events. The data of Kannel and coworkers[3] and DaSilva, Widmer, and Muller[35] are based on general population screening, while Begg and Richards[20] and Kallero[12] looked at patients referred to a specialist centre. In the Framingham epidemiological study over 14 years, subjects who developed claudication had a subsequent risk of developing nonfatal ischaemic heart disease almost two times higher in men and five times higher in women than those subjects who had not developed claudication.[3]

Table 1-5
Prevalence of Cerebrovascular Disease at Presentation to a
Doctor (Selected Studies)

First Author (Year of Publication)	Number of Patients	Method of Screening	Cerebro-vascular Diseases (%)
Begg[20] (1962)	198	Clinical history	0.5
DeWeese[31] (1977)	103	Clinical history	4
Malone[30] (1977)	180	Clinical history and clinical examination (including cervical bruit)	45
Hughson[27] (1978)	54	Clinical history	15
Szilagyi[19] (1979)	531	Clinical history ± angiography	13
Turnipseed[34] (1980)	160	Cervical bruit	44
		Noninvasive tests (Doppler)	52

Table 1-6
Incidence of Nonfatal Cardiac and Cerebrovascular
Complications

First Author (Year of Publication)	Number of Subjects	Follow-up (years)	Cardiac (%)	Cerebro-vascular (%)
Begg[20] (1962)	198	5–13	28.7	6.1
Kannel[3] (1970)	79	14	7.7	
DaSilva[35] (1985)	239	7–15	7.9	21
Kallero[36] (1985)	368	0.1–11.1	6.5	8

Kallero and coworkers showed that in their surgical series the incidence of nonfatal myocardial infarction was a half to a quarter of the incidence of fatal myocardial infarcts. By contrast the incidence of nonfatal cerebrovascular accidents was three to nine times the incidence of fatal strokes.[36]

DaSilva, Widmer, and Muller's study of early claudicants showed a similar inverse relationship between fatal and nonfatal events in the coronary and cerebral territories.[35] It is impossible to draw any definite conclusions about the incidence of nonfatal coronary and cerebrovascular events in claudicants from the presently available scanty data.

MORTALITY OF PATIENTS WITH CHRONIC LEG ISCHAEMIA

There is considerably better information on the incidence of fatal coronary or cerebrovascular events in claudicants. Table 1-7 summarises the results of three studies of newly developed claudicants (group A) and five nonsurgical studies of patients referred to hospital (group B). As usual, the majority of studies are surgical and the results in a selection of these is given (group C). Therefore, the patients studied in group C probably had more severe disease than a completely unselected group of claudicants. Considering the disparity in patient selection, there is a surprising degree of agreement about the overall mortality. After 5, 10, and 15 years of follow-up, the mean mortality rate in all the studies was approximately 30, 50, and 70% respectively. In nine of the studies the mortality in claudicants was compared to a parallel age and sex matched groups of the general population, who were not necessarily healthy and were only characterised by not having claudication. Figure 1-1 compares the survival of claudicants and the nonclaudicating general population in the nine studies. In the two studies by Eickhoff[37] and Bloor[14] the mortality rate has been calculated from the time of onset of claudication; in the other seven mortality is calculated from the time of presentation. In these seven studies the mortality of the claudicants was almost three times that of the general population after 10 years and almost twice as high at 15 years. Another way of looking at the data summarised in Fig. 1-1 is to conclude that the life expectancy of claudicants is about 10 years less than that of the general population.

The mortality can be further analysed in terms of coexisting risk factors. Probably the most important of these is smoking,[9] which in one study tripled the

Table 1-7
Total Mortality Rate

First Author (Year of Publication)	Number of Subjects	Follow-up (years)	Total Mortality Rate (%)						Cause of Death (as a percentage of total mortality)		
			5 Years		10 Years		15 Years				
			Patients	Matched Controls	Patients	Matched Controls	Patients	Matched Controls	Cardiac	Cerebro-vascular	Other Vascular Causes
Group A. General population screening											
Kannel[3] (1970)	79	14					M7.9 F4.1	2 1	48	9	13
Reunanen[8] (1982)	215	5	12.7	5.7					38		
Biland[38] (1985)	239	7–15			37	13			41	7	
Group B. Early and nonoperative series											
LeFevre[16] (1959)	500	5	43								
Bloor[14] (1961)	1476	4–10	21 28* 40	6.5 30	46 65* 80				60	17	8
Schadt[18] (1961)	362	9	24 46†		41 62†				63	12	6
Begg[20] (1962)	198	5–13	25.3	11	58.3	22			56	12	
Kallero[12] (1981)	193	8.5–11.5			48.7				35		7.6

Group C. *Reconstructive surgery series (selected studies)*

Study	n	Follow-up (yr)									
Hansteen[13] (1975)	307	8–16	30		50		63		50	17	13
DeWeese[31] (1977)	103	10	48		72				36‡	17	
Malone[30] (1977)	180	0–15	20	13	57	27	74	44	55	17	
Eickhoff[37] (1978)	144	10–20	29 / 15§		50 / 35§	18	70 / 56§	33	59	7	
Hughson[27] (1978)	160	5–8	M24¶ 52 / F14¶ 26	8 / 20 / 4 / 10							
Szilagyi[19] (1979)	531	0–15	56	5	75	8	94	10	57	15	3
Martinez[25] (1980)	376	3–13	21	10	52	20			46	7	
Crawford[26] (1981)	949	0–25	26		50		70		43	11	6
Hertzer[29] (1981)	256	6–11	20		40				55	7	5
Veith[40] (1981)	679	0–6	52								
Burnham[39] (1982)	415	15	30** / 30		45** / 70**		70** / 75**				
Schoop[41] (1982)	631	10	22	7	48	20 / 32 / 25					
Kallero[36] (1985)	368	0.1–11.1	M40 / F30	14 / 10	60 / 40				61	7	44

Note. M = men, F = women.
* Age groups 45–54, 55–64, and 65–74 years respectively.
† Presence or absence of diabetes mellitus.
‡ Myocardial infarction only.
§ From onset of claudication.
¶ Age groups 50–59 and 60–69 years.
** Aorto-iliac and femoro-popliteal bypass respectively.

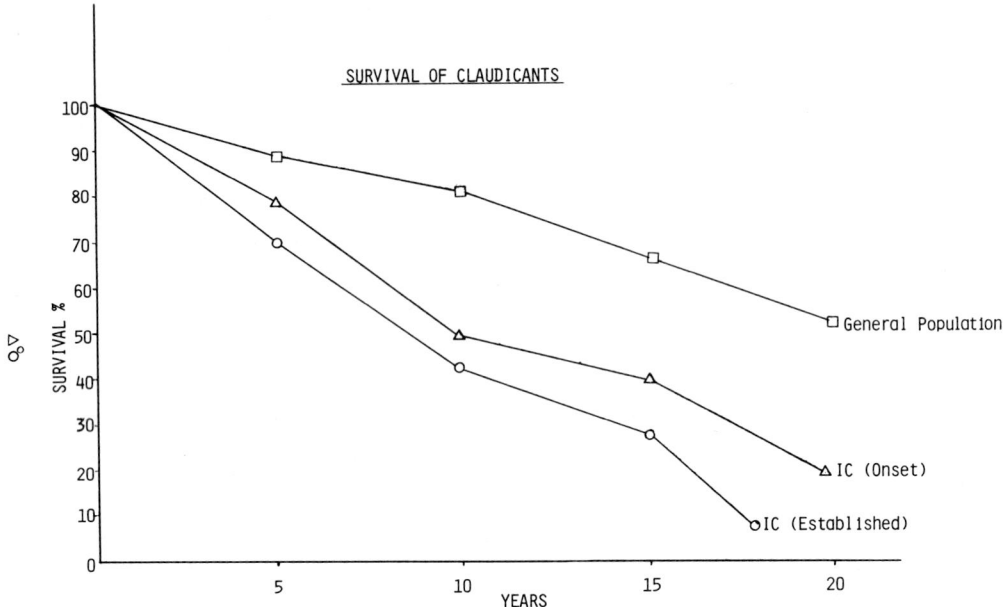

Fig. 1-1.   Survival of claudicants versus matched groups of general population.

mortality at 11 years.[38] The presence of diabetes is also of grave prognostic significance.[26, 29–31, 38] In Hertzer's study, about half of the nondiabetic patients survived 10 years but only one-third of the diabetics did so.[29] In the Malone, Moore, and Goldstone series the 10-year mortality rate in nondiabetics was about 50% compared to 100% in diabetics.[30] Hypertension has been shown to be an additional risk in three studies.[30, 31, 38] The presence of concomitant coronary or cerebrovascular disease is, as expected, a poor prognostic sign[26, 30, 31] and the five-year mortality in patients with associated coronary artery disease is three times that of patients with no evidence of coronary artery disease at entry.[26] In the Finnish study, the increased mortality in male claudicants seemed to be totally due to concomitant heart disease.[8] Analysis of the influence on mortality of the extent of the local disease in the legs is interesting. The presence of distal disease is a poor prognostic sign[25, 36, 37, 39] and the five-year mortality of men is doubled in the presence of popliteal trifurcation disease.[36] The mean survival of patients with aorto-iliac disease is 10.7 years compared to that of 7.2 years in patients with femoro-popliteal disease.[4] Severity of the symptoms and signs in the legs has been found to be one of the prognostic factors by DeWeese and Rob[31] and Crawford and coworkers[26] but not by Eickhoff.[37]

The importance of recognising the high mortality in claudicants was emphasised by Szilagyi in his analysis of the results of his surgical series. He found that after the fifth postoperative year, the annual mortality of the patients exceeded the annual rate of graft occlusion.[19] This not only suggests the possible need for reviewing the indications for surgery but also emphasises the need to concentrate as much on the prevention of the complications of atherosclerosis in other regions as on the prevention of graft occlusion, which is the traditional preoccupation of the vascular surgeon.

The analysis of the cause of death is rather surprising. In only about half of the cases was death thought to be due to myocardial ischaemia and in none of the 16 series was the incidence of cardiac death higher than 63%. The proportion of claudicants dying of cerebrovascular disease varied from 7 to 17% in the different series. In a surprising proportion of patients, approximately 10% on average in the different series, death was due to vascular events other than strokes or myocardial ischaemia. This group was composed mainly of ruptured aneurysms and visceral ischaemia.

CONCLUSIONS

Our present knowledge of the natural history of intermittent claudication is very incomplete, largely because of the lack of data on the majority of claudicants who never came to the attention of the vascular surgeon. Only the following very tentative conclusions, summarised in Fig. 1-2, can be drawn from the existing published evidence.

About 1.5% of men under 50 and 5% of men over 50 will have symptoms of leg ischaemia due to atheromatous disease. (The incidence in women is not much lower, but the disease seems to follow a more benign course.) In 75% of the men claudication will never become a very serious problem and no more than 5% are ever likely to require a major amputation. By contrast, the life expectancy of patients presenting with claudication is very much decreased due to atheromatous disease in other regions of the circulation. Compared to the general population, the claudicants' mortality is three times higher after 10 years and about two times higher at 15 years.

About 75% of the deaths will be due to atherosclerosis—50% in the coronaries, 15% in the cerebral region, and 10% in the abdomen. Patients with claudication,

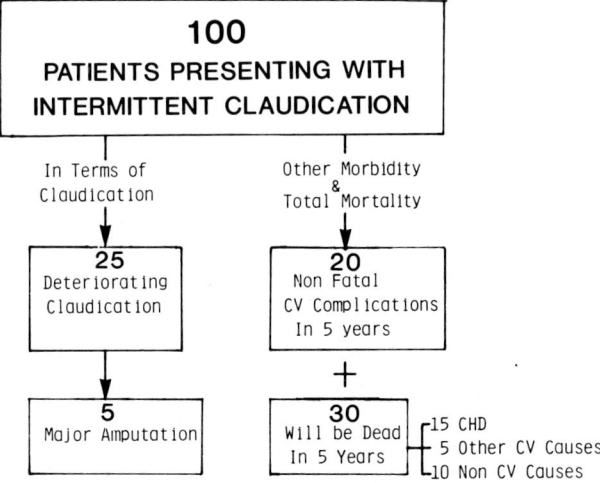

Fig. 1-2. Natural history of intermittent claudication.

even in the absence of other symptoms, are a very high risk group where active treatment aimed at modifying the progression and complications of atherosclerosis is particularly important.

REFERENCES

1. Widmer LK, Greensher A, Kannel WB: Occlusion of peripheral arteries—A study of 6400 working subjects. Circulation XXX:836, 1964
2. Allison RB, Rodriguez FL, Higgins EA, et al: Clinicopathologic correlations in coronary atherosclerosis. Four hundred and thirty patients studied with postmortem coronary angiography. Circulation XXVII:170, 1963
3. Kannel WB, Skinner JJ, Schwartz MJ, Shurtleff D: Intermittent claudication—Incidence in the Framingham study. Circulation XLI:875, 1970
4. Reid DD, Brett GJ, Hamilton PJS, et al: Cardiorespiratory disease and diabetes among middle aged male civil servants. Lancet i:469, 1974
5. Böthing S, Metelitsa VI, Barth W, et al: Prevalence of ischaemic heart disease, arterial hypertension and intermittent claudication and distribution of risk factors among middle-aged men in Moscow and Berlin. Cor Vasa 18:104, 1976
6. DeBacker G, Kornitzer M, Thilly C, Depoorter AM: The Belgian multifactor preventive trial in CVD. Design and methodology. Hart Bulletin 8:143, 1977
7. Richard JL, Ducimetiere P, Elgrishi I, Gelin J: Depistage par questionnaire le Linsuffisance coronarienne et de la claudication intermittente. Res Epid Med Soc Sante Pubique 20:735, 1972
8. Reunanen A, Takkunen H, Aromaa A: Prevalence of intermittent claudication and its effect on mortality. Acta Med Scand 211:249, 1982
9. Hughson WG, Mann JI, Garrod A: Intermittent claudication: Prevalence and risk factors. Br Med J 1:1379, 1978
10. Widmer LK, Biland L, DaSilva A: Risk profile and occlusive peripheral artery disease (OPAD), in Proceedings of the 13th International Congress of Angiology, Athens, 9–14 June 1985
11. Isacsson S: Venous occlusion plethysmography in 55 year old men—A population study in Malmo, Sweden. Acta Med Scand Suppl:537, 1972
12. Kallerö KS: Mortality and morbidity in patients with intermittent claudication as defined by venous occlusion plethysmography. A ten year follow up. J Chron Dis 34:455, 1981
13. Hansteen V, Lorentsen E, Sivertssen E, Bergan F: Long-term follow up of patients with peripheral arterial obliterations treated with arterial surgery. Acta Chir Scand 141:725, 1975
14. Bloor K: Natural history of arteriosclerosis of the lower extremities. Ann Roy Coll Surg Engl 28:36, 1961
15. Taylor GW, Calo AR: Atherosclerosis of arteries of lower limbs. Br Med J 1:507, 1962
16. LeFevre FA, Corbacioglu C, Humphries AW, DeWolfe VG: Management of arteriosclerosis obliterans of the extremities. JAMA 170:656, 1959
17. Jeurgens JL, Barker NW, Hines EA: Arteriosclerosis obliterans: Review of 520 cases with special reference to pathogenic and prognostic factors. Circulation XXI:188, 1960
18. Schadt DC, Hines EA, Jeurgens JL, Barker NW: Chronic atherosclerotic occlusion of the femoral artery. JAMA 175:937, 1961
19. Szilagyi DE, Hageman JH, Smith RF, et al: Autogenous vein grafting in femoropopliteal atherosclerosis: The limits of its effectiveness. Surgery 86:836, 1979
20. Begg TB, Richards RL: The prognosis of intermittent claudication. Scot Med J 7:341, 1962

21. Imparto AM, Kim G, Davidson T, Crowley JG: Intermittent claudication: Its natural course. Surgery 78:795, 1975

22. Ulrich J, Engell HC, Siggaard-Andersen J: A plethysmographic study of the spontaneous course of obliterative arterial disease in the lower leg. Scand J Clin Lab Invest 31 (Suppl 128):75, 1973

23. Eickhoff JH, Hansen HJB, Lorentzen JE: The effect of arterial reconstruction on lower limb amputation rate. Acta Chir Scand 502:181, 1980

24. McGrath MA, Graham AR, Hill DA, et al: The natural history of chronic leg ischaemia. World J Surg 7:314, 1983

25. Martinez BD, Hertzer NR, Beven EG: Influence of distal arterial occlusive disease on prognosis following aortobifemoral bypass. Surgery 88:795, 1980

26. Crawford ES, Bomberger RA, Glaeser DH, et al: Aortoiliac occlusive disease: Factors influencing survival and function following reconstructive operation over a twenty five year period. Surgery 90:1055, 1981

27. Hughson WG, Mann JI, Tibbs DJ, et al: Intermittent claudication: Factors determining outcome. Br Med J 1:1377, 1978

28. Hertzer NR, Beven EG, Young JR, et al: Coronary artery disease in peripheral vascular patients—A classification of 1000 coronary angiograms and results of surgical management. Ann Surg 199:223, 1984

29. Hertzer NR: Fatal myocardial infarction following lower extremity revascularization—Two hundred and seventy three patients followed six to eleven post-operative years. Ann Surg 193:492, 1981

30. Malone JM, Moore WS, Goldstone J: Life expectancy following aorto-femoral arterial grafting. Surgery 81:551, 1977

31. DeWeese JA, Rob CG: Autogenous venous grafts ten years later. Surgery 82:775, 1977

32. Vecht RJ, Nicolaides AN, Brandao E, et al: Resting and treadmill electrocardiographic findings in patients with intermittent claudication. Inter Angio 1:119, 1982

33. Brewster DC, Okada RD, Strauss HW, et al: Selection of patients for preoperative coronary angiography: Use of dipyridamol stress–thalium myocardial imaging. J Vasc Surg 2:504, 1985

34. Turnipseed WD, Berkoff HA, Belzer FO: Postoperative stroke in cardiac and peripheral vascular disease. Ann Surg 192:365, 1980

35. DaSilva A, Widmer LK, Muller HR: Cerebrovascular disease and occlusive peripheral artery disease (OPAD), in Proceedings of the 13th International Congress of Angiology, Athens, 9–14 June 1985

36. Kallero KS, Bergqvist D, Cederholm C, et al: Late mortality and morbidity after arterial reconstruction: The influence of arteriosclerosis in popliteal artery trifurcation. J Vasc Surg 2:541, 1985

37. Eickhoff JH: Survival after arterial reconstruction in arteriosclerosis obliterans of the lower limbs—Follow up after 10–20 years. Acta Chir Scand 144:17, 1978

38. Biland L, DaSilva A, Zemp E, Widmer LK: Occlusive peripheral artery disease (OPAD). Mortality and risk profile, in Proceedings of the 13th International Congress of Angiology, Athens, 9–14 June 1985

39. Burnham S, Johnson G, Gurri JA: Mortality risk for survivors of vascular reconstructive procedures. Surgery 92:1072, 1982

40. Veith FJ, Gupta SK, Samson RH, et al: Progress in limb salvage by reconstructive arterial surgery combined with new or improved adjunctive procedures. Ann Surg 194:386, 1981

41. Schoop W, Levy H: Lebenserwartung bei Mannern mit peripherer arterieller Verschlubkrankheit. Lebensversicherungsmedizin Heft 5:98, 1982

Wiley F. Barker

2

How Should We Prevent Progression of Atheroma?

The progression of atheroma should be considered under two headings: the problem as it pertains to the generalized process in the patient and the problem as it pertains to the recurrence of atheroma in the vessel upon which we have operated.

Much of the writing on the topic of management and prevention of human atherosclerosis in the medical literature is concerned with relatively common types of hyperlipidemia, and especially the congenital patterns, which are best described in the classifications of Frederickson and Levy.[1] Only type III and type IV forms have significant relationship to atherosclerosis, according to Buchwald.[2] Fogelman has offered a more practical classification which more conveniently fits with the patients seen by the vascular surgeon.[3] He divides hyperlipidemias into primary forms and secondary forms. The primary forms include those with a genetic component and those without (sporadic hyperlipidemias). The genetic forms are the polygenic forms in which an increased level of cholesterol and/or triglycerides occurs in a familial pattern, but the risk for atherosclerosis is not so great as in the polygenic forms, with an onset of disease which often occurs after the age of 60.

The monogenic forms include familial hypercholesterolemia, familial combined hyperlipidemia, familial hypertriglyceridemia, broad beta disease, and lipoprotein lipase deficiency. These disease forms account for no more than about 1% of the population, and because they often produce severe disease at an early age that is not amenable to surgery they will be considered no further here.

The patients with secondary hyperlipidemias represent the major problems and they include the diabetic patients who may have a hyperlipidemia caused by an overproduction phenomenon which is secondary to their disease; when these patients lose weight the defect tends to return toward normal. Subnormal lipoprotein lipase activity may be found in some diabetics who will benefit from treatment with insulin. In other circumstances, specific drugs may cause a hyperlipidemia, and this is amenable to cessation of the drug therapy.

VASCULAR SURGERY: ISSUES IN CURRENT PRACTICE
ISBN 0-8089-1839-7

The remainder of the population without specific forms of hyperlipidemia may also suffer from atherosclerotic disease, however, and it is the management of that group of patients that most concerns the vascular surgeon. There are few sadder situations than the patient who has undergone highly successful carotid or femoral artery surgery who shortly succumbs to myocardial ischemia from coronary atherosclerosis.

The nature of the disease in these patients is somewhat obscure; the majority of patients in a vascular surgical clinic are not grossly hyperlipidemic. Rather, their metabolic defect probably more closely involves the relatively low ratios of high-density lipoproteins (HDL) to low-density lipoproteins (LDL), a distortion which also occurs in the hyperlipidemic patients. Some agents or processes that seem to affect this ratio may be useful in therapy. Many of these agents or processes have come into use empirically, and their relationship to the atherosclerotic diathesis has been clarified only later. It has long been recognized, for instance, that there is a close relationship between arterial hypertension and accelerated atherosclerosis, and this is especially true when a hyperlipidemia is present.

The use of cigarettes has also been known to have an adverse effect, but the exact nature of that relationship is not clear. Seiffert has shown that rats who have been required to inhale cigarette smoke show spontaneous multicentric lesions in the arterial intima.[4] Greenhalgh has advocated the elimination of cigarette smoking on the basis of his experiences with failed reconstructions during the postoperative follow-up period, and found that the level of carboxyhemoglobin in the blood of failed reconstruction patients was significantly higher than that of successful bypass patients.[5]

Similarly, exercise has been advocated for the control or prevention of atherosclerosis, but the effects of exercise are not clear. Exercise may reduce symptoms and mortality from atherosclerotic disease, but this may be related more to the development of collateral circulation in response to demands on the heart and peripheral muscles than to any subtle metabolic effect. On the other hand, Fogelman[3] asserts that exercise decreases the VLDL (very low density lipoproteins) and LDL in some patients with hyperlipidemias, and raises the HDL levels in others—both effects are theoretically favorable. The effect on the patient with a relatively normal level of lipoproteins and only a modestly diminished HDL–LDL ratio is not clear, but is not likely to be unfavorable.

Dietary intake assumes a major role in therapy. It is very likely that the lipid abnormalities of the majority of the patients are simply related to the modern environment, including diet, tobacco, activity, stress, and the like. Weight reduction is essential in all forms of hyperlipidemia, and through many secondary mechanisms may be helpful in other patients. Regression of lesions may possibly occur under the severe dietary and exercise regimens but it is not a form of therapy that large numbers of patients will accept and remain compliant.

While a reduction in general caloric intake is probably the most important dietary maneuver, with that reduction should also go a reduction in the amount of saturated fatty acids in the diet. There is recent information suggesting that certain fish (especially salmon) oils contain a large amount of omega-3 fatty acids which tend to lower triglyceride levels and incidentally reduce platelet aggregation. Unfortunately the amount of fish one must eat to obtain the full effect becomes more than the usual patient can readily accept.

No matter how little dietary cholesteral is taken, the body can still manufacture cholesterol out of simple acetate radicals. This is fortunate, because cholesterol and its derivatives are essential in many of the critical functions of the body. Nonetheless, a reduction in the exogenous cholesterol is important because it is believed that "dietary" cholesterol alters the composition of HDL and causes it to behave like LDL.

Both estrogens and thyroid hormones have been implicated in the genesis of atherosclerosis on the basis of the recognized hypercholesterolemia and increased atherosclerosis seen in patients who do suffer from hyperthyroidism. The protective effect of estrogens on the female population is also a clinical observation, but the treatment of male atherosclerosis with estrogens has not had much popularity.

Diabetics are notoriously susceptible to atherosclerotic lesions, and the distal vessels of the lower limb especially concern the surgeon. Hyperlipidemias are common in diabetics because of the reasons outlined above, but in the past a large proportion of the diabetic's diet was composed of fats in order to avoid excessive carbohydrate intake. This dietary aberration should be avoided.

The use of alcohol has many considerations. In limited quantities alcohol increases HDL levels in most patients. There are exceptions to this statement, for in the type V hyperlipidemias, alcohol may act in just the reverse manner; however, type V patients are rarely a surgical consideration.

Control of hypertension by dietary, environmental, or pharmacologic means is advisable.

Many drugs have been advocated for the control of atherosclerosis. Niacin, which is needed in quantities 15–30 times as large as the dose, as a vitamin tends to produce a transitory inhibition of the mobilization of free fatty acids from fat tissue, a source for the hepatic production of VLDL. The effect is brief and there is a rebound phenomenon that may negate the transitory beneficial result. Furthermore, the drug is not easily tolerated in the large doses necessary for this metabolic effect.

Other agents that have been used include the cholestyramine and colestipol hydrochloride resins which bind bile acids in the gut, increasing their excretion and thus diminishing the cholesterol pool. Side effects of these agents make their protracted use difficult. Clofibrate has also been used to interfere with lipid metabolism at several points, but its overall effect has not been beneficial in prolonging life in hyperlipidemic patients. On the other hand, one new drug which may show promise is Mevinolin, a drug not yet released for general use in the United States. It inhibits the enzyme that regulates the biosynthesis of cholesterol.[6]

Fogelman puts these agents in perspective, however, when he states: "There is no evidence to prove that lowering plasma lipid levels by drug therapy will reduce the risk for atherosclerosis. Therefore, we reserve these agents for persons who have failed to normalize their lipid levels on diet alone and who are at high risk for premature atherosclerosis."[3] This statement takes the onus for complicated medical management from the shoulders of the surgeon and places it on those of the internist who should be his consultant in the management of the special patients at usual risk.

This section cannot be ended, however, without mention of two surgical procedures, neither of which is necessarily useful in the usual patient, but each of which may have special application.

In 1967, Buchwald described the use of distal intestinal bypass as an experimental attempt to alter the whole blood cholesterol in the rabbit,[7] and has since treated a large number of patients using this operation. His reported mortality in these high-risk patients, many of whom had prior myocardial infarcts, was less than 1%. The procedure consists of blind-end bypass of the terminal 200 cm or the distal one-third of the small intestine (whichever is greater), with the open distal end of the blind loop sutured into the cecum about 2 inches above the appendiceal stump. Scott has summarized the experimental and clinical background of this work.[8]

The other operation is the standard portacaval anastomosis which Starzl[9] applied to patients with type I glycogenosis (glucose-6-phosphatase deficiency). These patients also exhibited hyperlipidemia, which was greatly relieved by the operation. The operation was applied thereafter to a patient with homozygous type II hyperlipidemia. More than 30 patients have had portacaval shunt for this disorder with dramatic lowering of the cholesterol levels.[9] The physiologic effects of this procedure are not so well understood as to allow its performance except in centers in which careful protocols can be followed.

THE PREVENTION OF RECURRENCE OF ATHEROMA FOLLOWING ARTERIAL RECONSTRUCTION

The relative pessimism which the author has expressed with regard to the general management of atherosclerosis applies to a somewhat lesser degree to the management of the recurrent atherosclerosis.

In the earliest days of reconstructive vascular surgery patients were often told that since they had taken half a century to acquire the lesion in question, operative removal should give them another half a century of relief. That prognosis soon proved to be sadly wrong. In 1971 Szilagyi's presidential address to the North American Chapter of the International Cardiovascular Society in which he discussed the durability of aorto-iliac endarterectomy really demonstrated the lack of durability in his hands of the operation.[10] At about the same time the author had observed some unusually variable results in a specific group of 12 patients operated upon at the University of California at Los Angeles during a brief period. These patients showed most favorable anatomical prospects for a long-lasting successful aorto-iliac endarterectomy; they exhibited short terminal aortic and proximal iliac occlusions, with no evidence of disease in other sites, and strongly palpable pulses were present immediately after operation. On review of the records of these 12 patients it was found that there had been a variation in the amount of heparin which had been used, suggesting that the use of heparin was associated with the long survival without recurrent atherosclerosis. Most patients at the University of California at that time received 20,000–24,000 units of heparin a day for a week to 10 days after operation, but with increasing familiarity and possibly contempt for the established practice, some of the resident staff began to omit the use of postoperative heparin. Thus it was found that among the 12 patients there were eight patients who promptly showed recurrence and reaccumulation of atheroma, and whose lesions had the same appearance as those reported by Szilagyi. Five of these patients had had no heparin used at all, and three had had only very small doses for a day or two. On the other hand, the four patients who received full (or in one case intermediate) doses of heparin remained entirely free of atheroma in the site of operation (one for 14 years), although the general status of their atherosclerotic diathesis was manifest by occurrence of significant arterial obstructions in distant sites.[11]

In the earliest endarterectomies, heparin had been used by us as well as by many other surgeons postoperatively in an attempt to control thrombosis. In 1956 we had performed anatomical studies[12] that had shown that in the presence of heparin a new layer of endothelium was promptly (48 hours) laid down upon a bare medial wall after endarterectomy of the canine aorta. Without heparin, a thick layer of fibrous scar formed which required many weeks for complete endothelization. Comparable observations were made as well upon the scanty human material available. Review of that pathological material suggests the lesion seen was partly organizing thrombus, but it is hard to distinguish by light microscopy alone some of the material from myointimal fibroplasia. From a clinical point of view, however, the pragmatic answer was that the postoperative use of heparin was of no great value in preventing acute failures of the operation, and many surgeons experienced serious problems with hemostasis which led to its abandonment. Parenthetically, the author's experience indicated that there were no more hematomas either in absolute numbers or in severity when heparin was used.

Sabiston's work agreed with our concepts concerning the origin of the endothelial coverage in both prosthetic grafts and endarterectomies.[13]

Szilagyi's observations and the 12 patients mentioned above suggested laboratory experiments to us. Hyperlipidemic rabbits were found to heal endarterectomies with minimal fibrous thickening under the influence of heparin, whereas without heparin the recurrence of florid atheroma would nearly completely obstruct the iliac artery in 5–10 weeks.[14] Pilcher repeated similar rabbit experiments.[15] The beneficial effect was attributed to the lipid-lowering effect of heparin, but dextran was just as effective. Beyond this, however, it was also shown by these authors that if healing was allowed to progress for three to five weeks and then hyperlipidemia was induced, the relatively mature endothelium could by that time resist the hyperlipidemia and remain free of fat and cellular hypertrophy.

In retrospect, it is likely that the effect on platelet aggregation of these weak agents was at least as much responsible. The above unsophisticated and early experiments have some substantiation in the more carefully controlled work in the literature.

Subsequently, Ross and Glomsett reviewed the theories of atherogenesis and implicated the platelet as an agent which adhered to the site of an endothelial injury and could produce a mitogenic stimulus resulting in overgrowth of myointimal cells at that site. The first lesion to appear was a highly cellular one, consistent with which is now commonly recognized as myointimal fibroplasia. In the presence of hyperlipidemia, however, the hyperplastic lesion was apt to absorb lipids and become a typical atherosclerotic lesion.[16] To date, however, no consistent patterns proving clinical benefit from antiplatelet drugs other than heparin and dextran have been published.

Clinical surgical descriptions of similar processes have been made by many authors, including Cossman,[17] Gryska,[18] Imparato,[19] Sabiston,[20] Stephenson,[21] and Stoney.[22,23] Indeed, the bibliographic references concerning this aspect of the subject could fill this entire chapter.

The above discussion of healing of an endarterectomy has possible pertinence to the recurrence of atheroma, or of myointimal fibroplasia, at the site of any arterial wound. This becomes apparent at the suture lines joining plastic prosthetic material, or even homologous prostheses to the donor artery, for even a simple arteriotomy in the hyperlipidemic rabbit heals with an exuberant plaque of atheroma.[14]

Small's work indicates that the insoluble end-point of lipid metabolism in the atheromatous lesion is crystalline cholesterol; once it appears, it is almost impossible to mobilize it, and its soluble esters may be in the cell for some time prior to the appearance of grossly visible cholesterol.[24]

There is probably more than just the role of the lipids in this process, however. The initial concept expressed by Wylie[25] concerning the healing of an endarterectomy was that circulating monocytic "stem-cells" differentiated into the endothelium. Our observations[12] led us to believe that the endothelial cells appeared as a proliferating pannus at the edge of the endarterectomy as well as from the orifices of vasa vasorum. Poole's work,[13] as well as the studies by Mosely with electron microscopy,[26] agreed with that conclusion. Many other authors, however, have shown evidence that a circulating cell is the source of some of the endothelium. Lazzarini-Robertson showed that the endothelial cells lining an endarterectomy in male dogs who received transfusions from female donors belonged to the female donor.[27] Jordan suspended a fragment of gelatin-impregnated sponge in the arch of the aorta of a pig and found that all of the cellular elements of the arterial wall were soon represented in the cellular material that appeared in the Dacron;[28] and Kennedy showed that the endothelium in heart transplants that developed secondary atherosclerosis was derived from a biological source other than the original heart.[29] Lazzarini-Robertson suggested a difference between true intima and the pseudointima based on his observations of the difference in morphology and the apparent difference in susceptibility to atheroma.[30] He believed that by tissue culture of material obtained both at autopsy and at the time of reconstructive surgery he could identify two types of cells from the intima. Cyto-I cells are very active cells in a metabolic sense which take up lipids readily. Cyto-II cells are spindle-shaped cells with specific morphological differences which are much less active and are reluctant to take up lipids at the same lipid concentrations. Both strains of these cells were derived from the same sources. This study suggests a preview of the Benditts' monoclonal theory of smooth muscle cells and their differential participation in the formation of atheroma.[31]

In the first of several studies which have been published concerning the evolution of clot in thread in an arterial channel, Still placed a suture in the lumen of a rat carotid and saw the following sequence.[32] Platelets arrived and their disintegration paralleled the formation of fibrin. Mononuclear cells on the surface of the fibrin clot suggested the appearance of "pseudoepithelium." By the time six or eight days had passed the surface of the clot was covered with flat endothelial cells with what appeared to be granulation tissue beneath them. He also noted that at times platelets appeared to adhere to normal endothelium and that the endothelium thereafter disintegrated. This opens the question as to whether the schema of Ross and Glomsett[16] is correct—do the platelets cluster at the site of injured endothelium or do they adhere and cause that injury? This phenomenon of endothelial necrosis and repair has also been discussed by Wesolowski with regard to the lining of Dacron prostheses.[33]

In a clot which formed in a rabbit aorta after ligation Ts'ao found a migration of myointimal cells and believed that he could identify their conversion to either foam cells or to endothelial cells.[34] In his preparations are endothelial cells with concentrated patches of myofibrils which he suggests are recent "arrivals" undergoing differentiation in their final anatomic destination. Poole's 1971 study using light microscopy alone to follow the evolution of the clot on a suture in the rat aorta saw a sequence of healing in which thrombus with polymorphonuclear cells first arrived at the site of injury.[35] The polymorphonuclear cells soon became pycnotic and were replaced by healthy appearing monocytic cells which functioned as macrophages. New endothelium was seen as early as three days. It appeared that the macrophages were derived from their bloodstream, and they ingested the platelets at the site of their deposition. No new macrophages were recruited after the seven-day mark. It appeared that smooth muscle cells underwent "dedifferentiation" and migrated from a source in the media below. These observations by light microscopy should be confirmed by electron microscopy in order to purify the understanding of the cellular pedigree.

The different cell types may thus have different susceptibilities to blood lipids; from our experience one might hypothesize that the first layer of cells laid down so promptly not only protect against the deposition of mitogenic platelet accumulations but are also in themselves resistant to lipids. Cells of other pedigrees, from either the deeper layers of the arterial wall or from primitive circulating stem cells, may be the villains in primary atherosclerosis, and may be the source of secondary atherosclerotic changes as well.

A recent study in which endothelial protection was observed after the vein graft had been treated with alpha-methylprednisolone suggests another method of avoiding the cataract of changes described in previous pages.[36]

There are clues as to the localization of the atheromatous process as well. Texon has long been an advocate of a mechanical aspect to the localization of these lesions, especially at the bifurcation of vessels.[37] The usual human aortic bifurcation is not ideal from a hemodynamic point of view. In order to have no lessening of volume flow past a bifurcation, the sum of the cross-sectional areas of the limbs of the bifurcation should be 1.414 times the area of the parent vessel.[38] Since the early observations by Leriche,[39] and even the even earlier ones of Barth,[40] it has been observed that it was common to find the iliac branches much smaller than the expected aorta, and a ratio of 1:1.2 is not uncommon. Such a pattern implies an increase in the velocity of flow and an exchange of energy at the level of the arterial wall which could account for the aggregation of platelets and initiation of the atheromatous lesion. This might also have a practical application in human aortic surgery; reconstruction of an abnormal aortic bifurcation in the exact but incorrect hemodynamic pattern that it had originally may only be tempting prompt atherosclerotic recurrence.

Much study of human material by morphologic and histochemical methods will be required to answer the questions raised by this hypothesis and improve the management of our patients. There may be an infinite number of other tracks to follow. The majority of accepted studies in the literature deal with animal models which may not accurately reflect the human situation. Since in the United States alone there were 95,000 carotid endarterectomies performed in the year 1983,[41] and since it is anticipated that at least 5% will show a recurrence, it would appear that there should be abundant material available for the dedicated pathologist to pursue some of these studies in the human model, albeit that the human model may not have the precise controls and conveniences of some irrelevant animal models.

The role of tobacco appears important to most practicing surgeons and yet there has been little evidence that its use promotes the rate of atherosclerotic recurrence, except for the laboratory model of Seiffert[4] and the work of Greenhalgh.[5] Greenhalgh and others have gone so far as to recommend that patients who refuse to stop smoking be denied elective operation.

To the author it would appear that the best way to prevent recurrence of atherosclerosis in our patients consists of dietary restriction with regard to calories and cholesterol content, specific therapy for specific forms of hyperlipidemia, control of smoking and hypertension, and the protection of the healing artery by means of postoperative dextran and heparin, in appropriate sequence. It is hoped that the Symposium in London in 1986 will provide significant information better than that which we have at hand today.

REFERENCES

1. Frederickson DS, Levy RI: Familial hyperlipoproteinemia, in Stanbury JB, Wyngaarden JB, Frederickson DS (eds): The Metabolic Basis of Inherited Disease. New York, McGraw-Hill, 1972, pp 545–614
2. Buchwald H: The lipid clinic concept. Hosp Practice 5:119, 1970
3. Fogelman AM, Edwards PA, Haberland ME: Atherosclerosis: Pathology, pathogenesis, and medical management, in Moore WS (ed): Vascular Surgery: A Comprehensive Review. New York, Grune and Stratton, 1983, pp 45–52
4. Seiffert GF, Keown K, Moores WS: Pathologic effect of tobacco smoke inhalation on arterial intima. Surgical Forum 32:333, 1981
5. Greenhalgh RM, Laing SP, Cole PV, Taylor GW: Smoking and arterial reconstruction. Br J Surg 68:605, 1981
6. Fogelman AM: Atherosclerosis; Pathology, pathogenesis and medical management, in Moore WE (ed): Vascular Surgery: A Comprehensive Review 2 ed. New York, Grune and Stratton, 1986
7. Buchwald H, Moore RB, Varco RL: Ten year's clinical experience with partial ilial bypass in the management of the hyperlipidemias. Ann Surg 180:384, 1974
8. Scott HW Jr: Ilieal bypass in the control of hyperlipidemia and atherosclerosis. Arch Surg 113:62, 1978
9. Starzl TE, Putnam CW, Koep LJ: Portacaval shunt and hyperlipidemia. Arch Surg 62:71, 1978
10. Szilagyi DE, Smith RF, Whitney DG: The durability of aortoiliac endarterectomy: A roentgenologic and pathologic study of late recurrence. Arch Surg 89:827, 1964
11. Barker WF: Peripheral Arterial Disease 2 ed. Philadelphia, WB Saunders, 1975, p 155
12. Barker WF, Cannon JA, Zeldis LG, Ah-Tye P: Anatomical results of endarterectomy. Surgical Forum 6:266, 1956
13. Poole JCF, Sabiston DC Jr, Florey HW, Allison PR: Growth of endothelium in arterial prosthetic grafts and following endarterectomy. Surgical Forum 13:225, 1962
14. Barker WF, Barakonski A: The use of heparin and dextran in arterial reconstruction. Acta Chir Scand Suppl 387:97, 1968
15. Pilcher DB, Barker WF: Retardation of experimental atherosclerosis in endarterectomized arteries by the administration of dextran and heparin. Am J Surg 120:270, 1971
16. Ross R, Glomsett JA: The pathogenesis of atherosclerosis. N Engl J Med 295:309, 1976. Ibid 295:420, 1976
17. Cossman D, Callow AD, Stein A, Matsumoto G: Early restenosis after carotid endarterectomy. Arch Surg 113:275, 1978

18. Gryska PF: The development of atheroma in arteries subjected to experimental thromboendarterectomy. Surgery 45:655, 1959
19. Imparato AM: In discussion of Stoney RJ, String ST: Recurrent carotid stenosis. Surgery 80:705, 1976
20. Sabiston DC, Gutelius J, Vasko JS: Evaluation of endarterectomy in the presence of experimental hypercholesterolemia and atherosclerosis. Surgery 48:894, 1960
21. Stephenson SE Jr, Mann GV, Younger R, Scott HW Jr: Factors influencing the segmental deposition of atheromatous material. Arch Surg 84:49, 1962
22. Stoney RJ, String ST: Recurrent carotid stenosis. Surgery 80:705, 1976
23. Rapp JH, Qvarfordt P, Krupski WC, Ehrenfeld WK, Stoney RJ: Hypercholesterolemia and early restenosis after carotid endarterectomy. Presented at the Western Vascular Society, Laguna Nigel, California, 23–26 January 1986
24. Small DM: Cellular mechanisms for lipid deposition in atherosclerosis. N Engl J Med 297:873, 1977 and 297:924, 1977
25. Wylie EJ Jr: Personal communication, 1951
26. Mosely , Connel RS, Krippaehne WW: Healing of the canine aorta after endarterectomy. Ann Surg 180:329, 1974
27. Lazzarini-Robertson A: Discussion cited by Jordan GL: in Wesolowski SA, Dennis C (eds): Fundamentals of Vascular Grafting. New York, McGraw-Hill, 1963, pp 188
28. Jordan GL, Stumpf MM, Allen J, DeBakey ME, Halpert B: Gelatin-impregnated Dacron prosthesis implanted into the porcine thoracic aorta. Surgery 53:45, 1963
29. Kennedy LJ, Weissman IL: Dual origin in intimal cells in cardiac-allograft arteriosclerosis. N Engl J Med 285:884, 1971
30. Lazzarini-Robertson A: Some aspects of metabolism and ultrastructure of human and animal intimal lining, in Wesolowski SA, Dennis C (eds): Fundamentals of Vascular Grafting. New York, McGraw-Hill, 1963, pp 79–116
31. Benditt EP, Benditt JM: Evidence for a monoclonal origin of human atherosclerotic plaques. Proc Natl Acad Sci USA 70:1753, 1973
32. Still WJS: An electron microscopic study of the organization of experimental thromboemboli in the rabbit. Lab Invest 15:1492, 1966
33. Wesolowski SA, Seaman AR: Growth and differentiation of the endothelial lining of the vascular prosthesis by scanning electron microscopy. J Abd Surg 13:219, 1971
34. Ts'ao CH: Myointimal cells as a possible source of replacement for endothelial cells in the rabbit. Circulation Res 13:671, 1967
35. Poole JCF, Cromwell SB, Benditt RP: Behaviour of smooth muscle cells and formation of extracellular structures in the reaction of arterial walls to injury. Am J Path 62:391, 1971
36. Pearce JE, Dujovny M, Ho KL, Shrontz C, Ausman JI, Berman SK, Diaz FG: Acute inflammation and endothelial injury in vein grafts. Neurosurgery 17:626, 1985
37. Texon M: The hemodynamic basis of atherosclerosis. Further observations. The bifurcation lesion. Bull New York Acad Med 15:1942, 1976
38. McDonald DA: Blood Flow in Arteries. London, Edward Arnold, 1960, p 30
39. Leriche R: Des oblitérations artérielles hautes (oblitérations de la termination de l'aorte) comme causes des insuffisances circulatoires des membres inférieurs. Bull Mém Soc Chir (Paris) 49:1404, 1923
40. Barth (no initial): Observation d'une oblitération complète de l'aorte abdominale, recuille dans le service de M. Louis, suivie de réflections. Arch Gén Méd, Second Series 8:26, 1835
41. Rutkow IM, Ernst CB: An analysis of vascular surgical manpower requirements and vascular surgical rates in the United States. J Vasc Surg 3:74, 1986

A. Bollinger

3

Can Drugs Improve the Circulation in Arterial Disease?

INTRODUCTION

The natural course of atherosclerosis in the lower limbs is characterized by slow or rapid deterioration (stenosis or occlusion) followed by a slow and partial recovery (collateral development, improvement of altered metabolism). Gangrene and limb loss may occur if there is not enough time for recovery or if multilevel disease slowly induces severe ischaemia.

In this view drugs might be useful for the following therapeutic aims:

1. prevention of symptomatic disease in patients at increased risk;
2. prevention of recurrent stenoses or occlusions after procedures reopening the arterial lumen;
3. acceleration or improvement of recovery after disease manifestation or worsening (intermittent claudication);
4. reversal of rest pain or incipient gangrene.

In this article the possibilities offered by drug treatment in peripheral atherosclerosis are shortly reviewed. No attempt is made to describe the modes of action attributed to the different medicaments with "vasoactive properties". They include vasodilatation, alpha-adrenergic blockade, improvement of rheology, and enhancement of tissue oxidative potential. Antiplatelet drugs, anticoagulants, and fibrinolytic agents, however, are relatively well-defined compounds. The only agents potentially capable of reopening occluded blood vessels have fibrinolytic properties.

VASCULAR SURGERY: ISSUES IN CURRENT PRACTICE
ISBN 0-8089-1839-7

PRIMARY PREVENTION

The main risk factors established in epidemiological studies are cigarette smoking, diabetes, hypertension, and hypercholesterinaemia. Primary prevention is based on this knowledge. Whenever possible smoking should be eliminated. Drug treatment is indicated to influence the other risk factors. The usefulness of these measures results from intervention studies carried out during the last two decades.

SECONDARY PREVENTION

The main therapeutic aim is to slow down spontaneous progression of disease. If this goal is reached slightly symptomatic patients may lead an almost normal life without requiring invasive treatment. This is especially true in older people with low physical activity. Moreover, it is important to maintain the therapeutic effect obtained by reconstructive arterial surgery, transluminal angioplasty, or fibrinolysis. As in primary prevention, treatment should be directed against the *risk factors* present in an individual patient. Cessation of cigarette smoking improves the prognosis of peripheral vascular disease.[1] The beneficial effects of antihypertensive and hypocholesterolaemic treatment are less well documented with regards to patients with intermittent claudication, although femoral atherosclerosis is favourably influenced by drugs, lowering high blood cholesterol levels.[2] It must be borne in mind, however, that patients with lower limb involvement suffer or die often from cerebral or coronary atherosclerosis. Secondary prevention aims to reduce cardiovascular events in all vascular territories.

Two prospective, randomized, double-blind studies[3,4] have shown that the spontaneous progression of lower limb atherosclerosis is delayed by the antiplatelet drug aspirin (ASA) or by the combination of aspirin and dipyridamole (ASA-D). In comparison with placebo treatment the occlusion rate of femoral artery stenoses is decreased by ASA during 4.5 years from 58 to 20% and by ASA-D to 34%.[3] The effect of both regimens was significantly superior to placebo, but there was no significant difference between ASA and ASA-D. In a second trial[4] the same drugs inhibiting platelet function were given to 240 patients. The disease progression was assessed by a score system applied to arteriographic images[5] before beginning the treatment and after a follow-up of two years. The additive score as a measure of the severity of atherosclerotic lesions in the leg arteries showed a mean increase of 6.2 with placebo, 4.4 with ASA, and 2.2 with ASA-D. In this study only ASA-D induced a significant delay of spontaneous progression (lowest increase of mean additive score). The results of the two studies support the view that drugs influencing platelet activity are not only useful for secondary prophylaxis in cerebrovascular disease[6] but also in peripheral atherosclerosis.

Additional prospective studies conducted in a randomized and double-blind way[7,8] give evidence for a reduced recurrence rate after reconstructive surgery, especially after femoro-popliteal endarterectomy, if ASA or ASA-D are selected for secondary prevention. After two years the operated segment remained patent in 84% with ASA, in 76% with ASA-D, and in 58% with coumadine preparations. The difference between the ASA and the coumadine group was statistically significant ($p < 0.02$). The use of the antiplatelet drugs improves the long-term patency rate and permits use of endarterectomy as the treatment of first choice for femoro-popliteal occlusions. ASA has been shown to be helpful after carotid endarterectomy as well.[9] The ASA doses administered in all four trials mentioned was 1 g/day, those of dipyridamol 225 mg/day. Up to now there is no convincing evidence in peripheral arterial disease that lower doses are as effective as the high ones. A limitation for long-term administration of ASA is poor gastrointestinal tolerance. In one of the studies gastroduodenal ulcers developed in 5% of the patients.[8]

In conclusion, the data available at present suggest a favourable action of antiplatelet drugs for stabilizing the symptoms of peripheral vascular disease at an acceptable level of discomfort or for maintaining the results obtained by endarterectomy. A number of open questions remain. What drugs should be given after different bypass procedures or after peripheral transluminal angioplasty? Are there aspirin preparations with better gastrointestinal tolerance? What do new drugs like thromboxane-synthetase inhibitors or the serotonin antagonist ketanserin add to solve the problem?

INTERMITTENT CLAUDICATION

As has been pointed out, intermittent claudication of recent onset tends to become less disabling independently of the pharmacological agents given to the patient and provided that no additional stenoses or occlusions develop.

There is now considerable evidence that several drugs improve pain-free walking distance when compared with placebo. They include pentoxifylline,[10–15] naftidrofuryl,[16–20] cinnarizine,[21,22] flunarizine,[22–24] buflomedil,[25] cyclandelate,[26] and ketanserin.[27] For all these compounds a significant increase of walking capacity has been demonstrated in at least one controlled clinical trial. Several double-blind studies with positive results have been performed with some of these drugs, adding to objective documentation of the therapeutic value. However, one should proceed with caution before advising drug therapy on the basis of one positive controlled study alone. Some negative results have been gained with the drugs mentioned above, e.g., the large double-blind trial in the United States comparing pentoxifylline with placebo was negative in one of the centres involved.[11] Another example is ketanserin, with controversial data regarding prolongation of walking distance.[28] It should be added that the tendency of most authors to publish positive results and to forget the negative ones might contribute to a too optimistic view.

The knowledge that positive results may be obtained by "vasoactive" drugs increasing walking capacity is relatively new. On the basis of the data available in 1979 Coffman[29] denied any value of vasodilators for the treatment of intermittent claudication. Most of the experts agreed with him. One of the consequences was that the pharmaceutical companies started to abandon the denomination of vasodilator. Names like vasoactive substances, drugs promoting microcirculation or rheology, were created in many instances on doubtful grounds. On the other hand, the justified critical attitude stimulated some companies to plan controlled trials.

In spite of the positive results in double-blind studies demonstrating significant improvements of walking distance it is still open to question whether statistical significance also means clinical relevance.[30] The mean increases of walking distance observed in the various studies mentioned vary between 50 and 208%. These increases depend on the different selection of patients and on the techniques of investigation. They amount to 80–100% on the average. The alternative conservative therapy is physical training. If it is well conducted it permits one to augment the walking distance by 80–150%.[31, 32] Exercise treatment for intermittent claudication is at least as effective as drug therapy. It remains the therapy of first choice for improving walking distance. On the other hand, not all the patients are suited for physical exercise. Concomitant diseases like arthrosis may limit the walking capacity. In these cases the administration of vasoactive drugs seems justified. There are no convincing data proving that drug therapy added to physical training is more effective than training alone.

No conclusive studies are available comparing the efficacy of different compounds claimed to increase walking capacity. Moreover, combined effects would be desirable, e.g., a given drug could have a favorable influence on walking distance and provide protection against progression of atherosclerosis. At present, the antiplatelet or antithrombotic properties of pentoxifylline and ketanserin are being tested in controlled clinical trials.

REST PAIN AND GANGRENE

Reversing ischaemia which threatens a limb is the ideal goal of any therapy for arterial occlusive disease. However, it must be realized that skin capillaries in severely ischaemic digits may be empty of red blood cells.[33] In this situation with very low or abolished microvascular flow the drugs do not reach the region of interest. Naftidrofuryl improves tissue pH in patients with rest pain, but not in patients with incipient gangrene.[34]

A few studies indicate that naftidrofuryl[34, 35] and buflomedil[36] contribute to the treatment of severe ischaemia. This evidence, however, is not sufficient to advocate the use of these medicaments in patients in whom a more effective treatment seems possible. Reconstructive vascular surgery, peripheral transluminal angioplasty, and local fibrinolysis have to be considered before drug therapy is started. In the best situation drugs help to reverse severe ischaemia during some weeks, but the methods for restoring patency of main arteries allow an immediate and lasting success to be reached. Advanced disease will remain a domain of procedures which reopen the occluded vessels, at least in the near future. It is improbable that the use of prostacyclin and its derivatives will change this situation.

In some patients with severe ischaemia reopening of vessels by reconstructive vascular surgery, peripheral transluminal angioplasty, or local fibrinolysis is not possible. Then the administration of pharmacologic agents is a valid approach. Intraarterial therapy with prostacyclin or prostaglandin E_1 is now widely used.[37–41] These compounds have a potent vasodilator effect and inhibit platelet aggregation. In a high percentage of cases they relieve rest pain.[39, 41] With continuous intraarterial infusion of prostaglandin E_1 during several weeks major amputation could be avoided in 67% of rest pain or gangrene patients without diabetes and in 47% with diabetes.[39] Occasionally, the indwelling catheters lead to infection of the arterial wall and to formation of false aneurysms requiring resection. In another study with infusions lasting 72 hours only about half of the patients lost their limbs during a follow-up of two years.[38] These results should be compared to those obtained by optimal local care alone. In a report from the Aggertal Clinic[42] ulcerations on the feet due to peripheral atherosclerosis healed in 63% of patients. It seems, however, that many of these patients belonged to a group with chronic lesions and a relatively good prognosis. Nevertheless, a critical attitude is still advised[40] until new positive results with prostaglandins become available.

An important observation has been made by Pardy, Lewis, and Eastcott.[37] In their series the success of intraarterial prostaglandin therapy depended on the patency of the femoral artery. In cases with a palpable popliteal pulse the success rate was high, but was low in patients with occlusions of the femoral artery. Similar unpublished results have been obtained by our group using adenosin triphosphate by the intraarterial route. Severe ischaemia due to occlusions distal to the knee joint appears to be the best indication for drug therapy. The optimal applications are not yet established. Most workers prefer continuous or intermittent intraarterial infusions, others the intravenous route. Moreover, controversial data appear in the literature which concern the dosage and the duration of treatment.

FIBRINOLYTIC AGENTS

It is beyond the scope of this short review to evaluate the efficacy of fibrinolytic treatment, but a few words appear necessary to broaden the view of drug therapy. In Central Europe streptokinase and urokinase have been given in a systemic way to treat acute and subacute occlusions of limb arteries. Since systemic fibrinolysis often induces haemorrhagic complications leading to death in about 1% of the treated patients the tendency is towards local application of streptokinase or urokinase.[43] Instillation of the drug into the thrombi by appropriate catheters seems to offer the best way and permits reopening of underlying stenoses by the Grüntzig balloon catheter during the same intervention. Bleeding complications are rare because marked hypofibrinogenaemia does not occur. A further promising therapy has recently been introduced to dissolve acute coronary thrombi. Tissue plasminogen activators have the fascinating property of attacking thrombi, but attack circulating fibrinogen only to a minor degree. They have not yet been used in peripheral vascular disease.

REFERENCES

1. Jonason T, Ringquist I: Factors of prognostic importance for subsequent rest pain in intermittent claudication. Acta Med Scand 218:27, 1985
2. Barndt R, Blankenhorn DH, Crawford DW, Brooks SH: Regression and progression of early femoral atherosclerosis in treated hyperlipoproteinemic patients. Ann Int Med 86:139, 1977
3. Schoop W, Levy H, Schoop B, Gaentzsch A: Experimentelle und klinische Studien zu der sekundären Prävention der periopheren Arteriosklerose, in Bollinger A, Rhyner K (eds): Thrombozytenfunktionshemmer. Stuttgart, Thieme, 1983, p 49
4. Hess H, Mietaschk A, Deichsel G: Drug-induced inhibition of platelet function delays progression of peripheral occlusive arterial disease. Lancet I:415, 1985
5. Bollinger A, Breddin K, Hess H, et al: Semiquantitative assessment of lower limb atherosclerosis from routine angiographic images. Atherosclerosis 38:339, 1981

6. Canadian Cooperative Stroke Study Group: Randomized trial of therapy with platelet antiaggregants for threatened stroke. CMA J 122:293, 1980

7. Ehresmann U, Alemany J, Loew D: Prophylaxe von Rezidivverschlüssen nach Revaskularisationseingriffen mit Acetylsalicylsäure. Med Welt 28:1157, 1977

8. Bollinger A, Brunner U: Antiplatelet drugs improve the patency rates after femoropopliteal endarterectomy. Vasa 14:272, 1985

9. Fields WS, Lemak NA, Frankowski RF, Hardy RS: Controlled trial of aspirin in cerebral ischemia. Part II: Surgical group. Stroke 9:309, 1978

10. Bollinger A, Frei C: Double-blind study of pentoxifylline against placebo in patients with intermittent claudication. Pharmatherapeutica 1:557, 1977

11. Porter JM, Cutler BS, Lee BY, et al: Pentoxifylline efficacy in the treatment of intermittent claudication: Multicenter controlled double-blind trial with objective assessment of chronic occlusive arterial disease patients. Am Heart J 104:66, 1982

12. Porter JM, Baur GM: Pharmacologic treatment of intermittent claudication. Surgery 92:966, 1982

13. Ehrly AM: The effect of pentoxifylline on the deformability of erythrocytes and on the muscular oxygen pressure in patients with chronic arterial disease. J Med 10:331, 1979

14. Heidrich H: Vasoaktive Pharmaka bei peripheren arteriellen Durchblutungsstörungen. Dtsch med Wschr 110:1219, 1985

15. Rudofsky G, Brock F-E, Ulrich M, Nobbe F: Behandlung von Patienten mit arterieller Verschlusskrankheit (Stadium II) mit Pentoxifyllin. Med Klin 74:1093, 1979

16. Pohle W, Hirche H, Barmeyer J, et al: Doppelblindstudie mit Naftidrofuryl-Hydrogenoxalat bei Patienten mit peripheren arteriellen Verschlusskrankheit. Med Welt 30:269, 1979

17. Clyne CAC, Galland RB, Fox MJ, et al: A controlled trial of naftidrofuryl in the treatment of intermittent claudication. Br J Surg 67:347, 1980

18. Boobis LH, Bell PRF: Can drugs help patients with lower limb ischemia? Br J Surg 69(Suppl):17, 1982

19. Becker HM, Ehlert O, Häring R, et al: Wirksamkeitsnachweis von Dusodril-PI bei arterieller Verschlusskrankheit in einer multizentrisch angelegten Doppelblindstudie. Med Welt 30:1602, 1979

20. Maass U, Amberger H-G, Böhme H, et al: Nafidrofuryl bei arterieller Verschlusskrankheit: Kontrollierte multizentrische Doppelblindstudie mit oraler Applikation. Dtsch Med Wschr 109:745, 1984

21. Ellis F, Hyams DE: Vascular responses with cinnarizine to standard exercise in patients with intermittent claudication. Proc R Soc Med 70(Suppl 8):13, 1977

22. Staessen AJ: Treatment of circulatory disturbances with flunarizine and cinnarizine: A multicentre, double-blind and placebo-controlled evaluation. Vasa 6:59, 1977

23. Rudofsky G, Brock F-E, Ulrich M, Nobbe F: Clinical evaluation of flunarizine: Walking distance, ergometric performance, and hemodynamic and biochemical effects. Angiology 30:470, 1979

24. Schetz J, Bostoen H, Clement D, et al: Flunarizine in chronic obstructive peripheral arterial disease: a placebo-controlled double-blind, randomized multicentre trial. Curr Ther Res 23:121, 1978

25. Trübestein G, Balzer K, Bisler H, et al: Buflomedil bei arterieller Verschlusskrankheit. Dtsch Med Wschr 107:1957, 1982

26. Reich T: Cyclandelate: Effect on circulatory measurements and exercise tolerance in chronic arterial insufficiency of the lower limbs. J Am Ger Soc 25:202, 1977

27. De Cree J, Leempoels J, Genkens H, Verhaegen H: Placebo-controlled double-blind trial of ketanserin in treatment of intermittent claudication. Lancet II:775, 1984

28. Bounameaux H, Holditch T, Hellemans H, Berent A, Verhaeghe R: Placebo-controlled, double-blind, two-centre trial of ketanserin in intermittent claudication. Lancet II:1268, 1985

29. Coffman JD: Vasodilator drugs in peripheral vascular disease. N Engl J Med 300:713, 1979

30. Mahler F: Medikamentöse Behandlung der peripheren arteriellen Verschlusskrankheit. Schweiz Med Wschr 111:637, 1981

31. Clifford PC, Davies PW, Hayne JA, Baird RN: Intermittent claudication: Is a supervised exercise class worthwhile? Br Med J 280:1503, 1980

32. Mass U, Cachovan M, Alexander K: Einfluss eines kontrollierten Intervalltrainings auf die Gehstrecke bei Patienten mit Claudicatio intermittens, in Mahler F, Nachbur B (eds): Zerebrale Ischämie. Bern, Huber, 1984, p 356

33. Fagrell B: Vital capillaroscopy—A clinical method for studying changes of skin microcirculation in patients suffering from vascular disorders of the leg. Angiology 23:284, 1972

34. Meehan SE, Walker WF: Naftidrofuryl for severe ischemia: Assessment using skin pH micro-electrode measurements. Curr Med Res Op 7:690, 1982

35. Greenhalgh RM: Naftidrofuryl for ischemic rest pain: A controlled trial. Br J Surg 68:265, 1981

36. Fagrell B, Hermannsson IL: The effect of buflomedil on skin microcirculation in patients with severe skin ischemia, in Messmer K (ed): Microcirculation and Ischemic Vascular Disease. Acad Prof Inf Serv, 1981, p 285

37. Pardy BJ, Lewis JD, Eastcott HHG: Preliminary experience with prostaglandins E_1 and I_2 in peripheral vascular disease. Surgery 88:826, 1980

38. Negus D, Irving JD, Lewis J, et al: Intra-arterial prostacyclin in the management of lower limb ischemia. Inter Angio 3:49, 1984

39. Gruss JD, Vargas-Montano H, Bartels D, et al: Use of prostaglandins in arterial occlusive disease. Inter Angio 3:7, 1984

40. Vermylen J, Verstraete M, Verhaege RH: Clinical ineffectiveness of intraarterial or intravenous infusions of epoprostenol in patients with peripheral obliterative disease, stage III to IV. Inter Angio 3:73, 1984

41. Hossmann V, Anel H, Rücker W, Schrör K: Prolonged infusion of prostacyclin in patients with advanced stages of peripheral vascular disease: A placebo-controlled crossover study. Klin Wschr 62:1108, 1984

42. Rieger H, Reinecke B, Levy H: Früh- und Spätergebnisse konservativer Therapie bei Patienten mit peripheren arteriellen Durchblutungsstörungen im klinischen Stadium IV. Vasa-Suppl 12:124, 1984

43. Hess H, Ingrisch H, Mietaschk A, Rath H: Local low-dose thrombolytic therapy of peripheral arterial occlusions. N Engl J Med 307:1627, 1982

Peter Gloviczki
and Larry H. Hollier

4

Can Graft Occlusion be Prevented by Drugs?

During the past four decades, progress in vascular surgery has been attributed to a great extent to the development and continuous improvement of vascular grafting. Presently available graft materials enable replacement of large-caliber arteries with excellent long-term results; grafting of medium- and small-caliber vessels, however, continues to pose significant problems. In below-knee revascularization, results with vein grafts are superior to those obtained with prosthetic materials,[1] but good-quality autogenous veins are not always available and secondary morphologic changes in the wall may lead to failure of vein grafts as well. Endothelial injury, caused by mechanical manipulation and ischemic insult during surgery and by changes in luminal pressure, plays an important role in the development of secondary changes, subintimal fibrosis, and intimal hyperplasia. As a result of these changes and the progression of the underlying disease, 10-year patency of femoro-popliteal vein grafts was only 38 and 44% in two large studies.[2,3] The quality of the grafts was an important factor since patency half-life with good and excellent grafts 10.5 years, but with fair or poor veins was only 0.5 years. Thus, there exists a need for ways of improving patency of prosthetic grafts.

Patency of vascular grafts is determined by several factors, including the skill of the vascular surgeon, the type and characteristics of the graft material used, and a number of host-related factors such as hemodynamics, graft–host biocompatibility, and thrombogenic and atherogenic potentials of the host. Early occlusion is usually attributed to errors in surgical technique, to hemodynamic factors, and to the thrombogenic surface of the implanted graft, while late occlusion may be the result of progression of the underlying disease or the development of neointimal fibrous hyperplasia, usually more prominent at the distal anastomosis.

Unfortunately, even "ideal" grafts can fail because of host-related factors, many of which are still poorly understood and, therefore, difficult or impossible to control. There is, however, ample evidence now that some graft-related factors, especially surface thrombogenicity, can be effectively influenced by certain medications, primarily antiplatelet drugs, at least in the early perioperative period.

VASCULAR SURGERY: ISSUES IN CURRENT PRACTICE
ISBN 0-8089-1839-7

THROMBUS FORMATION IN VASCULAR GRAFTS

All grafts, with the possible exception of arterial autografts, have increased thrombogenicity when compared to the ideal endothelial surface of the native artery.[4]

Thrombus formation after graft placement starts with adherence of platelets to the thrombogenic surface of prosthetic grafts, to deendothelialized areas of vein grafts, and to sites of endothelial injury of the native artery of the anastomoses. Platelet adherence is enhanced by exposed subendothelial collagen, by von Willebrand's factor, by certain glycoproteins, and by fibrin. Platelet adhesion is followed by irreversible aggregation and release of vasoactive substances; these include platelet factor 3, which enhances thrombin formation, and serotonin, which results

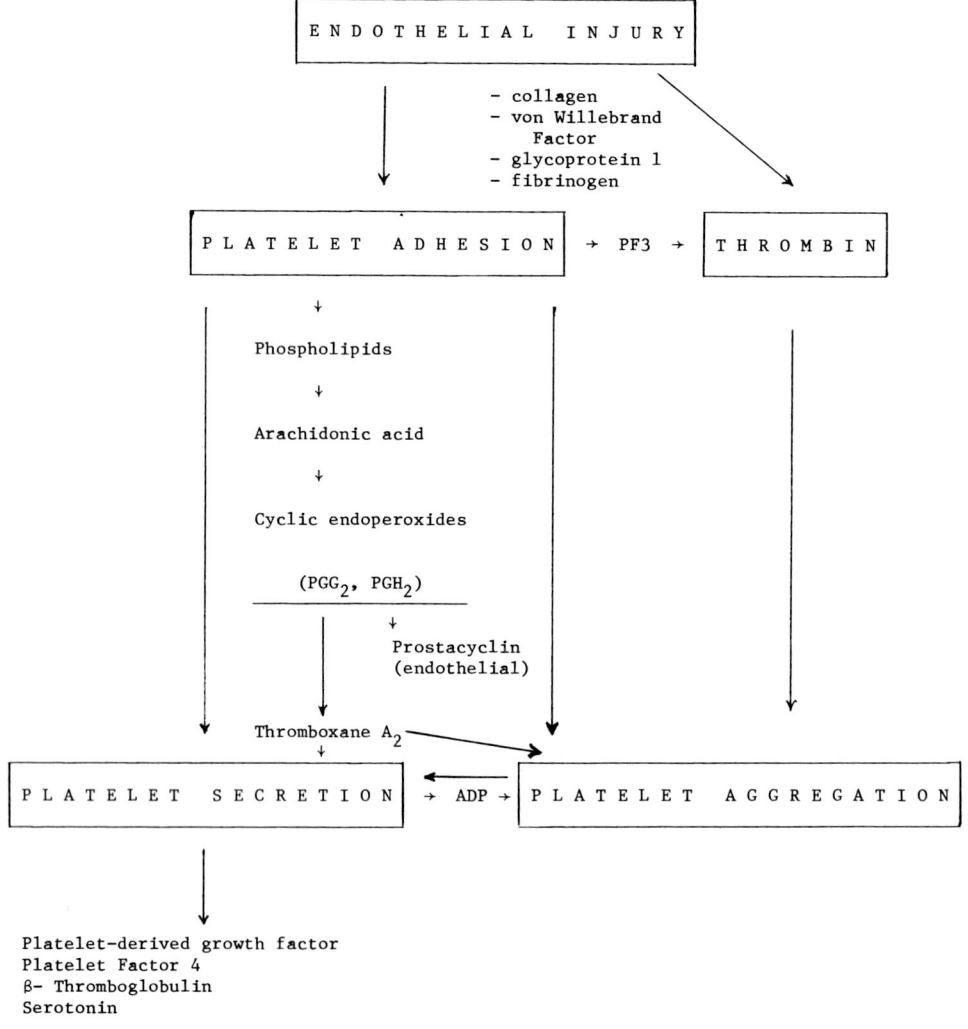

Fig. 4-1.   Mechanism of platelet activation in endothelial injury.

in vasoconstriction and release of different mitogenic factors, the most important being platelet-derived growth factor.

Activation of the arachidonic acid pathway and production of prostaglandins (Fig. 4-1) are of major importance in the development of intragraft thrombus. Thromboxane A_2, the active platelet prostaglandin, is a strong vasoconstrictor and promotes platelet aggregation and release. The other active prostaglandin, prostacyclin (PGI_2), is formed in vascular endothelium from cyclic endoperoxides, has a vasodilator effect, and inhibits platelet aggregation. Thus imbalance in the production of prostacyclin and thromboxane A_2 can lead to increased thrombogenicity and thrombus formation. Decreased prostacyclin production and increased thromboxane A_2 levels have been demonstrated even in the in situ vein grafts which are supposedly most "physiologic."[5] Prostacyclin production has been documented in the neointima of prosthetic grafts, but levels are inferior to those measured in the native artery[6] and thus help to explain the relative thrombogenicity of prosthetic grafts.

The role of leukocytes in the initial surface–blood interaction is still poorly understood. Adherence and activation have been observed in vein grafts,[5] and there is growing evidence that both platelet- and leukocyte-derived mitogenic factors play roles in the late proliferative changes of neointimal hyperplasia.

Hemodynamic factors, such as turbulent blood flow at the anastomotic areas or stasis due to narrowing of the lumen, play an important role in the formation and composition of thrombus. In the arterial circulation, a high-flow situation, the thrombus is usually "white thrombus" rich in platelets. "Red thrombus" containing mostly fibrin and red cells, however, may also develop in association with impeded flow or as an extension of occlusive white thrombus.

An activation of coagulation factors by the thrombogenic prosthetic graft, by certain conditions such as trauma, malignant tumors, sepsis, or by congenital or acquired deficiency of inhibiting factors, result in a hypercoagulable state and increased risk of graft thrombosis. A deficiency of antithrombin III, a potent inhibitor of thrombin and factor Xa, has been found in association with "unexplained" failure of vascular grafts.[7] Reduced antithrombin III activity has recently been reported in patients with early thrombosis of femoro-distal grafts.[8]

The tendency of recurrent thromboembolic disease and a deficiency in protein C seems now well established. Activated protein C is a potent anticoagulant that inhibits the coagulation cascade by selective inactivation of the active cofactors Va and VIIIa.[9]

NEOINTIMAL FIBROUS HYPERPLASIA

Besides progression of the underlying vascular disease, neointimal fibrous hyperplasia has been described as the most important case of late graft failure. First described by Imparato, Bracco, and Kim,[10] neointimal fibrous hyperplasia was found to be responsible for about one-third of the failures of distal limb revascularizations.

Neointimal hyperplasia develops at the site of endothelial injury where platelets adhere to exposed subendothelial collagen, aggregate, and release substances which induce migration and proliferation of fibroblasts and myofibroblasts (Figs 4-2 to 4-4). This trauma may be directly related to the surgical manipulation during

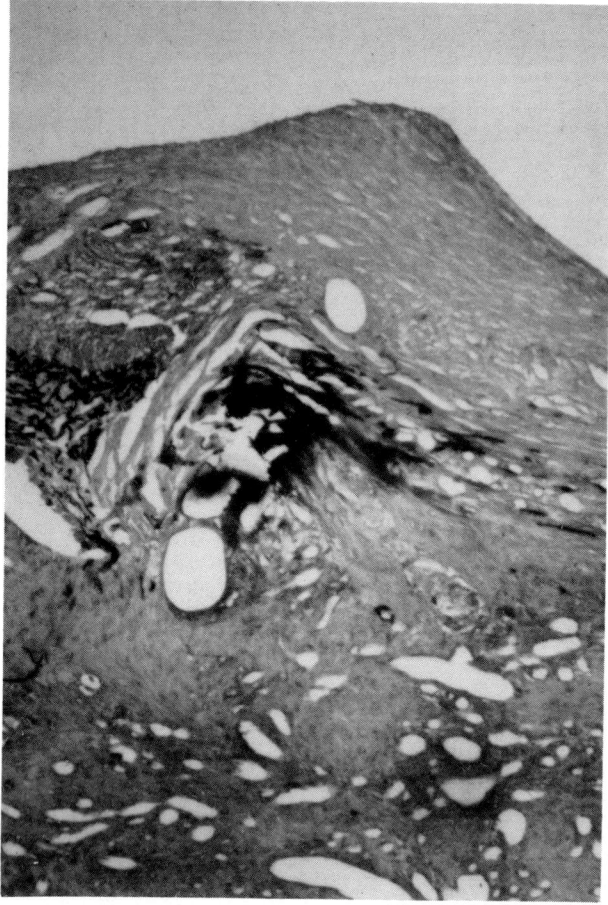

Fig. 4-2. Anastomotic intimal hyperplasia: vein graft (right) and femoral artery (left) anastomosis in dog at 30 days after implantation (hematoxylin-eosin stain, original magnification 100 ×). From Gloviczki P, Hollier LH, Dewanjee MK, et al: Quantitative evaluation of ibuprofen treatment on thrombogenicity of expanded polytetrafluoroethylene vascular grafts. Surgery 95:160, 1984. With permission.

implantation of the graft or caused by turbulent flow or mechanical mismatch between the graft and host vessel. The area of increased susceptibility is the site of the anastomosis—most frequently the distal one. Hagen and coworkers[11] made a distinction between neointimal hyperplasia in the distal arterial segment, dominated by the presence of smooth muscle cells, and neointimal hyperplasia within the graft, consisting mostly of fibroblasts and myofibroblasts. There is certainly an early type of neointimal plaque which forms within the graft and originates directly from initial surface thrombus. While the role of platelet reactivity in this form of intimal hyperplasia seems important, less well established is the direct relation between platelets and late intimal hyperplasia. It seems that myofibroblastic proliferation can develop not only as a result of mitogenic factors, originating from platelets and

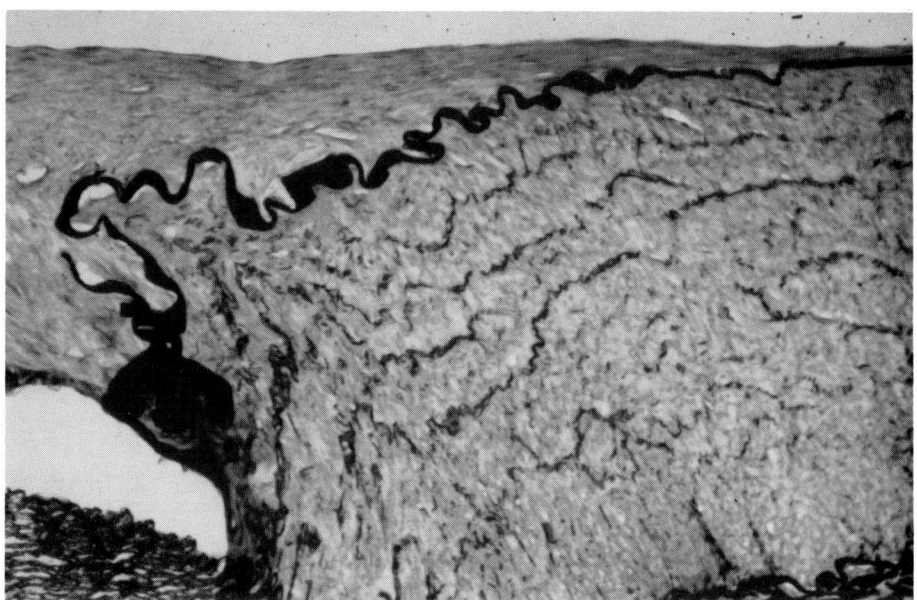

Fig. 4-3. Anastomotic neointimal fibrous hyperplasia of ePTFE femoral artery graft in an ibuprofen-treated animal at 30 days (Verhoeff's stain, original magnification 100 ×). From Gloviczki P, Hollier LH, Dewanjee MK, et al: Quantitative evaluation of ibuprofen treatment on thrombogenicity of expanded polytetrafluoroethylene vascular grafts. Surgery 95:160, 1984. With permission.

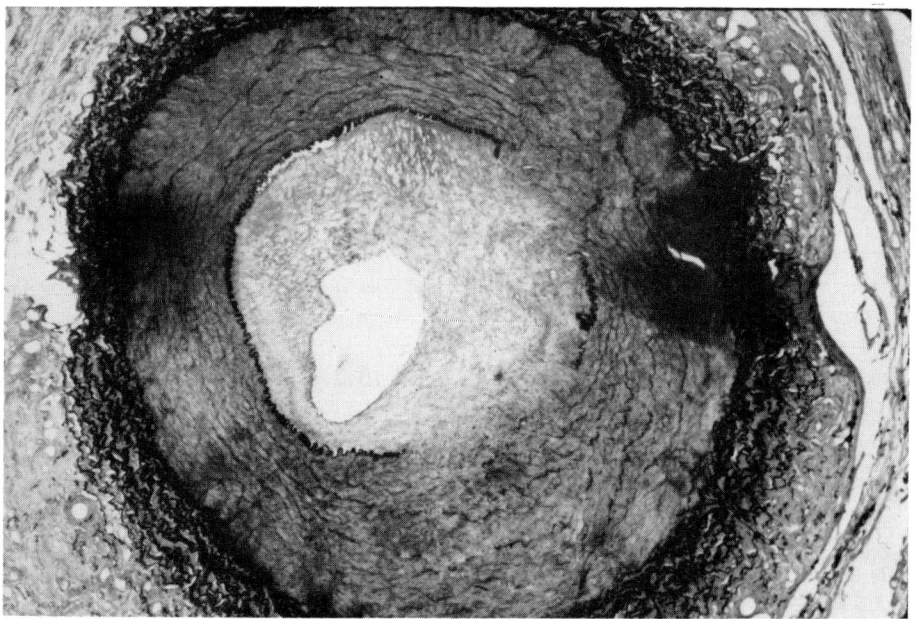

Fig. 4-4. Cross section of a femoral artery near the proximal anastomosis with ePTFE graft. Note the disruption of the internal elastic lamina, intimal fibrous hyperplasia, and significant narrowing of the lumen at 30 days following implantation (Verhoeff's stain, original magnification 20 ×). From Gloviczki P, Hollier LH, Dewanjee MK, et al: Quantitative evaluation of ibuprofen treatment on thrombogenicity of expanded polytetrafluoroethylene vascular grafts. Surgery 95:160, 1984. With permission.

probably leukocytes, but also as a response to changes in flow characteristics and arterial wall stress.[10] Experiments of Pomposelli and coworkers suggest that an increase in wall tension due to conformational stress at the anastomosis leads to neointimal fibrous hyperplasia.[12] On the basis of these findings, one can better understand why antiplatelet treatment is less effective in preventing these late proliferative changes in vascular grafts.

ANTITHROMBOTIC TREATMENT

Anticoagulants

Heparin, a natural mucopolysaccharide, that consists of sulfated D-glucosamine and D-glucoronic acid, prolongs clotting time by accelerating the inhibitory effect of antithrombin III against serine proteases, the most important being thrombin (factor IIa), but also factors Xa, IXa, XIa, XIIa, plasmin, and kallikrein.[13] In the presence of only 0.01 U/ml of heparin, the thrombin-inhibiting potential of 1 μg of antithrombin III increases 750 times.[14] In intravenous form, beef lung or porcine mucosal heparin has routinely been used intraoperatively during extracorporeal circulation in cardiac surgery and during aortic or peripheral arterial reconstructions to prevent thrombosis following aortic or arterial cross-clamping. It has been demonstrated that heparin can be used safely and effectively in the perioperative period, even with porous prosthetic grafts, without significant risk of major hemorrhage.[15] In vivo heparin has only minimal fibrinolytic activity; therefore, its main indication is prevention of intraoperative thrombus formation or the stabilization and prevention of propagation of developed acute thrombosis. There has been increased interest recently in studying the antimitogenic activity of heparin.[16]

Warfarin, a coumarin derivative, is an oral anticoagulant. Coumarin drugs are vitamin K antagonists and interfere with the synthesis of prothrombin, factors II, VII, IX, X, and protein C. Long-term anticoagulants failed to improve patency of lower extremity bypass grafts, though warfarin showed a beneficial effect in improving patency of aorto-coronary vein grafts at six months.[17] Long-time coumadin treatment is indicated in those patients who have antithrombin III deficiency and undergo distal revascularization of the extremity.

Anticoagulants are contraindicated in patients who have hemorrhagic diathesis, GI bleeding, a recent operation on the central nervous system, or have suspected intracranial bleeding or severe hypertension. The further disadvantage of these drugs is that regular laboratory monitoring is necessary to control drug levels.

Dextrans

Dextrans are low molecular weight polysaccharides, used primarily as plasma volume extenders. Because of their special rheologic effect, as well as their antiplatelet activity, both dextran 70 and dextran 40 have increasingly been used in patients with venous thrombosis as well as with acute and chronic arterial insufficiency. Dextrans decrease platelet adhesiveness and platelet aggregation. It has been demonstrated that they reduce blood viscosity and decrease surface thrombogenicity by changing the electron negativity of the surface as well as by a special coating effect.[18] Dextran also reduces factor VIII activity and increases clot lysability, and as a plasma volume expander it increases peripheral flow. In experiments, it improved patency of small-caliber arterial anastomoses[19] and arterial grafts.[20] The efficacy of dextrans in the prevention of deep venous thrombosis has been well established.[21] There is also increasing evidence that dextran, in doses of 500 to 1000 ml/day given in the early postoperative course, improves results of arterial reconstruction. In a randomized, multicenter study, dextran 40 (Rheomacrodex®) significantly improved early patency of difficult lower extremity bypasses. The overall one-week occlusion rate was 6.9% (5 of 73) in the treated group and 20.5% (17 of 83) in the control group. The one-month occlusion rate (15.3% versus 20.7%) was, however, not significantly different.[22] Clinical efficacy of dextran 40 seems to be better than dextran 70. Clinical results of Bergentz, Eiken, and Gelin[23] indicate that at least early occlusion of small-artery reconstructions could be avoided in patients who received perioperative dextran 40.

Though regular laboratory monitoring is not necessary for patients on dextran treatment, the drug is not completely without side effects. Fluid overload, pulmonary edema, and allergic or even anaphylactic reactions have been described.

Antiplatelet Medication

The most extensively studied group of antiplatelet agents is that which inhibits the enzyme cyclooxygenase necessary for conversion of arachidonic acid to cyclic endoperoxides (PGG_2, PGH_2). These drugs inhibit platelet thromboxane A_2 production but also inhibit endothelial prostacyclin synthesis. Fortunately, prostacyclin synthetase in endothelial cells is readily available; therefore, prostacyclin inhibition is not long lasting.

Aspirin irreversibly acetylates cyclooxygenase, and since anuclear platelets are unable to synthesize the enzyme, the effect lasts for the life span of the affected platelets. Large doses of aspirin theoretically may have thrombogenic action by inhibiting endothelial prostacyclin production; therefore, the maximum doses recommended are 325 mg t.i.d. No clinical study is available, however, which would prove a difference between low- and high-dose treatment.

Nonsteroidal, anti-inflammatory agents such as ibuprofen, sulfinpyrazone, and indomethacin inhibit cyclooxygenase only transiently; thus maintenance of adequate blood levels of these drugs is necessary for effective platelet inhibition.

Dipyridamole inhibits phosphodiesterase, thereby preventing the breakdown of cyclic adenosine 5'-monophosphate which interferes with intracellular calcium activation and decreases adherence of platelets. Dipyridamole seems to potentiate the effect of aspirin and, in several studies, the two drugs have been given together. Studies with selective thromboxane A_2 synthetase inhibitors are presently being undertaken but clinical trials are not yet available. These drugs do not inhibit endothelial prostacyclin production.

Quantitative evaluation of the effect of antiplatelet treatment on graft surface thrombogenicity is possible in experiments using several methods. Sauvage introduced the term "thrombotic threshold velocity" (TTV) which is calculated in vitro from the thrombus-free surface area of the harvested grafts.[4] He also demonstrated that antithrombotic treatment decreases TTV. Labeling platelets with indium-111 tropolone permits quantitative measurements of the thrombus deposited in prosthetic grafts. Preoperative and continuous postoperative administration of aspirin and dipyridamole diminished the number of autologous platelets labeled with indium-111 deposited in aorto-coronary vein grafts at 3, 7, and 30 days following implantation. Following complete endothelialization, the effect of antiplatelet treatment on platelet deposition was, however, not significant.[24]

Ibuprofen, started prior to clamping the artery, significantly ($p < 0.01$) reduced platelet deposition at three hours in canine ePTFE femoral grafts. Patency rates at 5 and 30 days were also better in the treated group ($p < 0.01$).[25] In a controlled-flow situation in the carotid model, we were able to reproduce these data when we compared ibuprofen to a new effective antiplatelet drug, calcium dobesilate (Fig. 4-5).[26] Several other experiments suggest that aspirin, alone or with dipyridamole, ibuprofen, and calcium channel blockers, like nifedipine, effectively decrease early thrombus deposition and improve early patency.[27–29] It seems, however, that for antiplatelet medication to be fully effective, the drug should be administered before the "first pass" of blood through the graft.

A number of studies show that at least early intimal thickening, which may be a direct result of early thrombus deposition, can be decreased with antiplatelet drugs.[11,27,30] Experimental studies of Metke and coworkers demonstrated that intimal thickening two to six weeks after surgery was decreased in vein grafts in dogs treated with aspirin and dipyridamole.[30] The pseudointima formed from surface thrombus following endarterectomy of the canine aorta could successfully be diminished by ibuprofen up to three weeks after surgery,[31] and a combination of

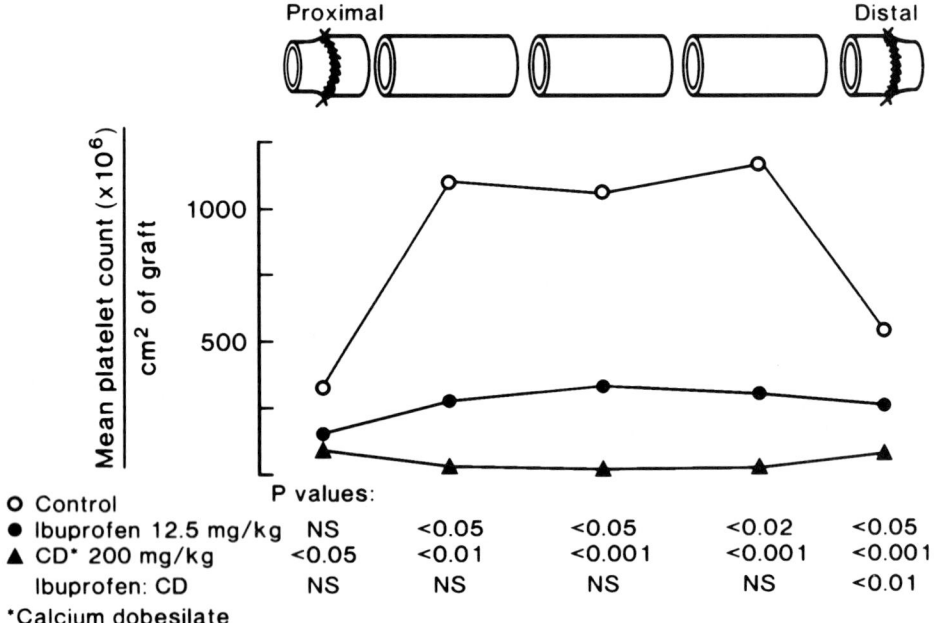

Fig. 4-5. Mean platelet deposition in canine carotid graft at three hours following implantation in control and treated animals. From Gloviczki P, Fowl RJ, Hollier LH, et al: Prevention of platelet deposition by ibuprofen and calcium dobesilate in expanded polytetrafluoroethylene vascular grafts. Am J Surg 150:589, 1985. With permission.

aspirin and persantine successfully diminished intimal hyperplasia in the baboon aorta distal to the implanted ePTFE graft.[11] Oblath and coworkers, with similar treatment, studied the formation of neointimal fibrous hyperplasia in knitted Dacron internal velour and ePTFE grafts, bypassing short segments of canine femoral arteries.[27] Medication was started prior to surgery and all 18 grafts in the treated group stayed patent at four months, compared to 60% patency in the control group ($p < 0.01$). There was evidence of anastomotic fibrous hyperplasia in 7 of 20 patent grafts. Hancock, Forshaw, and Kaye[28] found aspirin and dipyridamole effective in ePTFE coronary grafts with no patency at one month in the control group and 60% patency at six months in the treated group. In ePTFE micrografts implanted into rat aorta, ibuprofen treatment resulted in 100% patency at one month compared to 10% patency in the control group.[29] McCready, however, analyzed the amount of anastomotic intimal hyperplasia and pannus extension in canine ePTFE grafts but could not demonstrate a significant change after ibuprofen treatment.[32]

Some recent studies suggest that re-endothelialization would be inhibited by antiplatelet agents; therefore, healing of the anastomotic area might be delayed.[33] Experiments from our laboratory, however, did not confirm this, as ibuprofen did not retard endothelialization in endarterectomized canine aorta.[34] In ePTFE grafts implanted in the goat aorta, antiplatelet treatment with aspirin, dipyridamole, nifedipine, and ibuprofen resulted in no significant change in the rate of endothelialization.[32]

Chesebro and coworkers from the Mayo Clinic demonstrated the benefit of perioperative antiplatelet treatment on early patency of human aorto-coronary vein grafts.[35] Postoperative administration of aspirin and dipyridamole has been shown to be ineffective if treatment is not started prior to surgery,[36-38] although studies of low-dose aspirin[39] and ticlopidine,[40] started on the first postoperative day, did suggest early beneficial effects in the treated group at three and four months.

Clinical trials confirming the efficacy of antiplatelet treatment on patency of prosthetic grafts are sparse, although several studies are currently being conducted.

In a prospective study, Harjola, Meurala, and Frick[41] studied the early (10-day) patency following revascularization of patients treated with antiplatelet agents. A statistically significant difference between the combined aspirin- and dipyridamole-treated group could be demonstrated against the control group, though data about the type of grafts used in the 242 patients were not included. Also studied were 166 other patients after endarterectomy, but no data were given about late patency.

Veith and coworkers[42] reported a patency rate of 72% in ePTFE femoro-popliteal grafts compared to 59% in the control group. The difference in this non-randomized study was not statistically significant. Data of Green, Roedersheimer, and DeWeese[43] indicated improved patency for above-knee bypasses at 12 months if antiplatelet treatment was started preoperatively. Kohler and coworkers,[44] using aspirin and dipyridamole started postoperatively, were unable to demonstrate benefit in ePTFE grafts at 24 months following implantation.

The presently available clinical results correlate with early findings of the national cooperative antiplatelet study that we are currently undertaking to evaluate the effect of ibuprofen on patency of lower extremity ePTFE grafts. While in-hospital graft occlusion is almost four times higher in the control group, this difference between patency rates is no longer demonstrable at six months.

CONCLUSION

Anticoagulant drugs appear to have a limited role in the long-term management of patients with bypass grafts, except in patients with antithrombin III deficiency and selected patients with distal tibial grafts and poor runoff situations.

Experimental and clinical studies confirm the effectiveness of antiplatelet treatment in decreasing thrombus formation and improving early patency of grafts used for medium and small arterial replacement. It seems necessary to start antiplatelet treatment before graft placement to prevent the initial activation of platelets by the thrombogenic surface of the grafts and by the endothelial injury caused during implantation. Antiplatelet treatment does not seem to have a deleterious effect on the role of re-endothelialization of vascular grafts. Prospective studies to evaluate the results of grafts in patients on antiplatelet drugs are currently being undertaken, but it appears that graft- and host-related factors other than platelets play important roles in the development of neointimal fibrous hyperplasia and late graft occlusion. Future drug research must concentrate on finding both the optimal antithrombotic and antiproliferative medication to improve graft performance, though the major goal should be the control of underlying atherogenic process, the ultimate factor responsible for a significant number of late graft failures.

REFERENCES

1. Bergan JJ, Veith FJ, Bernhard VM, et al: Randomization of autogenous vein and polytetrafluoroethylene grafts in femoral-distal reconstruction. Surgery 92:921, 1982
2. Szilagyi DE, Hageman JH, Smith RF, et al: Autogenous vein grafting in femoropopliteal atherosclerosis: the limits of its effectiveness. Surgery 86:836, 1979
3. DeWeese JA, Rob CG: Autogenous venous grafts ten years later. Surgery 82:775, 1977
4. Sauvage LR, Walker MW, Berger K, et al: Current arterial prostheses: Experimental evaluation by implantation in the carotid and circumflex coronary arteries of the dog. Arch Surg 114:687, 1979
5. Bush HL Jr, Jakubowski JA, Curl GR, et al: The natural history of endothelial structure and function in arterialized vein grafts. J Vasc Surg 3:204, 1986
6. Sharp WV, Schmidt SP, Donovan DL: Prostaglandin biochemistry of seeded endothelial cells on Dacron prostheses. J Vasc Surg 3:256, 1986
7. Towne JB, Bernhard VM, Hussey C, et al: Antithrombin deficiency—A cause of unexplained thrombosis in vascular surgery. Surgery 89:735, 1981
8. Flinn WR, McDaniel MD, Yao JST, et al: Antithrombin III deficiency as a reflection of dynamic protein metabolism in patients undergoing vascular reconstruction. J Vasc Surg 1:888, 1984
9. Kazmier FJ: Thromboembolism, coumarin necrosis, and protein C. Mayo Clin Proc 60:673, 1985
10. Imparato AM, Bracco A, Kim GE: Intimal and neointimal fibrous proliferation causing failure of arterial reconstructions. Surgery 72:1007, 1972
11. Hagen P-O, Wang Z-G, Mikat EM, et al: Antiplatelet therapy reduces aortic intimal hyperplasia distal to small diameter vascular prosthesis (PTFE) in nonhuman primates. Ann Surg 195:328, 1982
12. Pomposelli F, Schoen F, Cohen R, et al: Conformational stress and anastomotic hyperplasia. J Vasc Surg 1:525, 1984

13. Bick RL: Disorders of Hemostasis and Thrombosis: Principles of Clinical Practice. New York, Thieme-Stratton, 1985, p 327
14. Yin ET: Effect of heparin on the neutralization of factor Xa and thrombin by the plasma alpha-2-globulin inhibitor. Thromb Diath Haemorrh 33:43, 1975
15. Collins GJ Jr, Rich NM, Clagett GP, et al: Heparin: Efficacy and safety after arterial operations. Arch Surg 116:1077, 1981
16. Clowes AW, Clowes MM: Kinetics of cellular proliferation after arterial injury. II. Inhibition of smooth muscle growth by heparin. Lab Invest 52:611, 1985
17. McEnany MT, Salzman EW, Mundth ED, et al: Effect of antithrombotic therapy on patency rates of saphenous vein coronary artery bypass grafts. J Thorac Cardiovasc Surg 83:81, 1982
18. Ross S, Ebert R: Microelectrophoresis of blood platelets and the effect of dextran. J Clin Invest 38:155, 1955
19. Sasamoto Y: Experimental studies on continuous local infusion of anticoagulants for reconstruction of small arteries. J Kumamoto Med Soc 44:839, 1970
20. Eiken O: Thrombotic occlusion of experimental grafts as a function of the regional blood flow. Acta Chir Scand 121:410, 1961
21. Bergentz S-E: Dextran prophylaxis of venous thromboembolism, in Bergan JJ, Yao JST (eds): Venous Problems. Chicago, Year Book Medical Publishers Inc, 1978, p 529
22. Rutherford RB, Jones DN, Bergentz S-E, et al: The efficacy of dextran 40 in preventing early postoperative thrombosis following difficult lower extremity bypass. J Vasc Surg 1:765, 1984
23. Bergentz SE, Eiken O, Gelin LE: Rheomacrodex in vascular surgery. J Cardiovasc Surg 4:388, 1963
24. Dewanjee MK, Tago M, Josa M, et al: Quantification of platelet retention in aorto-coronary femoral vein bypass graft in dogs treated with dipyridamole and aspirin. Circulation 69:350, 1984
25. Gloviczki P, Hollier LH, Dewanjee MK, et al: Quantitative evaluation of ibuprofen treatment on thrombogenicity of expanded polytetrafluoroethylene vascular grafts. Surgery 95:160, 1984
26. Gloviczki P, Fowl RJ, Hollier LH, et al: Prevention of platelet deposition by ibuprofen and calcium dobesilate in expanded polytetrafluoroethylene vascular grafts. Am J Surg 150:589, 1985
27. Oblath RW, Buckley FO Jr, Green RM, et al: Prevention of platelet aggregation and adherence to prosthetic vascular grafts by aspirin and dipyridamole. Surgery 84:37, 1978
28. Hancock JB, Forshaw PL, Kay MP: Gore-Tex (polytetrafluoroethylene) in canine coronary artery bypass. J Thorac Cardiovasc Surg 80:94, 1980
29. Claus PL, Gloviczki P, Hollier LH, et al: Patency of polytetrafluoroethylene microarterial prostheses improved by ibuprofen. Am J Surg 144:180, 1982
30. Metke MP, Lie JT, Fuster V, et al: Reduction of intimal thickening in canine coronary bypass vein grafts with dipyridamole and aspirin. Am J Cardiol 43:1144, 1979
31. Lovaas ME, Gloviczki P, Hollier LH, et al: Quantitative effects of antiplatelet therapy on healing of the endarterectomized canine aorta. Am J Surg 146:164, 1983
32. McCready RA, Price MA, Kryscio RJ, et al: Failure of antiplatelet therapy with ibuprofen (Motrin) to prevent neointimal fibrous hyperplasia. J Vasc Surg 2:205, 1985
33. Bomberger RA, DePalma RG, Ambrose TA, et al: Aspirin and dipyridamole inhibit endothelial healing. Arch Surg 117:1459, 1982
34. Rainwater LM, Plate G, Gloviczki P, et al: Morphologic quantitation of pseudointima and effects of antiplatelet drugs on vascular prostheses in goats. Am J Surg 148:195, 1984
35. Chesebro JH, Fuster V, Elveback LR, et al: Effect of dipyridamole and aspirin on late vein-graft patency after coronary bypass operations. N Engl J Med 310:209, 1984

36. Pantely GA, Goodnight SH Jr, Rahimtoola SH, et al: Failure of antiplatelet and anti-coagulant therapy to improve patency of grafts after coronary-artery bypass. A controlled, randomized study. N Engl J Med 301:962, 1979

37. Sharma GVRK, Khuri SF, Josa M, et al: The effect of antiplatelet therapy on saphenous vein coronary artery bypass graft patency. Circulation 68 (Suppl II):II-218, 1983

38. Brooks N, Wright J, Sturridge M, et al: Randomized placebo controlled trial of aspirin and dipyridamole in the prevention of coronary vein graft occlusion. Br Heart J 53:201, 1985

39. Lorenz RL, Weber M, Kotzur J, et al: Improved aortocoronary bypass patency by low-dose aspirin (100 mg daily). Effects on platelet aggregation and thromboxane formation. Lancet 1:1261, 1984

40. Chevigné M, David J-L, Rigo P, et al: Effect of ticlopidine on saphenous vein bypass patency rates: A double-blind study. Ann Thorac Surg 37:371, 1984

41. Harjola P-T, Meurala H, Frick MH: Prevention of early reocclusion by dipyridamole and ASA in arterial reconstructive surgery. J Cardiovasc Surg 22:141, 1981

42. Veith FJ, Gupta SK, Samson RH, et al: Progress in limb salvage by reconstructive arterial surgery combined with new or improved adjunctive procedures. Ann Surg 194:386, 1981

43. Green RM, Roedersheimer LR, DeWeese JA. Effects of aspirin and dipyridamole on expanded polytetrafluoroethylene graft patency. Surgery 92:1016, 1982

44. Kohler TR, Kaufman JL, Kacoyanis G, et al: Effect of aspirin and dipyridamole on the patency of lower extremity bypass grafts. Surgery 96:462, 1984

John A. Mannick, Anthony D. Whittemore,
Nathan P. Couch, and Walter Koltun

5

What Is the Place of Thrombolytic Therapy in Occluded Grafts?

The treatment of acute arterial thrombosis with thrombolytic agents has been described for many years. However, the systemic administration of thrombolytic agents, particularly streptokinase, the agent used in most early reports, was associated with a considerable risk of hemorrhagic complications. Dotter and coworkers in 1974[1] first reported the use of local intraarterial low-dose streptokinase in patients with arterial thrombosis in an attempt to reduce the hazards of the systemic administration of this agent. The stage was therefore set for clinical attempts to use this technique to lyse the thrombus in recently occluded arterial bypass grafts, particularly grafts in the lower extremities. Hargrove and coworkers in 1982[2] reported the use of local intraarterial low-dose streptokinase therapy in the treatment of eight patients with thrombosed vascular grafts, most in the femoro-popliteal or femorotibial position. Successful initial thrombolysis was achieved in five of the eight patients. A number of reports have subsequently been published describing the use of local streptokinase or urokinase infusions or systemic therapy with the same agents in patients with occluded bypass grafts.[3–10] The initial success rate of the thrombolytic therapy has varied greatly ranging from around 20 to 90% in various reports.

Depending upon the results achieved, the groups reporting experience with this technique have been enthusiastic about its usefulness in the treatment of thrombosed grafts, or have concluded as the authors of one recent publication that it is an idea "whose time has passed."[10] With these widely disparate opinions expressed in the medical literature, can one arrive at any conclusions as to the usefulness of thrombolysis in the patient with an occluded arterial graft?

In an attempt to answer this question, it is first necessary to consider the various thrombolytic agents currently available, the route of administration, the dose, the use of adjunctive anticoagulants, and finally the potential benefits and risk of thrombolytic therapy with the agents at present in clinical use.

49

Streptokinase, probably the most commonly used fibrinolytic agent, is an indirect activator of the native fibrinolytic system. It combines with plasminogen to form an activator complex which then cleaves other plasminogen molecules to form plasmin, the active thrombolytic agent. Urokinase, on the other hand, directly converts plasminogen to plasmin. Since urokinase is prepared from human urine or from cultures of human epithelial cells, it is a natural protein and is not recognized as a foreign substance by the immune system of the patient. Sensitivity reactions occur commonly, however, in patients receiving streptokinase, perhaps in 10–25% of such patients in an initial treatment course.[2–10] The feature which argues against urokinase use is its cost. Whereas streptokinase is relatively inexpensive, costing approximately $100 in the United States for a 24-hour course of local thrombolytic therapy, urokinase is quite expensive, costing approximately $5000 for the same period of local treatment.

A third natural fibrinolytic agent has recently become available for experimental clinical use. This is tissue-type plasminogen activator, one of the natural activators of the plasminogen–plasmin system, manufactured by recombinant DNA technique. This material has the theoretical advantage of activating only the plasminogen bound to thrombus, and therefore possibly reducing the hazard of hemorrhagic complications. Considerable success with this agent has been achieved in the lysis of recent coronary artery thrombi; however, its use in the treatment of thrombosed arterial grafts has not yet been sanctioned in the United States and we are aware of no reported series of patients with occluded grafts who have been treated with this agent. However, if thrombolytic therapy remains a viable option for the therapy of such patients, recombinant tissue-type plasminogen activator may very well become the thrombolytic agent of choice in the future.

The technique for the administration of the thrombolytic agent has been fairly well standardized over the past five years. The usual method is to introduce a catheter through a remote puncture site, usually the opposite groin in the case of an occluded femoro-popliteal or femoro-tibial graft, and then by fluoroscopic control to imbed the tip of the catheter in the occluding thrombus at the origin of the thrombosed graft. Streptokinase, if this agent is to be used, is infused at a dose of approximately 5000 units per hour without a prior bolus. Urokinase has been infused at varying rates by varying groups. The system utilized at our hospital is to administer an initial bolus of 60,000 units and then to infuse urokinase at 4000 units per minute over the first two hours and then at 2000 units per minute over the second two hours, followed by an infusion of 1000 units per minute subsequently.

There is debate as to whether or not concomitant anticoagulation with heparin should be utilized during the infusion of fibrinolytic agents. It was felt initially that this entailed an extra and unacceptable hemorrhagic hazard.[2] However, our own experience has been similar to that of Wolfson, Kumpe, and Rutherford[3] in that the concomitant use of intravenous heparin infusion during and after infusion of thrombolytic agents is associated with a higher success rate and no increased risk of bleeding or thromboembolic complications. The current regimen used at our institution is to administer heparin intravenously at the rate of approximately 1000 units per hour, beginning shortly after the thrombolytic therapy has been initiated. We believe that this has caused a reduction in re-thrombosis around the catheter as thrombolysis progresses more distally.

The major complication of thrombolytic therapy has been and continues to be hemorrhage, presumably on the basis of systemic thrombolysis in spite of the attempt to avoid systemic effects by the local administration of the thrombolytic agents. It is clear that circulating fibrinogen levels decrease in patients treated with local thrombolytic therapy in most reported series. We believe at present that it is probably of little value to monitor systemic fibrinogen levels and euglobulin lysis times and consider that any hemorrhagic complications that ensue are absolute indications for discontinuing therapy.

The duration of thrombolytic therapy is directly associated with hemorrhagic and other complications in most reports. While there are reports of successful thrombolysis after as many as five days of continuous thrombolytic therapy,[3] our experience, and that of most groups using this technique for thrombolysis of occluded grafts, is that partial success will be apparent within approximately 24 hours if it is to be achieved at all, and that persistence of therapy beyond 48–72 hours is seldom likely to yield a more favorable outcome. The incidence of hemorrhagic complications is also clearly related to the technique used in catheter introduction. Obviously only one arterial puncture site should be used and an introducer of the smallest possible caliber commensurate with successful infusion of the thrombolytic agent should be used, thus minimizing the diameter of the puncture site in the native artery. Obviously in the groin the arterial puncture should be below the inguinal ligament so that there is no opportunity for retroperitoneal hemorrhage from the puncture site. Axillary puncture sites have been successfully utilized, but again should be kept distal to the true axilla so that hemorrhage into the soft tissues in this area can be minimized.

Which patients, then, are candidates for thrombolytic therapy of occluded arterial grafts? Since hemorrhage remains a considerable hazard, it seems logical that thrombolytic therapy should be contraindicated in patients with a recent ischemic or hemorrhagic infarction of the central nervous system, patients with severe hypertension, patients with an open wound, patients with active bleeding from any site, patients with a coagulopathy, or patients who have had a surgical procedure within 10 days. It is also clear that since thrombolytic therapy takes many hours in order to achieve success, patients who enter with a thrombosed graft and a nonviable foot or lower extremity are candidates for immediate surgical exploration rather than thrombolytic treatment. However, a sizable number of patients with late occlusion of bypass grafts in the lower extremity will have an ischemic foot without loss of motion or sensation and it is in such individuals that a trial of thrombolytic therapy may be warranted.

While there is concern expressed in the literature about the advisability of thrombolytic therapy in patients with Dacron grafts because of evidence of extravasation of blood through the interstices of such a graft which had been in place for more than a year in one report,[2] other investigators report considerable success with thrombolytic therapy in chronically implanted Dacron prostheses without such hemorrhagic complications.[9] Obviously, the use of thrombolytic agents in a freshly implanted Dacron prosthesis would be contraindicated. Varying success rates with thrombolytic therapy have been reported in PTFE grafts. Our own experience is that such prostheses are clearly amenable to thrombolytic treatment.

Successful lysis of clotted grafts has been reported more than 30 days after occurrence of the thrombosis; however, we have had most success with thrombolytic therapy early, seven days or less, after graft occlusion.

Perhaps the patients with the greatest potential benefit from thrombolytic therapy are those with occluded autogenous vein grafts. It is clear from past experience that poor long-term results are the rule after operative thrombectomy of such grafts.[11] Several factors have perhaps contributed to this poor rate of success. These include intimal damage by the Fogarty balloon catheter, failure to remove adherent mural thrombus, and failure to identify all the areas of stenosis in the graft or the host vessel following operative thrombectomy and intraoperative angiography, and therefore failure to appropriately treat the lesions causing the graft thrombosis. Initial thrombolytic therapy in such occluded vein grafts will permit complete angiographic evaluation of the graft and clear-cut delineation of the cause of the graft failure. This should therefore permit adequate surgical therapy of the offending lesion or treatment by percutaneous transluminal angioplasty (PTA).

As noted in Table 5-1, the success rate for thrombolytic therapy of occluded arterial grafts in recent reports has varied greatly and hemorrhagic complications have been prominent in most reported series. An additional hazard of thrombolytic therapy mentioned in several reports has been distal embolization of clot during the course of thrombolysis. This clearly seems a major hazard in patients with limited runoff below a distal bypass. Our experience suggests that distal thrombus will also lyse in most instances with continued thrombolytic therapy. However, in an experience of this technique in 37 thrombosed grafts, we have encountered one patient with a distal embolus following graft thrombolysis which resulted in a below-knee amputation.

As noted in Table 5-2, the initial success rate at our own institution for thrombolytic therapy in 37 arterial grafts, the vast majority in the femoro-popliteal or femoro-tibial position, was 65% with a complication rate of 41%, mostly minor bleeding. However, a number of major complications occurred including hemorrhage requiring transfusion or surgical intervention in six patients, acute renal failure in three, and a death from myocardial infarction in one individual. Whether or not the latter event was in any way attributable to the thrombolytic treatment is unclear.

Of the patients with initial success with graft thrombectomy, 11 were not noted to have an obvious case of graft failure. All 11 patients had fabric prostheses. Six patients were treated with angioplasty of stenotic lesions of a vein graft or of the host artery and six were treated with surgical repair of stenotic lesions in the graft or native artery. Two amputations were performed in patients who had an initially successful thrombolysis and three amputations were performed in patients in whom thrombolysis was unsuccessful. Four patients in the unsuccessful group had surgical intervention, thrombectomy and graft repair, or replacement.

Our recent experience demonstrates a considerable difference between patients treated with urokinase and those treated with streptokinase, in terms of the success of the thrombolytic therapy and the incidence of hemorrhagic complications (Table 5-2). Of 17 grafts treated with local streptokinase therapy, 47% had initially successful thrombolysis with a complication rate of 47%, whereas 20 grafts treated with urokinase had an 80% initially successful thrombolysis with a complication rate of 35%. Thus, 16 of the 20 urokinase patients had their grafts reopened and of these only one came to an amputation, whereas only eight of the streptokinase patients had their grafts reopened and one amputation was again necessary in this subgroup. Overall, three amputations were necessary in the patients treated initially with strep-

Table 5-1

Reported Results of Intraarterial Thrombolytic Therapy
in Patients with Thrombosed Grafts

Authors	No. of Patients	Initial Success (%)	Significant Hemorrhagic Complications (%)
Hargrove et al 1982[2]	8	62	35
Dardik et al 1984[8]	16	30	3
Wolfson et al 1984[3]	9	78	3.7
Sicard et al 1985[7]	12	21	18
Hallett et al 1985[6]	8	75	14
Graor et al 1985[4]	43	70	12
Goldberg et al 1985[9]	10	90	50
Perler et al 1985[10]	10	30	10

tokinase and two amputations were necessary in the patients initially treated with urokinase. Since our experience with patent but stenotic vein grafts has shown that patch graft angioplasty of stenotic lesions has been much more durable in terms of long-term graft patency than percutaneous transluminal angioplasty applied to similar patients, we prefer in most instances to perform a patch graft angioplasty of a stenotic lesion demonstrated angiographically after successful thrombolytic therapy of a thrombosed vein graft in the lower extremity.

What is not clear is whether or not thrombolytic therapy and patch graft angioplasty of occluded vein grafts will permit long-term patency of such grafts. The theoretical advantages of this technique as compared with catheter thrombectomy of such grafts are unattractive, as noted above. However, not enough patients have been followed for a long-enough time to be certain that a high rate of long-term patency will result. We are encouraged, however, by the continued good function of several vein grafts treated in this fashion at the $2\frac{1}{2}$–3 year interval.

At present, our conclusion would be that thrombolytic therapy has a role in the treatment of patients with occluded arterial grafts who lack the contraindications noted above. These patients include those with one thrombosed limb of a well-incorporated aorto-femoral Dacron graft, certain patients with axillo-femoral and femoro-femoral grafts, as well as those with grafts in the lower extremities. Thrombolytic therapy has the advantage of allowing complete clearance of thrombus from the occluded prosthesis preoperatively, thus permitting accurate angiographic delineation of the probable cause of the prosthetic failure. This is particularly useful in patients with thrombosed vein grafts in whom catheter thrombectomy seldom yields

Table 5-2

Results of Present Series of Thrombosed Grafts
Treated with Thrombolytic Agents

Treatment	No. of Patients	Initial Success (%)	Hemorrhagic Complications (%)
Urokinase	20	80	15 (10 major)
Streptokinase	17	47	36 (24 major)
Total	37	65	

a successful long-term result. The advantages of the technique have to be weighed against the high incidence of hemorrhagic complications, most of which fortunately are minor.

REFERENCES

1. Dotter CT, Rosch J, Seaman AJ: Selective clot lysis with low-dose streptokinase. Radiology 111:31–37, 1974
2. Hargrove WC III, Barker CF, Berkowitz HD, Perloff LJ, McLean G, Freiman D, Ring EJ, Roberts B: Treatment of acute peripheral arterial and graft thromboses with low-dose streptokinase. Surgery 92:981–990, 1982
3. Wolfson RH, Kumpe DA, Rutherford RB: Role of intra-arterial streptokinase in treatment of arterial thromboembolism. Arch Surg 119:697–702, 1984
4. Graor RA, Risius B, Denny KM, Young JR, Beven EG, Hertzer NR, Ruschhaupt WF III, O'Hara PJ, Geisinger MA, Zelch MG: Local thrombolysis in the treatment of thrombosed arteries, bypass grafts, and arteriovenous fistulas. J Vasc Surg 3:406–414, 1985
5. Aldrich MS, Sherman SA, Greenberg HS: Cerebrovascular complications of streptokinase infusion. JAMA 253:1777–1779, 1985
6. Hallet JW Jr, Greenwood LH, Yrizarry JM, Pierson WP, Robison JG, Brown SB: Statistical determinants of success and complications of thrombolytic therapy for arterial occlusion of lower extremity. S, G & O 161:431–437, 1985
7. Sicard GA, Schier JJ, Totty WG, Gilula LA, Walker WB, Etheredge EE, Anderson CB: Thrombolytic therapy for acute arterial occlusion. J Vasc Surg 2:65–78, 1985
8. Dardik H, Sussman BC, Kahn M, Greweldinger J, Adler J, Mendes D, Svoboda J, Ibrahim IM: S, G & O 158:137–140, 1984
9. Goldberg L, Ricci MT, Sauvage LR, Paulson PS, Davis CC, Smith JC, Rittenhouse EA, Hall DG, Mansfield PB: Thrombolytic therapy for delayed occlusion of knitted Dacron bypass grafts in the axillofemoral, femoropopliteal and femorotibial positions. S, G & O 160:491–498, 1985
10. Perler BA, White RI Jr, Ernst CB, Williams GM: Low-dose thrombolytic therapy for infrainguinal graft occlusions: An idea whose time has passed? J Vasc Surg 2:799–805, 1985
11. Whittemore AD, Clowes AW, Couch NP, Mannick JA: Secondary femoral popliteal reconstruction. Ann Surg 193:35–42, 1982

PART II

Investigation

R. M. Greenhalgh, Susan Laing,
Mary Ellis, Jacqueline Walton,
Karen Baxter, and J. T. Powell

6

How Can We Detect Early Subclinical Disease?

This chapter will be concerned with the detection of early subclinical arterial disease. With the increasing use of noninvasive tests, arterial disease can be detected before it becomes symptomatic and frequently disease is found in an unexpected site as a chance finding. The possible significance of such findings is a major question in its own right but here we shall be concerned with the detection of subclinical or asymptomatic arterial disease. The discussion will fall into two main parts. First, when arterial disease is symptomatic in one part of the body efforts can be made to look for arterial disease in another site. Second, a search can be made for arterial disease in a completely asymptomatic patient—asymptomatic in respect of all of the arteries of the body. This second question implies a screening programme in the community and is an interesting spinoff from the noninvasive tests. We will first look at the detection of disease in other parts of the body in patients who present with symptomatic peripheral arterial disease in at least one leg in the arterial clinic.

DETECTION OF ARTERIAL DISEASE IN OTHER SITES IN PERIPHERAL ARTERIAL DISEASE PATIENTS

Coronary Artery Disease

Patients attending a peripheral arterial disease clinic undergo a thorough history and clinical examination and it is found that there is a past history of a cardiac condition in a significant number of patients. The precise percentage varies according to which clinician takes the history. Equally the prevalence of coronary artery disease in peripheral arterial disease patients is different, when assessed by history or electrocardiographic findings.

To illustrate this we have taken the most recent 88 consecutive patients presenting with symptoms of peripheral arterial disease and there was a clear history of

VASCULAR SURGERY: ISSUES IN CURRENT PRACTICE
ISBN 0-8089-1839-7

heart attack in 20% of this group. However, when a more careful history is taken of other symptoms of cardiac disease, including angina, cardiac dyspnoea, and so on, in addition to past history of myocardial infarction, a prevalence of 45% was recorded on history alone.

All patients then underwent a resting electrocardiogram (ECG) and 46% had evidence of previous myocardial infarction on an ECG at rest (Fig. 6-1). Exercise ECGs on a treadmill were then performed on those patients who had a normal ECG at rest. The patients were exercised until ischaemic changes occurred or until the heart rate had risen to 85% of the expected maximum heart rate for a patient of that age.[1] We found that 32% of patients were unable to exercise satisfactorily, usually by virtue of incapacitating intermittent claudication. A further 15% were shown to have an abnormal ECG on exercise which, added to the 46% with abnormal resting tests, gave a prevalence of 61%. Only 7% of the total were satisfactorily tested and shown to have a normal ECG both at rest and at exercise. From this very simple evaluation it can be seen that unsuspected myocardial disease can be detected and that it is present in at least 61% of the group and probably more, because the 32% who had such severe intermittent claudication that they could not walk will no doubt include patients with some coronary artery disease. Even the resting ECG showing 46% abnormalities is useful beyond the cursory history taking of myocardial infarction alone. It is not the purpose of this chapter to go into the significance of the findings nor what one should do. However, this high prevalence

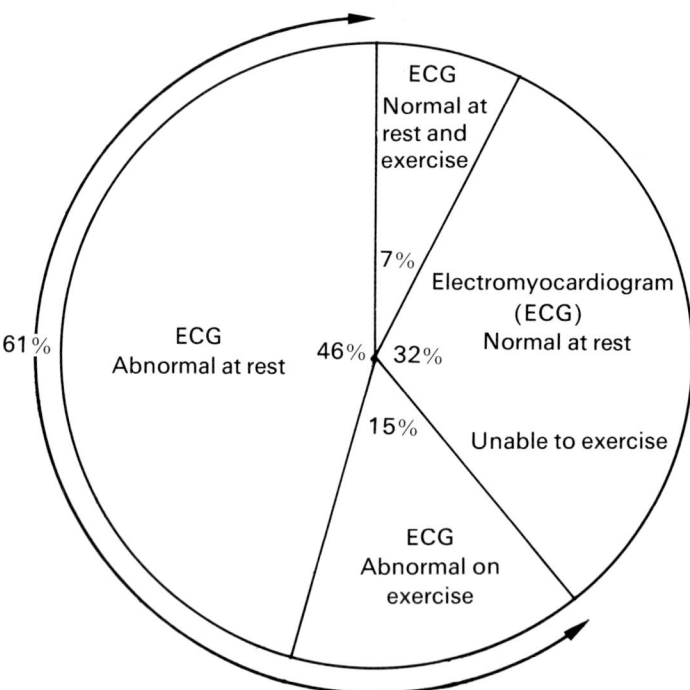

Fig. 6-1. Electrocardiograph findings at rest and after exercise on 88 peripheral arterial disease patients requiring surgery.

might be expected to influence the clinician in management of the peripheral arterial disease problem, either by performing coronary angiography and coronary artery bypass in some patients or, if not, at least monitoring patients thoroughly at the time of peripheral arterial reconstructive procedures.[2]

Carotid Artery Disease

Asymptomatic carotid artery disease may be suspected in peripheral arterial disease patients with a bruit,[3] but it can also be found in patients who do not have a bruit. In this section we shall review our recent findings of the prevalence of carotid artery disease in our peripheral arterial disease clinic whether the patient has a carotid bruit or not.

We have data on the most recent consecutive series of 352 peripheral arterial disease patients, 108 of whom were found to have a carotid bruit on one side or the other and 244 who had no carotid bruit at all (Table 6-1).

Patients with carotid bruit were examined with a Biosound duplex scanner and also Sonicaid "Vasoscan" (Fig. 6-2) and patients without a bruit a "Vasoscan" only. The "Vasoscan" is a continuous wave Doppler spectrum analyser and degrees of stenosis are ascribed according to peak frequencies; while it does not give any details of the quality of the vessel wall it is a useful screening instrument for rapid assessment of a large number of patients who could then be ascribed (on frequency analysis only) to have a degree of stenosis of less than 50% or greater than 50%. Unlike the duplex scanner this instrument is not able to detect minimal disease and roughenings in the artery wall for stenoses of less than 50%, but it can grade stenoses into smaller categories between 50 and 99% stenosis. The results in Table 6-1 for the nonbruit patients are based entirely upon the use of "Vasoscan", but the degree of stenosis for the bruit patients is based on "Vasoscan" and duplex scanning information. If anything, therefore, these findings underestimate the prevalence of subclinical or asymptomatic carotid artery disease, but any disease which is missed is most likely to be among those patients without bruit who have a stenosis of less than 50%.

There is always a problem when examining data in deciding whether to express results in terms of patients or sides (carotid arteries examined). We have displayed the data in both forms. Of the 352 patients, 87 were shown to have unilateral or bilateral stenosis of greater than 50%, a prevalence of 24.7%. There is, however, a striking difference between the bruit and nonbruit patients in terms of prevalence of carotid artery stenosis greater than 50%, being 51.8% for bruit and only 12.7% for nonbruit patients. From this it can be seen that the finding of a carotid bruit in the neck (which has for years alerted the clinician to the possibility of underlying carotid artery disease) does in fact have significance. In other words, approximately half of our series of patients with carotid bruits have a stenosis of greater than 50% in the underlying carotid artery, and this is much greater than where no bruit is found.

Looking at the problem in terms of carotid arteries examined rather than patients assessed, we have evaluated 704 carotid arteries recently in a consecutive series in our peripheral disease clinic. Of individual carotid arteries evaluated a total of 118 out of 704 were shown to have stenosis of greater than 50%, and once again significant stenosis occurs more commonly in the bruit patients (36.5%) than non-

Table 6-1
Carotid Artery Assessments on Patients Presenting with Peripheral Arterial Disease

	Total Patients	Bilateral <50% Stenosis	Unilateral or Bilateral >50% Stenosis	Total Carotids	Stenosis <50%	Stenosis >50%	Stenosis 50–79%	Stenosis 80–99%	Occluded
Bruit	108	52	56 (51.8%)	216	137	79 (36.5%)	70	5	4
Nonbruit	244	213	31 (12.7%)	488	449	39 (7.9%)	30	2	7
Total	352	265	87 (24.7%)	704	586	118 (16.7%)	100	7	11

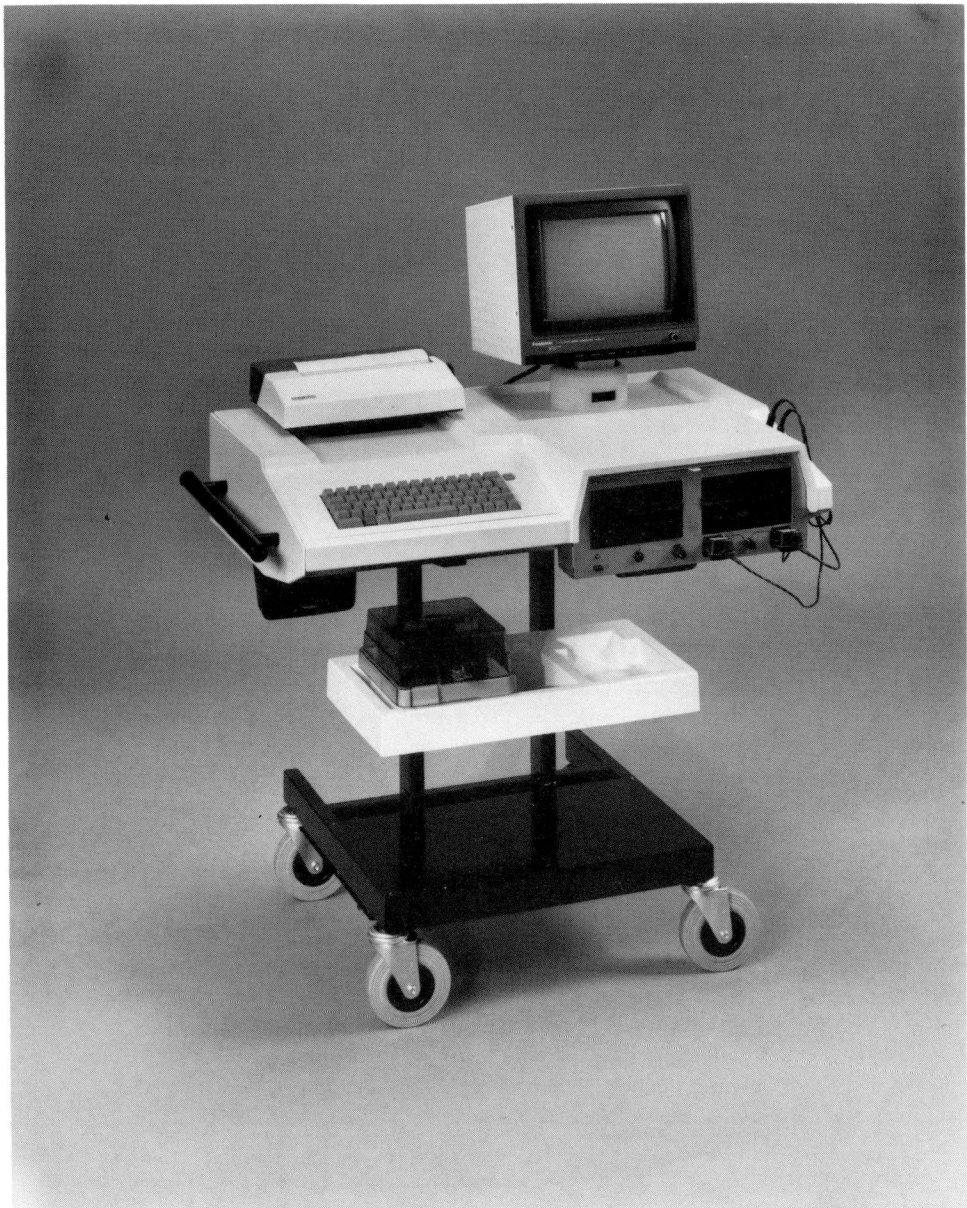

Fig. 6-2. Sonicaid "Vasoscan" continuous wave Doppler spectrum analyser.

bruit patients (7.9%). We then broke down the significant stenoses into groups of 50 to 79%, 80 to 99%, and occluded. As can be seen from Table 6-1, 11 internal carotid arteries were shown to be occluded in patients who had no symptoms of this whatsoever in their past history. This finding of previous "silent" occlusion of the internal carotid artery is not new and it remains a very foxing question of which tight stenoses are going to occlude without symptoms and which ones will occlude with development of disastrous stroke. The especially interesting group is therefore

Table 6-2
Asymptomatic Carotid Disease in Peripheral Arterial Disease Patients

	Number of Patients	Number of Patients Lost	Deaths	TIAs	Strokes	
					No Warning	With Warning
Bilateral asymptomatic bruit	44	8	16	6	3	2
Unilateral asymptomatic bruit	18	3	6	3	0	0
Total bruit patients	62	11	22	9	3	2
Nonbruit patients	62	5	14	2	3	0

that of 107 carotids with a stenosis between 50 and 99%. Particularly engaging are those seven with a tight stenosis of between 80 and 99%.

These data have shown without doubt that one can detect asymptomatic carotid artery disease in peripheral arterial disease patients whether there is a bruit or not in the neck. It is not our intention to go into detail in this chapter of what we do when we find these abnormalities. There is, however, a great need for us to know as much as we possibly can of the natural history of carotid artery disease to justify surgical intervention, particularly in the asymptomatic state. What is striking is what happens over a period of five years when bruit and nonbruit patients are followed (Table 6-2). A large number of deaths occurred and although transient ischaemic attacks occurred more commonly in bruit patients than in nonbruit (control) patients, stroke without warning occurred equally commonly in the bruit

Table 6-3
Deaths over Five Years of
Asymptomatic Carotid Artery Patients
with Symptomatic Peripheral Arterial Disease

	62 Bruit Patients	62 Nonbruit Patients
Range (months)	0.5–51	3–54
Mean time (months)	25	28
Myocardial infarction	13 (59%)	4 (28.5%)
Bronchopneumonia	2	2
Carcinoma	2	2
Uncertain	3	3
Fatal stroke	2	0
Other	0	3
Total	22	14

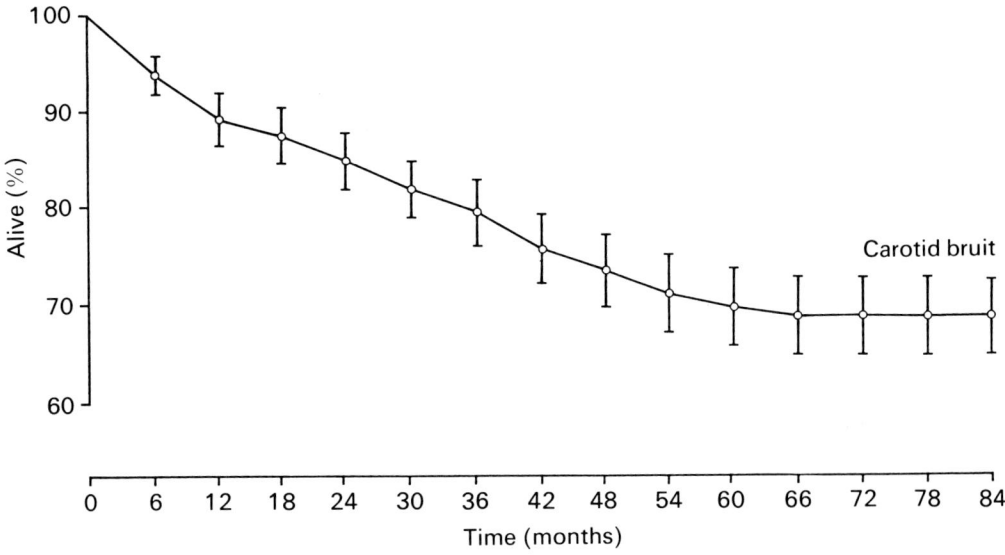

Fig. 6-3. Survival of peripheral arterial disease patients with carotid bruit.

and nonbruit groups. By stroke without warning we mean stroke which is not preceded by a transient ischaemic attack (TIA). TIAs certainly occurred more commonly with bruit than without bruit and when this occurred, patients were operated upon where appropriate. There remains a possibility that if this surgical intervention had not taken place at that stage, more strokes would have occurred. We were struck by the large number of patients who died over five years (Table 6-3) and noted that the majority of the patients died of a myocardial infarction (59% in the bruit group). This further underlines the coincidence of disease. These patients are symptomatically peripheral arterial disease patients and we have evaluated their carotid artery disease. Over the five years they have died of coronary artery disease in large numbers. Figure 6-3 is a life table analysis of our carotid bruit patients showing the expected attrition rate over a seven-year period, and this is no different for those patients with carotid bruit than no bruit and reflects the expected attrition rate of peripheral arterial disease patients of about 7% per year. In other words, about a third of our patients are dead within five years and the majority die of coronary artery disease.

The One-minute Exercise Test

We now turn to assess the prevalence of peripheral arterial disease among patients with symptomatic arterial disease in other sites such as the coronary arteries, carotid arteries, and in the contralateral lower limb. Much of this would not be possible were it not for the development of the one-minute exercise test.[4] This test was developed to assess patients after a period of standard exercise. The value of the ankle–brachial Doppler systolic pressure ratio has been known for some years[5] and the one-minute exercise test was devised as an extension of this for the detection of more minor degrees of disease in the arteries supplying the lower limbs. The claudication distance is an assessment of the patient but it is subjective and may fluctuate considerably between visits and does not correlate with any objective measurement.[6] Furthermore, it applies only to the most severely diseased limb such that claudication in one limb may "mask" the development of symptoms in the other less affected limb. The ankle pressure after exercise is a sensitive and objective assessment of haemodynamically important disease and thus has advantages over the claudication distance alone.

The one-minute exercise test as described[4] commences after the patients have rested for 10 minutes, after which the resting arm and ankle systolic pressures are measured using a Doppler probe and pressure cuff. After a period of exercise on a treadmill the patient is returned to bed. During the development of the test, patients were exercised for either one minute at 4 kilometres per hour, 1 minute at 6 kilometres per hour, 2 minutes at 4 kilometres per hour, or 2 minutes at 6 kilometres per hour (Fig. 6-4). It was found that for any given ankle pressure before exercise the pressure fell to the same value however far and fast the patient walked. The recovery

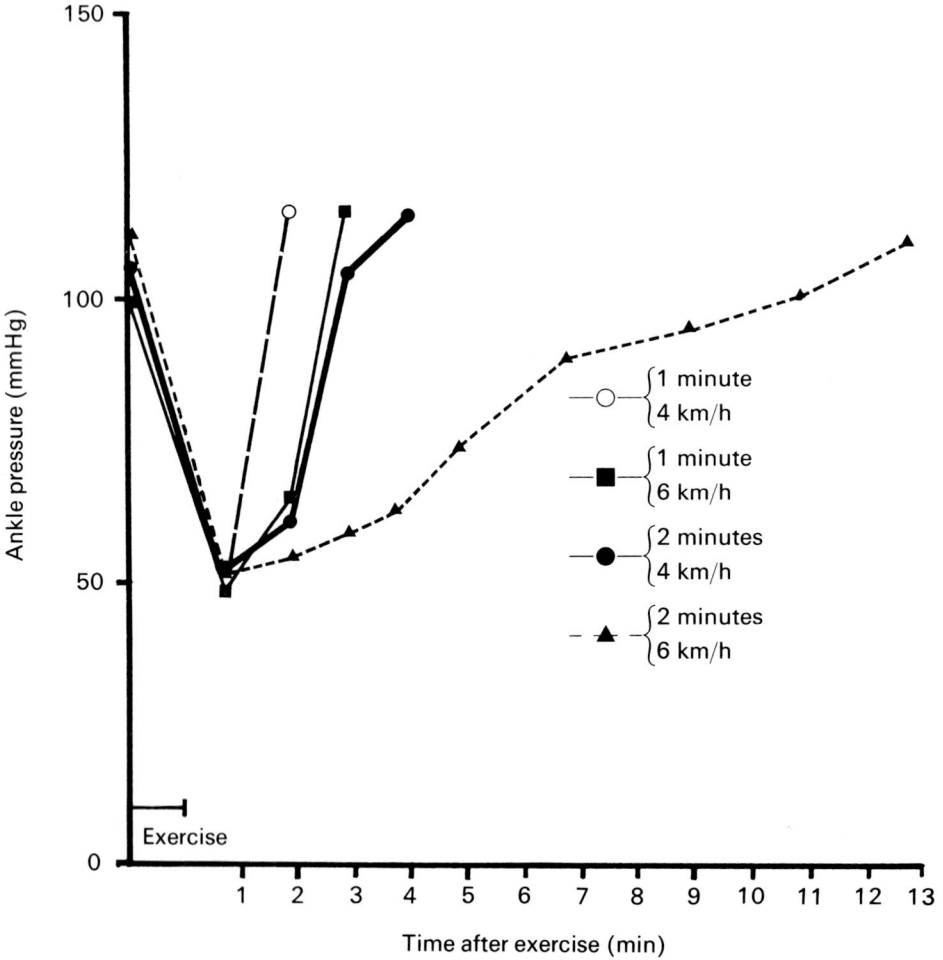

Fig. 6-4. Ankle pressure response to exercise.

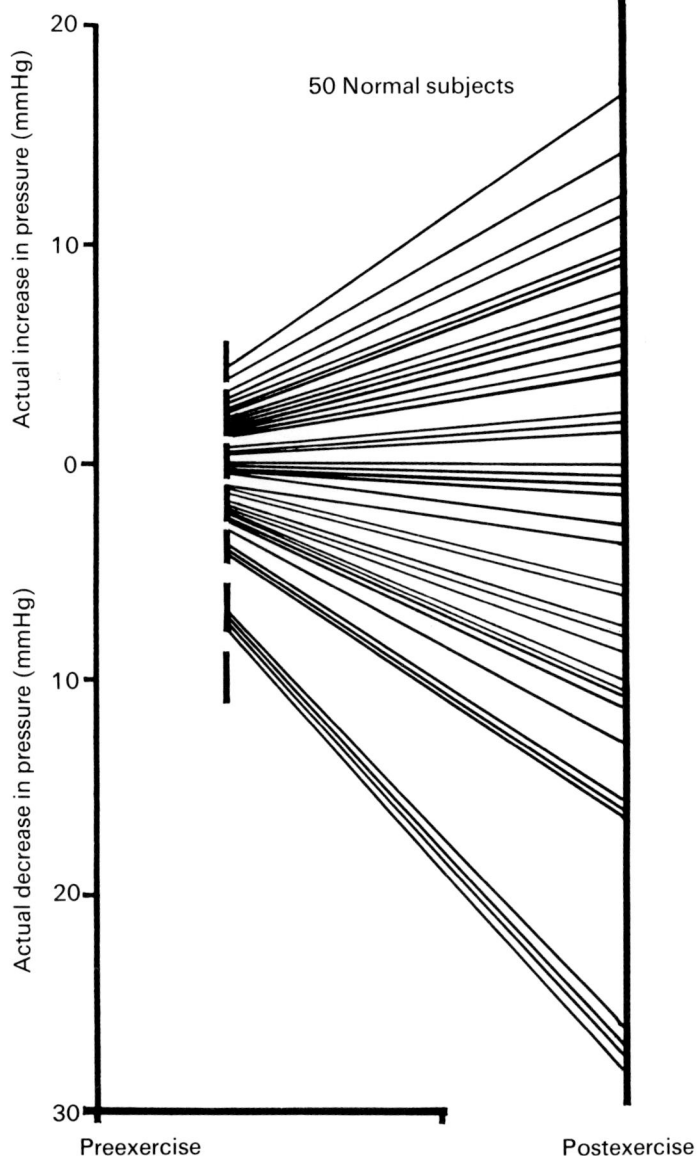

Fig. 6-5. Ankle pressure response of 50 normal subjects after the one-minute exercise test at 4 kilometres per hour on a 10 degree slope.

time was extended with an increased workload. Consequently, it was decided that all that was required to achieve the postexercise end-point was that the patient should walk for 1 minute at 4 kilometres per hour on a 10 degree slope and that the fall in pressure should be noted, the "one-minute exercise test."

It was next necessary to establish normal levels and a group of 67 healthy subjects (100 legs) form the control group; 18 were women and 49 men with an age range of 20–34 years. Peripheral arterial disease is rare in this age group and it was

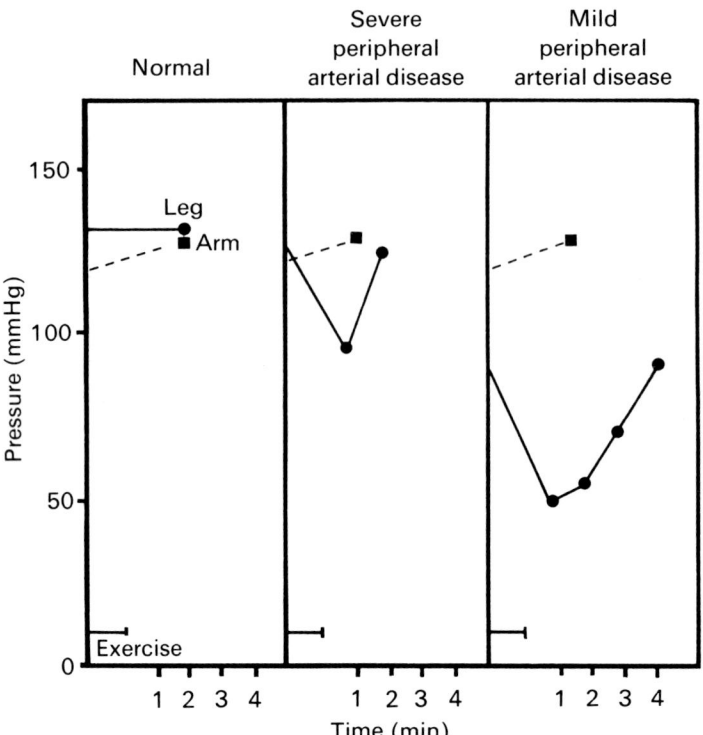

Fig. 6-6. Gradation of response of the one-minute exercise test with severity of disease.

unlikely that a subject with significant asymptomatic disease would inadvertently be included, but this was indeed possible. The resting ankle–brachial Doppler pressure ratio, pressure index (PI), was measured for the 100 legs and the one-minute exercise test was performed. The ankle pressure was measured 30 seconds after exercise and if both legs were examined the whole procedure was repeated for the second leg after a further 10-minute rest.

The mean resting PI was 1.23 ± 0.13 ($x \pm$ SD) with a range of 0.9–1.5 and 95% of the observations fell between 0.97 and 1.49. From these results a resting pressure index of less than 0.9 would be regarded as abnormal and we should aim to perform the one-minute exercise test only on those occasions when the resting pressure index was greater than 0.9.

The responses of 50 normal subjects to the standard exercise period are shown in Fig. 6-5. The mean preexercise ankle pressure was 140 ± 17.4 mmHg ($x \pm$ SD) and the mean postexercise pressure was 138 ± 19.9 mmHg. The change in ankle pressure following exercise was not significant. The ankle pressure change following exercise ranged from -27 to $+35$ mmHg and 95% of the postexercise results were between -25 and $+22$ mmHg. From these results a pressure fall of 30 mmHg was taken to be indicative of significant peripheral arterial disease.

This enabled subsequent recognition of normal from mild peripheral arterial disease from severe peripheral arterial disease (Fig. 6-6). In all, the arm pressure rises after a period of exercise. The resting pressure index is normal for the patients with mild peripheral arterial disease but reduced for patients with severe peripheral arterial disease. Mild peripheral arterial disease is detected only by the one-minute exercise test (Fig. 6-6) and applications of this test have proved to be most extensive.[7]

Prevalence of Peripheral Arterial Disease in Patients Admitted for Coronary Artery Bypass Graft Surgery

These patients were all awaiting coronary artery bypass surgery and had coronary artery disease demonstrated by angiography. Eighty consecutive patients (4 female and 76 male) were studied (six patients had symptoms of peripheral arterial disease and nine were unsuitable for testing on a treadmill because of the severity of their coronary artery disease.[7] Of the 65 remaining patients, 50 were evaluated. A history was taken and clinical examination performed, and the absence of both pedal pulses was regarded as indicative of significant peripheral arterial disease. The results are summarised in Fig. 6-7. Six of the 80 patients had symptoms of intermittent claudication and signs of peripheral arterial disease. The prevalence of symptomatic peripheral arterial disease in this group is thus 7.5%. Of the 50 patients assessed one had a reduced PI at rest and the ankle pressure response to exercise was abnormal in a further 18 patients; thus 38% of patients who were asymptomatic were shown to have functionally significant peripheral arterial disease, giving an overall prevalence of 42.7% of coronary artery disease patients (Fig. 6-8).

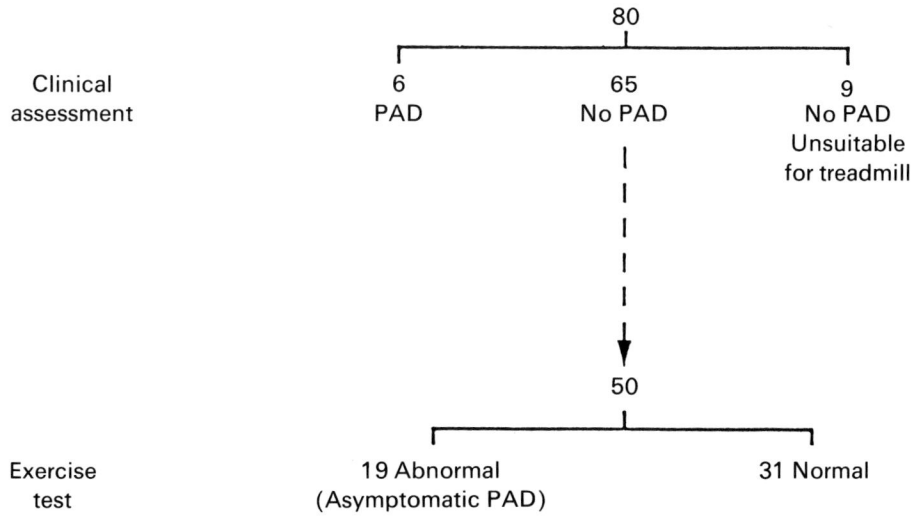

Fig. 6-7. Symptomatic and asymptomatic peripheral arterial disease in CABG patients.

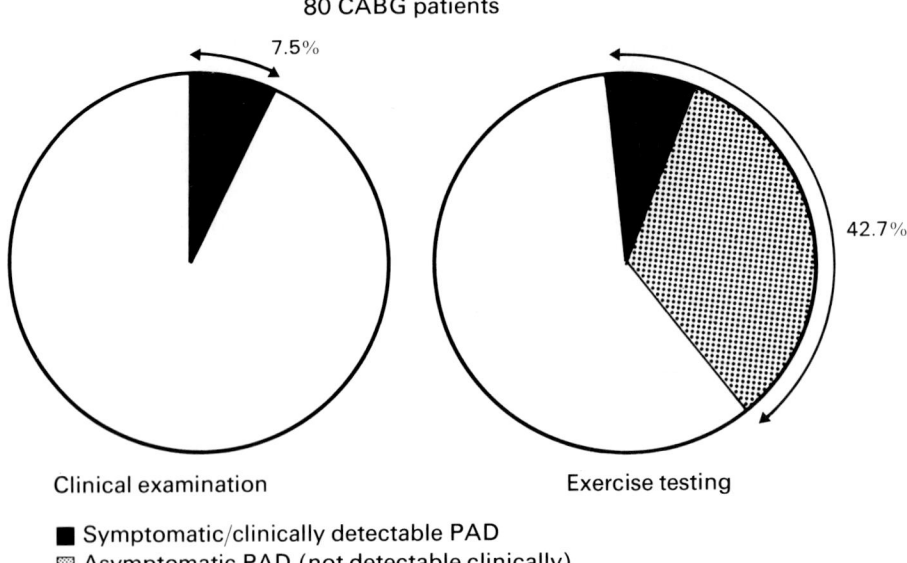

Fig. 6-8.   Prevalence of peripheral arterial disease in 80 patients undergoing CABG.

Peripheral Arterial Disease in Diabetic Patients

Similarly 219 consecutive diabetic patients (96 female and 123 male) aged 40 years and over were reviewed as before (Fig. 6-9). Twenty-four had symptoms and signs of peripheral arterial disease and an additional seven had arterial disease on clinical examination only, giving a total of 31 (14.2% with clinical disease) (Fig. 6-10). The remaining 188 patients (85.8%) had no symptoms or signs of peripheral

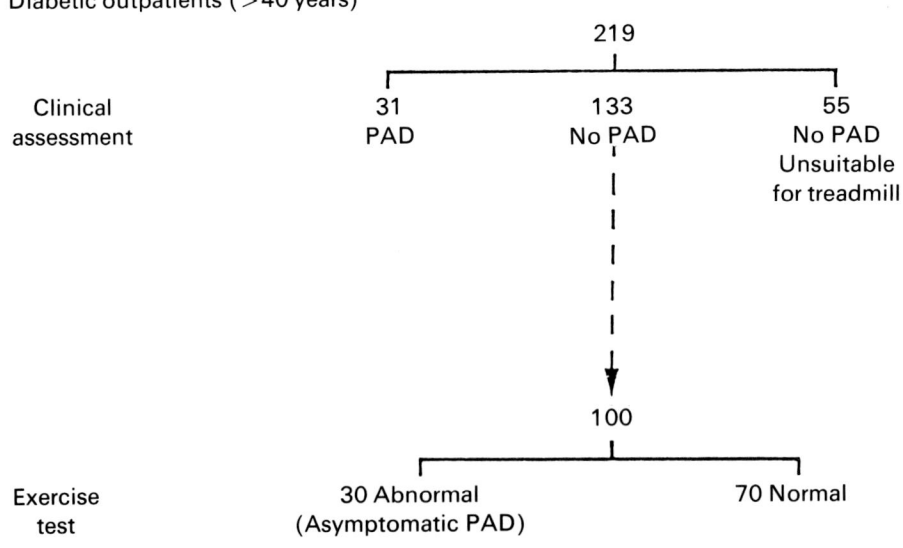

Fig. 6-9.   The prevalence of symptomatic and asymptomatic disease in diabetic patients.

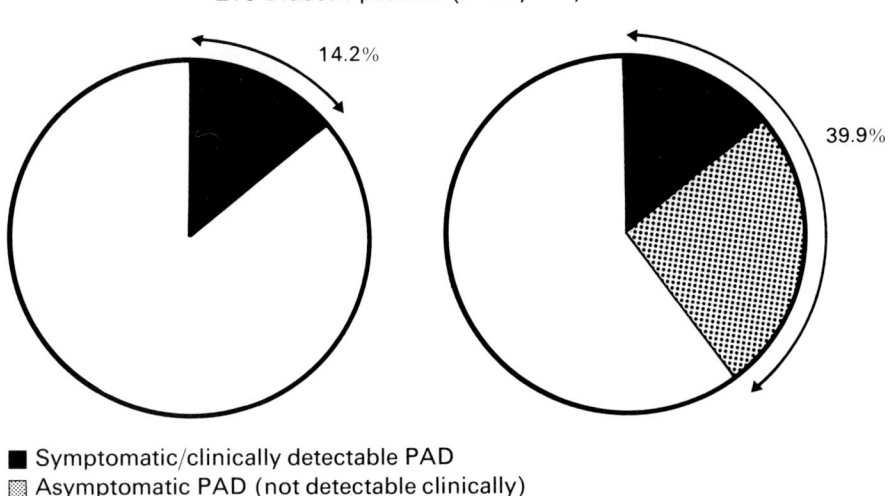

219 Diabetic patients (>40 years)

14.2%

39.9%

■ Symptomatic/clinically detectable PAD
▨ Asymptomatic PAD (not detectable clinically)

Fig. 6-10. Prevalence of peripheral arterial disease in 219 diabetic patients over 40 years of age.

arterial disease. Fifty-five of the patients without symptoms and signs of peripheral arterial disease were considered unsuitable for treadmill testing and of the remaining 133 patients (Fig. 6-9) 100 agreed to undergo treadmill testing.[7] Three of these had a reduced resting pressure index and a further 27 had an abnormal ankle pressure response to exercise. Thus 30% of the 85.8% (25.7%) with no symptoms or clinical signs of peripheral arterial disease had functionally significant disease detectable by noninvasive investigation. The overall prevalence of peripheral arterial disease in diabetics is thus 39.9% (Fig. 6-10). Again the addition of noninvasive tests to the investigation, and the one-minute exercise test in particular, revealed considerably more disease than suggested by clinical examination or Doppler resting tests alone.

SCREENING FOR SUBCLINICAL ARTERIAL DISEASE IN THE COMMUNITY

Screening for Abdominal Aortic Aneurysms: The "Dalby Study"

In the United Kingdom, sudden death which requires a Coroner's autopsy is found to be caused most commonly by myocardial infarction followed closely by fatal stroke. The third commonest cause of sudden death is a burst abdominal aortic aneurysm and so there has been interest in screening for abdominal aortic aneurysm so that surgery may be performed in good time. The vast majority of abdominal aneurysms are asymptomatic and a person is lucky if the aneurysm causes symptoms such as backache or diarrhoea to attract attention. At other times aneurysms may be found when patients see their doctor for some other trivial reason and a careful clinical examination is performed. In the "Dalby study" all hypertensive patients born in the period 1912 to 1931 who visited the Dalby Health Centre in 1980 were invited to a medical examination including ultrasonography of the abdominal aorta. Of the 264 patients, age range 50 to 70 years, 253 attended the clinical examination and 245 had an ultrasound. The patients were identified by means of the statistical computer scheme for patient care in the Dalby primary care district. It comprised 9% of all inhabitants in that age group. The scheme was described as an individually based computer system for the processing of statistical information about inhabitants and their contacts and health and medical care services.[8]

Clinical examination was performed including blood pressure measurement and abdominal palpation. This was followed by ultrasonography whereby the abdominal aorta was scanned longitudinally and transversly. The transverse scans were made at intervals of 2 cm covering the area from the diaphragm to aortic bifurcation. The diameter of the aorta was measured at the level of the renal arteries and the left renal vein. The abdominal aorta was considered normal when its diameter at the aortic bifurcation was identical with or smaller than at the renal arteries.

Of the 245 patients only one was shown to have an abdominal aortic aneurysm, a prevalence of 0.4%. This abdominal aortic aneurysm was not diagnosed at the clinical examination. Two clinically suspected abdominal aortic aneurysms were found to be negative after ultrasonography.

The prevalence of abdominal aortic aneurysm in this study is extremely low and it was thought that it would be higher in the hypertensive group of patients who would be expected to have a higher risk of arterial disease in general. On the contrary, in the age group 40–59 years, 21% of the male and 8% of the female hypertensives had suffered from stroke, coronary artery disease, or intermittent claudication at the time they were seen. Corresponding figures for those aged 60–69 were 36% for the male and 14% for the female group respectively. The low prevalence of abdominal aortic aneurysms in this high-risk group of patients is likely to be relevant. In summary, subclinical abdominal aortic aneurysm can certainly be detected but in this population study it did not seem to be worth the effort.

Screening for Peripheral Arterial Disease in Patients Seen for Inguinal Hernia

This study was performed to investigate the extent of symptomatic and asymptomatic peripheral arterial disease in a consecutive series of patients admitted for hernia repair.[7] The study comprised 165 consecutive patients (12 female, 153 male) admitted for herniorrhaphy. Symptoms and signs of peripheral arterial disease were found during routine clinical assessment in eight of the 165 (Fig. 6-11). Those with no symptoms or signs of peripheral arterial disease and suitable for treadmill testing were invited to participate in a more thorough noninvasive investigation. One hundred patients (6 female, 94 male) aged 61.1 ± 10.2 years agreed and were usually tested as outpatients after they had recovered from surgery. The mean ($\pm$SD) resting PI was 1.2 ± 0.14. Only one patient had a reduced pressure index but the ankle pressure response to exercise was abnormal in a further nine patients; thus 10 of 95.2% of patients who were asymptomatic were shown to have peripheral arterial

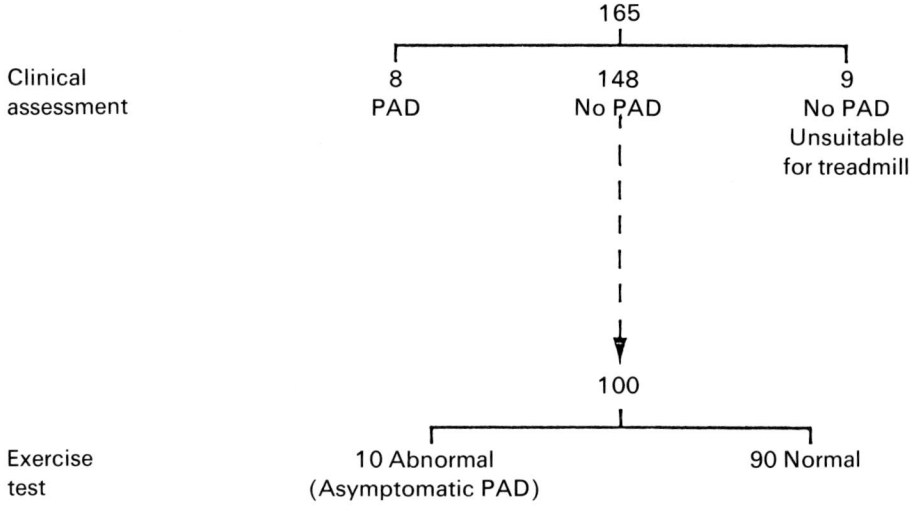

Fig. 6-11. Symptomatic and asymptomatic peripheral arterial disease in hernia patients.

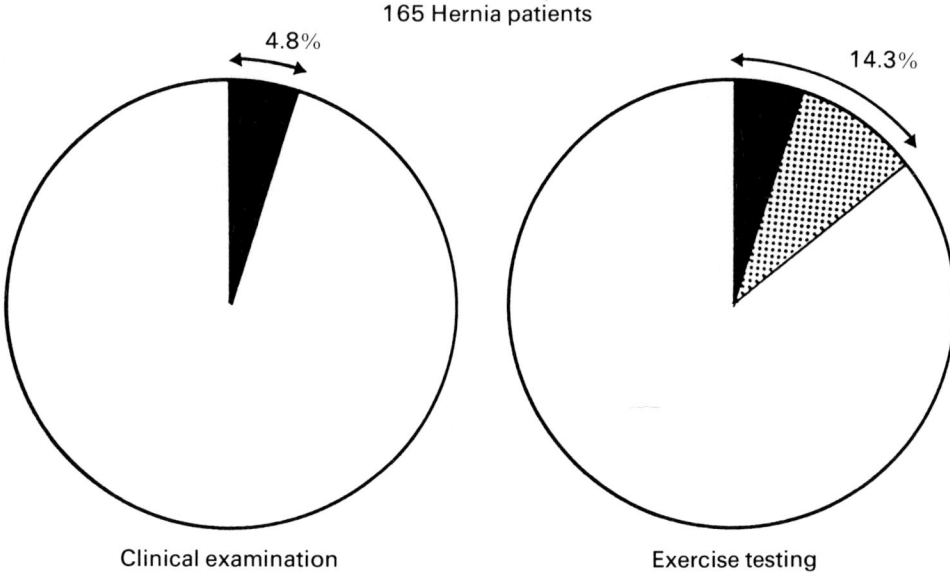

■ Symptomatic/clinically detectable PAD
▨ Asymptomatic PAD (not detectable clinically)

Fig. 6-12. The extent of symptomatic and asymptomatic peripheral arterial disease detectable using clinical assessment alone and noninvasive pressure measurements is shown in patients admitted for hernia repair.

disease by noninvasive tests. Adding this to the eight patients out of 165 found on clinical assessment (4.8%), the overall prevalence of symptomatic and asymptomatic peripheral arterial disease in hernia patients was 14.3% (Fig. 6-12).

The IBM Screening Study

One of us (KB) screened 109 healthy men and women in their sixth decade for asymptomatic arterial disease and plasma risk factors. With the cooperation of a local employer, IBM, we invited all the personnel between the ages of 50 and 60 to attend noninvasive arterial screening at the place of their work. Previous referral to hospital for heart and arterial disease excluded people from screening. The response rate was 90%. One person had diabetes mellitus and 14 were hypertensive, 11 of these on treatment.

The screening lasted approximately 45 minutes and was performed by a nurse technician. No clinical examination was, therefore, possible. A history, resting ECG, resting and one-minute exercise ankle Doppler testing, and "Vasoscan" Doppler examination of the carotids were performed.

The results are shown in Table 6-4. From these it can be seen that 11 people had an abnormal one-minute exercise test whereas none of the 109 had an abnormal resting pressure index. Two had symptoms suggestive of arterial disease on history, but it must be remembered that the investigator was not medically qualified and also patients with known symptoms who had been investigated at hospitals were excluded from this study. Only five had an abnormal resting ECG (one of whom had an abnormal one-minute test) and in only one was there a carotid lesion thought to represent a stenosis of approximately 50% in one of the internal carotid arteries. The summation of abnormalities is 16 out of 109, a prevalence of 14.7%. Clearly this community screening project would have been hopeless were it not for the one-minute exercise test. The yield from PI and carotid "Vasoscan" alone is really too small to justify it.

Progression of Asymptomatic Peripheral Arterial Disease

Thirty patients (8 women and 22 men), age range 38–72 years, underwent either aortic reconstruction (19) or femoro-popliteal surgery (11) and were completely free from symptoms in both legs after surgery. In addition the 30 patients had clinically normal legs and a normal pressure index at rest and a normal response to the

Table 6-4
Results of the IBM Screening Study

	History	Resting ECG	Carotid "Vasoscan"	Resting PI	One-minute Exercise Test	Summation
Normal	107	104	108	109	98	93
Abnormal	2*	5+	1	0	11+	16 (14.7%)

* One claudicant with abnormal one-minute exercise test and with TIAs and abnormal ECG and one with TIAs and abnormal ECG and one-minute exercise test. This latter person (+) accounts for the single ECG test overlap in the sample.

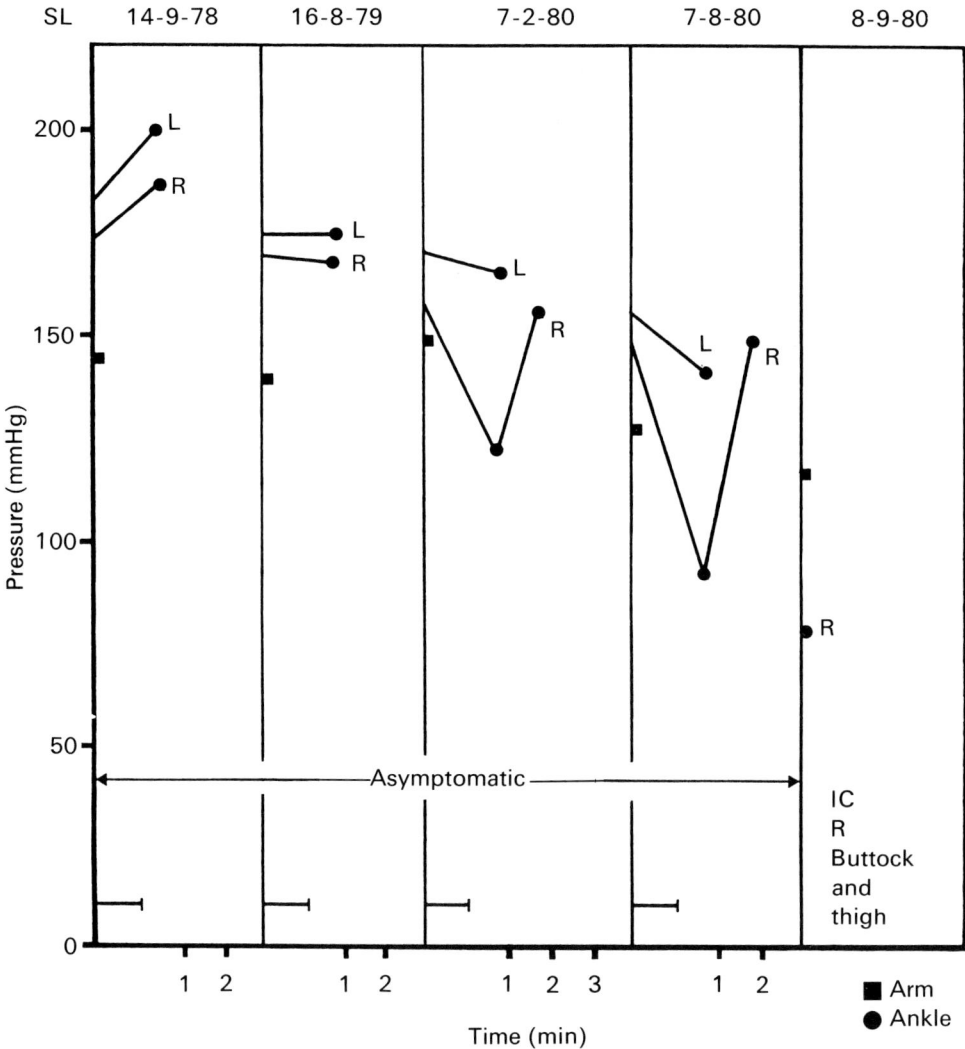

Fig. 6-13. Example of a patient successfully operated upon who became symptomatic again. There is a stage (on 7 February 1980 and 7 August 1980) when the exercise test falls more than 30 mmHg and is, therefore, abnormal while the patient remained asymptomatic.

one-minute exercise test. The patients were followed six monthly with clinical assessment and noninvasive evaluation for a minimum of three years. After three years 14 still had a normal ankle pressure response to exercise but the other 16 were abnormal. In four of these intermittent claudication had returned at the same time as the pressure response became abnormal. The others initially remained asymptomatic but within a year (as the ankle pressures worsened further) four more developed symptoms of intermittent claudication. Nine of the patients normal at three years were followed for four years. By this time five of them had developed an abnormal pressure response. Initially four were asymptomatic and one developed symptoms concurrently with the first abnormal test. Three more developed intermittent claudication within a year. The serial developments of an individual who developed an abnormal pressure response before recurrent symptoms is shown in Fig. 6-13.

The importance of the one-minute exercise test is stressed once again in that during a period when the patient was completely symptom free the exercise response was abnormal and the progression of disease could be inferred at this stage.

Summary

We have seen that it is indeed possible to detect subclinical asymptomatic arterial disease in a number of sites and recent developments in methodology could make screening in the community worthwhile for the first time. The one-minute exercise test has been shown to be quick and it has produced a useful yield in the screening studies. By contrast the resting pressure index and carotid testing and even resting ECG have yielded far fewer positives. The additional attraction of the one-minute test is that it enables progression of arterial disease to be monitored during the subclinical and asymptomatic stage.

CONCLUSIONS

When a patient develops arterial symptoms in one arterial system there is clearly an increased chance of arterial disease elsewhere in the body. With the range of noninvasive technology available at the present time a total body assessment of arteries by noninvasive techniques ought to be performed whenever a patient becomes symptomatic in one system. As we have seen, clinical disease can be detected frequently in other sites.

Whereas the Dalby study using ultrasound to detect abdominal aortic aneurysm in the community was somewhat disappointing, the use of the one-minute exercise test to detect disease in the community and to follow its progression would appear to have enormous future possibilities.

REFERENCES

1. Sheffield LT, Roitman D: Stress testing methodology. Prog in Cardiovasc Dis 14(1):33, 1976
2. Whittemore AD, Clowes AW, Hechtman HB, et al: Aortic aneurysm repair: Reduced operative mortality associated with maintenance of optimal cardiac performance. Ann Surg 192:414, 1980
3. Ellis MR, Greenhalgh RM: Management of asymptomatic carotid bruit. J Vasc Surg, 1986 (submitted)
4. Laing SP, Greenhalgh RM: Standard exercise test to assess peripheral arterial disease. Br Med J 280:13, 1980
5. Yao JST, Hobbs JT, Irvine WT: Ankle systolic pressure measurements in arterial disease affecting the lower extremities. Br J Surg 56:676, 1969
6. Yao ST, Needham TI, Gourmos C, Irvine WT: A comparative study of strain-gauge plethysmography and Doppler ultrasound in the assessment of occlusive disease of the lower extremities. Surgery 71:4, 1972
7. Laing SP: Assessment of symptomatic and asymptomatic peripheral arterial disease using a one minute exercise test. PhD Thesis, University of London, 1984
8. Lindholm L, Ejlertsson G, Forsberg L, Norgren L: Low prevalence of abdominal aortic aneurysm in hypertensive patients. A population study. Acta Med Scand 218(3):305, 1985
9. Laing SP, Greenhalgh RM: The detection and progression of asymptomatic peripheral arterial disease. Br J Surg :628, 1983

R. Eugene Zierler
and D. Eugene Strandness, Jr.

7

How Should Intraoperative and Postoperative Results Be Assessed?

INTRODUCTION

The rationale for the objective assessment of arterial surgery is to achieve the best possible functional result. Since the immediate result of an operation is determined mainly by technical factors, assessment must begin in the operating room. The purpose of intraoperative assessment is to detect technical errors at a time when they can be safely corrected, thereby avoiding ischemic complications and early failure of the reconstruction. After a successful operation, periodic evaluations of the reconstructed segment can minimize the risk of late failure. Postoperative assessment can identify problems related to the original procedure and progression of arterial disease in other areas. In either case, further operative intervention may be indicated.

The methods used for intraoperative and postoperative assessment must be safe, and they should provide objective physiologic or anatomic information on the arteries of interest. Intraoperative assessment techniques need to be simple, rapid, and readily applied in the operating room. For postoperative assessment, the methods should be inexpensive and noninvasive to facilitate serial follow-up evaluations.

This chapter will present the various methods available for assessing the results of arterial surgery and discuss the application of these methods to the evaluation of operations for lower extremity arterial disease and carotid endarterectomy.

INSTRUMENTATION AND METHODS

Imaging Methods

The methods for assessing the results of arterial surgery are based on either some type of anatomic imaging or flow detection. Although contrast arteriography is the standard imaging technique, arterial puncture and contrast injection are

VASCULAR SURGERY: ISSUES IN CURRENT PRACTICE
ISBN 0-8089-1839-7

associated with some risk.[1] Furthermore, this approach supplies no direct information on arterial flow. In spite of these disadvantages, arteriography still provides the most detailed anatomic information available, so the additional risk is justified in certain intraoperative and postoperative situations.[2,3] Arteriography also permits visualization of vessels outside the operative field. Comparisons with arteriography have generally been used to validate the other assessment techniques.

B-mode ultrasound is another imaging method that can be used to assess the arterial system.[4,5] The vessels within the operative field can be examined directly, and the same areas can usually be imaged transcutaneously in the postoperative period. Arteries are recognized by their characteristic B-mode appearance of bright wall echoes and a dark, sonolucent lumen. Atherosclerotic plaque may appear as a thickened segment of the arterial wall, and areas of calcification produce acoustic shadowing. Three types of arterial defects can be detected by intraoperative B-mode imaging: strictures, thrombi, and intimal flaps. In a series of over 450 vascular operations, Sigel and coworkers used B-mode ultrasound and found arterial defects in 32%.[6] However, in 22% of the operations the defects were not considered significant and no corrective action was taken. The presence or absence of a defect did not appear to influence the clinical outcome. This experience emphasizes that the interpretation of B-mode images is highly subjective, and most of the visualized defects do not require surgical repair. Thus, the extreme sensitivity of B-mode imaging in the detection of vascular defects can be a disadvantage. The method is also limited to evaluation of those vascular structures in the operative field. The main advantages of B-mode ultrasound in comparison to contrast arteriography are rapidity, ease of use, and elimination of the need for arterial puncture and contrast injection.

Flow Detection

Assessment methods that rely on flow detection include the electromagnetic flowmeter and Doppler ultrasound. The value of the electromagnetic flowmeter for intraoperative assessment is limited, since normal flowrates vary widely and many significant technical errors produce little or no flow reduction.[7,8] Doppler ultrasound has been used in the routine preoperative and postoperative evaluation of patients with arterial disease.[9] The intraoperative Doppler assessment provides an immediate and direct indication of blood flow in the exposed vessels without the additional risks of operative arteriography.

In vascular diagnosis, the Doppler effect refers to the frequency shift observed when ultrasound is reflected by moving blood cells. This frequency shift is directly proportional to blood velocity. Most Doppler instruments use transmitting frequencies in the range of 3–10 MHz. The lower frequencies are best suited for the transcutaneous examination of deeply located vessels, since low-frequency ultrasound penetrates tissue more effectively. However, for intraoperative assessment the Doppler probe is usually placed directly on the vessels, and tissue penetration is not a consideration.

There are two basic types of Doppler ultrasound: continuous and pulsed. When ultrasound is transmitted continuously, any blood cells moving through the beam will be detected, and the Doppler shifted signal will represent the entire flow profile of all vessels in the path of the beam. A pulsed Doppler uses short bursts of ultrasound to measure depth, in addition to flow.[10] With this system, blood flow is detected only at a discrete site, referred to as the sample volume. Thus, a pulsed Doppler can selectively evaluate center stream flow patterns and avoid superimposed signals from adjacent vessels. Continuous wave Doppler instruments are easy to use and quite adequate for the qualitative assessment of flow or indirect measurement of arterial pressure. Pulsed wave systems are better suited for quantitative signal processing methods such as spectral analysis.

The Doppler shifted signal can be amplifed to produce audible sounds. By listening to the quality of these sounds, an examiner can learn to distinguish between a smooth laminar flow signal and the harsh high-pitched signal associated with severe stenosis. However, this audible analysis may not be sensitive enough to detect the minor flow disturbances caused by minimal disease and technical errors. A more quantitative analysis of the Doppler signal can be based on analog waveforms generated by a zero-crossing detector.[11] The analog waveform reduces the entire Doppler signal to a single line that represents the change in Doppler shift frequency with respect to time (Fig. 7-1). While analog waveforms are subject to errors and artifacts, they are suitable for quantitative interpretation by methods such as the pulsatility index and the Laplace transform.[12,14]

Spectral analysis is an alternative method for processing Doppler signals that overcomes the limitations of the analog waveform.[14] A spectrum analyzer displays the entire frequency and amplitude content of the Doppler signal. In the Doppler spectrum, frequency is proportional to blood velocity and amplitude is proportional to the number of blood cells passing through the ultrasound beam. Spectra can be presented graphically with frequency on the vertical axis, time on the horizontal axis, and amplitude indicated by a gray-scale.

Arterial lesions cause flow disturbances that can be characterized by spectral analysis.[14] A laminar flow pattern is present in the center stream of a normal artery during systole. In this situation, all the blood cells have approximately the same speed and direction, so the corresponding pulsed Doppler spectrum shows a narrow band of frequencies. A wider band of frequencies is seen in diastole when the flow pattern is less uniform. Arterial wall irregularities and stenoses result in flow disturbances that produce spectra with a wider than normal range of frequencies and amplitudes. This abnormal widening of the frequency band is referred to as spectral broadening. Minor stenoses are associated with spectral broadening only; however, high-grade stenoses cause both spectral broadening and increases in the peak systolic frequency.

Pulsed Doppler spectral analysis can be used to evaluate the severity of arterial disease and document its progression. This method can also be applied intraoperatively to identify the flow disturbances produced by technical errors such as intimal flaps and intraluminal thrombi.[15] It is important to recognize that the flow disturbances created by stenoses and arterial wall defects are localized to the segment extending several vessel diameters distal to the lesion. Therefore, pulsed Doppler spectral analysis requires a direct examination of the arterial segment in question.

A continuous wave Doppler flow detector and pneumatic cuff can be used for the indirect, noninvasive measurement of arterial blood pressure.[9] Measurement of ankle systolic pressure is the most valuable test for assessing the lower limb arteries, since this single parameter reflects the status of the major arteries and collateral vessels from the abdomen to the ankle. The ratio of ankle systolic pressure to brachial systolic pressure, or the ankle–arm index, compensates for the normal varia-

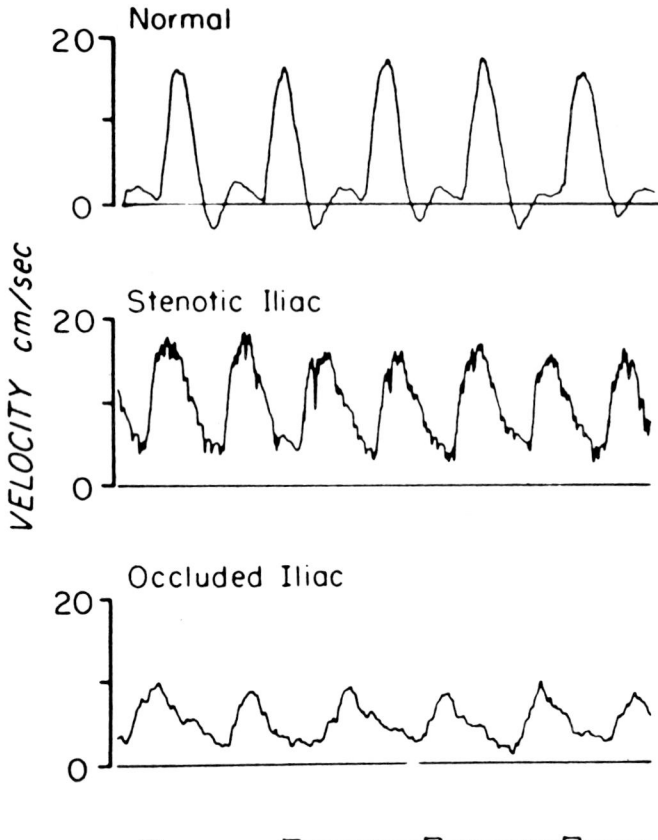

Fig. 7-1. Analog waveforms obtained from the common femoral artery with a continuous wave Doppler. The normal waveform is triphasic with a small reverse flow component (below the baseline). Iliac artery disease results in a monophasic, damped waveform. Velocity is proportional to Doppler shift frequency. From Strandness DE, Sumner DS: Hemodynamics for Surgeons. Orlando, Grune and Stratton, 1975, p 257. Reprinted with permission.

tion in central aortic pressure.[16] If the proximal arteries are normal, the ankle–arm index is greater than one, with a mean value of 1.11.[17] While the ankle–arm index does not discriminate between lesions at different anatomic levels, single-level occlusions are generally associated with indexes greater than 0.5 and multiple-level occlusions with indexes less than 0.5.[18]

The functional status of the lower limb arteries can be assessed by measurement of ankle systolic pressure before and after standard treadmill exercise.[19] In limbs with normal arteries, blood flow increases during exercise with little or no drop in ankle systolic pressure. However, in limbs with occlusive arterial disease the high-resistance collateral pathways prevent this normal response, and a decrease in ankle systolic pressure is observed with exercise. The magnitude of the immediate drop in ankle systolic pressure and the time for recovery to resting pressure are both proportional to the severity of occlusive disease. Exercise testing also permits an assessment of nonvascular factors that affect the ability to walk, such as musculo-skeletal and cardiopulmonary disease.

Duplex Scanning

The duplex scanner is an instrument that combines the previously described ultrasound methods of B-mode imaging and pulsed Doppler flow detection.[20] Until recently, duplex scanning was used primarily for the diagnosis of extracranial carotid artery disease; however, it is now being used successfully for examining the mesenteric, renal, and lower limb arterial systems.[21,22] With this technique, the B-mode image is used to identify the vessels of interest and assess their wall charac-teristics. The pulsed Doppler sample volume can then be placed within the imaged arteries and the center stream flow patterns evaluated by spectral analysis. By com-paring various spectral features with the results of contrast arteriography, sets of criteria have been established for classifying the degree of disease.[14] The develop-ment of small, maneuverable scan heads has facilitated the intraoperative use of duplex scanning. Thus, this instrument is now suitable for the preoperative evalu-ation, intraoperative assessment, and postoperative follow-up of patients having arterial surgery.

APPLICATIONS AND RESULTS

Doppler probes can be gas sterilized for intraoperative use, while B-mode and duplex scan heads are usually covered with a sterile plastic sheath. Only the probe or scan head and its connecting wires need to be brought into the operative field. The ultrasound transducers are placed directly on the external surface of the exposed arteries and acoustically coupled with blood or saline solution. When using Doppler instruments, optimal flow signals are obtained with a constant angle of approximately 60 degrees between the probe and the vessel wall. The noninvasive measurement of ankle systolic pressure can also be used to assess the immediate results of arterial surgery.[23,24] A sterile cuff and manometer may be required, depending on the location of the operative incisions. However, significant changes in pressure are only associated with major arterial lesions, so this method will not detect the small gradients caused by some technical errors.

At the conclusion of an arterial operation a rapid qualitative assessment can be performed by audible analysis of continuous wave Doppler signals.[25] The normal multiphasic arterial flow pattern is easily recognized. If an abrupt "water hammer" pulse is present or no flow signal is found, arterial occlusion is present. A harsh high-pitched signal is produced by the turbulence and increased flow velocity within an arterial stenosis. Distal to a stenotic area, the flow signal is low pitched and monophasic. The flow contributions of the various arteries in the operative field can be determined by compression and release of the vessels being evaluated. Abnormal flow patterns near anastomoses and endarterectomy end-points may indicate techni-cal errors. A more quantitative assessment of an arterial reconstruction can be obtained by pulsed Doppler and spectral analysis.

The routine postoperative assessment requires the facilities of a noninvasive

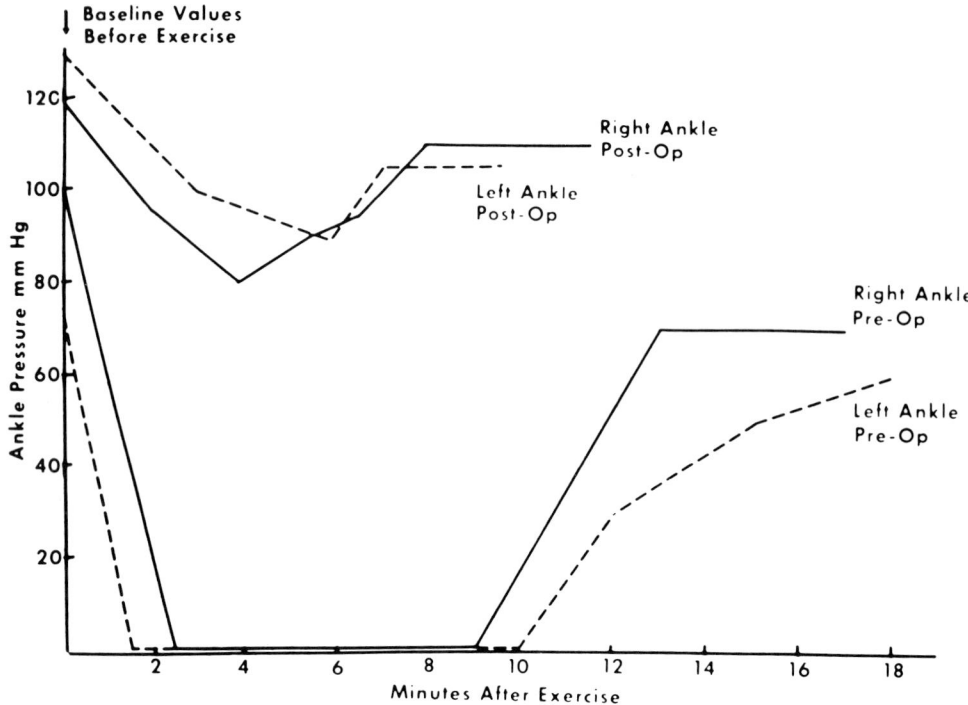

Fig. 7-2. Ankle pressure response to exercise before and after an aorto-femoral bypass graft. The preoperative response occurred after three minutes of treadmill exercise terminated due to bilateral calf claudication. Postoperative, the walking time was five minutes without development of symptoms. Although the result is considerably improved, it is still abnormal. From Strandness DE: Abnormal exercise responses after successful reconstructive arterial surgery. Surgery 59:325–333, 1966. Copyright © 1966, CV Mosby Company. Reproduced with permission.

vascular laboratory for measurement of ankle systolic pressures, exercise treadmill testing, and duplex scanning. After a successful arterial reconstruction, the ankle pressures are generally improved in comparison to the preoperative values.[26] A decrease in the ankle pressure later in the postoperative period may reflect either changes occurring in the reconstructed segment or progression of arterial disease at other sites. The treadmill exercise test is useful for documenting the status of patients who are improved after operation but still not returned to normal.[27] For example, the treadmill walking time may be significantly increased postoperatively, despite a persistent drop in ankle pressure (Fig. 7-2). Serial postoperative follow-up is recommended, since patency of a failing arterial reconstruction is best maintained by early identification and repair of the responsible lesion.

Aorto-femoral Bypass

The value of an intraoperative continuous wave Doppler assessment was evaluated by Keitzer and coworkers in 35 elective aortic operations.[28] These results were compared with 22 similar procedures in which a Doppler was not used. In the group assessed by Doppler, nine reoperations were performed in five patients to manage vascular complications; 15 reoperations were required in seven of the patients not having a Doppler assessment. The reoperation rate was significantly lower in the intraoperative assessment group.

Garrett and coworkers studied the value of intraoperative ankle pressure measurements for predicting the results of aorto-femoral bypass.[29] An increase of 0.1 or more in the ankle–arm index immediately following bypass correlated highly with relief of preoperative symptoms, and all the limbs that were not improved showed either no change in the ankle–arm index or a decrease. However, many of the limbs without a significant increase in the ankle–arm index also had symptomatic improvement. Baird and coworkers reported similar findings and concluded that failure of the ankle–arm index to increase during operation was not a reliable indication for immediate distal reconstruction.[30]

The late results of aorto-femoral bypass can be assessed by serial measurements of the ankle–arm index and response to treadmill exercise. Between 9 and 57% of patients having an aorto-iliac or aorto-femoral reconstruction do not obtain adequate relief of symptoms, and many of these patients will require subsequent distal bypass procedures.[31] Figure 7-2 shows the ankle pressure response to treadmill exercise before and after an aorto-femoral bypass graft. Although this patient was relieved of intermittent claudication, the ankle pressures still fall with exercise. In this case, the persistent abnormality is probably due to mild occlusive disease in the superficial femoral arteries. The specific locations of new or remaining lesions can be determined by duplex scanning or arteriography.

Femoro-popliteal and Femoro-tibial Bypass

Barnes and Garrett used the continuous wave Doppler method to assess the immediate results of 31 femoro-popliteal bypass operations.[24] When qualitative interpretation of the Doppler flow signals was compared to operative arteriography, no technical errors were identifed by either approach. Keitzer and coworkers reported a study in which 24 femoro-popliteal bypasses were performed with an intraoperative Doppler assessment and 14 were done without the Doppler assessment.[28] In the former group, two patients required three reoperations for vascular complications, while in the latter group 13 reoperations were necessary in six patients. These results are similar to those previously described for aortic operations, and a significant difference in favor of intraoperative Doppler assessment is apparent.

A 20-MHz pulsed Doppler system and spectrum analyzer were used by Bandyk, Zierler, and Thiele to assess the immediate results of 20 femoro-popliteal and 10 femoro-tibial bypass grafts.[15] The center stream spectra were evaluated for localized increases in peak systolic frequency and spectral broadening that could be associated with technical errors. Operative arteriography was also performed, and the lesions considered significant were intimal flaps larger than 2 mm, stenoses of greater than 30% diameter reduction, and intraluminal defects consistent with thrombus. Figure 7-3 shows a normal operative arteriogram and the corresponding spectra from a femoro-popliteal bypass graft. Spectral abnormalities were observed in five of the 30 bypass grafts and operative arteriography identified defects requiring immediate repair in three of the five. These defects consisted of one graft kink and two greater than 30% stenoses; the abnormal spectra in the two remaining

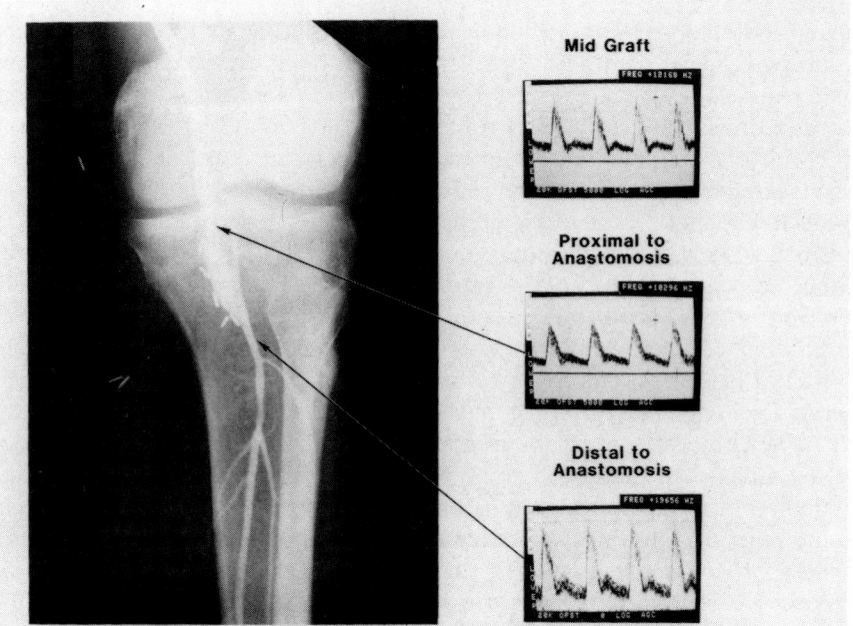

Fig. 7-3. Normal operative arteriogram and intraoperative spectra obtained after a reversed saphenous vein femoropopliteal bypass graft. There are no significant flow disturbances present in the region of the anastomosis. From Bandyk DF, et al: Detection of technical error during arterial surgery by pulsed Doppler spectral analysis. Arch Surg 119:421–428, 1984. Copyright © 1984, American Medical Association. Reproduced with permission.

grafts were caused by spasm and a 20% stenosis. No other significant defects were noted and none of the grafts occluded within one month after operation.

Pulsed Doppler spectral analysis has also been used for intraoperative evaluation of peak systolic and end-diastolic blood flow velocities.[32] When these parameters were measured in 24 femoro-popliteal and 42 femoro-tibial in situ saphenous vein bypass grafts, the mean peak flow velocity was greater in femoro-popliteal grafts (90 cm/sec) than in femoro-tibial grafts (68 cm/sec). Forward flow at the end of diastole, a reflection of low outflow resistance, was present in all successful grafts. Graft occlusion in the early postoperative period was associated with a peak systolic velocity of less than 40 cm/sec and absence of diastolic forward flow. A low flow velocity should prompt a complete arteriographic evaluation for technical problems such as anastomotic strictures, intact valves, and graft torsion. If no lesion can be found and there is little or no flow in diastole, bypass to a second distal artery can be considered to increase graft flow velocity.

The principles of postoperative assessment for bypass grafts in the leg are similar to those already discussed for aortic surgery. After a successful operation, the ankle pressure should be improved both at rest and after treadmill exercise.[26, 33] With vein grafts this increase in ankle pressure can occur gradually over days or weeks, presumably due to progressive dilation of the graft. A decrease in the ankle pressure during postoperative follow-up can be a sign of impending graft failure.[33, 34] When this occurs, further diagnostic and therapeutic procedures may be necessary to preserve graft function. A continuous wave Doppler or duplex scanner can also be used in the postoperative period to measure peak systolic and end-diastolic blood flow velocities.[32] The diastolic forward flow seen at operation in successful bypass grafts becomes less prominent during follow-up. Bandyke, Cato, and Towne found that a decrease in peak velocity to less than 45 cm/sec was consistent with an intrinsic graft lesion or progression of occlusive disease elsewhere.[32] In their series, 21% of grafts required revision in the postoperative period to maintain patency.

Carotid Endarterectomy

Neurologic complications of carotid endarterectomy are especially devastating to the patient and often irreversible. Thus, intraoperative assessment is particularly important for detection and correction of technical errors before serious neurologic sequelae develop. While routine operative arteriography has been advocated, this method has not been widely used because of the potential risks involved.[35, 36] In 1967 Blaisdell, Lim, and Hall reported a 25% incidence of unacceptable technical results in a study based on operative arteriography.[37] Subsequent experience with this approach indicates that unacceptable results occur in between 5 and 10% of operations.[7, 35–38]

Imaging with B-mode ultrasound avoids the risks of operative arteriography. The carotid bifurcation can be examined before and after endarterectomy to confirm complete removal of the plaque and look for technical problems (Fig. 7-4). In a series of 48 carotid endarterectomies evaluated with intraoperative B-mode imaging, Flanigan, Sigel, and Schuler observed defects in 13 (27%).[39] However, the defects

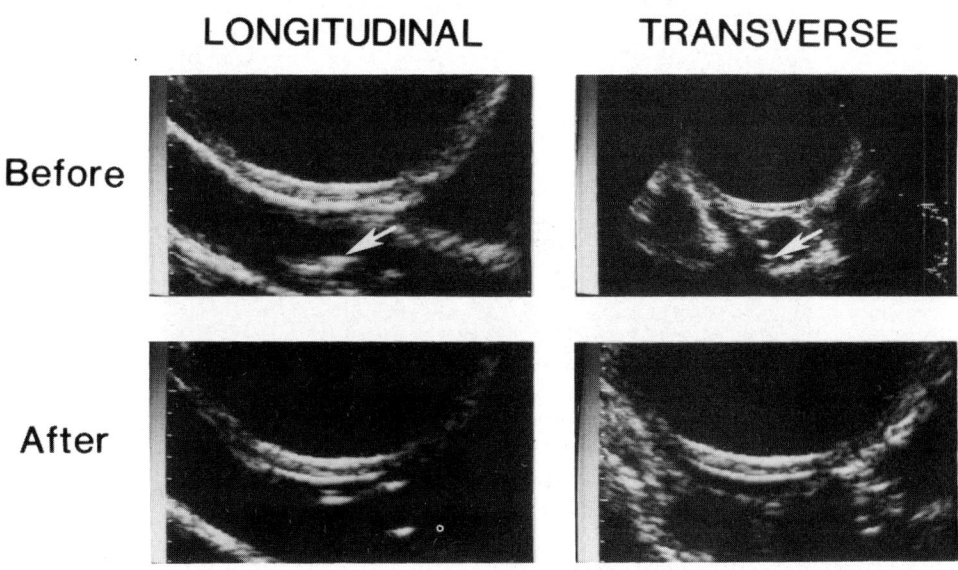

Fig. 7-4. Intraoperative longitudinal and transverse B-mode images of the carotid bifurcation taken before and after endarterectomy. Atherosclerotic plaque (arrows) can be visualized in the internal carotid prior to endarterectomy.

were considered minor in 11 cases, and only two (4%) were repaired. Thus, although B-mode imaging was extremely sensitive, the incidence of unacceptable technical results was similar to that found with operative arteriography.

Barnes and Garrett used audible interpretation of continuous wave Doppler signals to assess the results of 42 carotid endarterectomies.[24] The internal carotid signals were all considered normal, but three external carotids had obstructive signals. In these three cases, an intimal flap was removed from the external carotid artery and a satisfactory result was confirmed by repeat Doppler examination.

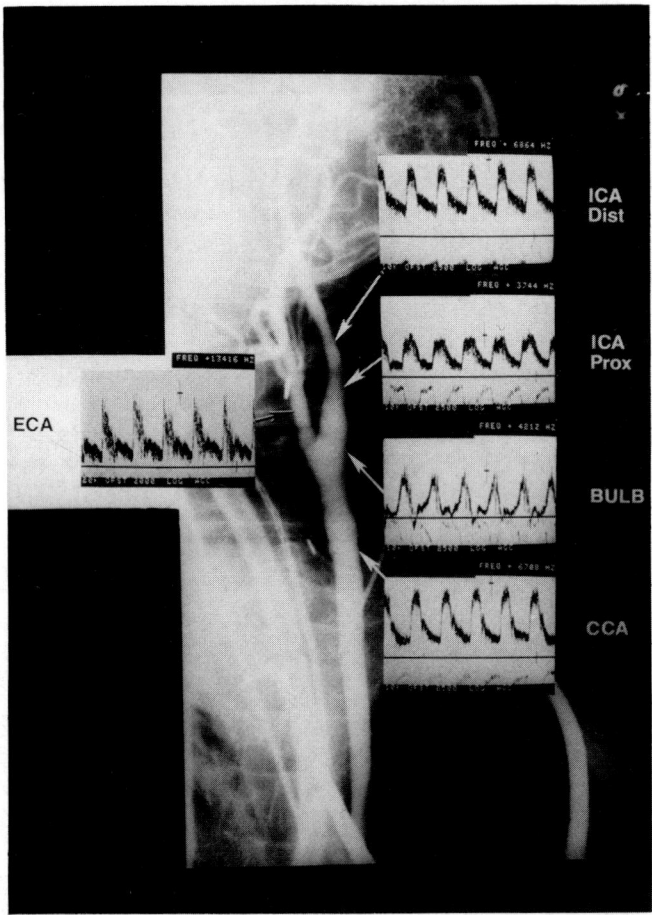

Fig. 7-5. Normal operative arteriogram and intraoperative spectra obtained after carotid endarterectomy. Spectra from the CCA, Bulb, and ICA all represent minimal flow disturbances; the ECA spectrum shows moderate spectral broadening. CCA = common carotid artery; ICA = internal carotid artery; ECA = external carotid artery; Prox = proximal; Dist = distal. From Zierler RE, et al: The use of frequency spectral analysis in carotid arterial surgery, in Bergan JJ, Yao JST (eds): Cerebrovascular Insufficiency. Orlando, Grune and Stratton, 1983, p 158. Reproduced with permission.

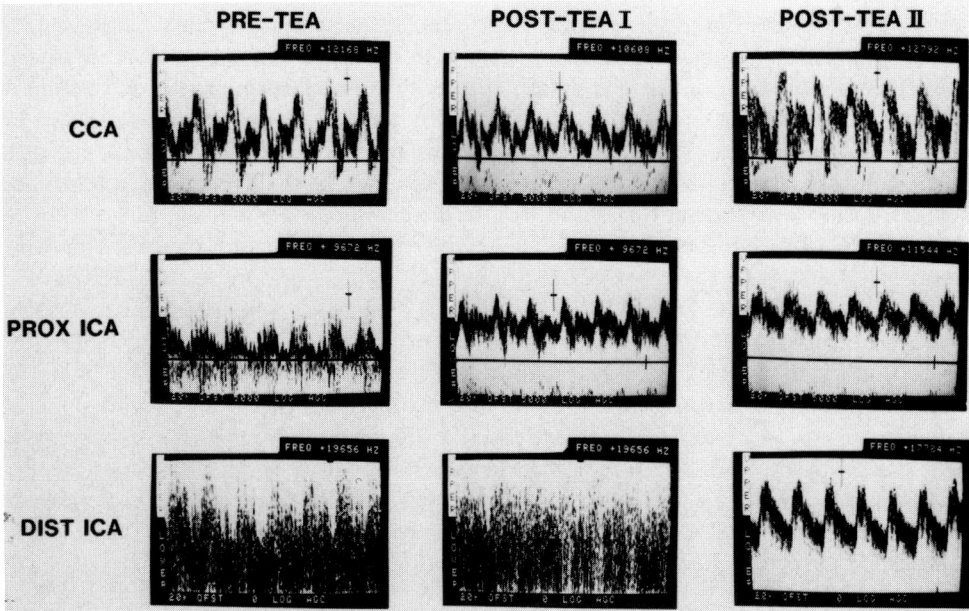

Fig. 7-6. Intraoperative pulsed Doppler assessment of carotid endarterectomy. Spectra before endarterectomy (PRE-TEA) immediately after endarterectomy (POST-TEA I), and after correction of a technical error (POST-TEA II). See text for explanation. CCA = common carotid artery; PROX ICA = proximal internal carotid artery; DIST ICA = distal internal carotid artery. From Zierler RE, et al: Duplex scan and frequency analysis in the evaluation of recurrent carotid stenosis, in Bergan JJ, Yao JST (eds): Reoperative Arterial Surgery. Orlando, Grune and Stratton, 1986, p 116. Reproduced with permission.

Zierler, Bandyk, and Thiele used spectral analysis of 20-MHz pulsed Doppler signals and operative arteriography to assess 50 carotid endarterectomies.[35] A normal operative arteriogram and the corresponding spectra are shown in Fig. 7-5. Flow disturbances consistent with technical errors were noted in seven internal carotids, and operative arteriography showed defects that required immediate repair in two of these arteries. No other technical errors were found and there were no neurologic complications in any of the patients studied. An example of the spectra produced by a technical error is given in Fig. 7-6. Before endarterectomy a severe flow disturbance is present in the distal internal carotid artery. This flow disturbance is still evident on the Doppler assessment immediately after endarterectomy, and operative arteriography revealed a stenosis at the distal end of the arteriotomy. After repair of the lesion by patch angioplasty, the internal carotid spectra are significantly improved.

Duplex scanning has been used to determine the incidence of recurrent stenosis after carotid endarterectomy.[40,41] While symptomatic recurrent stenosis occurs in less than 5% of patients, it is now recognized that many recurrent stenoses are asymptomatic, and the overall incidence by noninvasive testing is between 9 and 19%.[40–45] Nicholls and coworkers used duplex scanning and spectral analysis to serially evaluate 134 patients having 145 carotid endarterectomies.[41] During a mean postoperative follow-up period of 18 months, progression to a stenosis of greater than 50% diameter reduction occurred in 32 of the 145 carotid arteries. However, seven of these postoperative stenoses became less severe on serial examinations, resulting in a 17% incidence of persistent high-grade recurrent stenosis. Most of these recurrent lesions developed within 10 months of operation. The spectra from a recurrent stenosis that became less severe during the follow-up period are shown in Fig. 7-7. There was a significant difference in the incidence of recurrent stenosis according to sex, with 41% of the females and 15% of the males being affected. Late strokes occurred in four patients and transient ischemic attacks in six, but there was no clear relationship between these neurologic symptoms and recurrent carotid stenosis.

Recurrent stenoses developing in the early postoperative period are usually smooth fibrous lesions that do not tend to ulcerate or progress to occlusion.[46] Stenoses that occur for several years or more after endarterectomy are more likely to resemble primary atherosclerotic plaque. The treatment of recurrent carotid stenosis is controversial. Since the early lesions rarely produce symptoms and may regress, it seems appropriate to follow these patients with noninvasive testing. Even late recurrent stenoses appear to have a relatively benign natural history, making the role prophylactic reoperation uncertain. If a patient has symptoms that are clearly related to a recurrent stenosis, reoperation should be considered.

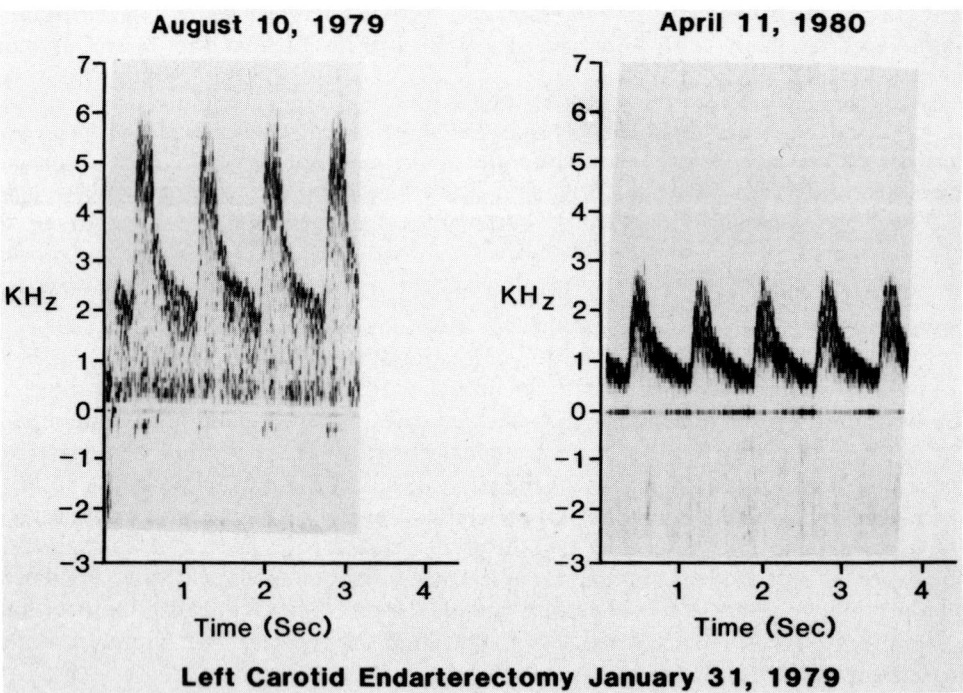

Fig. 7-7. Spectra from an early postoperative stenosis that regressed. The examination shown on the left, six months after endarterectomy, is characteristic of a high-grade stenosis with elevated peak systolic frequency and spectral broadening. On the right, a repeat study eight months later (14 months postoperatively) is consistent with less than 50% internal carotid stenosis. From Zierler RE, et al: Carotid artery stenosis following endarterectomy. Arch Surg 117:1408–1415, 1982. Copyright © 1982, American Medical Association. Reproduced with permission.

CONCLUSIONS

The primary reason for assessing arterial surgery is to achieve and maintain the best functional result in the individual patient. A secondary purpose is to provide an objective means for evaluating various procedures in order to improve the surgical treatment of arterial disease. Ultrasound is the basis for imaging and flow-detection methods that are ideally suited for both intraoperative and postoperative assessment. The B-mode imaging and pulsed Doppler techniques for intraoperative assessment can detect relatively minor arterial defects that may not need correction. This results in a high sensitivity (low false–negative rate) and a low specificity (high false–positive rate). These methods also require considerable skill and interpretation by the examiner. The ultrasound assessment could be used to select patients for operative arteriography. A low false–negative rate is important for a screening test to insure that significant defects will not be overlooked and operative arteriography will only be performed in those patients most likely to benefit from it. Operative arteriography is still the standard method for intraoperative assessment, and it is the only way to directly evaluate vessels outside the operative field.

The postoperative assessment of arterial surgery requires the same physiologic noninvasive tests that have been used for evaluating the location and severity of arterial disease in preoperative patients. Contrast arteriography should be reserved for those patients who are being considered for further surgical procedures. Arterial reconstruction can relieve ischemic symptoms and prevent amputations, but it has no direct effect on the atherosclerotic disease process. Therefore, patients having arterial surgery require lifelong follow-up of both their reconstructed vessels and their native arteries.

REFERENCES

1. Zierler RE: Intraoperative Doppler techniques for arterial evaluation. Seminars in Ultrasound 6:73–84, 1985
2. Courbier R, Jausseran M, Reggi M: Detecting complications of direct arterial surgery. Arch Surg 112:1115–1118, 1977
3. Dardik H, Ibrahim IM, Koslow A, et al: Evaluation of intraoperative arteriography as a routine for vascular reconstructions. Surg Gynecol Obstet 147:853–858, 1978
4. Sigel B, Coelho JCU, Flanigan DP, et al: Ultrasonic imaging during vascular surgery. Arch Surg 117:764–767, 1982
5. Lane RJ, Appleberg M: Real-time intraoperative angiosonography after carotid endarterectomy. Surgery 92:5–9, 1982
6. Sigel B, Machi J, Anderson KW, et al: Operative ultrasonic imaging of vascular defects. Seminars in Ultrasound 6:85–92, 1985
7. Hobson RW, Rich NM, Wright CW, et al: Operative assessment of carotid endarterectomy—Internal carotid arterial back pressure, carotid arterial blood flow, and carotid arteriography. Am Surg 41:693–610, 1975
8. Dean RH, Yao JST, Stanto PE, et al: Prognostic indicators in femoropopliteal reconstruction. Arch Surg 110:1287–1293, 1975
9. Zierler RE, Strandness DE: Ultrasonic techniques of lower extremity arterial diagnosis, in Zwiebel WJ (ed): Introduction to Vascular Ultrasonography. Orlando, Grune and Stratton, 1982, pp 252–272

10. Baker DW: Pulsed ultrasonic Doppler blood flow sensing. IEEE Trans Sonics Ultrasonics 17:170–173, 1970

11. Johnston KW, Marozzo BC, Cobbold RSC: Errors and artifacts of Doppler flowmeters and their solution. Arch Surg 112:1335–1342, 1977

12. Thiele BL, Bandyk DL, Zierler RE, et al: A systematic approach to the assessment of aortoiliac disease. Arch Surg 118:477–481, 1983

13. Baird RN, Bird DR, Clifford PC, et al: Upstream stenosis—Its diagnosis by Doppler signals from the femoral artery. Arch Surg 115:1316–1322, 1980

14. Zierler RE, Roederer GO, Strandness DE: The use of frequency spectral analysis in carotid artery surgery, in Bergan JJ, Yao JST (eds): Cerebrovascular Insufficiency. Orlando, Grune and Stratton, 1983, pp 137–163

15. Bandyk DF, Zierler RE, Thiele BL: Detection of technical error during arterial surgery by pulsed Doppler spectral analysis. Arch Surg 119:421–428, 1984

16. Yao JST, Hobbs JT, Irvine WT: Ankle systolic pressure measurements in arterial diseases affecting the lower extremities. Br J Surg 56:676–679, 1969

17. Yao JST: Hemodynamic studies in peripheral arterial disease. Br J Surg 57:761–766, 1970

18. Sumner DS, Strandness DE: The relationship between calf blood flow and ankle blood pressure in patients with intermittent claudication. Surgery 65:763–771, 1969

19. Strandness DE, Zierler RE: Exercise ankle pressure measurements in arterial disease, in Bernstein EF (ed): Noninvasive Diagnostic Techniques in Vascular Disease, 3 ed. St Louis, CV Mosby Co, 1985, pp 575–583

20. Strandness DE: Echo–Doppler (duplex) ultrasonic scanning. J Vasc Surg 2:341–344, 1985

21. Jager JA, Langlois Y, Roederer GO, et al: Noninvasive assessment of lower extremity ischemia, in Bergan JJ, Yao JST (eds): Evaluation and Treatment of Upper and Lower Extremity Circulation Disorders. Orlando, Grune and Stratton, 1984, pp 97–121

22. Jager KA, Fortner GS, Thiele BL, et al: Noninvasive diagnosis of intestinal angina. J Clin Ultrasound 12:588–591, 1984

23. Williams LR, Flanigan DP, Schuler, JJ, et al: Intraoperative assessment of limb revascularization by Doppler-derived segmental blood pressure measurements. Am J Surg 144:578–579, 1982

24. Barnes RW, Garrett WV: Intraoperative assessment of arterial reconstruction by Doppler ultrasound. Surg Gynecol Obstet 146:896–900, 1978

25. Mozersky DJ, Sumner DS, Barnes RW, et al: Intraoperative use of a sterile ultrasonic flow probe. Surg Gynecol Obstet 136:279–280, 1973

26. Strandness DE, Bell JW: Ankle pressure responses after reconstructive arterial surgery. Surgery 59:514–516, 1966

27. Strandness DE: Abnormal exercise responses after successful reconstructive arterial surgery. Surgery 59:325–333, 1966

28. Keitzer WF, Lichti EL, Brossart FA, et al: Use of the Doppler ultrasonic flowmeter during arterial vascular surgery. Arch Surg 105:308–312, 1972

29. Garrett WV, Slaymaker EE, Heintz SE, et al: Intraoperative prediction of symptomatic result of aortofemoral bypass from changes in ankle pressure index. Surgery 82:504–509, 1977

30. Baird RJ, Feldman P, Miles JT, et al: Subsequent downstream repair after aorta-iliac and aorta-femoral bypass operations. Surgery 82:785–793, 1977

31. Sumner DS, Strandness DE: Aortoiliac reconstruction in patients with combined iliac and superficial femoral arterial occlusion. Surgery 84:348–355, 1978

32. Bandyk DF, Cato RF, Towne JB: A low flow velocity predicts failure of femoropopliteal and femorotibial bypass grafts. Surgery 98:799–809, 1985

33. Sumner DS, Strandness DE: Hemodynamic studies before and after extended bypass grafts to the tibial and peroneal arteries. Surgery 86:442–452, 1979

34. Blackshear WM, Thiele BL, Strandness DE: Natural history of above- and below-knee femoropopliteal grafts. Am J Surg 140:234–241, 1980

35. Zierler RE, Bandyk DF, Thiele BL: Intraoperative assessment of carotid endarterectomy. J Vasc Surg 1:73–81, 1984

36. Anderson CA, Collins GJ, Rich NM: Routine operative arteriography during carotid endarterectomy: A reassessment. Surgery 83:67–73, 1978

37. Blaisdell FW, Lim R, Hall AD: Technical result of carotid endarterectomy—Arteriographic assessment. Am J Surg 114:239–246, 1967

38. Rosental JJ, Gaspar MR, Mavius HJ: Intraoperative arteriography in carotid thromboendarterectomy. Arch Surg 106:806–808, 1973

39. Flanigan DP, Sigel B, Schuler JJ: Intraoperative ultrasonic carotid artery imaging, in Bergan JJ, Yao JST (eds): Cerebrovascular Insufficiency. Orlando, Grune and Stratton, 1983, pp 343–352

40. Zierler RE, Bandyk DF, Thiele BL, et al: Carotid artery stenosis following endarterectomy. Arch Surg 117:1408–1415, 1982

41. Nicholls SC, Phillips DJ, Bergelin RO, et al: Carotid endarterectomy—Relationship of outcome to early restenosis. J Vasc Surg 2:375–381, 1985

42. Turnipseed WD, Berkoff HA, Crummy A: Postoperative occlusion after carotid endarterectomy. Arch Surg 115:573–574, 1980

43. Salvian A, Baker JD, Machleder HI, et al: Cause and noninvasive detection of restenosis after carotid endarterectomy. Am J Surg 146:29–34, 1983

44. Glover JL, Bendick PJ, Dilley RS, et al: Restenosis following carotid endarterectomy—Evaluation by duplex ultrasonography. Arch Surg 120:678–684, 1985

45. Keagy BA, Edrington RD, Poole MA, et al: Incidence of recurrent or residual stenosis after carotid endarterectomy. Am J Surg 149:722–725, 1985

46. Rapp J, Stoney R: Recurrent carotid stenosis, in Bernhard VM, Towne JB (eds): Complications in Vascular Surgery, 2 ed. Orlando, Grune and Stratton, 1985, pp 763–773

I. B. Faris
and H. J. Duncan

8

The Assessment of Critical Skin Ischaemia

Critical ischaemia can be defined as a degree of ischaemia such that there is a high risk that amputation will be required if the ischaemia is unrelieved. The fulfilment of this criterion is the principal indication for arterial reconstruction in the limb. However, it may be difficult on clinical grounds to determine if critical or "limb-threatening" ischaemia is present. This may be illustrated by two examples.

1. Patients with early rest pain. The question is whether survival of the limb is threatened in this group of patients who have been regarded as the most suitable candidates for lumbar sympathectomy. In reported series of the results of arterial reconstruction for "threatened limb" it is found that amputation does not inevitably follow closure of the reconstruction. One explanation (among several) for this phenomenon is that the patient did not have critical ischaemia when submitted to operation.
2. Patients with ulcers or gangrene of the foot. In these circumstances the question is: "Will this lesion heal spontaneously or following local amputation?"

An incorrect answer to this question may result in two possible harmful outcomes for the patient. On the one hand, if the blood supply is adequate, arterial reconstruction may be performed where local amputation, e.g., of a toe or forefoot, would have been sufficient. On the other hand, there may be several futile attempts at local amputation in the presence of severe ischaemia. These problems are particularly likely to occur in diabetic subjects when the presence of neuropathy means that there is no ischaemic pain which requires early relief, either by reconstruction or major amputation.

The laboratory assessment of acute ischaemia is an important issue which has not been addressed adequately in the literature. It is conventional to regard the limb as threatened if there is ischaemic rest pain, muscle weakness, or loss of sensation in the distal part of the limb. However, there has been a trend to treat conservatively many of these patients, and our experience with thrombolytic therapy had indicated

VASCULAR SURGERY: ISSUES IN CURRENT PRACTICE
ISBN 0-8089-1839-7

that most limbs with these signs will survive at least 8–12 hours until the circulation improves.[1] This remains an important unresolved issue.

In addition to determining the appropriate treatment for individual patients, the development of an agreed definition of critical ischaemia would aid communication between authors who wish to compare results with other surgeons. This problem has been addressed recently and suggestions made for objective criteria to identify critical ischaemia.[2] The guidelines are that critical ischaemia is likely if the ankle systolic pressure is lower than 40 mmHg if the skin is intact or lower than 60 mmHg if necrosis is present.

It is the purpose of this chapter to review the published data from which objective definitions of critical ischaemia might be derived.

ANKLE BLOOD PRESSURE

If this measurement gave adequate information there would be no need to look for alternatives because the simplicity of the method means that it can be used easily in ward, emergency room, or operating theatre. The method gives reasonable discrimination between clinical groups of patients[3] and forms the basis of the suggested definition of critical ischaemia.[2] These results may be expressed as the absolute value of the ankle systolic pressure or as the ankle–arm ratio systolic pressure (pressure index, PI). The method is also reasonably precise,[4-6] although the amount of variation may make it hazardous to predict the outcome on a single reading. The pressure index should change by more than 0.15 before it is regarded as significant.

There are, however, two major disadvantages to the method:

1. Arterial calcification may mean that the recorded level of ankle pressure is falsely high. We have evidence that this applies across the whole range of ankle pressures and not just in those patients with incompressible vessels.[7]
2. The ankle pressure takes no account of the effect of disease of the arteries of the foot which may be important, particularly in diabetic subjects.[8]

In this and the following sections considering reported results, conventional clinical criteria have been used viz. a limb was considered threatened if rest pain ulceration or gangrene were present. The usual starting point has been to attempt to specify a level of ankle pressure below which severe ischaemia is likely and local healing is unlikely to occur.[9] This has been reported by a number of authors.[10-19] It has been suggested that the absolute pressure gives a better discrimination than the PI.[10] Reported series have given critical values of 35–70 mmHg and PI 0.43–0.6 with correct predictions in 14–100%. There have been several reports that a higher pressure is needed for healing in diabetics than in nondiabetics,[12,17,20] although this has not been the finding in all reports.

TOE BLOOD PRESSURE

The measurement of toe blood pressure[21,22] does not incur the objections raised for the ankle pressure measurements. The measurement is made closer to the site of any lesions and thus will be influenced by disease in the foot. In addition, incompressible vessels are not encountered in the digits. The reproducibility of the measurement has been stated to be similar to that of ankle pressure measurements,[23, 24] but a recent report[6] suggests that it is much less reproducible. Measurement of toe pressure is technically more demanding than estimation of ankle pressure. In particular, the end-point may be difficult to determine, particularly at low levels of pressure in the digital arteries. If the great toe has been amputated or is gangrenous, measurements can be made on the remaining toes,[25] although this may require different cuffs or pulse detectors.

There have been several studies which have compared the toe pressure and the clinical state of the patient.[26, 27] A toe pressure of less than 30 mmHg correctly predicted severe ischaemia in 56–95% of cases, while higher levels predicted milder clinical disease in 75–86% of patients.

In the same series where comparison with ankle pressure is possible[27] the respective correct predictions were 69 and 53%. Thus it appears that a high (greater than 60 mmHg) ankle pressure is less good in predicting mild disease than a high toe pressure (greater than 30 mmHg), although the prediction of severe disease is similar with both tests.

The results have also been expressed in different ways:[24, 28] patients with rest pain had a toe blood pressure of 25 and 0–10 mmHg and patients with ulceration or gangrene 10 and 10–20 mmHg, although the range in each case was 0–60 mmHg. If the toe pressure is expressed as a ratio it has been found that patients with a toe–arm ratio of less than 0.07 had an 82% risk of amputation[24] and patients with severe ischaemia had a toe–arm ratio of 0.2 (mean) and a toe–ankle ratio of 0.26 (mean).[29]

There have been a number of studies which have compared the ability of toe and ankle pressure levels to predict the healing or failure of amputation of forefoot or toes.[11, 12, 26, 30–33] The critical level of toe pressure chosen has been 30–40 mmHg. The results of prediction of failure of healing fall into two groups: one with poor results (55–69% correct) and another with better results (85–100% correct). However, successful healing was correctly predicted in 86–100% (median 91%). In the same patients the ankle pressure (at a critical level of 50–80 mmHg) correctly predicted failure in 50–100% (median 80%) and success in 55–92% (median 71%). It appears therefore that both toe and ankle pressures are probably equivalent in the prediction of failure, but toe pressure measurements are better in the prediction of successful healing of a local amputation.

The observation that a high ankle pressure does not protect against failure of healing is analogous to the finding that a high ankle pressure may be found in severe clinical disease (vide supra). Part of the explanation may be false elevation of the ankle pressure in diabetics.

ISOTOPE CLEARANCE TEST

This method allows the measurement of pressure and flow distally in the foot. The method involves the intradermal injection of a small dose of radioisotope mixed with a vasodilator drug in order to eliminate the effect of local neurons or humoral factors.[34] External counter pressure is applied over the isotope depot until clearance of the isotope ceases. The pressure required to stop the clearance is called the skin perfusion pressure (SPP) and in normal subjects is close to mean arterial pressure,[35]

Table 8-1
Percent healing at various levels
of SPP and SVR. (Data from
Duncan and Faris[39])

		SPP	
	< 40	40–50	> 50
SVR < 1000	21	56	81
> 1000	0	0	31

and probably represents the local arterial perfusion pressure. From the relationship between pressure and clearance a variable can be obtained which has the same dimensions as vascular resistance and is called the skin vascular resistance (SVR).[36] This method has been applied previously to the predictions of healing of above- and below-knee amputation.[37, 38] We have used it to predict the healing of gangrene or ulcers of the foot.[39] In 106 patients, at a critical level of SPP of 40 mmHg, a prediction of failure of healing was correct in 85% and a prediction of healing was correct in 62%. In a subgroup of diabetic patients the corresponding results were 95 and 85%. The SVR at a critical level of 1000 u predicted failure in 83% and success in 63%. However, when the two criteria are combined, better discrimination was obtained (see Table 8-1).

It is our hypothesis that a raised SVR is related to the presence of micro-angiopathy, whether caused by diabetes or hypertension, and we have produced the following evidence in support:

1. The SVR was increased in diabetic and hypertensive patients who developed ulcers and gangrene in the foot.[39]
2. The SVR and SPP were independent predictors of healing of the foot in patients with ulcers or gangrene.[39]
3. The SVR was raised in patients with Martorell's ulcers of the leg.[40]
4. The SVR was raised in a group of diabetic patients with retinopathy compared with a matched group without retinopathy.[7]
5. Preliminary studies have suggested that the level of the SVR is related to the degree of histological evidence of microangiopathy in the skin (unpublished).

The measurement of the SPP provides evidence about the blood supply of the foot which is as valuable as that obtained by other methods, e.g., toe blood pressure. However, the SVR cannot be obtained by other methods and is probably an important independent predictor of outcome. This method has the additional advantage that it requires an easily available, cheap, isotope (^{99m}Tc as pertechnetate) in low dose (100 microcuries) and the counting equipment is inexpensive.

ISOTOPE PERFUSION SCANNING

This method[41] involves the intraarterial injection of radioactive tracer and imaging of the accumulated isotope in the legs with a gamma camera. The activity of the isotope around the ulcer is compared with the activity in the ulcer ("ulcer ratio"). If there is hyperaemia, indicating that healing is likely, there will be more isotope in the area around the ulcer. The critical level of the ulcer ratio was given as 3.5. It has been applied to patients with skin ischaemia and ulcers.[42] In 40 patients a prediction of failure of healing was correct in 89% and of successful healing in 86%. Using a slightly different critical level for the ulcer ratio (2.5) Johnson and Patten[15] predicted correctly in 84 and 92% of cases respectively. Shionoya and coworkers[43] studied the blood flow velocity in the foot by following the activity of technecium which had been injected intraarterially. They found that the movement of tracer was slower in patients with ischaemia and that this was reversible following surgery.

These methods have not been used widely, perhaps because of the need for a large gamma camera and its associated facilities.

PULSE VOLUME RECORDING

This method involves the application of cuffs at various sites in the limb. The cuffs are filled with known volumes of air at standard pressures and the oscillations in pressure produced in the cuffs by the underlying arteries are amplified and recorded. Extensive results have been reported by Raines and coworkers.[17] However, the reproducibility of this test has been found less satisfactory than ankle pressure measurements.[6] A pulse volume recording which showed minimal or no pulsation correctly predicted rest pain, ulceration, or gangrene in 75% of cases. More normal recordings indicated an absence of severe disease in 73% of cases. These results are comparable to those obtained for toe and ankle pressures.

TRANSCUTANEOUS MEASUREMENT OF OXYGEN TENSION (PtcO$_2$)

This has been widely used in the care of infants and has recently been investigated in the assessment of patients with ischaemic limbs. The measurement is made with the electrode heated to 43–44°C to produce maximal local vasodilation. The transcutaneous oxygen tension will reflect the cutaneous blood flow which, under these conditions, varies with the local arterial perfusion pressure.[44] Thus the PtcO$_2$ should be closely related to the SPP (vide supra). There is a good correlation between PtcO$_2$ measurements and Doppler pressure recordings,[45–47] but a poor correlation between PtcO$_2$ and toe blood pressure measurements has been reported.[48]

A number of reports have given information about the levels of PtcO$_2$ at various sites in the limb in patients with varying degrees of ischaemia.[45,47–55] In the foot, the ranges of values given for PtcO$_2$ in normal subjects is 38–70 mmHg. The most commonly quoted mean value is about 60 mmHg with a standard deviation which varies between 3 and 12 in different reports. Thus the normal range is probably 50–70 mmHg. In patients with claudication the PtcO$_2$ mean value in the foot is between 45 and 52 mmHg with a wider standard deviation than in normal subjects. Thus there are likely to be many patients with claudication who have a PtcO$_2$ in the normal range.

In patients with rest pain or gangrene, the level of PtcO$_2$ is lower, the reported mean values being 3–35 mmHg. The method has also been used to predict amputation healing. The critical level appears to be 40 mmHg.[46, 54]

It appears that the use of the PtcO$_2$ measurement is at about the same stage as the ankle pressure measurements were 10 years ago: the range of values expected in normal subjects and patients have been described but there is still overlap between the groups.

OTHER METHODS

A variety of other methods has been described for the measurement of the skin circulation, although none has come to be widely used. Jogestrand and Bergland[28] compared five of these in a small series of patients without finding evidence of clear superiority for any single measurement. The methods used were toe blood pressure measurement, skin temperature recording, analysis of the toe pulse wave,[56] vital capillary microscopy,[57] and dynamic fluorescein angiography.[58]

Recently the results have been given of a test which attempts to measure perfusion pressure by determining the height of elevation of the foot at which capillary flow returns during reactive hyperaemia.[59] This provided better prediction of healing than Doppler ankle pressures. The local pressure which was critical for healing was about 40 cm of blood.

The method of laser Doppler flowmetry has also been used to study the circulation in the skin.[60] There remains uncertainty about the depth of the vessels from which the signals are obtained, and it is not known if the signal reflects total skin blood flow or capillary (nutrient) flow. In addition it is affected by skin pigmentation and cannot be calibrated for blood flow measurement.

RECOMMENDATIONS

The following section summarises the data provided which help to define critical skin ischaemia. The evidence suggests that the critical values quoted indicate comparable degrees of clinical disease.

The critical values are:
Ankle systolic pressure: 50–60 mmHg
Toe systolic pressure: 30 mmHg
Isotope clearance: skin perfusion pressure 40 mmHg
                       skin vascular resistance 1000 u
Isotope perfusion scanning: ulcer ratio 2.5–3.5
Pulse volume recording (foot): minimal or no pulsation
Transcutaneous oxygen tension (foot): 40 mmHg

The tests which measure criteria reflecting the blood supply to the foot have given reasonably consistent results; a blood pressure of 30–40 mmHg in the forefoot is the critical level. A strong case can be made for use of one of the methods which assess the circulation distal to the ankle. The advantages and disadvantages of each have been discussed above. All the tests are dependent on experienced operators but each (except isotope scanning) can be performed easily and repeated as necessary. The test(s) chosen will depend on the experience of the laboratory assistants and the equipment available.

REFERENCES

1. Ferguson LJ, Faris I, Robertson A, et al: Intra-arterial streptokinase therapy for acute limb ischaemia. J Vasc Surg, 1986 (in press)
2. Jamieson CW: Editorial. The definition of critical ischaemia of a limb. Br J Surg 69:S2, 1982
3. Yao ST: Haemodynamic studies in peripheral arterial disease. Br J Surg 57:761, 1970
4. Baker JD, Dix D: Variability of Doppler ankle pressures with arterial occlusive disease: An evaluation of ankle index and brachial-ankle pressure gradient. Surgery 89:134, 1981
5. Yao, JST, Flinn WR, Bergan JJ: Noninvasive vascular diagnostic testing: Techniques and clinical applications. Prog in Cardiovasc Dis 26:459, 1984
6. Osmundson PJ, O'Fallon WM, Clements IP, et al: Reproducibility of noninvasive tests of peripheral occlusive arterial disease. J Vasc Surg 2:678, 1985
7. Duncan HJ: MD Thesis, University of Adelaide, 1986
8. Faris I: Small and large vessel disease in the development of foot lesions in diabetics. Diabetologia 11:249, 1975
9. Sumner DS: Presidential address: Noninvasive testing of vascular disease—Fact, fancy, and future. Surgery 93:664, 1983
10. Ouriel K, Zarins CK: Doppler ankle pressure: An evaluation of three methods of expression. Arch Surg 117:1297, 1982
11. Baker WH, Barnes RW: Minor forefoot amputation in patients with low ankle pressure. J Thor Cardiovasc Surg 133:331, 1977
12. Carter SA: The relationship of distal systolic pressures to healing of skin lesions in limbs with arterial occlusive disease with special reference to diabetes mellitus. Scand J Clin Lab Invest 31:239, 1973
13. Faris, I, Duncan HJ: Skin perfusion pressure in the prediction of healing in diabetic patients with ulcers or gangrene of the foot. J Vasc Surg 2:536, 1985
14. Gibbons GW, Wheelock FC, Siembieda C, et al: Noninvasive prediction of amputation level in diabetic patients. Arch Surg 114:1253, 1979
15. Johnson WC, Patten DH: Predictability of healing of ischemic leg ulcers by radioisotopic and Doppler ultrasonic examination. Am J Surg 133:485, 1977
16. Nicholas GG, Myers JL, DeMuth WE: The role of vascular laboratory criteria in the selection of patients for lower extremity amputation. Ann Surg 196:469, 1982
17. Raines JK, Darling RC, Buth J, et al: Vascular laboratory criteria for the management of peripheral vascular disease of the lower extremities. Surgery 79:21, 1976
18. Strandness DE: The use and abuse of the vascular laboratory. Surg Clin N Am 59:707, 1979
19. Verta MJ, Gross WS, van Bellen B, et al: Forefoot perfusion pressure and minor amputation for gangrene. Surgery 80:729, 1976
20. Wagner FW: Transcutaneous Doppler ultrasound in the prediction of healing and the selection of surgical level for dysvascular lesions of the toes and forefoot. Clin Orthop Rel Res 142:110, 1979
21. Gundersen J: Segmental measurements of systolic blood pressure in the extremities including the thumb and great toe. Acta Chir Scand Suppl:426, 1972
22. Nielsen PA, Bell G, Lassen NA: The measurements of digital systolic blood pressure by strain gauge technique. Scand J Clin Lab Invest 29:371, 1972

23. Nielsen PA, Bell G, Lassen NA: Strain gauge studies of distal blood pressure in normal subjects and in patients with peripheral arterial disease. Analysis of normal variation and reproducibility and comparison to intra-arterial measurements. Scand J Clin Lab Invest 31:103, 1973

24. Paaske WP, Tønnesen KH: Prognostic significance of distal blood pressure measurements in patients with severe ischaemia. Scand J Thor Cardiovasc Surg 14:105, 1980

25. Hirai M, Kawai S, Ohta T, et al: Measurement of blood pressure in all toes in arterial occlusive disease of the leg. Angiology 33:418, 1982

26. Ramsey DE, Manke DA, Sumner DS: Toe blood pressure: A valuable adjunct to ankle pressure measurement for assessing peripheral arterial disease. J Cardiovasc Surg 24:43, 1983

27. Tønnesen KH, Noer I, Paaske W, et al: Classification of peripheral occlusive arterial disease based on symptoms, signs and distal blood pressure measurements. Acta Chir Scand 146:101, 1980

28. Jogestrand T, Berglund B: Estimation of digital circulation and its correlation to clinical signs of ischaemia—A comparative methodological study. Clin Physiol 3:307, 1983

29. Vincent DG, Salles-Cunha SX, Bernhard VM, et al: Noninvasive assessment of toe systolic pressures with special reference to diabetes mellitus. J Cardiovasc Surg 24:22, 1983

30. Holstein P, Noer I, Tønnesen KH, et al: Distal blood pressure in severe arterial insufficiency, in Bergan JJ, Yao JST (eds): Gangrene and Severe Ischaemia of the Lower Extremities. New York, Grune and Stratton, 1978, p 95

31. Bone GE, Pomajzl MJ: Toe blood pressure by photoplethysmography: An index of healing in forefoot amputation. Surgery 89:569, 1981

32. Barnes RW, Thornhill B, Nix L, et al: Prediction of amputation wound healing. Arch Surg 116:80, 1981

33. Schwartz JA, Schuler JJ, O'Connor RJA, et al: Predictive value of distal perfusion pressure in the healing of amputation of the digits and the forefoot. Surg Gynaecol Obstet 154:865–869, 1982

34. Lassen NA, Holstein P: Use of radioisotopes in assessment of distal blood flow and distal blood pressure in arterial insufficiency. Surg Clin N Am 54:39, 1974

35. Duncan H, Faris I: Evaluation of an isotope washout technique to measure skin vascular resistance and skin perfusion pressure: Influence of age, site and arterial surgery. Clin Sci, 1986 (in press)

36. Faris IB, Lassen NA: Increased vascular resistance in vasodilated skin an indicator of diabetic microangiopathy? Cardiovasc Res 16:607, 1982

37. Holstein P, Sager P, Lassen NA: Wound healing in below-knee amputations in relation to skin perfusion pressure. Acta Orthop Scand 50:49, 1979

38. Holstein P, Dovey H, Lassen NA: Wound healing in above-knee amputations in relation to skin perfusion pressure. Acta Orthop Scand 50:59, 1979

39. Duncan JH, Faris IB: Skin vascular resistance and skin perfusion pressure as predictors of healing of ischemic lesion of the lower limb: Influences of diabetes mellitus, hypertension and age. Surgery (in press)

40. Duncan HJ, Faris IB: Martorell's hypertensive ischemic leg ulcers are secondary to an increase in the local vascular resistance. J Vasc Surg 2:581, 1985

41. Siegel ME, Siemsen JK: A new noninvasive approach to peripheral vascular disease: Thallium-201 leg scans. Am J Roentgenol 131:827, 1978

42. Siegel ME, Giargiana A, Rhodes BA, et al: Perfusion of ischemic ulcers of the extremity. Arch Surg 110:265, 1975

43. Shionoya S, Hirai M, Kawai S, et al: Hemodynamic study of ischemic limb by velocity measurement in foot. Surgery 90:10, 1981

44. Eickhoff JH, Jacobsen E: Correlation of transcutaneous oxygen tension to blood flow in heated skin. Scand J Clin Lab Invest 40:761, 1980

45. Clyne AC, Ryan J, Webster JHH, et al: Oxygen tension on the skin of ischemic legs. Am J Surg 143:315, 1982
46. White RA, Nolan L, Harley D, et al: Noninvasive evaluation of peripheral vascular disease using transcutaneous oxygen tension. Am J Surg 144:68, 1982
47. Matsen FA, Wyss CR, Pedegana LR, et al: Transcutaneous oxygen tension measurement in peripheral vascular disease. Surg Gynec Obstet 150: 525, 1980
48. Borzykowski J, Krahenbuhl B: Measurement of pedal transcutaneous oxygen tension to follow up lower limbs arterial occlusive disease. Vasa 11:137, 1982
49. Franzeck UK, Talke P, Bernstein EF, et al: Transcutaneous PO_2 measurements in health and peripheral arterial occlusive disease. Surgery 91: 156, 1982
50. Hauser CJ, Shoemaker WC: Use of a transcutaneous PO_2 regional perfusion index to quantify tissue perfusion in peripheral vascular disease. Ann Surg 197:337, 1983
51. Bongard O, Krahenbuhl B: Pedal blood flow and transcutaneous PO_2 in normal subjects and in patients suffering from severe arterial occlusive disease. Clin Physiol 4:393, 1984
52. Wyss CR, Matsen FA, Simmons CW, et al: Transcutaneous oxygen tension measurements on limbs of diabetic and nondiabetic patients with peripheral vascular disease. Surgery 95:339, 1984
53. Byrne P, Provan JL, Ameli FM, et al: The use of transcutaneous oxygen tension measurements in the diagnosis of peripheral vascular insufficiency. Ann Surg 200:159, 1984
54. Dowd GSE, Linge K, Bentley G: Transcutaneous PO_2 measurement in skin ischaemia. Lancet 1:48, 1982
55. Katsamouris A, Brewster DC, Megerman J, et al: Transcutaneous oxygen tension in selection of amputation level. Am J Surg 147:510, 1984
56. Megibow RS, Megibow SJ, Pollack H, et al: The mechanism of accelerated peripheral vascular sclerosis in diabetes mellitus. Am J Med 15:322, 1953
57. Fagrell B: Vital capillary microscopy. Scand J Clin Lab Invest Suppl:133, 1973
58. Lund F: Fluorescein angiography of the skin in diagnosis, prognosis and evaluation of therapy in peripheral vascular disease, in Proceedings 9th European Conference on Microcirculation, Antwerp July 1976. Bibl Anat No 16 257, Karger, Basel
59. Gilfillan RS, Leeds FH, Spotts RR: The prediction of healing in ischemic lesions of the foot. A comparison of Doppler ultrasound and elevation reactive hyperemia. J Cardiovasc Surg 26:15, 1985
60. Nilsson GE, Tenland T, Oberg PA: Evaluation of a laser Doppler flowmeter for measurement of tissue blood flow. IEEE Trans Biomed Eng 27:597–604, 1980

Eugene F. Bernstein

9

How Does a Vascular Laboratory Influence Management of Arterial Disease?

The diagnosis and management of peripheral arterial occlusive disease have been based on a careful history, physical examination, and arteriography, which, in expert hands, provide the basis for an excellent level of patient care. However, the development of the vascular laboratory has provided an additional modality for the management of such problems. First, it provides an objective appraisal that raises each physician's level of information to that of the expert. Second, it quantitates the functional disability due to arterial disease, permitting the physician to balance these measured variables with the patient's complaints. For instance, it aids in the distinction between the true claudication and pseudoclaudication due to neurologic causes and orthopedic causes. Third, the benefits of any therapeutic maneuvers may be objectively assessed, and changes in condition may be monitored serially. Finally, laboratory data now offer the most reliable predictive indices regarding the eventual outcome of potential surgical maneuvers.

Although the noninvasive vascular laboratory also has clearly established itself in the management of patients with cerebrovascular and venous thrombotic disease, it is in the study of peripheral arterial disease that the laboratory has proved to be most valuable. A finite number of techniques have evolved, requiring relatively modest equipment and technologic expertise and yielding data that are sensitive, accurate, reproducible, and important in diagnosis and clinical management. Some of the essential equipment includes blood pressure cuffs of appropriate widths, mercury strain gauge plethysmography, and Doppler velocity probes. A pulse volume recorder, segmental plethysmograph, treadmill, computer-automated interpreter, and Duplex scanner will also provide useful information.

Since the measurements are simple to perform and straightforward in their interpretation, a technician or nurse may obtain very significant information in a few minutes in the physician's office or outpatient clinic. Thus, the data may be immediately available to the practicing surgeon and rapidly integrated into the daily decision-making process.

VASCULAR SURGERY: ISSUES IN CURRENT PRACTICE
ISBN 0-8089-1839-7

The goals of the peripheral arterial examination are to detect, quantitate, predict, and monitor significant peripheral arterial disease. This capability includes the potential of wide-scale screening of asymptomatic patient populations to obtain data regarding the natural history, prevalence, and incidence of the disease and to correlate peripheral arterial disease with the presence, extent, and progression of atherosclerosis in other organs, such as the heart and brain.

The objective data provided by the noninvasive vascular laboratory identify the location and extent of disease. In addition, the data are useful in predicting the likelihood of operative mortality, operative success, and late mortality, and therefore may significantly influence the surgeon's recommendation regarding the appropriateness of operative therapy. Finally, both intraoperative and postoperative monitoring with noninvasive techniques are useful in documenting the success of operative procedures and detecting suboptimal repairs at an early moment when revision is easier to accomplish.

This review includes a survey of the current standard techniques for examination of the peripheral arterial system of the lower extremity and summarizes available data concerning the applications of these techniques to common clinical management problems in peripheral vascular disease.

HISTORICAL BACKGROUND OF THE VASCULAR LABORATORY

Lower extremity pressure measurements were first described by Naumann[1] and used by Winsor in patients with arterial disease.[2] In 1965, Strandness and Bell described the use of pressure measurements in the lower extremities with a mercury strain gauge as a useful technique for the study of peripheral arterial occlusive disease.[3] Winsor was also the first to perform segmental plethysmography for lower extremity arterial insufficiency.[4,5] Although the Doppler principle was first adapted to the study of velocity patterns in arteries by Satomura in 1959,[6] it was not until Strandness began to apply it to peripheral vascular disease that the first significant noninvasive patient studies were undertaken.[7,8] The earliest measurements of distal pressure drops with exercise were reported by Ejrup[9] and Winsor,[10,11] but this approach did not become clinically popular until Sumner and Strandness identified the relationship between calf blood flow and the exercise ankle blood pressure in patients with intermittent claudication.[12]

TECHNIQUES FOR STANDARDIZED MEASUREMENTS IN PERIPHERAL ARTERIAL DISEASE

Tests with the Limb at Rest

Segmental Blood Pressure

Stenosis or occlusion of a major artery to the lower extremity will result in diminished pressure and flow distal to the lesion, and this may be detected and quantified by noninvasive methods. Measurements in the lower extremity are very analogous to those used for the usual brachial systolic blood pressure, with special concerns about the width of the pressure cuff and the method used to detect resumption of the blood flow distal to the cuff. Pressures are usually measured at the upper thigh, above the knee, below the knee, above the ankle, and at the second toe of both legs simultaneously. Segmental blood pressure data may be analyzed either by determining the pressure gradient between any two sites in an extremity or by comparison with systolic pressure in the arm (the pressure index or ratio). In addition, one may compare pressures in one leg with those in the other.

At one time, the ankle pressure measurement or ankle–arm ratio was considered an adequate screen for the presence of disease and a reliable indicator of the magnitude of the problem. However, artifacts in ankle blood pressure measurements are frequent and may be serious.[13–16] Rigid tibial arteries, particularly in association with calcification and severe diabetes mellitus, prevent these vessels from being compressed readily by the cuff. Therefore, higher cuff pressures must be used than the actual intraarterial blood pressure, resulting in an overestimation of the ankle blood pressure. For this reason the ankle blood pressure may appear to be normal or even elevated in patients with significant disease and should not be used as the sole measurement for screening purposes. Rather, a complete segmental blood pressure profile should be obtained.

The upper thigh pressure measurement is also subject to artifacts in the presence of significant occlusive lesions between the thigh cuff and the distal sensor, which is usually at the ankle or toe. Significant stenosis between the groin or ankle decreases the apparent thigh pressure measurement. Such thigh pressure artifacts can falsely suggest the presence of nonexistent aorto-iliac disease. These artifacts can be detected on the basis of a normal palpable femoral arterial pulse and normal femoral arterial Doppler velocity tracings.[17] In interpreting thigh pressure data, one must realize that normal upper thigh pressure measurements do not identify or quantitate isolated disease of the profunda femoris artery.

Table 9-1
Ratio of Leg–Arm Arterial Pressure in Patients with Peripheral Arterial Occlusive Disease

Functional Index	Normal Subjects	Group I (Localized Aorto-iliac Obstruction)	Group II (Localized Femoro-popliteal Obstruction)	Group III (Combined Aorto-iliac and Femoro-popliteal Obstruction)
Segmental blood pressure				
Upper thigh/arm	1.34 ± 0.27	0.720 ± 0.25*†‡	1.263 ± 0.39†	0.970 ± 0.34*‡
Above knee/arm	1.32 ± 0.23	0.698 ± 0.24*	0.915 ± 0.39*	0.794 ± 0.32*
Below knee/arm	1.26 ± 0.24	0.621 ± 0.21*	0.728 ± 0.30*	0.606 ± 0.28*
Above ankle/arm	1.08 ± 0.10	0.571 ± 0.18*	0.513 ± 0.28*	0.478 ± 0.31*

From Fronek A, Bernstein EF: Noninvasive Studies in Peripheral and Cerebrovascular Disease. San Diego, University of California Medical Center, 1977.
* $p < 0.01$ in comparison with normal subjects.
† $p < 0.01$ between groups I and II.
‡ $p < 0.01$ between groups I and III.
$\pm$ Standard deviation.

Despite the limitations just described, the segmental blood pressure profile is the single most reliable and quantitative measurement in the study of peripheral arterial occlusive disease in the resting state. Table 9-1 presents a summary of data based on a large laboratory experience that indicates how these measurements can be used to distinguish various levels of peripheral arterial obstruction. A leg segment–arm ratio greater than 0.85 is considered normal. Ratios between 0.6 and 0.8 are consistent with claudication; measurements between 0.4 and 0.6 are consistent with rest pain; and ratios of less than 0.4 are generally associated with limb-threatening complications, including ulceration and gangrene. When thigh and calf cuffs measuring 17.5 cm are used these figures are decreased by 0.05 to 0.1.

Correlations between ankle systolic pressures measured at rest and angiographic diagnosis have been published by Carter, indicating the range of measurements seen in patients presenting with intermittent claudication and threatened limb loss.[18] Diabetes is common in patients with limb loss, and diabetic patients tend to have higher measured ankle systolic pressures than nondiabetics under these circumstances, at least in part because of the increased rigidity of their arteries.

Pulse Volume Recording

The pulse volume recorder (PVR) is a quantitative segmental air plethysmograph that utilizes cuffs placed at the thigh, calf, and ankle.[19,20] The amplitude of the pulse volume recording is related to the local blood pressure, segmental arterial compliance, and number of arterial vessels in the involved segment, as well as to the degree of arteriosclerotic occlusive disease present. The amplitude of the calibrated pulse volume recorder tracing has proved to have a clear relationship to the degree of peripheral arterial occlusive disease, and the available data base permits correlating the likelihood that presenting symptoms are due to arterial disease, as well as the likelihood that arterial skin lesions in the foot will heal spontaneously (Table 9-2). Raines has developed a scheme for the localization of disease using both segmental pressure and pulse volume recording information.[20]

The pulse volume recorder can be used to obtain segmental pressure data, and both pressure and pulse volume information are generally used in arriving at diagnoses. It is conceivable that pulse volume data may provide additional diagnostic information in patients with normal and even abnormally elevated arterial pressure data due to increased arterial wall stiffness. However, this possibility has yet to be documented.

Doppler Velocity Measurements

The directionally sensitive Doppler velocity probe can reveal a great deal of information concerning the presence, localization, and degree of peripheral arterial disease, depending upon the sophistication of the instrumentation and the knowledge and training of the observer. This instrument is far more sensitive to the training and skill of the operator than any of the other equipment in common use in examining peripheral arterial disease. As a result, the information obtained is not as well standardized, with a variety of different techniques for examination, analysis, and interpretation proposed by various investigators.

The level of utilization of Doppler signals may include (1) simple subjective analysis of the audible signal, (2) a proportionate analysis, including such derived functions as the pulsatility index, damping factor, transit time, acceleration time, and turbulence factor,[21-25] and (3) a quantitative analysis with emphasis on the peak forward velocity, reverse velocity, acceleration, and deceleration (Table 9-3).[26, 27]

Table 9-2
Classification of Peripheral Arterial Disease by
Pulse Volume Recording (PVR) Data

A. Definition of PVR categories

	Chart Deflection (mm)	
PVR Category	*Thigh and Ankle*	*Calf*
1	>15	>20*
2	>15	>20†
3	5–15	5–20
4	<5	<5
5	Flat	Flat

B. Criteria for evaluation of rest pain

	Unlikely	Probable	Likely
Ankle pressure (mmHg)			
Nondiabetic	>55	35–55	<35
Diabetic	>80	55–80	<55
Ankle PVR category			
Nondiabetic and diabetic	1,2,3	3,4	4,5

C. Criteria for limiting claudication

	Unlikely	Probable	Likely
Postexercise ankle pressure (mmHg)	>50	>50	>50
Postexercise ankle PVR category	2.3	4	4.5

D. Criteria for the prediction of lesion healing without surgery

	Unlikely	Probable	Likely
Ankle pressure (mmHg)			
Nondiabetic	>65	55–65	<55
Diabetic	>90	80–90	<80
Ankle PVR category			
Nondiabetic and diabetic	1,2,3	3	4.5

From Raines JK, Darling RC, Buth J, et al: Vascular laboratory criteria for the management of peripheral vascular disease of the lower extremity. Surgery 79:21, 1976. With permission.
* With reflected wave.
† Without reflected wave.

Duplex Scanning

Strandness and his colleagues have pioneered the use of the Duplex scanner in lower limb arterial disease.[28] The B-mode image is used to identify obvious stenoses and to guide the placement of the Doppler probe in a center stream site and at a

Table 9-3
Arterial Velocity in Patients with Peripheral Arterial Occlusive Disease

Sensitive Velocity Discriminating Functions in Occlusive Disease	Normal Subjects	Localized Aorto-iliac Obstruction	Localized Femoro-popliteal Obstruction	Combined Aorto-iliac and Femoro-popliteal Obstruction
Peak forward velocity (cm/sec)				
Femoral artery	40.7 ± 10.9	25.8 ± 9.4*	30.3 ± 15.4*	20.9 ± 11.2*
Posterior tibial artery	16.0 ± 10.0	13.4 ± 11.5	13.3 ± 6.6	11.7 ± 8.2*
Dorsalis pedis artery	16.8 ± 5.7	14.7 ± 6.4†	11.4 ± 9.2*†	6.9 ± 6.5*
Deceleration (cm/sec^2)				
Femoral artery	250.9 ± 60.0	122.9 ± 75.6*	181.0 ± 117.0*†	91.0 ± 70.7*
Posterior tibial artery	129.8 ± 75.7	79.2 ± 62.4†	77.2 ± 89.9*†	43.0 ± 40.2*
Dorsalis pedis artery	137.9 ± 54.5	79.9 ± 50.8*†	71.8 ± 55.9*†	28.9 ± 20.8*
Peak velocity/mean velocity				
Femoral artery	4.8 ± 1.6	3.1 ± 1.1*	3.6 ± 0.8*†	2.7 ± 0.8*
Posterior tibial artery	4.8 ± 2.5	3.0 ± 0.8†	2.8 ± 1.1*†	2.1 ± 0.8*
Dorsalis pedis artery	6.0 ± 4.1	3.4 ± 1.5†	2.6 ± 0.9*†	2.0 ± 0.7*

From Fronek A, Bernstein EF: Noninvasive Studies in Peripheral and Cerebrovascular Disease. San Diego, University of California Medical Center, 1977.

± Standard deviation.

* $p < 0.01$ in comparison with normal subjects.

† $p < 0.01$ between groups I or II and III.

Table 9-4
Comparison of Duplex Scanning Results with
Conventional Arteriography

Results of Duplex Scan		Distribution According to Conventional Arteriography				
% Stenosis	No. of Arteries	Normal	1–19%	20–49%	50–99%	Total Occlusion
Normal	97	**88**	7	1	1	
1–19	124	19	**80**	15	9	1
20–49	39	1	6	**21**	11	
50–99	41		3	1	**36**	1
Total Occlusion	37			1	3	**33**

constant angle with respect to the vessel axis (preferably 60 degrees). Spectral analysis of the Doppler signal is performed by a real-time fast-Fourier transform (FFT) spectrum analyzer. Mean velocity values and standard deviations have been obtained, and criteria for disease classification derived, using (1) the overall wave-form contour, (2) peak systolic velocity, and (3) spectral broadening. An analysis of the initial experience suggests that the method is highly sensitive (96%), and permits categorizing the degree of stenosis into one of five degrees, and also can localize the anatomic level of disease very accurately (Table 9-4), although the specificity of the method is only fair (81%). Thus, the technique may play a special role in identifying and quantitating ileo-femoral disease, selecting patients for angioplasty and monitoring the results of bypass surgery.

Power Frequency Spectrum Analysis

An additional approach to Doppler spectral analysis has been developed by Fronek in which the power (or amplitude) of the Doppler signal is plotted as a function of frequency, or power frequency spectrum analysis (PFSA).[29] This method

Table 9-5
Frequency Bandwidth of 50% ($f_{50\%}$) Changes Prior to and
After Occlusion

	No. of Limbs	Preocclusion	10–15 sec	45–60 sec	90–105 sec
Control group	19	1935 ± 542	3827 ± 1327	2504 ± 1194	2496 ± 1084
Isolated disease group					
A-I-CF > 50%	28	1038 ± 401	1288 ± 662	1200 ± 575	1034 ± 571
SFA > 50%	14	1903 ± 471	2747 ± 1437	2706 ± 1403	2745 ± 1530
Multilevel disease group					
A-I-CF > 50%	28	1062 ± 387	1231 ± 739	1238 ± 457	1150 ± 476
SFA > 50%					
A-I-CF < 50%	16	2111 ± 582	2810 ± 573	3126 ± 1303	2558 ± 786
SFA > 50%					

All data shown as mean ± 1 SD (standard deviation).

has been used at rest and combined with reactive hyperemic stress, and analyzed for peak frequency (f_{max}) and the bandwidth at 50% of peak amplitude ($f_{50\%}$). This test has been able to distinguish hemodynamically significant lesions from less significant ones (Table 9-5). The change of $f_{50\%}$ was a very sensitive indicator.

Tests under Stress

It seems reasonable that tests that duplicate or mimic the stress of walking should be used to enhance the sensitivity of noninvasive measurements. Two such stress tests are in general use at the present time: postexercise ankle blood pressure and postocclusive reactive hyperemia.

Postexercise Ankle Blood Pressure

Strandness described a treadmill exercise test in which the patient's maximal walking time, lowest level of subsequent ankle blood pressure reduction, and time for the ankle blood pressure to return to normal are measured.[7, 8, 30] These correlate well with the degree of intermittent claudication, both clinically and angiographically. The technique duplicates the conditions under which the patient's symptoms occur and provides quantitative data.

The postexercise ankle pressure is the standard stress test in use in most vascular laboratories at the present time. However, the data are somewhat subjective, since the patient can indicate when the pain precludes continued walking. In addition, the treadmill exercise test is limited to the data provided by the worst leg, since the patient must stop exercising as a result of that limitation. Generalized or regional neuromuscular or orthopedic disabilities also may limit or prevent the application of this test.

Postocclusive Reactive Hyperemia

In contrast to the limitations of the postexercise treadmill ankle pressure test, postocclusive reactive hyperemia measurements are objective, quantitative, and quick. Each leg is independently evaluated. Reactive hyperemia is generally stimulated by the application of a blood pressure cuff to the calf (or thigh), with a suprasystolic pressure for four (or five) minutes. Upon release of cuff compression, measurements of ankle pressure,[31-38] the reappearance time of toe pulsation,[39-41] or mean Doppler femoral artery velocity can be measured (Table 9-6).[42, 43] The first index seems to be the most specific and the last the most sensitive but least specific. Mahler and coworkers have documented the equivalence of the postocclusive reactive hyperemia test to exercise ankle pressures in normal controls and marathon runners.[44] The mean femoral artery velocity, the postocclusive reactive hyperemia response, and the toe pulse reappearance time clearly separate the normal patient from the abnormal, and separate the patient with single-segment aorto-iliac or femoro-popliteal disease from the individual with multilevel arterial occlusive disease (Table 9-7).

Table 9-8 summarizes a classification of peripheral arterial occlusive disease and includes criteria for the diagnosis of small artery disease when the segmental pressures and Doppler velocity measurements are normal.

Table 9-6
Reactive Hyperemia in Patients with Peripheral Arterial Occlusive Disease

	Normal Subjects	Localized Aorto-iliac Obstruction	Localized Femoro-popliteal Obstruction	Combined Aorto-iliac and Femoro-popliteal Obstruction
Postocclusive reactive hyperemia				
Maximal velocity increase (% of mean)	209.7 ± 95.5	136.9 ± 111.9†‡	47.6 ± 53.5*†	42.7 ± 59.8*‡
Recovery time ($T_{1/2}$) (sec)	26.4 ± 8.6	46.9 ± 21.9*	63.7 ± 50.8	41.3 ± 21.4*
Toe pulse reappearance time (sec)	0.2 ± 0.09	7.2 ± 4.04*§	3.7 ± 3.67‡	45.3 ± 5.51*‡§
Reappearance of ½ control amplitude (sec)	3.4 ± 0.84	23.9 ± 6.65*§	26.5 ± 12.71*‡	71.2 ± 5.53*‡§

From Fonek A, Bernstein EF: Noninvasive Studies in Peripheral and Cerebrovascular Disease. San Diego, University of California Medical Center, 1977.

* $p < 0.05$ in comparison with normal subjects.
† $p < 0.01$ between aorto-iliac and femoro-popliteal obstruction.
‡ $p < 0.05$ between femoro-popliteal and multilevel obstruction.
§ $p < 0.01$ between aorto-iliac and multilevel obstruction.
± Standard deviation.

Table 9-7

Distinction between Single-segment Aorto-iliac and Multilevel
Arterial Occlusive Disease

Measurement	Isolated Aorto-iliac Lesions	Combined Aorto-iliac and Femoro-popliteal Disease
Upper thigh pressure ratio	0.72 ± 0.25	0.97 ± 0.34*
Velocity deceleration, posttibial artery (cm/sec²)	79.2 ± 62.4	43.0 ± 40.2*
Postocclusive reactive hyperemia (%)	137 ± 112	43 ± 60*
Pulse reappearance time (sec)	23.9 ± 4.0	71.2 ± 5.5*

* $p < 0.01$.

Table 9-8

Summary of the Relative Value of Noninvasive Tests for the
Diagnosis of Peripheral Arterial Occlusive Disease

Test	Normal	Large-artery Disease*	Diffuse Small-artery Disease
1. Segmental pressure ratio (all leg segments/arm)	≥1	<0.9	≥1
2. Doppler arterial flow velocity	Normal	↓	Normal
3. Postocclusive reactive hyperemia (% of control)	>100	<80	<80
4. Toe pulse reappearance time (sec)	<5	>5	>5

From Fronek A, Bernstein EF: Noninvasive Studies on Peripheral and Cerebrovascular Disease. San Diego, University of California Medical Center, 1977.
* In addition, the approximate anatomic level of significant large-artery disease may be localized by the segmental pressure ratio and Doppler velocity data.

PREDICTIONS OF OPERATIVE SUCCESS

A number of investigators have demonstrated the value of the noninvasive tests in predicting the likelihood of success of conventional vascular reconstructive procedures and primary amputations.[45]

Aorto-femoral bypass represents the single most common and effective operation for dealing with peripheral arterial insufficiency, with a long-term patency rate exceeding 90%. Nevertheless, 10–30% of patients subjected to this procedure continue to have disabling symptoms. To some degree this failure of symptomatic control represents the misapplication of aorto-femoral bypass to patients with pseudoclaudication from neuroorthopedic causes, which should be ruled out by a careful evaluation of the symptom complex and a standard preoperative vascular laboratory screening test. However, in addition, there is the difficult problem of multisegmental occlusive disease in which the decision to perform proximal or distal arterial reconstruction may be contingent on the constellation of angiographic and vascular laboratory data.

The earliest correlation of preoperative vascular laboratory information with the results of aorto-femoral bypass was published by Bone in 1976 and included angiographic and hemodynamic data from 42 patients.[46] The value of the thigh pressure index (TPI) was emphasized as critical in predicting the success of surgery. All 22 limbs with a TPI of 0.85 or less were improved following aorto-femoral bypass. In contrast, only 63% of patients with a TPI greater than 0.85 were clinically improved. Thus the authors emphasized that the development of a pressure gradient between the measurements taken at the brachial artery and those at the proximal thigh demonstrated significant aorto-femoral occlusive disease and a high likelihood of successful surgery.

Unfortunately, when similar data were analyzed by Sumner and Strandness[12] the original conclusions of Bone were not confirmed. In the Sumner series, 36% of the patients with poor results had preoperative TPI of less than 0.85. Sumner suggested that the upper TPI failed primarily because such pressures are subject to significant measurement artifacts, a finding confirmed by the clinical studies of Franzeck and coworkers[14] and experimental studies of Bernstein and coworkers.[13] Additional data attempting to use thigh pressure measurements in the prediction of success following aorto-femoral graft for multilevel occlusive disease have recently been presented by Brewster[47] using a cutoff index of 0.6. In this more difficult group of patients, a TPI of 0.6 or less was associated with a good outcome in 83% of patients, whereas an index of greater than 0.6 was associated with a good outcome in only 65%.

Another pressure index was developed by Sumner and Strandness,[12] using the thigh-to-ankle pressure gradient to identify those patients with significant disease distal to the groin. This test, the index of runoff resistance (IRR), is calculated as thigh pressure minus ankle pressure divided by brachial pressure. In their study, essentially all patients with monosegmental aorto-iliac disease and a low IRR (less than 0.2) improved after surgery. However, none of the indices measured by these researchers were reliable in predicting the results of aorto-femoral bypass in patients with multilevel disease. Confirmation of these data was subsequently reported by Bernstein.[48] An IRR of less than 0.2 predicted success correctly in 91% of the patients. However, an index greater than 0.2 was associated with failure in only 26%. Thus a large number of patients with significant distal obstructive disease benefited from aorto-femoral bypass. The IRR was also evaluated by Brewster[47] in patients with multilevel disease where it also appeared to have significant predictive value, with a low index predicting success in 89% and a high index indicating failure correctly in 38%.

An alternative approach to the assessment of aorto-iliac disease was investigated by Thiele,[49] who analyzed the ability of the femoral pulsatility index (FPI), based on the femoral velocity waveform, to evaluate the hemodynamics of the aorto-iliac segment. The FPI was calculated from the waveform by digitizing the envelope to obtain the mean amplitude and the peak-to-peak range. An FPI of 4 was determined to be critical. In comparison with the direct measurement of femoral artery pressures (FAP) before and after an injection of papaverine, the FPI correctly identified aorto-iliac disease in 92% of 64 limbs studied, as well as in 92% of 36 limbs with combined aorto-iliac and distal disease. However, a negative FPI (less than 4) was not as good in identifying the absence of aorto-iliac disease in the face of occlusive disease of vessels distal to the inguinal ligament. Of 26 limbs with multisegmental disease studied in which the FPI was greater than 4, 25 limbs were hemodynamically normal for a sensitivity of 92%. However, of 55 limbs with an FPI value of less than 4 and combined aorto-iliac and distal disease, only 33 were abnormal. Therefore, the specificity of the FPI in combined disease was only 51%.

In addition, these studies only confirmed the ability of the FPI to identify hemodynamically significant aorto-iliac disease, but did not attempt to correlate the preoperative laboratory findings with eventual clinical symptom relief.

A plethysmographic correlation to the IRR was developed by O'Donnell and named the *FP omega*.[50] This measurement represents the difference between the femoral and popliteal pulse volumes as measured by the pulse volume recorder (PVR). Using a cutoff criterion of 0.2, the technique was capable of predicting success in 81% of patients, and failure was predicted accurately in 92% of a selected group of patients with multilevel disease. Although the series is small (40 limbs), the data suggest that this is an impressive preoperative noninvasive predictive index.

Finally, Bernstein[48] has reported the value of the toe pulse reappearance time (TPRT/2)[39] in identifying those patients in whom aorto-femoral bypass is most likely to be a clinical success. With a TPRT/2 less than 10 seconds, every patient was significantly improved by surgery, and with a TPRT/2 of less than 20 seconds, 98% of the patients were improved. However, the ability of the test to predict late failures was not adequately described.

Table 9-9
Toe Pulse Reappearance Time (TPRT) as a Predictor
of the Success of Aorto-femoral Bypass

TPRT/2 (sec)	Asymptomatic (%)	Late deaths (%)
0–10	63	0
0–20	56	3
20–60	27	7
>60	13	21
>90	10	25

Because of the difficulties in identifying a single noninvasive measurement with significant predictive capability, Bernstein also evaluated the combination of the ankle pressure index (API) and the TPRT/2 in 74 limbs with multilevel disease. These criteria identified a group of patients in whom clinical success could be predicted with 100% accuracy and another group in which failure was predicted with a 43% likelihood.

Another effort at using multiple test data to discriminate between potential success and potential failure was published by Brewster,[47] who identified five variables that were independent predictors of clinical outcome after aorto-femoral bypass including femoral pulse, the angiogram, IRR, and intraoperative PVR.

Using this model, 86% of outcomes were predicted correctly. This assessment, although identifying a variety of key predictive factors, was not much more accurate than several of the independent indices that have been discussed previously. In addition, only one vascular laboratory index, the IRR, was among the important indices.

Frustration with the noninvasive approaches has led to the use of semi-invasive techniques that generally involve femoral artery pressure measurements before and after the intraarterial injection of papaverine, as originally developed by Sako[51] and Brener.[52] Brewster confirmed the value of FAP measurements, using a cutoff index of a 10% change in pressure following femoral artery injection of papaverine as an indicator of significant proximal disease.[47] Based on these criteria, in 66 limbs with multilevel disease the test was 91% accurate in predicting success and 60% accurate in predicting failure. Flanigan,[53] using a similar test but relying on a 15% femoral pressure drop after papaverine, reported 100% success in separating eventual clinical symptomatic relief from clinical failure in 20 limbs. Use of these semi-invasive techniques during angiography does not significantly add to the cost or morbidity of the preoperative patient workup. However, femoral puncture techniques are not as useful as a completely noninvasive approach that could be applied to evaluate patients who may not need simultaneous angiography and could be repeated following interventions such as balloon angioplasty or with symptom persistence or recurrence after surgery.

In addition to the value of individual pressure measurements, Bone emphasized the importance of the number of segmental pressure gradients distal to the groin. In extremities in which no abnormal preoperative pressure gradients were measured distal to the femoral artery, all extremities were symptomatically improved by aorto-femoral bypass.[46] Of those limbs with a single gradient greater than 30 mmHg of mercury, 76% obtained symptomatic relief. However, with two abnormal preoperative pressure gradients, the likelihood of success was only 29%, and all of these differences were statistically significant. These findings were confirmed in an additional review by Garrett[54] in which the series was enlarged with essentially identical results. However, Sumner and Strandness were unable to confirm the selectivity of this pressure classification.[12] Bernstein evaluated a similar classification, dividing patients into those with pure aorto-iliac disease, one additional disal pressure gradient, and two additional gradients.[48] The data indicated a stepwise decreasing likelihood of symptom relief from aorto-femoral bypass that reached a statistically significant level only in those patients with two gradients below the groin. Thus this classification was not more successful in identifying potential surgical failures than other efforts based on pressure measurements.

In summary, pressure-based noninvasive indices identify individuals in whom a high likelihood of surgical success can be predicted. However, they are not as capable of isolating future failures. Velocity-based information is essentially equal. PVR and TPRT data appear to offer greater accuracy, but the initial reports of success await future confirmation from other researchers.

INTRAOPERATIVE MONITORING

Garrett measured the API in 72 symptomatic extremities undergoing aorto-femoral bypass as an indicator of eventual symptomatic relief.[54] In this report, if the intraoperative API increased more than 0.1 during surgery, the eventual likelihood of clinical relief of symptoms was 100%. Patients with increases in the intraoperative API ranging from 0 to 0.1 generally had significant improvement in symptoms. All patients who failed to have any increase in their API during surgery reported no significant symptomatic improvement from the procedure. Similar results were reported by O'Donnell using both Doppler systolic ankle pressure and segmental plethysmography.[50] Whereas a significant increase in either the API or PVR amplitude suggests a technical success of the procedure and its absence indicates that a search for technical misadventure should be undertaken, the surgeon's inability to detect a significant increase in either of these indices after a technically satisfactory procedure does not necessarily harbor failure. Kozloff has documented the fallibility of postoperative Doppler ankle pressures in a group of patients with limb-threatening ischemia.[55] An increase in the ankle-to-arm pressure index was a reliable predictor of success, but its absence in the early postoperative period, particularly in patients with occluded superficial femoral arteries, did not necessarily signify eventual clinical failure. Twenty limbs with occluded superficial femoral arteries did not demonstrate a significant increase until three hours postoperatively. However, within 24 hours, the ankle–arm pressure ratio should significantly exceed the preoperative value if the procedure has provided adequate revascularization.

Brewster has also commented on the value of intraoperative monitoring of the PVR cuffs.[47] In his experience, in patients with multilevel occlusive disease, an improved intraoperative PVR amplitude was associated with eventual clinical and hemodynamic success in 63 out of 65 limbs (97%). However, a lack of improvement was also associated with eventual clinical success in 48% of these patients. Thus the conclusions of Kozloff and coworkers[55] using the ankle measure were confirmed by Brewster and coworkers[47] for the PVR amplitude. Satiani, Hayes and Evans also compared the postoperative ankle pressure measurement within the first five days after surgery with the eventual clinical result.[56] In their experience the absence of an improvement of the ankle-to-brachial artery index of at least 0.1 within the first five postoperative days did not predict a clinical failure in seven of eight limbs. O'Hara also reported the value of the PVR amplitude intraoperatively in detecting 15 instances of technical problems in approximately 400 arterial reconstructive procedures.[57]

FEMORO-POPLITEAL BYPASS

In 1975 Dean correlated the late results of femoro-popliteal reconstruction with the API in 115 patients.[58] Intraoperative blood flow and angiographic runoff patterns were also correlated with graft patency. An 83% success rate was associated with patients in whom the preoperative API exceeded 0.4, and the success rate successively declined with decreasing API. If the API was less than 0.2, the success rate was only 9%. In a later review of this index by Corson, all but one of the early failures were in limbs with a preoperative API greater than 0.5.[59] However, late failures occurred in patients throughout the range of ankle pressures and the ankle pressure measurement was not as well correlated with eventual success as in the Dean study.

No additional data dealing with the clinical results of femoro-popliteal or femoro-tibial bypass have been published. However, several groups are currently evaluating a number of preoperative vascular laboratory indices with eventual clinical success in these patient groups, and new data should become available in the near future.

SUMMARY

In this review of the current status of the vascular laboratory in the management of peripheral artery disease, the major emphasis has been upon those tests that have become well established and documented, including resting pressure, pulse volume measurements, velocity studies including the Duplex scanner and spectral analysis, and three stress measurements—exercise ankle pressure, postocclusive reactive hyperemia, and the toe pulse reappearance time. Additional technology that may have application to peripheral arterial disease includes photoplethysmography, transcutaneous oxygen tension, laser–Doppler velocimetry, fluorescein angiography, infrared thermography, and transcutaneous electromagnetic flowmetry. These techniques, which are currently in development and experimental trial, were not discussed but are likely to provide significant additional information.

The future role of the vascular diagnostic laboratory in the area of peripheral arterial occlusive disease appears clear. It has already become a standard resource of the community hospital and tertiary referral center. Its functions will become more and more generally accepted with time as newly graduating physicians who have been exposed to this technology enter the practice of medicine. It should permit obtaining an evaluation of all patients at the expert level, aid in the education of all physicians concerned with peripheral arterial disease, and play an important part in guaranteeing a higher level of patient care than has heretofore been available.

REFERENCES

1. Naumann M: Der Blutdruck in der Arterie dorsalis pedis in der Norm und bei Kreislaufstorungen. L Keslaufforsahg 31:513, 1933
2. Winsor T: Influence of arterial disease on the systolic blood pressure gradients of the extremity. Am J Med Sci 220:117, 1950
3. Strandness DE Jr, Bell JW: Peripheral vascular disease. Diagnosis and objective evaluation using a mercury strain gauge. Am Surg 161:1, 1965
4. Harpman HL, Winsor T: The plethysmographic peripheral vascular study. J Int Coll Surg 30:425, 1958
5. Winsor T: The segmental plethysmograph. Angiology 8:87, 1957
6. Satomura, S: Study of flow patterns in peripheral arteries by ultrasonics. J Acoust Sci Jpn 15:151, 1959
7. Strandness DE Jr: Abnormal exercise responses after successful reconstructive arterial surgery. Surgery 59:325, 1966
8. Strandness DE Jr, McCutcheon EP, Rushmer RR: Applications of a transcutaneous Doppler flowmeter in evaluation of occlusive arterial disease. Surg Gynecol Obstet 122:1039, 1966
9. Ejrup B: Tonoscillography after exercise in peripheral arterial disease and coarctation of aorta. Am Heart J 35:41, 1948
10. Winsor T: Peripheral Vascular Diseases. Springfield, Ilinois, Charles C Thomas, 1959, p 178
11. Winsor T, Hyman C, Payne JH: Exercise and limb circulation in health and disease. Arch Surg 78:184, 1959
12. Sumner DS, Strandness DE: Aortoiliac reconstruction in patients with combined iliac and superficial femoral arterial occlusion. Surgery 84:348, 1978
13. Bernstein EF, Witzel TH, Stotts JS, et al: Thigh pressure artifacts with noninvasive techniques in an experimental model. Surgery 89:319, 1981
14. Franzeck UK, Bernstein EF, Fronek A: The effect of sensing site on the limb segmental blood pressure determination. Arch Surg 116:912, 1981
15. Gipstein RM, Coburn JW, Adams DA, et al: Calciphylaxis in man. A syndrome of tissue necrosis and vascular calcification in 11 patients with chronic renal failure. Arch Intern Med 136:1273, 1976

16. Lazarus SM, Albo D Jr, Welling D, et al: Doppler ankle pressures and stiff arteries, in Diethrich EB (ed): Non-invasive Cardiovascular Diagnosis. Baltimore, University Park Press, 1978, p 127

17. Fronek A, Coel M, Bernstein EF: The importance of combined multisegmental pressure and Doppler flow velocity studies in the diagnosis of peripheral arterial occlusive disease. Surgery 84:804, 1978

18. Carter SA: Response of ankle systolic pressure to leg exercise in mild or questionable arterial disease. N Engl J Med 287:578, 1972

19. Darling RC, Raines JK, Brener JJ, et al: Quantitative segmental pulse volume recorder: A clinical tool. Surgery 72:873, 1972

20. Raines JK, Darling RC, Buth J, et al: Vascular laboratory criteria for the management of peripheral vascular disease of the lower extremity. Surgery 79:21, 1976

21. Gosling RG, King DH: Ultrasonic angiology, in Harcus AW, Adamson L (eds): Arteries and Veins. Edinburgh, Churchill Livingstone, 1975, pp 61–98

22. Johnston KW, Taraschuk I: Validation of the role of pulsatility index in quantitation of the severity of peripheral arterial occlusive disease. Am J Surg 131:295, 1976

23. Johnston KW, Maruzzo BC, Taraschuk IC: Fourier and peak-to-peak pulsatility indices—quantitation of arterial occlusive disease, in Taylor DEM, Whamond D (eds): Noninvasive Clinical Measurement. Tunbridge Wells, England, Pitman Medical Publishing, 1977

24. Johnston KW, Maruzzo BC, Cobbold RSC: Errors and artifacts of Doppler flowmeters and their solution. Arch Surg 112:1335, 1977

25. Nicolaides AN, Gordon-Smith JC, Dayandas J, et al: The value of Doppler blood velocity tracings in the detection of aortoiliac disease in patients with intermittent claudication. Surgery 80:774, 1976

26. Fronek A, Coel M, Bernstein EF: Quantitative ultrasonographic studies of lower extremity flow velocities in health and disease. Circulation 53:957, 1976

27. Fronek A, Johansen K, Dilley RB, et al: Noninvasive physiological tests in the diagnosis and characterization of peripheral arterial occlusive disease. Am J Surg 126:205, 1973

28. Jager KA, Richetts HJ, Strandness DE Jr: Duplex scanning for the evaluation of lower level arterial disease, in Bernstein EF (ed): Noninvasive Diagnostic Technique in Vascular Disease, 3 ed. St Louis, CV Mosby Co, 1985, pp 619–631

29. Harward TRS, Bernstein EF, Fronek A: The value of power frequency spectrum analysis in the identification of aortoiliac artery disease (in press)

30. Strandness DE Jr, Sumner DS: The relationship between calf blood flow and ankle blood pressure in patients with intermittent claudication. Surgery 65:763, 1969

31. Baker JD: Post stress Doppler ankle pressures. Arch Surg 113:1171, 1978

32. Baker JD: Reactive hyperemia: A simple approach to stress testing of the lower extremity. Proceedings of the San Diego Symposium on Noninvasive Diagnostic Techniques in Vascular Disease, University of California at San Diego, 1979, p 67

33. Delius W: Hamodynamische Untersuchungen uber den systolischen Blutdruck und die arterielle Durchblutung distal von arteriellen Gefassverschlussen an den unteren Extremitaten. Z Kreis 58:319, 1969

34. Dornhorst AC, Sharpey-Schafer EP: Collateral resistance in limbs with arterial obstruction: Spontaneous changes and effects of sympathectomy. Clin Sci 10:371, 1951

35. Hummel BW, Hummel BA, Mowbry A, et al: Reactive hyperemia vs treadmill exercise testing in arterial disease. Arch Surg 113:95, 1978

36. Johnson WC: Doppler ankle pressure and reactive hyperemia in the diagnosis of arterial insufficiency. J Surg Res 18:177, 1975

37. Myrhe HO: Reactive hyperemia of the human lower limb. Vasa 4:227, 1975

38. Wilbur BG, Olcott A: A comparison of three modes of stress on Doppler ankle pressure, in Diethrich EB (ed): Non-invasive Cardiovascular Diagnosis. Baltimore, University Park Press, 1977, p 137

39. Fronek A, Coel M, Bernstein EF: The pulse reappearance time—an index of overall blood flow impairment in the ischemic extremity. Surgery 81:376, 1977

40. Fronek A, Coel M, Bernstein EF: Post-occlusive hyperemia and the toe-pulse reappearance time in the evaluation of arterial occlusive disease, in Bernstein EF (ed): Noninvasive Diagnostic Techniques in Vascular Disease. St Louis, CV Mosby Co, 1978

41. Guiterrez TZ, Gage AA: Toe pulse study in the diagnosis and evaluation of the severity of ischemic arterial disease of the lower extremity. Proceedings of the San Diego Symposium on Non-invasive Diagnostic Techniques in Vascular Disease, 1979, p 68

42. Fronek A, Bernstein EF, Dicus RB: Transcutaneously monitored post-occlusive reactive hyperemia in man and its significance. Fed Proc 31:379, 1972

43. Fronek A, Johansen K, Dilley RB, et al: Ultrasonographically monitored post-occlusive reactive hyperemia in the diagnosis of peripheral arterial occlusive disease. Circulation 48:149, 1973

44. Mahler F, Loen L, Johansen KH, et al: Post-occlusive and post-exercise flow velocity and ankle pressures in normals and marathon runners. Angiology 27:721, 1976

45. Bernstein EF: The predictive value of noninvasive testing in peripheral vascular disease, in Bernstein EF (ed): Noninvasive Diagnostic Techniques in Vascular Disease, 3 ed. St Louis, CV Mosby Co, 1985, pp 614–618

46. Bone GE, Hayes AC, Slaymaker EE, et al: Value of segmental limb blood pressures in predicting results of aortofemoral bypass. Am J Surg 132:733, 1976

47. Brewster DC, et al: Aortofemoral graft for multilevel occlusive disease. Arch Surg 117:1593, 1982

48. Bernstein EF, Rhodes GA, Stuart SH, et al: The toe pulse reappearance time in prediction of aortofemoral bypass success. Ann Surg 193:201, 1981

49. Thiele BL, et al: A systemic approach to the assessment of aortoiliac disease. Arch Surg 118:477, 1983

50. O'Donnell TF, Lahey SJ, Kelly JJ, et al: A prospective study of Doppler pressures and segmental plethysmography before and following aortofemoral bypass. Surgery 86:120, 1979

51. Sako Y: Papaverine test in peripheral arterial disease. Surg Forum 17:141, 1966

52. Brener BJ, et al: Measurement of systolic femoral arterial pressure during reactive hyperemia. Circulation 50 (Suppl):259, 1974

53. Flanigan DP, et al: Hemodynamic evaluation of the aortoiliac system based on pharmacologic vasodilation. Surgery 93:709, 1983

54. Garrett WV, Slaymaker EE, Heintz SE, et al: Intraoperative prediction of symptomatic result of aortofemoral bypass from changes in ankle pressure index. Surgery 82:504, 1977

55. Kozloff L, et al: Fallibility of postoperative Doppler ankle pressures in determining the adequacy of proximal arterial revascularization. Am J Surg 139:326, 1980

56. Satiani B, Hayes JP, Evans WE: Prediction of distal reconstruction following aortofemoral bypass for limb salvage. Surg Gynecol Obstet 151:500, 1980

57. O'Hara PJ, et al: The value of intraoperative monitoring using the pulse volume recorder during peripheral vascular reconstructive operations. Surg Gynecol Obstet 152:275, 1981

58. Dean RH, Yao JST, Stanton PE, et al: Prognostic indicators in femoropopliteal reconstructions. Arch Surg 110:1287, 1975

59. Corson JD, Johnson WE, Logerfo FW, et al: Doppler ankle systolic blood pressure: Prognostic value in vein bypass grafts of the lower extremity. Arch Surg 113:932, 1978

Mary Paula Colgan
and David S. Sumner

10

How Does a Vascular Laboratory Influence Management of Venous Disease?

The optimum management of any vascular problem depends on accurate diagnosis and a precise assessment of associated physiologic aberrations. Those conditions commonly classified under the rubric of "venous disease" are among the most challenging faced by the vascular physician. Included in this group of diseases are superficial and deep venous thrombosis, pulmonary embolism, varicose veins, and chronic venous insufficiency. Not only have vascular laboratories contributed to the diagnosis of these conditions, but they have also furnished the means for identifying physiologic defects in need of correction and have provided objective methods for evaluating the efficacy of therapeutic endeavors.

ACUTE VENOUS THROMBOSIS

In the field of venous disease, the vascular laboratory has had its greatest impact on the diagnosis of acute deep venous thrombosis (DVT). It was this malady that first commanded the attention of those working in the area of noninvasive technology and has generated the most interest subsequently. The fallibility of clinical diagnosis and the reluctance to use phlebography created a climate conducive to the acceptance of a new modality—less invasive and more readily available than phlebography but more accurate than clinical assessment.

Although the patient presenting with an acutely swollen, painful, cyanotic limb with good peripheral pulses probably has DVT, it is well recognized that the likelihood of a false negative or false positive clinical diagnosis of DVT approaches 50% when the signs and symptoms are less flagrant.[1-3] None of the many clinical tests that have been proposed, including those of Lowenberg, Ramirez, Provan, Pratt or Homan, have proved reliable. Phlebography, on the other hand, is highly sensitive and specific when carefully performed by skilled and interested radiologists. Although it remains the "gold standard" for examining the venous system, it is not without risks and limitations. Unfortunately, the required combination of skill and interest is not universally available in X-ray departments. Even when these requirements are met, observer variation in interpreting phlebograms is about 10%.[4] Moreover, phlebography is expensive, time consuming, employs sophisticated and bulky equipment, and cannot be used at the patient's bedside. Some areas—most notably, the soleal sinuses and profunda femoris and pelvic veins—are often inadequately visualized. The study itself may be painful, and the contrast material carries a small but finite risk of causing allergic reactions, inducing venous thrombosis, and producing skin necrosis if extravasation occurs.[5]

For these reasons, or perhaps because of clinical hubris, many patients have been and continue to be diagnosed as having DVT or, alternatively, have been cleared of the diagnosis without having undergone any form of objective testing. Prentice, Lowe, and Forbes, in a recent survey of 358 consultants in Scotland, found that 47% relied on clinical observation alone in making the diagnosis of DVT.[6] We recently surveyed the practice in our Midwestern community and were gratified to find that only 3% of patients hospitalized with the diagnosis of DVT were diagnosed and treated without the benefit of objective tests. Noninvasive tests were employed in 40%, phlebography in 33%, and both examinations in 24%. The results 10 years ago would have been entirely different. We feel that the emphasis on objective diagnosis engendered by the introduction of vascular laboratory facilities has been responsible for this favorable trend.

Methods

Noninvasive methods used to diagnose DVT in the vascular laboratory include Doppler ultrasonography; impedance, strain-gauge, or air plethysmography; phleborheography; thermography; and B-mode or duplex ultrasonic scanning. The ^{125}I-fibrinogen uptake test and other similar tests employing radionuclides are only slightly more "invasive." All of these methods are described extensively in other publications, and the details need only be summarized here.

Doppler ultrasonography detects abnormalities in venous flow patterns caused by an obstructing thrombus: reduced or absent flow, absence of phasic flow, decreased or absent augmentation of flow produced by leg compression, and increased flow in surface veins. The method is widely applicable and can be used on virtually any patient in any clinical setting. It does, however, demand of the examiner considerable skill, experience, and flexibility. Although the technique is most accurate for detecting venous obstruction proximal to the popliteal level, thrombi within the posterior tibial vein can often be recognized.[7]

The principle underlying venous volume plethysmography is the same regardless of the sensor used. Although the strain-gauge plethysmograph (SGP) and air plethysmograph (PVR) have their advocates, the impedance plethysmograph (IPG) has emerged as the most popular instrument. A pneumatic cuff placed around the thigh is inflated to 50 mmHg, impeding venous return; the resulting changes in limb volume are recorded by a plethysmographic sensor applied to the calf. The magnitude of calf volume expansion produced in response to inflation of the pneumatic cuff is plotted on a graph against the rate at which blood leaves the calf when the cuff is deflated. A discriminant line separates normal limbs from limbs with proximal venous obstruction, which display reduced calf volume expansion and venous outflow. The IPG has the virtue of simplicity and demands less skill and experience than the Doppler. It is, however, insensitive to calf vein thrombosis.

Phleborheography (PRG) uses six air-filled cuffs to sense volume changes in the foot; lower, mid, and upper calf; thigh; and thorax. The lower two cuffs serve a dual function: recording and compression. Small volume changes in the limbs, synchronous with respiration, occur normally but are absent in legs with venous occlusion. Rapid sequential compression of the foot or lower-calf cuffs propels a bolus of blood up the leg. In normal limbs, this sudden surge of blood is transmitted easily by the low-resistance venous system, and no expansion of the limb occurs; however in the presence of impaired outflow, the veins are transiently congested causing the limb to expand. The phleborheograph is perhaps somewhat more cumbersome than either the IPG or Doppler. Like these instruments, it is most sensitive to proximal venous obstruction but may detect some calf vein thrombi.

The physiologic tests (Doppler, IPG, and PRG) are sensitive only to total or near total venous occlusion involving the main channel veins. Free-floating thrombi, attached only at the valve sinuses, are likely to be missed, and thrombi confined to the profunda femoris, internal iliac, or intramuscular veins cannot be detected. Precise anatomic location of clots is difficult or impossible with these devices, and extrinsic compression (caused by tumors, hematomas, etc.) cannot be distinguished from intrinsic obstruction.

An increasing number of laboratories are using B-mode ultrasonography to survey the veins of the lower extremity.[8, 9] Under ideal conditions, thrombi can be visualized in the major deep veins of the thigh and calf, including the profunda femoris vein and perforating veins. It is even possible to recognize thrombi in the intramuscular sinuses. Nonobstructive free-floating thrombi can be seen. Venous flow can be visualized or assessed with a pulsed Doppler (when a duplex device is used). While B-mode and duplex scanning offer many potential advantages, the instruments are expensive, each examination is time consuming, and the technician must be highly skilled. Its role remains undefined but will probably be complementary to other more simple devices.

The ^{125}I-fibrinogen uptake test (FUT) involves the relatively atraumatic injection of labeled fibrinogen, which is incorporated into developing thrombi. Abnormal concentrations of radioactivity may be recognized only after a delay of 18–72 hours. Although the test is extremely sensitive to thrombi in their formative stage, well-established clots may not be labeled. Moreover, all thrombi—including extravascular thrombi associated with trauma and small, clinically insignificant venous thrombi—are detected. False positive results may also be found in limbs with infection, edema, or arthritis. The test is most applicable to the study of the calf and lower thigh veins. Because of increased background counts due to the presence of large arteries and the proximity of the bladder, detection of thrombi within the proximal thigh or pelvic veins is unreliable. To avoid some of these shortcomings, ^{111}In labeled platelets or ^{99}Tc labeled streptokinase, urokinase, or plasmin are being investigated.[10]

Acute venous thrombi may raise the temperature of the overlying skin by 0.5–1.2°C, providing the rationale for thermographic scanning. Early reports are encouraging, but the technique has not yet been widely evaluated.[11]

Table 10-1
Accuracy of Noninvasive Tests for Suspected DVT

Test	Number of Studies	Sensitivity	Specificity	Remarks
Doppler	1273	93%	91%	Above knee only[54]
	2060	84%	88%	Above and below knee[12]
IPG	2561	93%	94%	Above knee[12]
PRG	886	97%	94%	Mostly above knee[12]

Accuracy

Data regarding the accuracy of the more commonly used methods for diagnosing DVT are listed in Table 10-1. These data are summarized from reports in which test results were compared with phlebographic findings.[12] There have been few prospective studies, and almost all have involved examinations on patients in whom DVT had been suspected on clinical grounds. It is likely, therefore, that the tests appear to be more sensitive than they really are. Moreover, figures for the IPG relate only to clots proximal to the popliteal vein, and those for the PRG are derived from populations with a low incidence of calf vein thrombi. Nevertheless, it appears that—in good hands—all the physiologic tests are reasonably accurate for detecting proximal venous thrombosis in symptomatic patients.

Preliminary results with B-mode or duplex scanning have been encouraging. Oliver reports a sensitivity of 90% and specificity of 95%,[9] and Hannan and coworkers, a sensitivity of 95% and specificity of 89%.[13]

Table 10-2
Accuracy of ^{125}I-Fibrinogen Uptake Test[12]

Clinical Problem	Number of Studies	Sensitivity	Specificity
Symptoms of DVT	654	56%	84%
Prospective screening	718	90%	96%

The ^{125}I-FUT is considerably less accurate in symptomatic limbs, but is useful as an adjunct to other noninvasive tests to increase diagnostic accuracy, especially for thrombi located below the knee (Table 10-2).

Application

All patients suspected of having DVT should first be examined with one or more of the noninvasive tests (Fig. 10-1).[14,15] If the results are unequivocally abnormal, appropriate treatment can be instituted without further study; if they are definitely normal, no further diagnostic methods are necessary. If, however, the results are equivocal, additional studies must be performed. Phlebography affords the most direct way of arriving at an answer in doubtful cases, but other approaches are possible. When calf vein thrombosis is suspected, the ^{125}I-FUT may be employed, or the noninvasive test initially used may be repeated daily or at suitable intervals

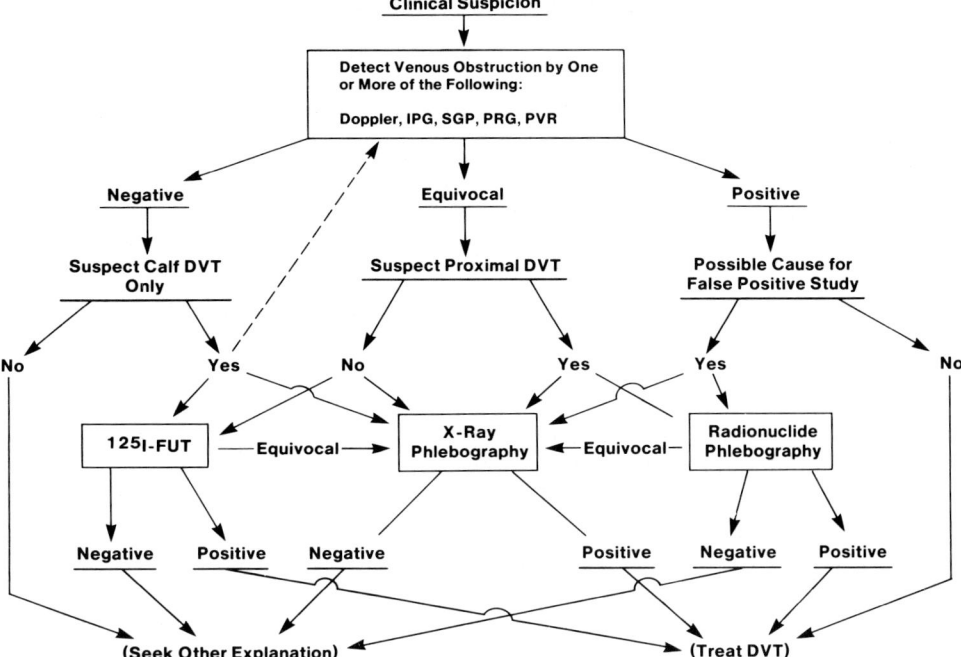

Fig. 10-1. An approach to the noninvasive diagnosis of acute DVT. From Sumner DS: Approach to diagnosis and monitoring of venous disease, in Rutherford RB (ed): Vascular Surgery, 2 ed. Philadelphia, Saunders, 1984, pp 167–184.

for a maximum of two weeks.[16] Potentially dangerous extension from the calf to the thigh veins should be detected by the approach. When the noninvasive findings are consistent with proximal venous obstruction, but other potentially confounding conditions coexist (trauma, tumors, etc.), radionuclide or conventional phlebography should be performed.

Several studies substantiate the validity of this or similar diagnostic algorithms. Wheeler and coworkers followed 1074 patients with negative IPG results who received no treatment.[17] None of this group suffered a fatal pulmonary embolus; only 1% developed a pulmonary embolus; and only 0.4% returned with symptoms suggestive of deep venous thrombosis. Hull and coworkers report that it is safe to withhold treatment when the IPG remains negative for 14 days.[16] Patients with false negative results, in whom the thrombi were confined to the calf veins, remained asymptomatic at three months without treatment. Similarly, Stallworth, Plonk, and Horne followed 593 patients with negative PRG findings and found that 0.2% suffered a pulmonary embolus and only 0.5 developed postphlebitic swelling, despite the fact that none were treated with anticoagulants.[18]

Noninvasive tests are ideal for documenting the results of therapy.[19] For example, the process of clot lysis with thrombolytic agents can be followed conveniently with noninvasive surveys.[20] In particular, the B-mode devices may be singularly appropriate for this purpose. Similarly, the results of venous thrombectomy can be evaluated noninvasively.[21, 22] In the past, such studies have shown a high incidence of residual or recurrent obstruction and valvular incompetence.

PERIOPERATIVE ASYMPTOMATIC DEEP VENOUS THROMBOSIS

The ^{125}I-FUT has called attention to the astonishing frequency with which thromboses develop in leg veins during the perioperative period. About 30% of all patients undergoing major surgery will develop clots that can be detected by this method.[23] While most of these clots remain asymptomatic and are of little immediate consequence, some will propagate and embolize. Pulmonary embolism is responsible for about one-fifth of postoperative deaths.

There are three ways of dealing with this problem. One can await the development of clinical signs and symptoms of DVT or pulmonary embolism and then institute the appropriate diagnostic and therapeutic measures; all patients at risk can be treated with low-dose heparin, intermittent compression, or other prophylactic measures; or all patients can be studied pre- and postoperatively to detect and treat asymptomatic thrombi. Although the latter approach is intellectually appealing, it is not only logistically difficult but is also prohibitively expensive.[24, 25] As an alternative, noninvasive studies could be applied only to those patients known to be at particularly high risk for pulmonary embolism. This group would include elderly patients; those with serious medical diseases, carcinoma, trauma, or a history of previous thromboembolism; and those undergoing operations plagued with a high incidence of DVT.

While the ^{125}I-FUT has provided most of the information relative to perioperative DVT, the majority of clots detected by this method probably require no treatment. Furthermore, the test may overlook proximal venous thrombi, from which most fatal emboli arise. Repeated testing is required to identify potentially dangerous clot propagation. Prospective studies with the Doppler identify unsuspected DVT in only about 2–5% of postoperative patients, suggesting that this modality overlooks many clots that would have been detected by the ^{125}I-FUT.[26, 27] It should, however, identify occlusive clots in the proximal veins and can be used in almost all clinical situations. The IPG has similar sensitivity but is more limited in its applicability, since it is difficult to use in patients who have undergone hip or leg surgery.[28] Both of these methods, unfortunately, are likely to overlook nonocclusive thrombi—the very ones that might break away to cause a fatal embolus.

In summary, therefore, the vascular laboratory has contributed to our knowledge of the incidence of perioperative DVT and is invaluable as a means of assessing the efficacy of prophylactic measures but has a limited and uncertain role in surveying patients during the perioperative period.

PULMONARY EMBOLISM

The vascular laboratory can play an important, albeit adjunctive role in the diagnosis of pulmonary embolism. As in the case of DVT, the clinical impression is frequently erroneous; thus, all clinical diagnoses deserve objective confirmation. Perfusion lung scans are adequately sensitive (few false negatives) but are insufficiently specific (many false positives). When a concomitant ventilation scan is mismatched and a "high-probability" perfusion scan is obtained, the positive predictive value approaches 90%. Unfortunately, more often than not some doubt persists regarding the diagnosis even after a ventilation–perfusion scan. In this event, the patient should be subjected to noninvasive testing for DVT. Findings indicative of DVT— although not diagnostic of pulmonary embolism—increase the probability that the patient has suffered an embolism. At any rate, the required treatment for DVT and pulmonary embolism are essentially the same. If the noninvasive test is negative, pulmonary angiography should be performed. Approximately 50% of patients with negative noninvasive tests and an abnormal lung scan will have a negative pulmonary angiogram.

It must be emphasized, however, that a negative noninvasive test does not rule out pulmonary embolism. While Sasahara, Sharma, and Parisi[29] found that 90% of patients with negative IPGs had negative angiograms and that 90% with positive IPGs had positive angiograms, Cheely and coworkers[30] found abnormal Doppler flow patterns in only 23% of patients with angiographically demonstrable pulmonary emboli. Other authors report positive noninvasive findings in about 50–60% of patients in whom the diagnosis of pulmonary embolism has been established.[31,32]

RECURRENT DEEP VENOUS THROMBOSIS

The patient with a previous history of DVT who returns with symptoms suggestive of recurrent DVT presents a difficult diagnostic problem. Since less than 30% of these patients will actually have new thrombus formation, it is incumbent upon the physician to make an accurate diagnosis.[33,34] Many of these patients suffer the effects of chronic venous insufficiency; others have any of a number of conditions that are commonly confused with DVT; and still others may be the victims of "thromboneurosis," a particularly pernicious and often iatrogenically generated fear of venous disease and pulmonary embolism. Unfortunately, phlebography may be inconclusive owing to the presence of residual disease and multiple collaterals.

An unequivocally normal noninvasive study essentially eliminates the possibility of recurrent DVT (within the limitations previously described). Hull and coworkers found that only 10% of such patients with a normal IPG had active thrombosis as demonstrated by a positive ^{125}I-FUT.[33] If the patient has been studied previously, and a Doppler survey or B-mode reveals new areas of thrombosis, or the IPG or PRG findings have deteriorated, recurrent disease is likely; however, a positive test for venous occlusion in a new patient or a test that demonstrates no change is inconclusive. These patients should undergo phlebography. If the X-ray picture is also indeterminate, a ^{125}I-FUT should be performed. It is safe to withhold anticoagulation in patients in whom noninvasive testing reveals no evidence of obstruction. Venous incompetence in the absence of obstruction does not demand new treatment aside from those measures that are appropriate to the treatment of chronic venous insufficiency.

SUPERFICIAL THROMBOPHLEBITIS

Finding an inflamed, tender, firm "cord" or "knot" along the course of a super-ficial vein is usually sufficient to establish the diagnosis of superficial thrombophle-bitis. Occasionally, however, other conditions, such as cellulitis or lymphangitis, may mimic superficial venous thrombosis. The Doppler or B-mode scan can be used to examine the involved area.[35] If the underlying vein is occluded, the diagnosis is confirmed, but if the underlying vein is patent, another inflammatory process is responsible. Of more importance is the use of noninvasive testing to rule out con-comitant DVT. This is particularly so when the thrombotic process has progressed to the sapheno-femoral junction. Anticoagulation is necessary if there is any deep vein involvement; otherwise, the superficial phlebitis can be managed with local heat or anti-inflammatory agents. Ligation of the sapheno-femoral junction or anti-coagulation should be considered when the physical examination or noninvasive tests indicate that the occlusion process has reached the sapheno-femoral junction.

CHRONIC VENOUS INSUFFICIENCY

Chronic venous insufficiency is far easier to recognize clinically than acute DVT. The typical picture of ankle edema, brawny induration, stasis dermatitis, pig-mentation, and ulceration in the gaiter area is often sufficiently characteristic to establish the diagnosis. Nevertheless, lymphedema, chronic inflammation, metabolic disorders, cardiac failure, autoimmune diseases, neoplasia, allergic phenomena, and traumatic ulcers can occasionally cause confusion. Although the symptoms of venous claudication are usually easily differentiated from those of arterial or neuro-genic claudication, the diagnosis may sometimes be unclear. The vascular labor-atory serves to confirm the diagnosis of chronic venous insufficiency, defines the nature of the physiologic abnormality responsible for the symptoms and signs, and helps direct the course of therapy.

The hallmark of chronic venous insufficiency is the presence of valvular incom-petence in the deep veins of the legs, with or without associated venous obstruction. The tests required, therefore, differ somewhat from those used to diagnose DVT.

Methods

Doppler ultrasonography is particularly well suited for identifying valvular incompetence. A Valsalva maneuver or manual compression of the limb above the site of the Doppler probe causes the immediate closure of all competent valves, and no reflux flow will occur. If, however, the valves proximal to the Doppler probe are incompetent, retrograde flow will be detected. By interrogating the major deep veins of the thigh and calf, the technician can localize the site or sites of valvular incompe-tence. The presence of incompetent perforating veins can be detected if superficial venous reflux is prohibited by a tourniquet placed around the calf above the site of interrogation.[36, 37] Unfortunately, localization of the perforating veins is imprecise.

Recently, B-mode or duplex scanning has been used for the same purpose.[13] Retrograde flow can often be "seen" in incompetent veins when the image is clear. It is frequently possible to visualize valve cusps, determine the extent of damage, and observe their function directly. The ability to identify a specific vein permits precise interrogation of venous flow characteristics. These devices may also permit accurate localization of incompetent perforators.

Retrograde flow can also be demonstrated by a variety of plethysmographic techniques.[38] A mercury strain-gauge plethysmograph (SGP) encircling the calf will detect venous reflux in limbs with damaged valves when a pneumatic cuff placed around the thigh is suddenly inflated. During this test, antegrade flow is prohibited by an upper thigh cuff that is inflated to a suprasystolic pressure.

More useful are those tests that evaluate the function of the calf muscle pump and the rapidity of venous filling in the dependent extremity after cessation of exercise.[39-42] These examinations are performed with the patient sitting or standing. To record venous volume, a mercury strain-gauge plethysmograph (SGP) is placed around the calf, a photoplethysmograph (PPG) is attached to the medial side of the leg just above the malleolus, or the foot is immersed in a simple water plethysmograph (foot volumetry). The patient is then requested to perform a series of five calf contractions or, alternatively, the calf is compressed a similar number of times. Normally, these maneuvers will cause the limb volume to decrease rapidly by about 2% of its original size as blood is displaced proximally. If the function of the calf muscle pump is impaired, the extent of limb volume reduction will be decreased. Limb volume may actually rise when there is associated venous obstruction. In legs with competent valves, the limb slowly returns to its preexercise volume as the veins are refilled by inflow through arteries and capillaries. Normally, the refilling time exceeds 20 seconds. When the proximal valves are incompetent, blood refluxes down the leg rapidly returning the limb to the preexercise volume. By placing narrow tourniquets at the ankle, below-knee, and above-knee levels, one can determine whether the reflux is the result of incompetent saphenous veins, perforating veins, or major deep veins (Fig. 10-2).

The "gold standard" of venous reflux studies is the direct measurement of venous pressure.[43] This is usually accomplished with a manometer connected by a plastic tube to a small needle inserted into a superficial vein of the foot. Since venous volume and pressure are closely related, the responses are similar to those observed plethysmographically. Pressure management has the advantage of being quantitative, but is invasive and more cumbersome than the plethysmographic methods.

Conventional ascending phlebography may be useful for localizing sites of venous obstruction, revealing the extent of collateral development, and identifying damage to venous valves. To determine the presence and extent of venous reflux, retrograde phlebography is required. Not only is this somewhat technically demanding, but also the results are not quantitative. Reflux throughout the femoral and superficial femoral systems may be normal.[44]

Application

When chronic venous insufficiency is suspected or when the physiologic abnormalities of this disease require clarification, noninvasive testing with the Doppler, SGP, or PPG should be performed.[14, 15] If evidence of deep venous valvular incompetence, venous obstruction, or both is obtained, the diagnosis is verified; in most

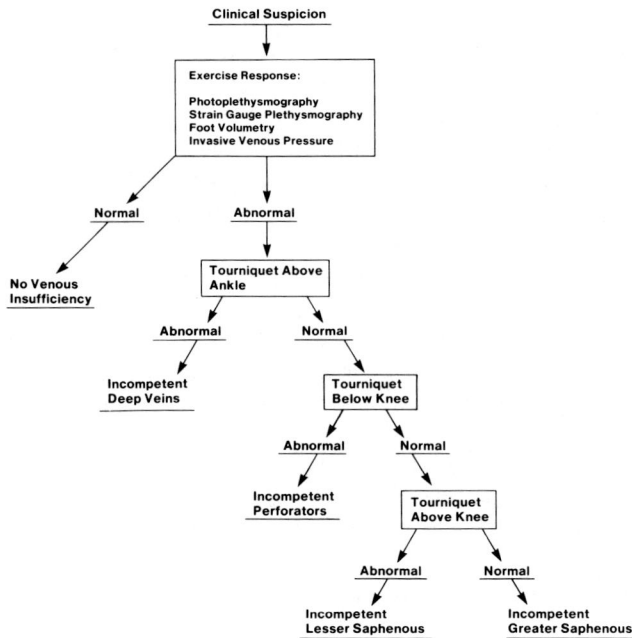

Fig. 10-2. Algorithm for localizing venous valvular incompetence. From Sumner DS: Approach to diagnosis and monitoring of venous disease, in Rutherford RB (ed): Vascular Surgery, 2 ed. Philadelphia, Saunders, 1984, pp 167–184.

cases, no further studies need be performed (Fig. 10-3). If doubt remains, phlebography may be required, but this rarely proves necessary.

When incompetent perforators are located, one may elect to perform subfascial ligation. A Linton or Cockett procedure, both of which permit extensive visualization of perforators, can be undertaken with no further investigation. In the event that proximal venous valvular incompetence is detected and plethysmographic studies indicate significant reflux, venous valvular reconstruction may be considered, provided the major deep veins are all patent. In order to define the anatomy, determine the technical feasibility of surgery and to plan the operative approach, preoperative ascending and descending phlebograms are required. Localized obstruction, confined to the iliac or superficial femoral veins, can be identified noninvasively. If the condition produces disabling venous claudication, a venous bypass graft may afford symptomatic relief. Again, phlebograms must be obtained prior to operative intervention. Patients with pure venous claudication, in contrast to those with arterial claudication, have normal (noninvasively determined) ankle pressures and no drop in ankle pressure following treadmill exercise.

In our experience, few patients with the postthrombotic syndrome are candidates for reconstructive venous surgery. Noninvasive studies reveal that obstruction or valvular incompetence is too widespread to benefit significantly from a localized procedure.[45] Most patients are treated quite satisfactorily by elastic support, Unna boots, and elevation. An occasional patient will require skin grafting of ulcers, with or without excision of the ulcer bed or perforator ligation.

Vascular laboratory findings are helpful prognostically. The development of stasis ulcers appears to be more closely related to incompetence of the popliteal and below-knee veins than to proximal venous valvular insufficiency.[45,46] Limbs in which plethysmographic studies reveal severe reflux or marked obstruction to venous outflow have a poor prognosis. Identification of these patients should stimulate the prompt institution of prophylactic measures to prevent the development, progression, or recurrence of lipodermatosclerosis and skin breakdown.

Noninvasive follow-up of patients in whom venous reconstructive operations have been performed is an important function of the vascular laboratory. Plethysmographic studies of venous reflux, ambulatory venous pressure measurements, and descending phlebography have demonstrated physiologic improvement in some—but not all—limbs that have undergone valvuloplasty, valve transplantation, or valve transposition.[47] Follow-up studies in many of these patients, however, have shown a disappointing return to the previously abnormal hemodynamic state. Careful physiologic monitoring is not only essential for evaluating the results of reconstructive procedures, but it should also assist the surgeon to design better or more appropriate operations and improve patient selection.

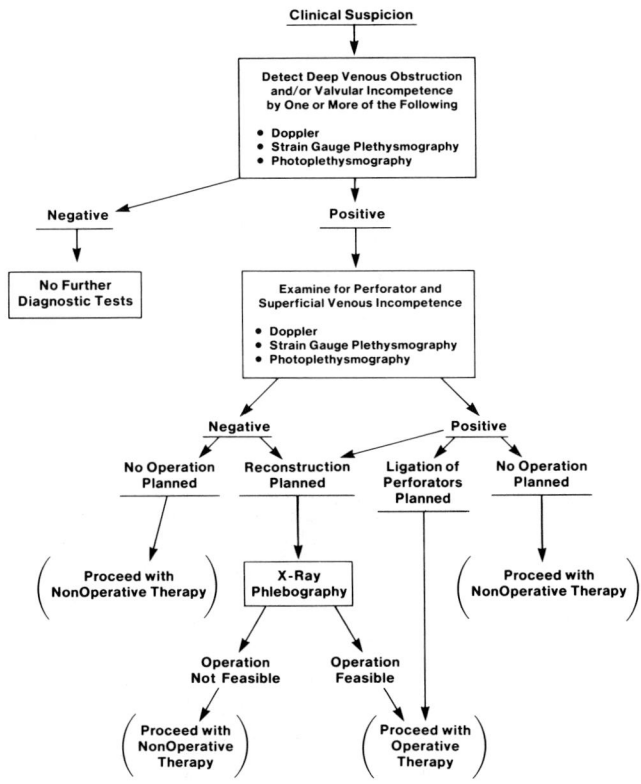

Fig. 10-3. An approach to the diagnosis of chronic venous insufficiency. From Sumner DS: Approach to diagnosis and monitoring of venous disease, in Rutherford RB (ed): Vascular Surgery, 2 ed. Philadelphia, Saunders, 1984, pp 167–184.

VARICOSE VEINS

Although varicose veins are easily recognized by visual inspection and careful palpation of the leg, the vascular laboratory can help identify their etiology and may provide information pertinent to their management (Figs 10-3 and 10-4). The first responsibility of the examining physician is to determine whether the varices are "primary" or "secondary." Secondary varices develop as collaterals in response to deep venous disease, the presence of which is easily recognized by examination with any of the methods previously discussed. Therefore, to classify varicose veins as primary, the superficial veins must be incompetent and the deep venous system, normal. Discovery of concomitant deep venous disease dictates the course of further investigation and management.

Primary varicosities involving the greater saphenous and tributary veins are usually associated with incompetence of the sapheno-femoral and ilio-femoral valves.[48] If these valves are found to be competent by Doppler examination, another source of venous reflux should be sought. Occasionally, the culpable valves may be in the vulvar or gluteal systems. A few patients with incompetent ilio-femoral valves will have a competent valve at the sapheno-femoral junction, in which case reflux into the distal saphenous system occurs via an incompetent thigh perforator. These findings are of value when operative therapy is planned. For example, if the sapheno-femoral junction is competent, ligation and stripping at this level is unnecessary.

In a few patients with a long history of varicose veins, superficial venous ulceration may occur in the absence of deep venous disease.[49] Identification of these

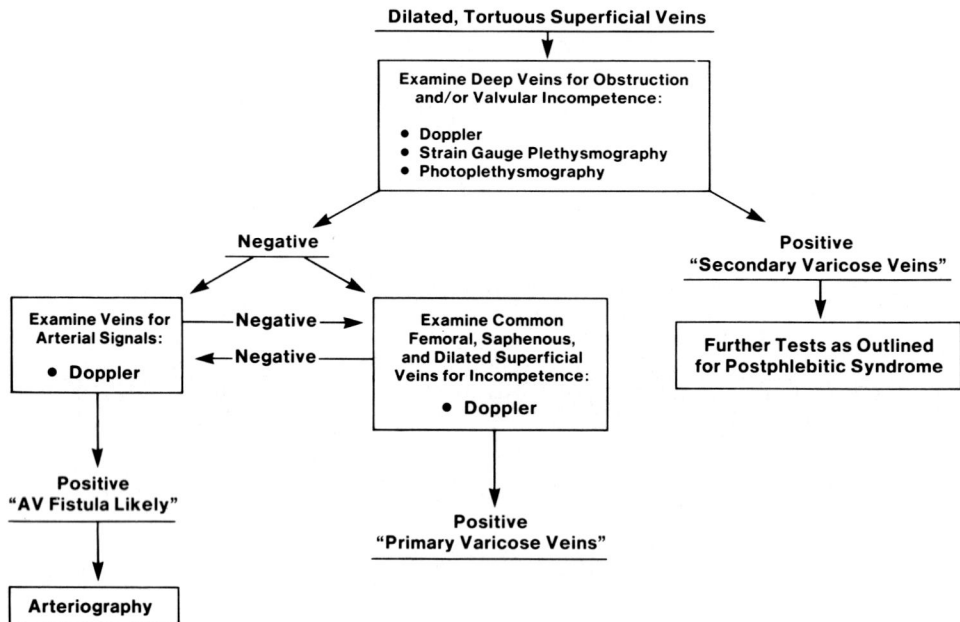

Fig. 10-4. Algorithm for noninvasive study of varicose veins. From Sumner DS: Approach to diagnosis and monitoring of venous disease, in Rutherford RB (ed): Vascular Surgery, 2 ed. Philadelphia, Saunders, 1984, pp 167–184.

individuals is important, since their ulcers respond favorably to simple ligation and stripping procedures or to compression sclerotherapy.

Unilateral varicose veins, especially in young people, may be secondary to an occult arterio-venous fistula—usually of the congenital variety. Excessive blood flow in the superficial varices—as revealed by Doppler studies—or the discovery of "arterial" flow signals in the veins should alert the examiner to this possibility.[50] Arteriography may be required to establish the diagnosis.

NATURAL HISTORY OF VENOUS DISEASE

Venous thrombosis is a dynamic disease. Clots may lyse, propagate, break off and embolize, organize and become adherent, or recanalize. Few investigators have made a serious attempt to follow venous disease objectively; consequently, our knowledge of the functional changes that follow an episode of DVT remains imperfect. Functional abnormalities are not easily characterized phlebographically. Moreover, the limitations of X-ray studies prohibit its widespread use for studies of this sort. Prospective studies using noninvasive methods are feasible and should help answer many of the lingering questions.[51–53]

CONCLUSION

The development of easily used, widely available, and accurate noninvasive methods has secured a place for the vascular laboratory in the diagnosis, management, and follow-up of venous disease. Noninvasive testing is rapidly becoming the preferred method for diagnosing DVT, relegating phlebography to a secondary role, and displacing the fallible clinical assessment. In all other facets of venous disease, the noninvasive laboratory offers valuable supplementary information. As new techniques are developed, some of the mysteries surrounding this most baffling and therapeutically recalcitrant vascular problem promise to be resolved.

REFERENCES

1. Haeger K: Problems of acute deep venous thrombosis, I. The interpretation of signs and symptoms. Angiology 20:219, 1969
2. Nicolaides AN, Kakkar VV, Field ES, Renney JTG: The origin of deep venous thrombosis: A venographic study. Br J Radiol 44:653, 1971
3. O'Donnell TF, Abbott WM, Athanasoulis CA, Millan VG, Callow AD: Diagnosis of deep venous thrombosis in the outpatient by venography. Surg Gynecol Obstet 150:69, 1980
4. McLachlan MSF, Thomson JG, Taylor DW, Kelly ME, Sackett DL: Observer variation in the interpretation of lower limb venograms. Am J Roentgenol 132:227, 1979
5. Albrechtsson U, Olsson CG: Thrombosis following phlebography with ionic and non-ionic contrast media. Acta Radiol (Diagn) (Stockh) 20:46, 1979
6. Prentice AG, Lowe GDO, Forbes CD: Diagnosis and treatment of venous thromboembolism by consultants in Scotland. Br Med J 285:630, 1982

7. Sumner DS, Lambeth A: Reliability of Doppler ultrasound in the diagnosis of acute venous thrombosis both above and below the knee. Am J Surg 138:205, 1979

8. Sullivan ED, Peter DJ, Cranley JJ: Real-time B-mode venous ultrasound. J Vasc Surg 1:465, 1984

9. Oliver MA: Duplex scanning in venous disease. Bruit 9:206, October 1985

10. Edenbrandt C, Nilsson J, Ohlin P: Diagnosis of deep venous thrombosis by phlebography and ^{99m}Tc-plasmin. Acta Med Scand 53:59, 1982

11. Nilsson E, Sunden P, Zetterquist S: Leg temperature profiles with a simplified thermographic technique in the diagnosis of acute venous thromboses. Scand J Clin Lab Invest 39:171, 1979

12. Wheeler HB, Anderson FA Jr: Can noninvasive tests be used as the basis for treatment of deep vein thrombosis?, in Bernstein EF (ed): Noninvasive Diagnostic Techniques in Vascular Disease, 3 ed. St Louis, Mosby, 1985, pp 805–818

13. Hannan LJ, Stedje KJ, Skorcz MJ, Karkow WS, Flanagan LD, Cranley JJ: Venous imaging of the extremities: Our first twenty-five hundred cases. Bruit 10:29, January 1986

14. Sumner DS: Approach to diagnosis and monitoring of venous disease, in Rutherford RB (ed): Vascular Surgery, 2 ed. Philadelphia, Saunders, 1984, pp 167–184

15. Barnes RW: Algorithms for diagnosis and therapy of venous thromboembolism, in Bernstein EF (ed): Noninvasive Diagnostic Techniques in Vascular Disease, 3 ed. St Louis, Mosby, 1985, pp 797–804

16. Hull RD, Hirsh J, Carter CJ, et al: Diagnostic efficacy of impedance plethysmography for clinically suspected deep-vein thrombosis. A randomized trial. Ann Int Med 102:21, 1985

17. Wheeler HB, Anderson FA Jr, Cardullo PA, Patwardhan NA, Jian-Ming L, Cutler BS: Suspected deep vein thrombosis. Management by impedance plethysmography. Arch Surg 117:1206, 1982

18. Stallworth JM, Plonk GW Jr, Horne JB: Negative phleborheography: Clinical followup in 593 patients. Arch Surg 116:795, 1981

19. Kakkar VV, Lawrence D: Hemodynamic and clinical assessment after therapy for acute deep vein thrombosis. A prospective study. Am J Surg 150(4A):54, 1985

20. Kupper CA, White GC, Burnham SJ: Streptokinase therapy for deep vein thrombosis: The role of noninvasive testing. Bruit 6:17, June 1982

21. Barnes RW, Miller EV: Late venous hemodynamics following thrombectomy for iliofemoral venous thrombosis. Vasc Surg 12:228, 1978

22. Hallböök T, Göthlin J: Strain gauge plethysmography and phlebography in diagnosis of deep venous thrombosis. Acta Chir Scand 137:37, 1971

23. Kakkar V: The diagnosis of deep vein thrombosis using the ^{125}I-fibrinogen test. Arch Surg 104:152, 1972

24. Salzman EW, Davies GC: Prophylaxis of venous thromboembolism. Analysis of cost effectiveness. Ann Surg 191:207, 1980

25. Hull R, Hirsh J, Sackett DL, Stoddart G: Cost effectiveness of primary and secondary prevention of fatal pulmonary embolism in high-risk surgical patients. Can Med Assoc J 127:990, 1982

26. Barnes RW: Prospective screening for deep vein thrombosis in high risk patients. Am J Surg 134:187, 1977

27. Reilly MK, McCabe CJ, Abbott WM, Brewster DC, Moncure AC, Reidy NC, Darling RC: Deep venous thrombophlebitis following aortoiliac reconstructive surgery. Arch Surg 117:1210, 1982

28. Satiani B, Tetalman MC, Van Aman M, Evans WE: Deep vein thrombosis following aortic surgery: Prospective evaluation of I^{125} fibrinogen and impedance plethysmography. Am Surg 45:507, 1979

29. Sasahara AA, Sharma GVRK, Parisi AF: New developments in the detection and prevention of venous thromboembolism. Am J Cardiol 43:1214, 1979

30. Cheely R, McCartney WH, Perry JR, Delany DJ, Bustad L, Wynia VH, Griggs TR: The role of noninvasive tests versus pulmonary angiography in the diagnosis of pulmonary embolism. Am J Med 70:17, 1981

31. Alexander RH, Folse R, Pizzorno J, Conn R: Thrombophlebitis and thromboembolism: Results of a prospective study. Ann Surg 180:883, 1974

32. Barnes RW, Kinkead LR, Wu KK, Hoak JC: Venous thrombosis is suspected pulmonary embolism: Incidence detectable by Doppler ultrasound. Thromb Haemost 36:150, 1976

33. Hull R, Carter CJ, Jay RM, Ockelford PA, Hirsch J, Turpie AG, Zielinsky A, Gent M, Powers PJ: The diagnosis of acute, recurrent deep vein thrombosis: A diagnostic challenge. Circulation 67(4):901, 1983

34. Barnes RW, Turley DG, Quereshi GD, Fratkin MJ: Objective diagnosis of recurrent deep vein thrombosis. Thromb Haemost 46:168, 1981

35. Barnes RW, Wu KK, Hoak JC: Differentiation of superficial thrombophlebitis from lymphangitis by Doppler ultrasound. Surg Gynecol Obstet 143:23, 1976

36. Folse R, Alexander RH: Directional flow detection for localizing venous valvular incompetency. Surgery 67:114, 1970

37. Miller SS, Foote AV: The ultrasonic detection of incompetent perforating veins. Br J Surg 61:653, 1974

38. Barnes RW, Collicott PE, Mozersky DJ, Sumner DS, Strandness DE Jr: Noninvasive quantitation of venous reflux in the postphlebitic syndrome. Surg Gynecol Obstet 136:767, 1973

39. Abramowitz HB, Queral LA, Flinn WR, Nora PF Jr, Peterson LK, Bergan JJ, Yao JST: The use of photoplethysmography in the assessment of venous insufficiency: A comparison to venous pressure measurements. Surgery 86:434, 1979

40. Kempczinski RF, Berlatzky Y, Pearce WH: Semi-quantitative photoplethysmography in the diagnosis of lower extremity venous insufficiency. J Cardiovasc Surg 27:17, 1986

41. Fernandes é Fernandes J, Horner J, Needham T, Nicolaides A: Ambulatory calf volume plethysmography in the assessment of venous insufficiency. Br J Surg 66:327, 1979

42. Thulesius O: Foot volumetry, in Bernstein EF (ed): Noninvasive Diagnostic Techniques in Vascular Disease, 3 ed. St Louis, Mosby, 1985, pp 828–833

43. Kriessman A: Ambulatory venous pressure measurements, in Nicolaides AN, Yao JST (eds): Investigation of Vascular Disorders. New York, Churchill Livingstone, 1981, pp 461–477

44. Thomas ML, Keeling FP, Ackroyd JS: Descending phlebography: A comparison of three methods and an assessment of the normal range of deep vein reflux. J Cardiovasc Surg 27:27, 1986

45. Moore DJ, Himmel PD, Sumner DS: Distribution of venous valvular incompetence in patients with the postplebitis syndrome. J Vasc Surg 3:49, 1986

46. Shull KC, Nicolaides AN, Fernandes é Fernandes J, Miles C, Horner J, Needham T, Cooke ED, Eastcott HHG: Significance of popliteal reflux in relation to ambulatory venous pressure and ulceration. Arch Surg 114:1304, 1979

47. Johnson ND, Queral LA, Flinn WR, Yao JST, Bergan JJ: Late objective assessment of venous valve surgery. Arch Surg 116:1461, 1981

48. Folse R: The influence of femoral vein dynamics on the development of varicose veins. Surgery 68:974, 1970

49. Hoare MC, Nicolaides AN, Miles CR, Shull K, Jury RP, Needham T, Dudley HAF: The role of primary varicose veins in venous ulceration. Surgery 92:450, 1982

50. Bingham HG, Lichti E: Use of ultrasound transducer (Doppler) to localize peripheral arteriovenous fistulae. Plast Reconstr Surg 46:151, 1970

51. Sandager G, Bartel P, Blackburn D, Flinn WR, Yao JST: Venous hemodynamics after acute deep venous thrombosis. Bruit 6:25, September 1982

52. Mahler DK, Foldes MS, Hayes AC, Halstuk K, Littooy FN, Baker WH: Followup of old deep venous thrombosis by Doppler ultrasound and strain gauge plethysmography. Bruit 6:30, June 1982

53. Strandness DE Jr, Langlois Y, Cramer M, Randlett A, Thiele BL: Long-term sequelae of acute venous thrombosis. JAMA 250:1289, 1983

54. Sumner DS: Doppler ultrasound, in Hirsh J (ed): Methods in the Diagnosis of Venous Thrombosis and Pulmonary Embolism. Edinburgh, Churchill Livingstone (in press)

Andrew N. Nicolaides, A-Majeed Salmasi
and Tansukh N. Sonecha

11

How Aggressively Should We Screen a Patient for Coexistent Lesions?

INTRODUCTION

Most patients with chronic arterial disease seen by the vascular surgeon or internist present with lower limb ischaemia, cerebrovascular, or aneurysmal disease. The surgical techniques that deal with such patients were developed during the first era of vascular surgery. The development of noninvasive screening techniques including computerised tomography in the 1970s resulted in a better selection of patients for arteriography and surgery, and provided better means by which we could study the natural history of vascular disorders. We have now entered a third era characterised by our ability to detect the presence of, to grade, and follow up asymptomatic arterial disease not only in the cerebrovascular, aorto-iliac, and distal lower limb circulation but also the coronary circulation. As a result of this ability we are witnessing a change in the values attributed to various risk factors and in our understanding of the balance of risks, i.e., nonoperative versus operative management. This is because subgroups of patients with asymptomatic and symptomatic atherosclerotic disease at high risk can be identified. Such subgroups are now being recognised as responsible for the overall perioperative mortality of 2–5% and the three-year mortality of 30–40% found in patients undergoing peripheral vascular reconstruction, the majority of deaths being the result of myocardial infarction and stroke.[1–16]

In contrast to the above, the management of ischaemic heart disease, in terms of short- and long-term results has improved dramatically in the last 15 years. The overall perioperative mortality of aorto-coronary bypass in many centres is now less than 2% and the five-year survival is greater than 90%.[17–21] A question, often asked, is how, despite the advent of aorto-coronary bypass surgery, advances in vascular surgical and anaesthetic techniques, and availability of intensive care units for postoperative care, the same degree of success has not been attained in patients undergoing peripheral vascular reconstructive surgery. This is because in the absence of noninvasive cardiac investigations, the presence of concomitant coronary artery disease has often been overlooked by the vascular surgeon, and the cardiac status of the patient has been less than adequately evaluated before peripheral vascular reconstructive procedures; it can also be due to uncertainty about the significance of asymptomatic cervical bruit and the doubtful value of screening patients for cerebrovascular disease.

The purpose of this chapter is to outline the most recent information about the incidence of both overt and occult cardiac disease in patients with peripheral arterial disease, the incidence of occult cerebrovascular disease in patients with lower limb ischaemia, the noninvasive tests that can be used to select the high-risk patients for the further invasive cardiac and cerebrovascular investigations, and the potential benefit of coronary reconstruction and carotid endarterectomy that justifies such an aggressive investigational approach.

INCIDENCE OF ISCHAEMIC HEART DISEASE IN PATIENTS WITH PERIPHERAL ARTERIAL DISEASE

Atherosclerosis is a systemic disorder that may affect several blood vessels in different organs simultaneously. The patient with peripheral arterial disease, whether lower limb atherosclerotic, extracranial cerebrovascular, or aneurysmal arterial disease, is particularly likely to have concomitant coronary disease. Although the patient may present with symptoms such as claudication, transient ischaemic attacks (TIAs), or angina, which indicate disease predominantly in one area, it does not follow that other sites are free from atheroma. The incidence of coronary artery disease in patients with claudication varies from 25 to 90% depending on the patient selection and diagnostic method used.[22-30]

Our routine assessment of the severity of lower limb ischaemia includes measurement of ankle pressures at rest and after exercise on a horizontal treadmill at 4 km/h. We have used conventional 12-lead ECG monitoring at rest and during the test in 100 consecutive patients. A total of 62% had ECG resting and/or postexercise ECG changes indicating ischaemic heart disease. During the exercise test 20% developed severe myocardial ischaemia and yet only three patients developed angina.[29]

In another series of 1000 consecutive patients, coronary artery disease was clinically suspected in 52% of 263 presenting with abdominal aortic aneurysm, 56% of 381 with lower limb ischaemia, and 57% of 169 with cerebrovascular disease.[23] However, when routine coronary angiography was performed in all 1000 patients, only 18% were found to have normal coronary arteries, indicating the presence of occult coronary disease in a very large number. Severe coronary disease representing a high risk of myocardial infarction, but correctable, was found in 25%. Severe but inoperable disease because of diffuse distal coronary disease or impaired left ventricular function was present in only 6%. More specifically, severe disease was present in 36% of patients with aortic aneurysm, in 32% of patients with cerebrovascular disease, and in 28% of patients with lower limb ischaemia. It cannot be overemphasised that a high incidence of severe three-vessel coronary disease was found in all ages: it was present in 22% of patients of less than 50 years, in 24% of the age group 50–59, in 30% of the age group 60–69, and in 41% of patients older than 70 years. Although myocardial revascularisation was indicated in 34% of 554 patients with a history of myocardial infarction or ECG changes demonstrating ischaemic heart disease, it was also indicated in 14% of 446 patients who had a negative history and a normal ECG.

INDICATORS OF CARDIAC RISK AND THE EFFECT OF AORTO-CORONARY BYPASS ON RISK

Indicators of Cardiac Risk

The clinical spectrum of atherosclerotic coronary disease is extremely broad and the risk of myocardial infarction or death is affected by whether the patient is asymptomatic, had prior myocardial infarction, stable angina, unstable angina, or has already undergone aorto-coronary bypass grafting. It has already been indicated that absence of cardiac symptoms does not mean the absence of coronary disease. This is more so in patients whose exercise tolerance is limited by claudication. Established "risk factors" for long-term development of coronary artery disease such as smoking, hyperlipidaemia, hypertension, and glucose intolerance do not predict perioperative myocardial infarction.[31] However, age, history of previous myocardial infarction, presence of congestive cardiac failure, or premature ventricular contractions are factors that correlate with life-threatening and fatal complications.[31]

In patients with previous myocardial infarction who undergo major noncardiac surgery, the more recent the infarction the greater is the perioperative morbidity and mortality. Major surgery performed during an episode of acute myocardial infarction carries a mortality of 90%; if performed within six months or less after myocardial infarction the cardiac mortality is 23%. With infarction occurring more than six months before noncardiac surgery, the risk gradually declines and eventually levels off at about 2.5%.[31]

Whereas the operative risks in patients with myocardial infarction are known, they are poorly defined in patients with angina pectoris. A surgical mortality from 0 to 17% has been reported in patients with angina undergoing noncardiac operations.[32] Most studies have not indicated the type of angina pectoris present despite the fact that the prognosis is different in different categories. Patients with stable angina with a normal ECG at rest and during exercise have the same operative risk as patients of the same age without angina; patients with stable angina and ischaemic changes on the exercise ECG have a moderate risk and patients with angina at rest constitute a major risk.

The presence or absence and type of angina, and ECG changes with exercise are relatively easy to determine in patients who present with cerebrovascular disease, but may be more difficult to elicit in patients with lower limb ischaemia. A carefully taken history may reveal that the patient had a myocardial infarct in the past. Some patients may recall having angina which disappeared when claudication developed or when the claudication distance became shorter; they often say that the angina has been "cured". Although these findings are good indicators of the presence of coronary disease, they are relatively crude or even poor indicators of risk. At one end is the patient who had an infarct several years earlier as a result of disease in one coronary only, with a well-developed collateral circulation; the risk in such a patient is low. At the other end of the spectrum is the patient who had claudication for years, is now well adapted to a life style requiring relatively little exercise and who has developed severe stenoses in all three coronary arteries (left anterior descending, circumflex, and right) or even in the left main stem. Although the latter may have no symptoms referable to the heart and the resting ECG may be normal, that patient would be at high risk of myocardial infarction.

We now know that the distribution and severity of coronary atheroma and the condition of the left ventricle are the most important determinants of cardiac morbidity and mortality available. We also know that patients with good results after aorto-coronary bypass (i.e., relief of angina and preservation of good left ventricular function) have a life expectancy close to the general population of the same age[10] and can undergo major operations without increased risk.[33-35]

Effect of Aorto-coronary Bypass on Risk

Of 873 patients with known coronary artery disease who underwent noncardiac surgery at Emory University Hospital in 1976, 48 had an acute myocardial infarction within three months of operation. In contrast, of 53 patients who had aorto-coronary bypass prior to noncardiac surgery only one of them had a perioperative myocardial infarct.[36] In another series, 358 patients with prior myocardial revascularisation underwent subsequent major noncoronary surgery. The subsequent operation was vascular in 232 patients with 1.3% mortality, general surgical in 13 with 0.9% mortality, and thoracic in 43 with no deaths.[37] It seems that successful revascularisation of the myocardium before subsequent surgery reduces operative morbidity and mortality. However, the risk of the bypass procedure should be included in the overall mortality and morbidity.

Another benefit from aorto-coronary bypass is the improvement in long-term survival. A number of reports suggest that an overall five-year actuarial survival of 90% may be expected for cardiac patients who had myocardial revascularisation.[19-21] In 77 patients who presented with TIAs and ischaemic heart disease and had carotid endarterectomy, a 20% three-year mortality was observed. In contrast, only a 3.5% mortality was observed at three years in 135 patients who presented with TIAs and ischaemic heart disease and subsequently had carotid endarterectomy and aorto-coronary bypass.[38] Similarly, Bernstein reported a 5% five-year mortality in patients who had carotid endarterectomy and aorto-coronary bypass surgery. However, in those who had carotid endarterectomy only or carotid endarterectomy plus peripheral vascular surgery without aorto-coronary reconstruction the mortality was 23 and 31% respectively.[39]

The five-year survival of patients with peripheral arterial disease quoted by Hertzer is as follows: 22% in patients with severe inoperable lesions; 43% in nonoperated patients with severe correctable coronary artery disease; 64% in those with advanced but compensated coronary lesions (two-vessel coronary disease) for which bypass was not thought to be necessary; 72% in patients with severe, correctable coronary disease who had received myocardial revascularisation; and 85% among those having normal coronary arteries or mild to moderate disease.[40]

Because of the above, a mortality of 20–30% at three years in patients with peripheral arterial disease is no longer acceptable and, as stated by Hertzer, "referral of a patient for peripheral vascular reconstructive surgery is the golden moment for the diagnosis of associated coronary artery disease; such a moment may never occur again in his life time".[41]

INCIDENCE OF ASYMPTOMATIC CEREBROVASCULAR DISEASE IN PATIENTS WITH LOWER LIMB ISCHAEMIC AND ANEURYSMAL DISEASE

Community studies of patients over 45 years in Framingham,[42] Evans County,[43] and Minnesota[44] have revealed a 4–5% incidence of bruit over the carotid bifurcation. The Framingham study showed that bruits were present twice as often in older people (over the age of 64) than in younger subjects (45–55 years) and the incidence was also twice as high in those with hypertension or diabetes.

Asymptomatic cervical bruits occur in approximately 20% (16–32%) of patients undergoing peripheral vascular reconstruction[45–48] and 10% (3–20%) of patients undergoing aorto-coronary bypass operation.[45, 46, 49–51] Unfortunately, the bruit corresponds poorly to the presence and severity of carotid artery disease. This is because not all cervical bruits arise at the carotid bifurcation and of those that do, some are from the external carotid artery. Also a stenosis greater than 85% may not produce a bruit because the flow may be too low to cause turbulence.[47, 51] A study comparing bruits with arteriographic changes[52] showed that 15% of patients with a tight stenosis had no bruit; that 24% of patients with internal carotid artery occlusion did have a bruit, presumably from an associated external carotid stenosis; and that 44% of patients with a minimal disease had a bruit if the opposite side was severely diseased, presumably because of turbulence produced by compensatory increased flow. Another arteriographic study showed that a bruit was present in only 50% of patients with stenosis greater than 20% and in 39% of patients with internal carotid occlusion.[53] It has been calculated that in patients undergoing aorto-coronary bypass because of the low prevalence of disease and the poor sensitivity and specificity of the sign, the predictive value of a bruit for significant disease (> 50% stenosis) is less than 15%.[54]

Two angiographic studies are available in asymptomatic patients undergoing peripheral vascular reconstruction or aorto-coronary bypass. In the first which consisted of 169 patients with cervical bruits, stenosis greater than 50% of lumen diameter was demonstrated in 47% of arteries with bruits; an additional 5% of arteries with bruits showed occlusion.[55] In the second study, Hertzer and coworkers found that cervical bruits were present in 11% of patients with aortic aneurysms and in 25% of patients with lower limb ischaemia. Since all these patients went on to have carotid arteriography, it was possible to show that internal carotid stenosis was present in about 60% of patients with a unilateral bruit and 85% of those with bilateral bruits, the stenosis being greater than 75% in about one half of the cases. Of the total 139 patients with incidental asymptomatic cervical bruits who had carotid angiography, internal carotid stenosis of 75–90% in diameter was found in 27%, stenosis of more than 90% was present in 6%, and occlusion in 11%.[56]

THE RISK OF ASYMPTOMATIC CEREBROVASCULAR DISEASE

Pathologic Changes in Relation to Risk

It is only recently that the changes in carotid arteries which may lead to a transient ischaemic attack (TIA), reversible ischaemic neurological deficit (RIND), or stroke have become clear. The most common site for disease is a plaque at the origin of the internal carotid artery. Pathological studies show that the larger the plaque, the more likely it is to cause symptoms[57, 58] and arteriographic studies show that the more severe the stenosis, the greater is the risk of stroke rather than TIA.[59] It appears that symptoms are often precipitated by acute haemorrhage into an atherosclerotic plaque or fracture of the plaque. This can cause disruption of its intimal surface so as to allow clot or cholesterol debris to discharge as emboli into the cerebral circulation. Sudden swelling of the plaque or release of contents onto the surface can cause occlusion from thrombosis.[57, 58] However, the size of the intimal defect, the amount of atheromatous debris discharged, and the likely damage to the brain are unpredictable. Nevertheless, these findings explain why internal carotid artery disease develops at varying rates; some lesions remain unchanged for years while others progress from mild disease to 90% stenosis or occlusion within weeks or months.[58, 60]

Although the extracranial internal carotid artery is the most frequent site for atherosclerosis, disease in the intracranial internal carotid or middle cerebral arteries is not uncommon and is even more likely to cause stroke, particularly if in "tandem" with extracranial disease.[53, 61] It has been reported in one study that arteriography showed intracranial carotid stenosis associated with extracranial disease in 29% of patients with TIAs and no less than 90% of those with a stroke.[53]

Although most hemispheric symptoms can be properly attributed to embolism, some patients suffer TIAs or stroke from diminished perfusion resulting from tight stenosis or occlusion. The diameter of the internal carotid artery needs to be reduced to 75% of the normal size before flow starts to fall. Even then, there is a considerable reserve before diminished flow causes hypoxia.[62] The severity of ischaemia depends on the adequacy of the Circle of Willis to provide collateral flow and, in turn, the state of the other carotid and the vertebro-basilar arteries. The cerebral vascular bed has a well-developed homeostatic mechanism and can maintain a constant blood flow by vasodilatation. Such vasodilatation which lowers the vascular bed resistance achieves this by producing pressure gradients across the stenoses and collateral vessels. However, in the presence of maximum vasodilatation a fall in blood pressure which may be the result of myocardial ischaemia or an episode of cardiac arrhythmia may cause acute hypoperfusion and hypoxia. Carotid endarterectomy has been performed by the author in several patients with severe internal carotid stenosis who presented with TIAs as a result of documented cardiac arrhythmias uncontrolled by medication. There have been no further TIAs after operation although the arrhythmias continued to occur. The fact that cerebral blood flow was at the lower level of normal and that there was maximum vasodilatation in these patients had been demonstrated by cerebral blood flow measurements using radioactive xenon before and after inhalation of CO_2. It was found that the normal response of increased cerebral flow in response to CO_2 inhalation was absent.

Risk in Patients with Asymptomatic Cervical Bruit

In both the Framingham and Evans County Studies[42, 43] a bruit predicted that the risk of subsequent stroke was about 2% per year. This was two to four times more than that expected in comparable subjects without bruits, the difference being rather greater in older or hypertensive patients. Both studies showed that the bruit was associated with a comparable increased risk of myocardial infarction. Bernstein's review (based on 1790 patients from seven recent publications) indicated that the stroke rate in subjects with an asymptomatic bruit was less than 1% per year.[63]

The risk of perioperative stroke in patients with asymptomatic cervical bruit undergoing peripheral vascular reconstruction is not any higher. A recent review of the available literature (five papers[45, 46, 64–66]) by Hart and Easton[67] indicated that cervical bruits do not effectively identify subgroups of asymptomatic peripheral vascular reconstruction patients at risk of perioperative stroke. In fact, the incidence of perioperative stroke in these asymptomatic patients was 1% (2/206) in patients with bruits and 1% (9/1102) of patients without bruits. In the same review, Hart and Easton indicated that in patients undergoing aorto-coronary bypass graft operations the incidence of perioperative stroke increased from 3% in patients without bruits to only 7% in patients with bruits[67] (aggregate data from four papers[45, 46, 49, 68]).

Risk in Patients with Asymptomatic Internal Carotid Stenosis

Considering all patients with stenosis, irrespective of severity, the risk of future stroke is probably little more than that for a bruit. The results of several clinical studies of patients with asymptomatic internal carotid disease treated conservatively have produced variable results.[64, 69–71]

The wide discrepancy in outcome may be because the groups of patients described were selected and quite different. For example, studies in which oculoplethysmography was used should have included a large number of patients with high-grade stenosis, and we now know that this is a most important factor associated with an increased risk (see below). Bernstein's review (668 patients from nine papers) indicates that the overall risk of stroke in patients with stenosis of the internal carotid artery is well under 2% per year.[63]

There is no evidence that in patients undergoing peripheral vascular reconstruction, the presence of asymptomatic unilateral or bilateral internal carotid stenosis increases the overall risk of stroke significantly.[45, 46, 67] Aggregate figures show a 2.5% (5/200) incidence of stroke in patients without internal carotid stenosis and a 5% (4/85) in patients with stenosis as detected by Doppler ultrasound. Data from three studies[45, 46, 68] in patients undergoing coronary artery bypass graft operations indicate little increase in the incidence of stroke in the presence of internal carotid stenosis (4%—14/524) as compared with patients without stenosis (3%—14/524). One exception has been Kartchner and McRae's study using oculoplethysmography (OPG) in a group of patients undergoing coronary revascularisation or peripheral vascular reconstruction, which demonstrated an increase in stroke rate from 1% when OPG was negative to 17% when OPG was positive.[72]

Recently it has become increasingly clear that whereas patients with mild to moderate disease run a relatively benign course, those with a tight stenosis or large plaque are at much higher risk. A Canadian study of 500 patients reported that where Doppler studies showed a stenosis less than 75%, the risk of stroke was only 2% per year, whereas in those with stenosis greater than 75% the risk of stroke was 15% per year.[73]

A study at St Mary's Hospital, London, identified a small subgroup at very high risk. One hundred and fifty-two patients with asymptomatic cervical bruits were followed for 2–6 years (mean 3 years) after noninvasive assessment using supraorbital Doppler, carotid phonoangiography, and oculoplethysmography. These patients had presented with symptoms of lower limb or myocardial ischaemia. Overall, there was a 9.8% incidence of cerebrovascular symptoms. During the follow-up period nine patients developed TIAs and six suffered a stroke. In three of the latter, the stroke was fatal. The noninvasive tests defined three grades of disease: internal carotid stenosis less than 50% (all three tests negative), 50–75% (CPA positive, i.e., duration of bifurcation bruit >0.70 of systole, SOD and OPG negative), and greater than 75% (SOD and OPG positive). Of those patients with stenosis less than 50%, none developed symptoms; of those with stenosis 50–75%, 10% developed TIAs and 7% had a stroke without prior warning; and of those who had a stenosis greater than 75%, 29% developed TIAs or stroke without warning. This study also showed that a haematocrit greater than 45% increased the risk of late symptoms from less than 5% to more than 50%. Other factors which increased the risk of stroke were bilateral severe carotid disease and associated vertebrobasilar disease.

A study from Seattle in which duplex scanning was used to study the natural history of asymptomatic patients showed that although the overall risk of stroke was less than 2% per year, the risk of developing symptoms in patients with stenosis greater than 80% rose to 35% by 6 months and 46% by 12 months. Only one-third progressed at all during the study, but 8% progressed from less than 50% to more than 50% stenosis and 10% progressed to more than 80%, and these patients were at high risk.[60]

Similarly, Sumner has found a 20% incidence of stroke at five years in patients with internal carotid stenosis greater than 50%.[74]

The Effect of Carotid Endarterectomy on Risk

The risk of stroke in patients with internal carotid stenosis and hemispheric TIAs is approximately 33% at five years (18 publications, 1826 patients reviewed by Bernstein[63]). Since carotid endarterectomy in these patients can be performed by many centres with an average mortality of 2%, a perioperative stroke rate of less than 5%, and a late stroke rate of less than 2% per year,[63] it has become the accepted method of treatment.

Although the risk of carotid endarterectomy (perioperative and long-term results) in patients with TIAs and internal carotid stenosis is many times less than the risk of nonoperative therapy and carotid endarterectomy is the accepted method of management of such patients even in the presence of coexisting lower limb ischaemia or coronary artery disease, this is not the case with patients with asymptomatic cervical bruit.

Prophylactic carotid endarterectomy in patients with asymptomatic cervical bruit who were candidates for peripheral vascular reconstruction[45,65,75,76] was associated with a perioperative stroke rate of 5% (range 0–10%) and a mortality rate of 2%. Similarly, prophylactic carotid endarterectomy in 97 patients who were candidates for coronary artery revascularisation was associated with a 4% (range 3–6%) incidence of perioperative ischaemia and a 3% mortality.[77–79] When the carotid endarterectomy was performed simultaneously with the coronary artery bypass operation in 490 patients the stroke rate was 5%.[77–80]

If prophylactic carotid endarterectomy were to be of value in preventing perioperative stroke in patients who are candidates for peripheral vascular reconstruction or coronary surgery it should be performed in patients in which the risk of stroke without carotid endarterectomy is considerably higher than 5%. This is not the case if one considers all patients with asymptomatic cervical bruit or internal carotid stenosis greater than 50% in diameter (see above), and therefore such patients should not be considered for prophylactic carotid endarterectomy.[67] Not only does it not diminish the incidence of a subsequent perioperative stroke, but, as stated above, it carries a considerable mortality: 2% in patients who are candidates for peripheral vascular reconstruction and 3% in patients for coronary surgery.

The long-term benefit of carotid endarterectomy in patients with peripheral vascular disease is a separate issue. A subgroup of patients with asymptomatic cervical bruit or internal carotid stenosis has now been identified with a risk of stroke (at three years) greater than 25%. These are patients with internal carotid stenosis greater than 75%. The risk is probably higher in the presence of similarly severe contralateral stenosis or vertebro-basilar disease. A number of randomised studies (medical versus surgical therapy) are now in progress, and the results will not be available for several years. In the meantime, the author believes that such patients should be identified and considered for prophylactic carotid endarterectomy by centres that have a low perioperative complication rate. The perioperative mortality rate is 1% or less and the perioperative stroke rate 2% or less (13 publications, 734 patients reviewed by Bernstein[63]). In addition, such centres should be able to assess the state of the coronary arteries, identifying patients with severe three-vessel coronary disease or left main stem stenosis. The author believes that if perioperative mortality were to be minimized in these high-risk patients carotid endarterectomy should be done after the coronary bypass operation (see below).

WHAT ARE THE AIMS OF SCREENING PATIENTS FOR COEXISTING LESIONS?

Patients with symptomatic peripheral arterial disease should be investigated so that a high-risk subgroup of patients with severe correctable coronary artery disease should be identified. Such a subgroup carries a 10% perioperative risk when vascular reconstruction is undertaken.[40] This risk is very low (1–1.5%) after myocardial revascularisation and the patient's five-year survival is increased from 43 to 72%.[40, 81–83]

Patients who present with symptomatic cardiac or peripheral arterial disease but without symptomatic cerebrovascular disease should be screened so that patients with internal carotid stenosis greater than 75% are identified. Because the long-term risk of stroke in such patients is greater than 25% they should be considered for carotid endarterectomy. Patients with less severe lesions should be followed up so that those with rapid progression would be detected.

Patients who present with angina or symptomatic carotid disease should also be screened for early asymptomatic aneurysmal or lower limb occlusive disease. Such disease may become apparent by producing symptoms after the angina is relieved by aorto-coronary bypass grafting. In addition, noninvasive screening will indicate to the cardiac surgeon which is the most ischaemic limb and which long saphenous vein should be preserved. Early detection of such disease may also offer the possibility of applying medical prophylaxis or even percutaneous transluminal angioplasty before arterial occlusion occurs.

HOW SHOULD WE SCREEN PATIENTS FOR COEXISTING LESIONS?

Routine panangiography as practised by Hertzer and his coworkers at the Cleveland Clinic has been instrumental in indicating the high incidence of coexisting asymptomatic disease, and especially the natural history of high-risk patients with correctable disease and the beneficial effect of surgical procedures on this risk.[40] Unfortunately, routine panangiography is expensive and not practical. The development of noninvasive tests in the 1970s has revolutionised the investigation of patients with lower limb arterial and carotid disease so that today only patients selected with the view to vascular reconstruction on the basis of the history, clinical examination, and noninvasive screening are admitted to hospital for angiography. The advent of intravenous digital subtraction angiography (DSA) means that in many patients even angiographic images can now be obtained without hospitalisation. Although the development of noninvasive cardiac investigations has lagged behind by at least 10 years, tests are now available that can identify patients with silent ischaemic heart disease and quantitatively assess its severity so that only patients at high risk would be considered for angiography.

The noninvasive screening tests available to assess the arteriopath irrespective of presentation that are used by the author are duplex scanning, ankle pressures, the one-minute treadmill test, ECG chest wall mapping stress test, and transcutaneous aortovelography. The above are performed routinely in most patients unless the presence of severe disease is obvious or there are contraindications. They should be supplemented in selected cases by ambulatory ST segment (Holter) monitoring, two-dimensional echocardiography, and dipyridamole–thallium imaging. The rational use of these tests implies the availability of a noninvasive vascular laboratory, enthusiastic cardiology and radiology departments, cardiac surgeons, neurologists, and above all the spirit of teamwork.

Duplex Scanning

The noninvasive cerebrovascular tests that were developed in the 1970s (supraorbital Doppler, oculoplethysmography, oculopneumoplethysmography, carotid phonoangiography, Doppler imaging) have now been superseded by duplex scanning. This is because most of these techniques could detect internal carotid stenosis greater than 50% or greater than 75% but could not grade the degree of stenosis accurately. Duplex scanning which can do the latter has provided the means of studying the progression of disease and eventually the identification of high-risk patients.[60] In view of the clinical decisions that can be made on the basis of such grading (see below) duplex scanning has become an essential investigation in patients of all vascular departments. Because the vascular surgeon should be by now familiar with this technique it will not be described here. The novice is referred elsewhere.[84]

Ankle Systolic Pressures and Doppler Velocity Tracings

Ankle systolic pressures and Doppler velocity tracings (of the common femoral, dorsalis pedis, and posterior tibial arteries) will establish the presence of lower limb arterial disease (ankle pressure less than 80% of the brachial pressure) and Doppler velocity tracings will help localize it. In the presence of an ankle pressure which is greater than 80% of the brachial pressure, the one-minute treadmill test will detect the presence and severity of early atherosclerotic disease affecting the lower limbs.[85] Because this is a standard test (one minute on a 10% inclined treadmill at 4 km/h) the decrease in ankle pressure at the end of the test is a quantitative measure of the severity of the disease. It has been shown to be a reproducible test that can follow the progression of early asymptomatic disease[85,86] and can be performed safely in patients with coexisting asymptomatic cardiac disease, or even mild to moderate angina.[87] This test will unmask early asymptomatic disease or document disease that will produce claudication after aorto-coronary bypass grafting would enable a patient to walk further than the limit imposed by the angina.

The cardiac surgeon should not excise the long saphenous vein from the more ischaemic limb in order to avoid wound-healing problems and leave the vein as a potential graft for lower limb vascular reconstruction in the future. In such patients with severe lower limb disease the author advises and practises elective aortography prior to coronary grafting so that in the event of acute lower limb ischaemia in the immediate postoperative period the latter can be dealt with promptly. It has been found to be very difficult to do an emergency arteriogram in the first 24 hours after coronary revascularisation while the patient is in the intensive care unit.

ECG Chest Wall Mapping Stress Test

The details of this test and its validation have been described elsewhere.[88] In our initial study, chest wall mapping of ST segment changes, inverted U waves, and Q waves using 16 electrocardiographic electrodes was performed at rest, during and after bicycle ergometry in 150 patients presenting with chest pain suggestive of angina. All patients underwent coronary angiography. The principle of this test is based on the observation that ECG changes obtained with an electrode at a point on the chest wall reflect changes in the myocardium immediately deep to that point. The position of the leads was such that they would reflect changes in the three main coronary artery territories, providing spatial information. Electrodes were placed in four vertical rows of four. Four were just to the right of the sternum to provide information about the right coronary territory; four were just to the left of the sternum and four along the anterior axillary line, providing information about the LAD/diagonal territory; four were on the back 6 cm medial to the posterior axillary line, providing information about the circumflex coronary territory. By using multiple criteria (ST segment depression, Q waves at rest, and the appearance of inverted U waves) the accuracy was improved. The presence or absence of appreciable coronary artery disease ($>50\%$ stenosis) was detected with a sensitivity of 98% and a specificity of 88%. The identification of lesions in individual coronary arteries was also possible: there was a sensitivity of 98% and a specificity of 88% for lesions of the left anterior descending or main diagonal artery; a sensitivity of 71% and a specificity of 85% for lesions of the right coronary artery; and a sensitivity of 86% and a specificity of 80% for lesions of the circumflex artery. The absence of appreciable coronary artery disease and the presence of single, double, or triple-vessel disease was predicted correctly in 70% of patients. Errors occurred in 25% of patients because the disease was missed or falsely diagnosed in one coronary artery. Errors in more than one vessel occurred in only 5% of patients. Left main stem coronary disease present in 11 patients was in every case demonstrated as disease of LAD/diagonal and circumflex territories.

Subsequently, we applied this test in claudicants. We have found that although these patients cannot exercise adequately on a treadmill, they do better on a bicycle. An average increase of heart rate to 82% of the expected maximum was produced. We have found that one-third of patients with claudication and no known cardiac disease have a positive effort test and in one-third of the latter the test reveals the presence of three-vessel coronary disease. Patients with three-vessel disease and patients with two-vessel disease including LAD/diagonal and circumflex disease are selected for coronary angiography and left ventriculography.[89]

Transcutaneous Aortovelography (TAV)

An indication of LV function is provided by the change in stroke volume in response to exercise which can be easily measured with transcutaneous aortovelography.[90] A 2 MHz continuous wave Doppler probe is applied at the suprasternal notch and directed in such a way that the beam insonates the aortic arch tangentially. The position of the probe is adjusted so that the maximum signal is obtained which is then processed by frequency analysis and displayed as a sonogram (frequency versus time). The area under the maximum frequency envelope is directly proportional to stroke volume and any changes in stroke volume as a result of exercise can be measured with an error of less than 5%.[91] The technique has been validated by comparison to simultaneous invasive measurements performed during cardiac catheterisation.[92–94] In our initial clinical study[90] we used TAV to determine changes in stroke volume on exercise in two groups of individuals. Group I consisted of 20 normal volunteers and 14 patients with atypical chest pain, who had normal left ventricular function and coronary arteriograms. Group II consisted of 44 patients who had $>50\%$ stenosis in one, two, or three coronary arteries. Aortic velocity was recorded before and immediately after maximum tolerated exercise using a bicycle ergometer. An increase in the average area (stroke volume) under the aortic velocity–time curve exceeding 5% (range 7–40%) was shown by all the subjects in group I and 16 in group II who had an ejection fraction $>60\%$ calculated from the left ventriculogram. In 22 patients from group II with ejection fraction $<60\%$, the average area (stroke volume) decreased by 5–36%. The increase in cardiac output in these patients was the result of increase in heart rate rather than increase in stroke volume.

We are now using this test to assess left ventricular function in patients with peripheral vascular disease. It provides information about the effect of exercise and we believe it is quantitatively superior to two-dimensional echocardiography which is performed at rest. It is also less invasive, simpler, and less expensive than the currently available radionuclide methods which use the gated pool technique.

Ambulatory Holter Monitoring[95,96]

Spontaneous or exertional chest pain, if accompanied by ST segment shift on a frequency modulated (FM) system, may help to substantiate the diagnosis of coronary artery disease. The frequency and magnitude of the ST segment changes with or without pain may indicate its severity. The monitoring can be done while the patient is at home or at work without the need for a hospital stay. An exercise ECG stress test and ambulatory ST segment (Holter) monitoring should be regarded as complimentary to each other. In addition, the frequency and type of arrhythmias will be documented.

Two-dimensional Echocardiography[97-99]

In the presence of CAD, assessment of the left ventricular (LV) function is as important as the information about the anatomical distribution of coronary artery lesions in arriving at a decision on optimum management. There are several non-invasive methods of evaluation of left ventricular status of which two-dimensional echocardiography is one of the least invasive.

Extensive tomographic sampling of LV dimensions, shape, and regional wall motion allows detection of segmental dysfunction, ventricular aneurysm, and estimation of the LV ejection fraction. The other cardiac chambers and great vessels can also be assessed together with the morphology and mobility of heart valves. These features are important in identification of underlying cardiac disorders such as mitral valve disease, mural thrombus, bacterial endocarditis, atrial myxoma, or cardiomyopathy, which are often a source of peripheral arterial embolisation.

Dipyridamole–Thallium Scanning[100,101]

The test is based on the principle that thallium-201 distributes uniformly through the normally perfused left ventricular myocardium. Established old infarcts appear as "cold spots". During myocardial ischaemia, such as induced by exercise, an underperfused area is not exposed to the isotope due to redistribution of blood, and is also detected as a "cold spot". Subsequently, when another image is obtained at rest the "cold spot" disappears provided the myocardial ischaemia is reversible. This thallium redistribution as a result of exercise is a marker for relative hypoperfusion of viable myocardium, whereas a persistent defect suggests that an established infarct is present.[100,101] Thallium redistribution is a strong predictor of future myocardial infarction.[102,103] Thallium imaging in combination with maximal coronary vasodilatation induced by intravenous dipyridamole instead of exercise has been shown to have a sensitivity and specificity for the detection of coronary disease comparable to that of exercise thallium imaging.[104-107]

In a recent study of stable patients scheduled for lower limb revascularisation who were suspected of having coronary disease because of a history of myocardial infarction, previous angina, or abnormal ECG, preoperative thallium imaging was performed.[108] All 20 patients with normal results on a dipyridamole–thallium study had an uneventful clinical course, whereas half (8 of 16) of the patients with thallium redistribution had a perioperative ischaemic event. There were no cardiac ischaemic events in 12 patients with persistent defects only.[108]

This test is the method of choice for screening patients who cannot exercise because of severe lower limb ischaemia (see below).

CLINICAL APPLICATIONS

Illustrations of the practical application of some of the tests described and examples of clinical decisions that can be made in different groups of patients are given in the flowcharts below. It cannot be overemphasised that these flowcharts are an oversimplification of the actual decision-making process because other risk factors such as the presence of additional nonvascular disease and age have not been taken into account. This is deliberate because the aim of this paper is to demonstrate how the noninvasive tests could be used to aid in the management rather than discuss the management of patients with complicated vascular problems. Even in the presence of full angiographic investigation (cerebrovascular, coronary, and lower limb) in many of these patients with multilevel disease the clinical decisions are difficult. Presentation of such cases at special rounds and discussion by a team consisting not only of vascular surgeons but also neurologists, neuro-radiologists, cardiologists, anaesthesiologists, and cardiac surgeons have been found to be very helpful. The flowcharts below are the result of such joint clinical decisions on many patients investigated and treated by the author during the last five years.

Patients Who Are the Candidates for Elective Lower Limb Vascular Reconstruction without Symptoms of Cardiac or Extracranial Cerebrovascular Disease and Normal Carotid Vessels or with Less Than 75% Internal Carotid Artery Stenosis on Duplex Scanning (Fig. 11-1)

In a series of 100 such patients the ECG chest wall mapping stress test using bicycle ergometry will be found to be positive in 45 because of ECG changes and negative in 30 because of a normal ECG, even when the heart rate exceeds 75% of the expected maximum; it will be inconclusive in 25 patients because although the ECG will be normal the heart rate will not rise above 75% of the expected maximum. This will be because of severe claudication limiting the exercise (16 patients) or beta-blocking agents administered usually for hypertension which suppress the heart rate (9 patients). The ECG stress test should be repeated after stopping or decreasing the beta-blocking agents. Alternatively, the dipyridamole–thallium test can be performed. Patients with thallium redistribution (positive test) have jeopardized viable myocardium and should be considered for preoperative coronary angiography (5 patients).

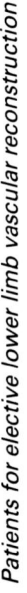

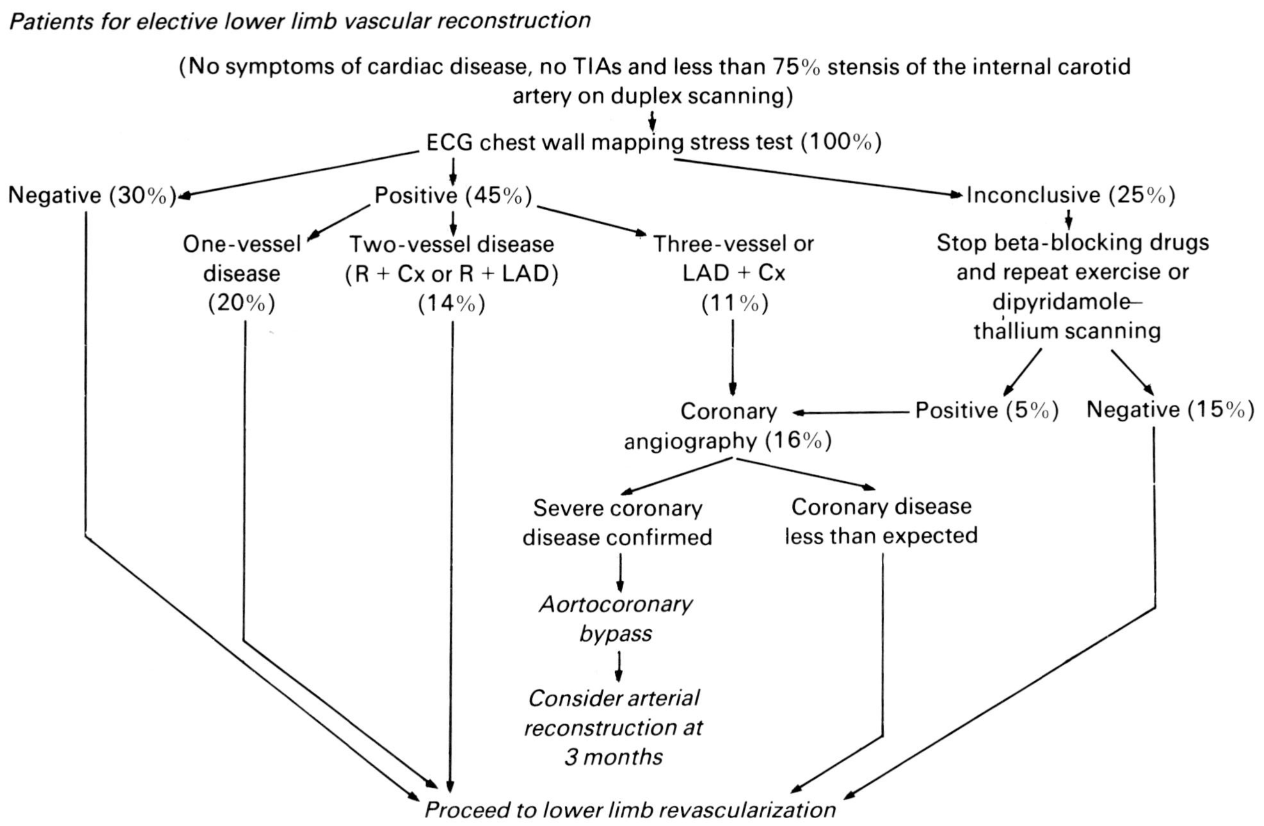

Patients for elective lower limb vascular reconstruction

(No symptoms of cardiac disease, no TIAs and less than 75% stensis of the internal carotid artery on duplex scanning)

ECG chest wall mapping stress test (100%)

Negative (30%)

Positive (45%)

One-vessel disease (20%)

Two-vessel disease (R + Cx or R + LAD) (14%)

Three-vessel or LAD + Cx (11%)

Inconclusive (25%)

Stop beta-blocking drugs and repeat exercise or dipyridamole–thallium scanning

Positive (5%)

Negative (15%)

Coronary angiography (16%)

Coronary disease less than expected

Severe coronary disease confirmed

Aortocoronary bypass

Consider arterial reconstruction at 3 months

Proceed to lower limb revascularization

Fig. 11-1. Procedure followed by the author in the management of patients who are candidates for elective lower limb vascular reconstruction. It demonstrates how the ECG chest wall mapping stress test and dipyridamole–thallium scanning can select a high-risk group (16%) for coronary angiography. R = right coronary artery, LAD = left anterior descending coronary artery, Cx = circumflex coronary artery.

149

Coronary angiography will also be performed when three-vessel coronary disease or when coexisting disease of the LAD and circumflex coronary arteries is indicated by the ECG stress test (11 patients). The combination of disease in the LAD and circumflex territories as indicated by the stress test is potentially dangerous because it may be the manifestation of left main stem stenosis. Thus a total of only 16% of patients will be selected for coronary angiography.

When the ECG stress test is negative and when it indicates one-vessel or two-vessel disease other than the LAD and circumflex (i.e., right and LAD or right and circumflex), the proposed vascular reconstruction is undertaken without resort to coronary angiography. When transcutaneous aortovelography (TAV) performed in the latter patients with two- or one-vessel coronary disease indicates a poor or moderately decreased left ventricular function Swan–Ganz monitoring is indicated during the vascular reconstructive procedure.

After aorto-coronary bypass grafting the claudication distance invariably increases markedly and many patients become asymptomatic. The reason for this has not yet been fully explained but evidence is accumulating that it is the result of improved left ventricular function and substitution of the beta-blocking agents with alternative function and substitution of the beta-blocking agents with alternative antihypertensive therapy. We have demonstrated in several such patients with superficial femoral artery occlusion that the following sequence of events occurs on exercise: myocardial ischaemia (ECG changes) followed by a decrease in stroke volume (on TAV) and cardiac output immediately followed by calf pain which stops them before they develop chest pain. It has been demonstrated that in patients who have angina and normal lower limb arteries that the ECG ischaemic changes produced by exercise may precede the onset of angina by as long as three minutes. For these reasons full reassessment of the lower limb circulation should be undertaken at approximately three months after the aorto-coronary bypass. As a result of this assessment many patients may be spared from an unnecessary vascular operation.

Patients for Elective Lower Limb Vascular Reconstruction without Symptoms of Cerebrovascular or Cardiac Disease and without Three-vessel or LAD and Circumflex Coronary Disease on ECG Chest Wall Mapping Stress Test (Fig. 11-2)

Duplex scanning performed routinely in patients for elective lower limb vascular reconstruction will detect and grade carotid disease. In patients with normal carotids and patients with internal carotid stenosis less than 75% in diameter vascular reconstruction is undertaken. However, patients with carotid stenotic lesions are followed up with duplex scanning at four-monthly intervals so that rapid progression of the disease or the development of a tight stenosis will be detected.

Patients with more than 75% internal carotid stenosis have an intravenous DSA and if the severity of the disease is confirmed they are considered for carotid endarterectomy prior to vascular lower limb reconstruction, although the carotid operation is performed in order to prevent a possible future stroke (long term) rather than a perioperative stroke. Unfortunately, information about the perioperative stroke rate in the presence of severe internal carotid stenosis is not yet available.

Patients for elective lower limb vascular reconstruction

(No symptoms of cerebrovascular disease and absence of three-vessel or LAD and circumflex coronary disease)

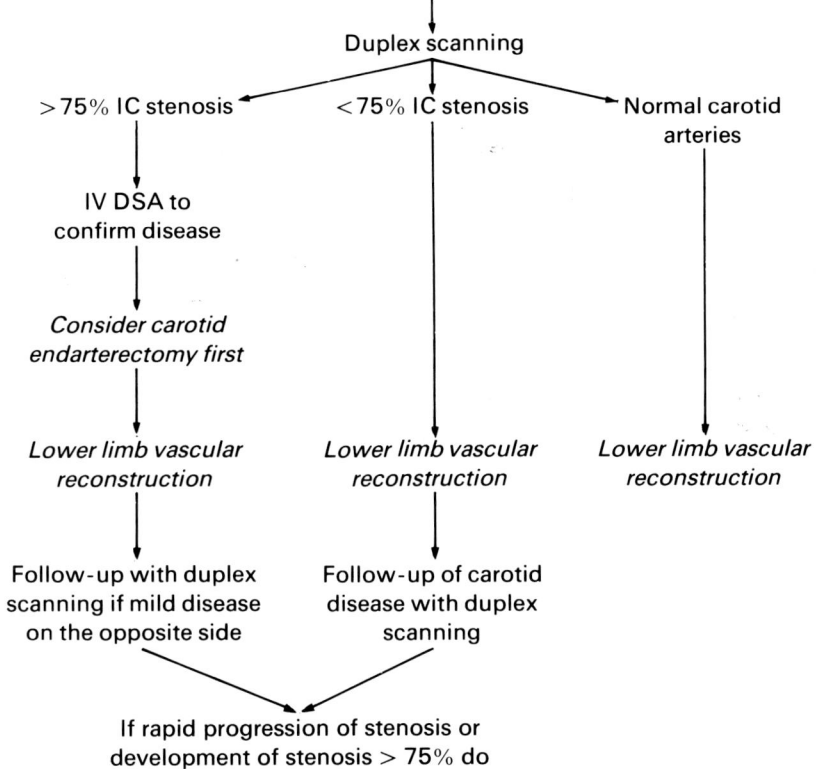

Fig. 11-2. Flowchart demonstrating how duplex scanning of the carotid arteries may influence the management of patients who are candidates for lower limb vascular reconstruction.

After carotid endarterectomy and lower limb reconstruction, duplex scanning is performed at regular intervals if any stenosis (<75%) of the opposite side exists.

Patients Presenting with TIAs and Internal Carotid Stenosis (Fig. 11-3)

Patients with internal carotid stenosis and TIAs involving the ipsilateral cortical hemisphere are candidates for carotid endarterectomy. An ECG stress test indicating severe three-vessel or LAD circumflex coronary disease would be an indication for coronary angiography, and if severe three-vessel coronary disease with good left ventricular function or left main stem stenosis is confirmed aorto-coronary bypass surgery should be considered.

In the absence of claudication, the presence or absence of cardiac symptoms is a useful indicator of risk. If the patient does not have angina or if angina is stable the carotid endarterectomy should be done first. However, in the presence of angina

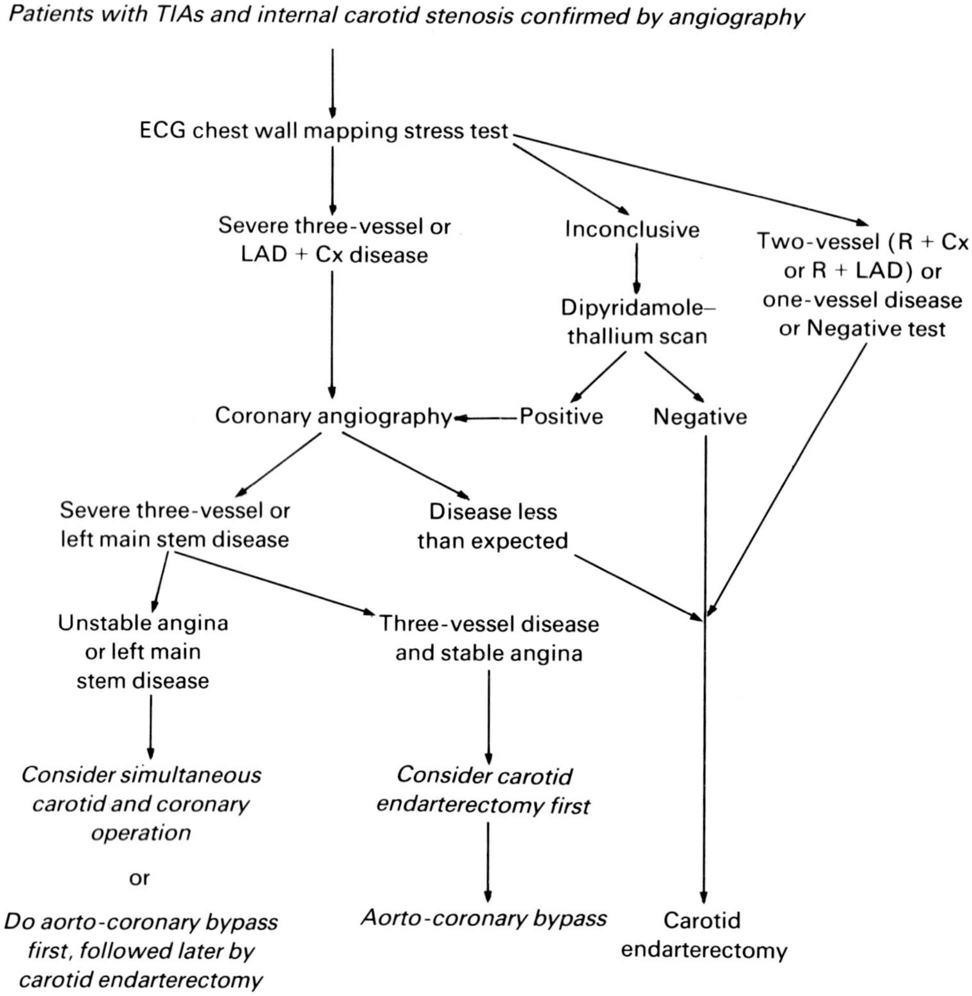

Patients with TIAs and internal carotid stenosis confirmed by angiography

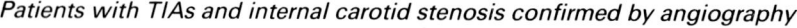

ECG chest wall mapping stress test

Severe three-vessel or
LAD + Cx disease

Inconclusive

Two-vessel (R + Cx
or R + LAD) or
one-vessel disease
or Negative test

Dipyridamole–
thallium scan

Coronary angiography ◄——— Positive   Negative

Severe three-vessel or
left main stem disease

Disease less
than expected

Unstable angina
or left main
stem disease

Three-vessel disease
and stable angina

*Consider simultaneous
carotid and coronary
operation*

or

*Do aorto-coronary bypass
first, followed later by
carotid endarterectomy*

*Consider carotid
endarterectomy first*

Aorto-coronary bypass   Carotid
endarterectomy

Fig. 11-3. Flowchart demonstrating how the ECG chest wall mapping stress test may influence the management of patients who are candidates for carotid endarterectomy because of TIAs.

at rest or severe left main stem lesions without angina, usually because the exercise is limited by severe claudication, the possibility of doing both the carotid endarterectomy and the aorto-coronary bypass under the same anaesthetic should be considered. In extreme cases of severe unstable angina and left main stem stenosis the author has reversed the order by doing an aorto-coronary bypass first and the carotid endarterectomy two weeks later.

Patients with Angina Who Are Candidates for Aorto-coronary Bypass Surgery (Fig. 11-4)

At our hospital all patients who are candidates for aorto-coronary bypass surgery are screened with duplex scanning irrespective of the presence or absence of cervical bruit. It has already been stated that bruits are unreliable indicators of risk and many patients with severe internal carotid stenosis do not have a bruit, or may have a bruit in the less severely stenosed opposite side.

Aorto-coronary bypass surgery is performed in the absence of carotid disease or in the presence of stenosis less than 75%. However, all patients with such stenoses are followed up with duplex scanning at four-monthly intervals. Subsequent rapid progression or stenosis greater than 75% is an indication to consider the patient for carotid endarterectomy.

In the presence of unilateral internal carotid stenosis (75–85%) which is asymptomatic, aorto-coronary bypass surgery will be done and the patient will be considered for carotid endarterectomy at a later date. This will be particularly so in the absence of vertebral artery disease and a normal CAT brain scan.

However, in the presence of severe bilateral carotid disease or severe unilateral disease with associated vertebral disease one should consider doing the carotid endarterectomy first, provided the angina is stable. This decision would be easier in the presence of silent infarcts on the ipsilateral side of the CAT brain scan. In the presence of unstable angina or left main stem disease both operations could be done under the same anaesthetic.

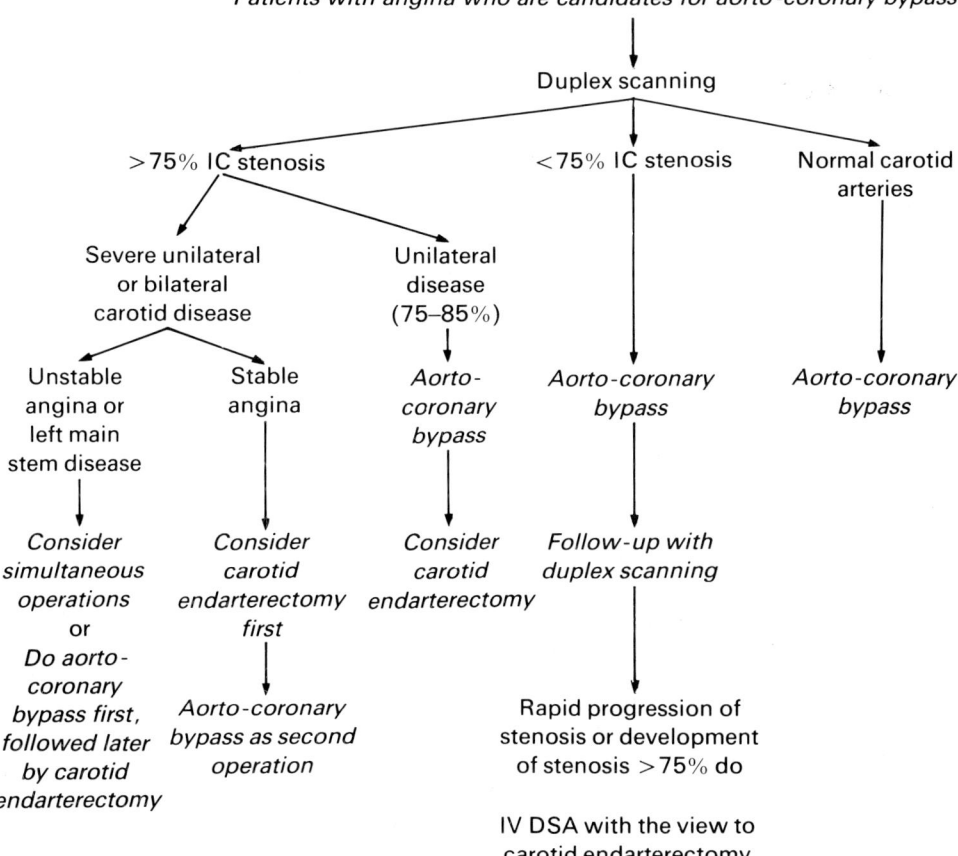

Fig. 11-4. Flowchart demonstrating how duplex scanning may influence the management of patients with angina who are candidates for aorto-coronary bypass operation.

REFERENCES

1. Cooley DA, Wakasch DC: Techniques in Vascular Surgery. Philadelphia, London, Toronto, WS Saunders and Co, 1979, p 261

2. Jamieson WRE, Jancesz TM, Miyagishima RT, Gerein A: Influence of ischaemic heart disease on early and late mortality after surgery for peripheral occlusive vascular disease. Circulation 66:92, 1982

3. Crawford ES, Bomberger RA, Glaeser DH, et al: Aortoiliac occlusive disease: Factors influencing survival and function following reconstructive operation over a twenty-five year period. Surgery 90:1055, 1981

4. Burnham NR, Johnson G, Gurri JA: Mortality risks for survivors of vascular reconstructive procedures. Surgery 92:1072, 1982

5. Hertzer NR: Fatal myocardial infarction following lower extremity revascularisation. 273 patients followed 6 to 11 postoperative years. Ann Surg 193:492, 1981

6. Bergan JJ, Veith FJ, Berhard VM, et al: Randomisation of autogenous vein and polytetrafluoroethylene grafts in femoral-distal reconstruction. Surgery 92:921, 1982

7. DeBakey ME, Crawford ES, Morris GC, et al: Late results of vascular surgery in the treatment of arteriosclerosis. J Cardiovasc Surg 5:473, 1964

8. Minken SL, DeWeese JA, Southgate WA, et al: Aortoiliac reconstruction for atherosclerotic occlusive disease. Surg Gynec Obstet 126:1056, 1968

9. Couch NP, Lance FC, Crane C: Management and mortality in resection of abdominal aortic aneurysms. Am J Surg 199:408, 1970

10. Lawrie, GM, Morris GC: Factors influencing late survival after coronary bypass surgery. Ann Surg 187(6):665, 1978

11. Veith FJ, Gupta S, Samson R, et al: Progress in limb salvage by reconstructive arterial surgery combined with a new or improved adjunctive procedure. Ann Surg 194:386, 1981

12. DeWeese JA, Rob CG: Autogenous venous grafts. Ten years later. Surgery 82:775, 1977

13. DeWeese JA, Rob CG, Satran R, et al: Results of carotid endarterectomy for transient ischaemic attacks. Five years later. Ann Surg 178:258, 1973

14. Szilagyi DE, Smith RF, DeRusso FJ, et al: Contribution of abdominal aortic aneurysmectomy to prolongation of life. Ann Surg 164:678, 1966

15. Szilagyi DE, Hageman JH, Smith FR, et al: Autogenous vein grafting in femoropopliteal atherosclerosis; the limits of its effectiveness. Surgery, 86:836, 1979

16. Thompson JE, Austin DJ, Patman RD: Carotid endarterectomy for cerebrovascular insufficiency; long term results in 592 patients followed up to thirteen years. Ann Surg 172:663, 1970

17. Julian DG: Coronary artery bypass surgery: The European prospective randomised study. Implications for management after infarction. Texas Heart Institute J 9:483, 1982

18. CASS Principal Investigators and their associates: Coronary artery surgery study (CASS): A randomised trial of coronary artery bypass surgery. Survival data. Circulation 68:939, 1983

19. Loop FD, Cosgrove DM, Lytle BW, Golding LR: Life expectancy after coronary artery surgery. Am J Surg 141:665, 1981

20. Loop FD, Cosgrove DM, Lytle BW, et al: An 11 year evolution of coronary artery surgery (1967–1978). Ann Surg 190:444, 1979

21. Hall RJ: Coronary artery bypass: Facts and figures. Texas Heart Institute J 9(4):478, 1982

22. O'Donnell TF, Callow AD, Willet C, et al: The impact of coronary artery disease on carotid endarterectomy. Ann Surg 198(6):705, 1983

23. Hertzer NR, Bevan EG, Young JR, et al: Coronary artery disease in peripheral vascular patients. A classification of 1000 coronary angiograms and results of surgical management. Ann Surg 199(2):223, 1984

24. Cutler BS, Wheeler HB, Paraskos JA, Cardyllo PA: Assessment of operative risk with electrocardiographic exercise testing in patients with peripheral vascular disease. Am J Surg 137:484, 1979

25. Gage AA, Bhayana JN, Baler V, Hook N: Assessment of cardiac risk in surgical patients. Arch Surg 112:1488, 1977

26. McCabe CJ, Reidy NC, Abbot WM, et al: The value of electrocardiogram monitoring during treadmill testing for peripheral vascular disease. Surgery 89(2):183, 1981

27. Koramees A, Bundin T: Continuous electrocardiographic recordings at examination of walking capacity in patients with intermittent claudication. J Cardiovasc Surg 509:12, 1976

28. Kanazawa M, Rose H, Vyden JK, et al: The importance of cardiac monitoring in treadmill claudication testing. Prac Card 7:48, 1981

29. Vecht RJ, Nicolaides AN, Brandao E, et al: Resting and treadmill electrocardiographic findings in patients with intermittent claudication. Int Angio 1(2):119, 1982

30. Carroll RM, Rose HB, Vyden J, et al: Cardiac arrhythmias associated with treadmill claudication testing. Surgery 83:284, 1978

31. Goldman L, Caldera DL, Southwick FS, et al: Cardiac risk factors and complications in non-cardiac surgery. Medicine 57:357, 1978

32. Salene DN, Homans DG, Ismer IM: Management of cardiac disease in the general surgical patient. Current Problems in Cardiology, 5(2):22, 1980

33. Scher K, Tice DA: Operative risk in patients with previous coronary bypass. Arch Surg 111:807, 1976

34. McCollum CH, Gareia Rindale R, Graham JM, DeBakey M: Myocardial infarction revascularisation prior to subsequent major surgery in patients with coronary artery disease. Surgery 81:302, 1977

35. Edwards WH, Mulheim JL, Walker WE: Vascular reconstructive surgery following myocardial revascularisation. Ann Surg 197:653, 1978

36. Wells PH, Kaplan JA: Optimal management of patients with ischaemic heart disease for non-cardiac surgery by complimentary anaesthesiologist and cardiologist interaction, in Curriculum in Cardiology. CV Mosby Co, 1981, pp 1029–1037

37. Crawford ES, Morris GS, Howell JF, et al: Operative risk in patients with previous coronary artery bypass. Ann Thorac Surg 26:215, 1978

38. Ennix CG Jr, Lawrie GM, Morris GC Jr, et al: Improved results of carotid endarterectomy in patients with symptomatic coronary disease: An analysis of 1546 consecutive carotid operations. Stroke 10:122, 1979

39. Bernstein EF, Humber PB, Collins GM, et al: Life expectancy and late stroke following carotid endarterectomy. Ann Surg 198:80, 1983

40. Hertzer NR, Young JR, Beven EG, et al: Late results of coronary bypass in selected peripheral vascular patients. 5 year survival according to age and clinical cardiac status. Cleveland Clinic Q (in press)

41. Hertzer NR: Personal Communication, 1985

42. Wolf PA, Kannel WB, Sorlie P, McNamara P: Asymptomatic carotid bruit and risk of stroke. JAMA 245:1442, 1981

43. Heyman A, Wilkinson WE, Heyden S, et al: Risk of stroke in asymptomatic persons with cervical arterial bruits. New Engl J Med 302:838, 1980

44. Sandok BA, Whisnaut JP, Furlan AJ, Mickell JL: Carotid artery bruits. Prevalence survey and differential diagnosis. Mayo Clinic Proc 57:227, 1982

45. Barnes RW, Liebman PR, Marszalek PB, et al: The natural history of asymptomatic carotid disease in patients undergoing cardiovascular surgery. Surgery 90:1075, 1981

46. Turnispeed WD, Berkoff HA, Belzer FO: Postoperative stroke in cardiac and peripheral vascular disease. Ann Surg 192:365, 1980

47. Hennerici M, Anlich A, Sandmann W, et al: Occurrence of asymptomatic extracranial arterial bruits. Stroke 12:750, 1981

48. Jain KM, Hobson RW, Jamil Z, et al: Clinical screening of preoperative patients for carotid occlusive disease by oculoplethysmography. Am Surg 46:679, 1980

49. Martin WRW, Hashimoto SA: Stroke in coronary bypass surgery. Canadian J Neurol Sci 9:21, 1982

50. Coffey CE, Masey EW, Roberts KR, Curtis SE, Jones RH: Natural history of neurologic complications following coronary artery bypass grafting. Neurol 32(2):186, 1982 (Abstr)

51. Carman LC: The preoperative patients with an asymptomatic cervical bruit. Med Clin North Am 63:1335, 1979

52. Pessin MS, Panis W, Prager RJ, Millan VG, Scott RM: Auscultation of cervical and ocular bruits in extracranial carotid occlusive disease: A clinical and angiographic study. Stroke 14:246, 1983

53. Theile BL, Strandness DE: Distribution of intracranial and extracranial arterial lesions in patients with symptomatic cerebrovascular disease, in Bernstein EF (ed): Noninvasive Diagnostic Techniques in Vascular Surgery, 3 ed. St Louis, CV Mosby Co, 1985, pp 316–322

54. Keagy BA, Battaglini JW, Lucas CL, Thomas DD, Wilcox BR: Identification of internal carotid artery stenosis in coronary artery bypass candidates. South Med J 76:996, 1983

55. David TE, Humphries AW, Young FR, et al: A correlation of neck bruits and arteriosclerotic carotid arteries. Arch Surg 107:729, 1973

56. Hertzer NR, Bevan EG, Young JR, et al: Incidental asymptomatic carotid bruits in patients scheduled for peripheral vascular reconstruction: Results of cerebral and coronary angiography. Surgery 96:535, 1984

57. Lusby RJ, Ferrell LD, Ehrenfeld WK, Stoney RJ, Wylie EJ: Carotid plaque haemorrhage. Its role in production of cerebral ischaemia. Arch Surg 117:1479, 1982

58. Persson AV, Robichaux WT, Silverman M: The natural history of carotid plaque development. Arch Surg 118:1048, 1983

59. Harrison MJG, Marshall J: Prognostic significance of severity of carotid atheroma in early manifestations of cerebrovascular disease. Stroke 13:567, 1982

60. Roederer GO, Langlois YE, Jager KA, Primozich JF, et al: The natural history of carotid arterial disease in asymptomatic patients with cervical bruits. Stroke 15:605, 1984

61. Marzewski DJ, Furlan AJ, St Louis P, Little JR, et al: Intracranial internal carotid artery stenosis: Long term prognosis. Stroke 13:821, 1982

62. Gibbs JM, Wise RJS, Leenders KL, Jones T: Evaluation of cerebral perfusion reserve in patients with carotid artery occlusion. Lancet 1:310, 1984

63. Bernstein EF: The clinical spectrum of ischaemic cerebrovascular disease, in Bernstein EF (ed): Noninvasive Diagnostic Techniques, 3 ed. St Louis, CV Mosby Co, 1985, pp 301–315

64. Treiman RL, Foran RF, Cohen JL, et al: Carotid bruit: A follow up report on its significance in patients undergoing an abdominal operation. Arch Surg 114:1138, 1979

65. Carney WI, Stewart WB, DePinto DJ, et al: Carotid bruit as a risk factor in aortoiliac reconstruction. Surgery 81:567, 1977

66. Evans WE, Cooperman M: The significance of asymptomatic unilateral carotid bruits in perioperative patients. Surgery 85:521, 1978

67. Hart RG, Easton JD: Management of cervical bruits and carotid stenosis in perioperative patients. Stroke 14:290, 1983

68. Breslau PJ, Fell G, Ivey TD, et al: Carotid arterial disease in patients undergoing coronary artery bypass operations. J Thorac Cardiovasc Surgery 82:765, 1981

69. Thompson JE, Garret WV, Talkington CM, Patman RD: The use of operation for asymptomatic bruits, in Delaney JP, Varco RL (eds): Controversies in Surgery II. Philadelphia, WB Saunders, 1983, pp 131–137

70. Archie FP: The case against prophylactic carotid endarterectomy. Surgery 95:739, 1984

71. Batson RC: The case for prophylactic carotid endarterectomy. Surgery 95:742, 1984

72. Kartchner MM, McRae LP: Guidelines for noninvasive evaluation of asymptomatic carotid bruits. Clin Neurosurg 28:418, 1981

73. Chambers BR, Norris JW: The case against surgery for asymptomatic carotid stenosis. Stroke 15:964, 1984

74. Sumner DS: Personal Communication, 1985

75. Jain KM, Hobson RW, Jamil Z, et al: Clinical screening of preoperative patients for carotid occlusive disease by oculoplethysmography. Am Surg 46:679, 1980

76. Lefrak EA, Guinn GA: Prophylactic carotid artery surgery in patients requiring a second operation. South Med J 67:185, 1974

77. Hertzer NR, Loop FD, Taylor PC, et al: Staged and combined surgical approach to simultaneous carotid and coronary vascular disease. Surgery 84:803, 1978

78. Mehigan JT, Buch WS, Pipkin RD, et al: A planned approach to coexistent cerebrovascular disease in coronary artery bypass candidates. Arch Surg 112:1043, 1977

79. Bernhard VM, Johnson WD, Peterson JJ: Carotid artery stenosis. Association with surgery for coronary artery disease. Arch Surg 105:837, 1972

80. Robertson JT, Auer NJ: Extracranial occlusive disease of the carotid artery, in Youmans JR (ed): Textbook of Neurological Surgery. Philadelphia, WB Saunders, 1981

81. Diehl JT, Cali RF, Hertzer NR, et al: Complications of abdominal aortic reconstruction. An analysis of perioperative risk factors in 557 patients. Ann Surg 197:49, 1983

82. Hertzer NR, Arison R: Cumulative stroke and survival ten years after carotid endarterectomy. J Vasc Surg 2:661, 1985

83. Hertzer NR, Loop FD, Taylor PC, et al: Combined myocardial revascularisation and carotid endarterectomy. J Thorac Cardiovasc Surg 85:577, 1983

84. Bernstein EF: Noninvasive Diagnostic Techniques, 3 ed. St Louis, CV Mosby Co, 1985

85. Laing S, Greenhalgh RM: Standard exercise test to assess peripheral arterial disease. Brit Med J, 1:13–16, 1980

86. Laing S, Greenhalgh RM: Detection and progression of asymptomatic peripheral arterial disease. Brit J Surg 70:628, 1983

87. Nicolaides AN: Unpublished data, 1986

88. Salmasi AM, Nicolaides AN, Vecht RJ, et al: Electrocardiographic chest wall mapping in the diagnosis of coronary artery disease. Brit Med J 2:9, 1983

89. Nicolaides AN: The diagnosis and assessment of coronary artery disease in vascular patients. J Vasc Surg 2:501, 1985

90. Nicolaides AN, Salmasi SN, Salmasi AM, et al: Transaortic velography (TAV) in the assessment of left ventricular function of patients with coronary artery disease. Brit J Surg 70:696, 1983

91. Light LH: Noninvasive ultrasonic technique of observing flow in the human aorta. Nature 224:1119, 1969

92. Cross G, Light LH: Noninvasive intrathoracic blood velocity measurement in the assessment of cardiovascular function. Biomed Engin 9:464, 1974

93. Sequeira RF, Light LH, Cross G, Raftery EB: Transcutaneous aortovelography: A quantitative evaluation. Brit Heart J 38:443, 1976

94. Brotherhood J, Cross G, Hanson GC, et al: Transcutaneous aortovelography as a measure of central blood flow. J Physiol 381:4, 1978

95. Allen RD, Gettes LS, Phala C, Avington D: Painless ST segment depression in patients with angina pectoris. Chest 69:467, 1976

96. Kennedy HI, Caralis DG: Ambulatory electrocardiography. A clinical perspective. Ann Intern Med 87:729, 1977

97. Reichek N: Uses and abuses of two-dimensional echocardiography. Int J Cardiol 1:221, 1982

98. Tortoledo FA, Quinones MA, Fernandez GC: Quantification of left ventricular volumes by two-dimensional echocardiography. A simplified and accurate approach. Circulation 67:579, 1983

99. Schnitger I, Gordon EP, Fitzgerald PJ, Poop RL: Standardized intracardiac measurements of two-dimensional echocardiography. Am J Cardiol, 2:934, 1983

100. Bodenheimer MW, Banka VS, Fooshee CM, Helfant RH: Comparative sensitivity of the exercise electrocardiogram, thallium imaging and stress radionucelide angiography to detect the presence and severity of coronary heart disease. Circulation 60:1270, 1979

101. Becker LC: Diagnosis of coronary artery disease with exercise radionucelide imaging. State of the art. Am J Cardiol 45:1301, 1980

102. Brown KA, Boucher CA, Boucher CA, Okada RD, et al: Prognostic value of exercise thallium-201 imaging in patients presenting for evaluation of chest pain. J Am Coll Cardiol 9:994, 1983

103. Gibson RS, Watson DD, Craddock GB, et al: Prediction of cardiac events after uncomplicated myocardial infarction: A prospective study comparing predischarge exercise thallium-201 scintigraphy and coronary angiography. Circulation 68:321, 1983

104. Leppo JA, O'Brien J, Rothendler JA, Getchell JD, Lee VW: Dipyridamol thallium-201 scintigraphy in the prediction of future cardiac events after acute myocardial infarction. N Engl J Med 310:1014, 1984

105. Albro PC, Gound KL, Westcott RJ, Hamilton GW, et al: Noninvasive assessment of coronary stenosis by myocardial imaging during pharmacologic coronary vasodilation. III Clinical trial. Am J Cardiol 42:751, 1978

106. Brown BG, Josephson MA, Petersen MA, et al: Intravenous dipyridamole combined with isometric handgrip for near maximal acute increase in coronary flow in patients with coronary artery disease. Am J Cardiol 48:1077, 1981

107. Leppo JA, Boucher CA, Okada RD, Newall JB, Strauss HW, Pohost GM: Serial thallium-201 myocardial imaging following dipyridamole infusion: Diagnostic utility in detecting the coronary stenosis and relationship to regional wall motion. Circulation 66:649, 1982

108. Boucher CA, Brewster DC, Darling RC, Okada RD, Strauss HW, Pohost GM: Determination of cardiac risk by dipyridamole–thallium imaging before peripheral vascular surgery. New Engl J Med 312:389, 1985

John J. Bergan, James S. T. Yao, William R. Flinn,
Walter J. McCarthy III, Madeleine R. Fisher,
and Robert L. Vogelzang

12

Value of Digital Subtraction Angiography, Magnetic Resonance Imaging, and Computed Tomography Scanning in Vascular Surgery

Improved methods of vascular imaging are considerably extending the surgeon's sensibilities in diagnosis of vascular conditions. Fortunately, these new techniques also involve less invasion of the patient and decrease the chance for iatrogenic injury to vessels. As each generation of imaging techniques develops, the images themselves become sharper, the separation of structures more precise, and the utility to vascular surgeons increases. What follows is an overview of the present status of three new methods of diagnostic imaging: digital subtraction angiography (DSA), magnetic resonance imaging (MRI), and computed tomography (CT) scanning.

DIGITAL SUBTRACTION ANGIOGRAPHY

Originally, intravenous DSA was developed to replace standard intraarterial angiographic procedures with a safer, less invasive technique. Early success with intravenous DSA spawned the hope that intraarterial injections would be totally replaced.[1] Now, after considerable experience and even extension of intravenous arterial visualization beyond the cerebral vasculature to other areas of the body, it is clear that replacement of intraarterial procedures with intravenous DSA is still an unfulfilled promise. The two limitations to DSA at present are the quality of the arterial image, which is inferior to conventional arteriography, and field size, which at present is usually restricted to approximately 25 cm, although newer angiographic equipment may possess field sizes up to 35 cm. The repeated injections of contrast media required bring the total contrast volume up to the level of conventional arteriography.

The ability to obtain an arterial image from an intravenous injection has an obvious advantage in allowing outpatient arteriography to be performed, but move-

VASCULAR SURGERY: ISSUES IN CURRENT PRACTICE
ISBN 0-8089-1839-7

ment of the patient distorts the subtraction and enhancing capacity of the instrumentation and produces artifacts and blurring of images. Thus, interpretation may be difficult, impossible, or erroneous. Abdominal images also may be distorted by overlying intestinal peristalsis. In addition, intracerebral vessels and arteries below the trifurcation in the leg are seen poorly.

In a study of the impact of DSA on carotid evaluation at the University of Minnesota, it was found that the use of traditional noninvasive tests was reduced from 100 to 36%, and conventional arteriograms from 29 to 4%.[2] Conventional arteriograms were done chiefly for compelling indications with regard to the patient symptomatology and negative or inadequate DSA. The cost of evaluation was increased somewhat in patients being treated medically but was reduced greatly in those patients having surgery.

The issue of quality of the study was important in evaluating the impact of DSA. Anderson and Fischer[2] reviewed the relevant literature and reported the rate of definitely inadequate DSA studies as varying from 4 to 42% of cases. They also called attention to the fact that DSA does not display intracranial arterial lesions well, and it is known that as many as 20% of patients undergoing carotid surgery have abnormal findings present in the intracranial vasculature. Whether such findings alter management decisions is undetermined, however. Most surgeons feel that coexistence of intracranial carotid disease does not influence the outcome in patients undergoing carotid endarterectomy.[3]

In the Mayo Clinic review of DSA and conventional arteriography, 25% of the studies were incomplete, and the authors concluded that while DSA examinations of acceptable quality did accurately depict atherosclerotic lesions, the studies were deficient for detection of intracranial vascular disease, and 5% of the patients had management decisions changed by intracranial findings.[4]

Attempts have been made to improve the quality of intracranial visualization.[5,6] However, Modic and coworkers[6] found that in 22% of cases, there was a significant chance of misinterpreting the results of the studies and in 13%, the angiogram was not diagnostic. It was felt that, when combined with computed tomography, DSA could replace conventional angiography for determining preoperative extent and vascularity of tumors and in postoperative evaluation of aneurysm surgery and procedures designed to ablate arterio-venous malformations.

In a study from the Massachusetts General Hospital, complications of intravenous DSA were examined.[7] A total of 55 complications occurred in 37 patients. Six of 17 central nervous system complications were major and transient, while one was major and permanent. Two of 35 systemic complications were major and permanent. Patients with multisystem disease and with a history of angina were thought to be at high risk for complications in this study.

It has become apparent to most workers in the field that the true application of DSA is in imaging of intraarterial contrast. In contradistinction to intravenous DSA, intraarterial DSA can decrease the time of examination, reduce contrast load, and by the use of smaller-diameter catheters, decrease arterial puncture site complications. One study compared intravenous DSA with intraarterial injection.[8] Of the intravenous DSA images 60% were adequate, 96% of the intraarterial DSA images were good, and 100% of the conventional arteriography images were acceptable. The accuracy of intraarterial DSA was significantly greater than that of intravenous techniques and was comparable to that of conventional arteriography.

Intraarterial DSA required less contrast injection (84 ml versus 144 ml). Complications of intraarterial and intravenous DSA were similar but lower than with conventional arteriography.

Inevitably, DSA has been used in peripheral arteriography, as well as in the evaluation of the cerebral vasculature.[9] At the University of Wisconsin, a study of 142 patients was carried out, in which 107 general angiography patients were studied and 35 neuroangiography patients were included.[9] Intraarterial DSA was found to have the advantages of less contrast injection, a reduced need for selective arterial catheterization, lower film cost, and shortened examination time, but the limitations of the technique when compared to standard film anteriography included reduced spatial resolution, limited field size, and an inability to conduct simultaneous biplane examinations. These authors concluded that DSA should not be used when a high degree of spatial resolution is required.

It was hoped that intravenous DSA could replace the timed intravenous pyelogram in detection of renovascular hypertension.[10] However, in a study from Vanderbilt University, it was concluded that the sensitivity of 87% and specificity of 87% was not as great as would be desired. In fact, there was a high false–positive rate, and troubles with the subtraction artifact, quantum noise, relatively low spatial resolution, and the Mach effect were limiting factors.

Digital subtraction angiography is of value in the postoperative evaluation of a variety of patients undergoing vascular surgery. It has provided excellent visualization of the reconstructed renal artery[11] and in the lower extremities, graft patency of even small complex grafts is easily evaluated.[12] Occlusions distal to the reconstructions can be identified and patient acceptance is excellent in these patients, who have already undergone conventional arteriography prior to the surgical event. Other uses of DSA have been in the mycotic aneurysms of intravenous drug abusers,[13] in pediatric angiography,[14] and in evaluation of extremity trauma.[15]

MAGNETIC RESONANCE IMAGING

Magnetic resonance imaging (MRI) has been available to vascular surgeons only since the early 1980s. The cardiovascular system is superbly delineated with magnetic resonance as a result of the inherent natural contrast between flowing blood and the walls of the cardiac chambers and blood vessels. At present, the quality of the images and spatial resolution vary depending upon the different manufacturers of the MR imagers. Overall image quality is continually being improved, but there is a marked limitation of the utility of this technique in the vascular system because of excessive respiratory and vascular motion. Magnetic resonance imaging of the vascular system does, however, hold tremendous promise due to its ability to visualize vessels well without contrast and to image vessels in multiple planes of section, and the superior soft tissue contrast when compared to CT.

Both the venous and arterial systems have been evaluated with MRI. Venous thrombosis,[16] congenital venous anomalies,[17] aortic aneurysms[18,19] (Fig. 12-1), and aortic dissections[20,21] have been accurately studied with MRI. In aortic dissections, the intimal flap is seen, and the true and false lumens are usually identified. Magnetic resonance may be the modality of choice in the assessment of chronic dissections. It is more difficult to evaluate the acute dissection, since critically ill patients cannot be adequately monitored during MRI examination.

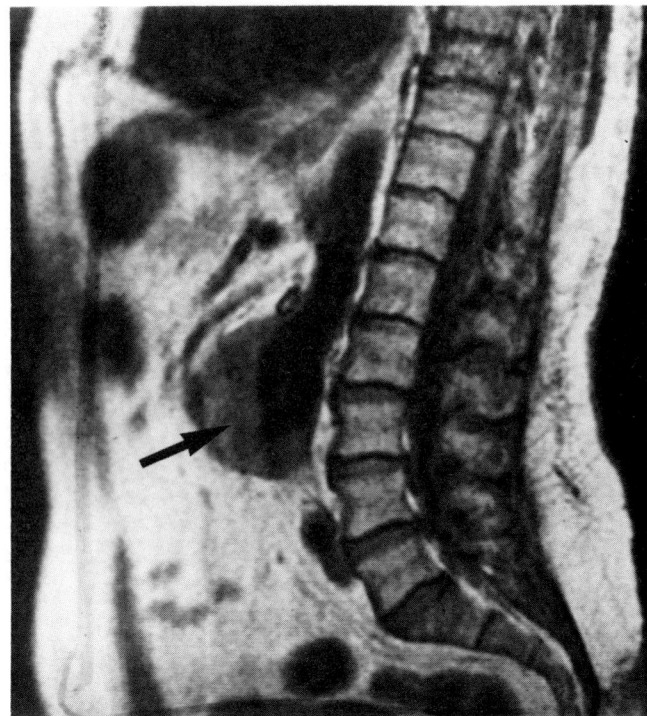

Fig. 12-1. Abdominal aortic aneurysm. This sagittal MRI through the abdomen obtained with a short TR/TE sequence demonstrates an infrarenal abdominal aortic aneurysm (arrow), partially filled with thrombus.

In a study of the first 1000 consecutive examinations (predominately of the head) at the Mayo Clinic, vascular disease was suspected in 62 patients.[22] The MRI revealed vascular lesions in 49 of these. The chief findings in patients with vascular abnormalities were infarcts, arterio-venous malformations, and aneurysms. Identification of subdural hematomas and intracerebral hematomas, as well as sinus thrombosis, indicated the utility of this technique in evaluating the central nervous system.

Evaluation of MRI imaging in the study of abdominal aortic aneurysms has been reported from various centers, including Vancouver[23] and Munich.[24] In one study,[23] the aorta, renal arteries, and iliac arteries were clearly identified in all normal patients but in only 10 of 13 patients with aneurysms. The three studies which poorly defined relevant structures were early in the experience of this group. Another study[18] showed delineation of the renal arteries in each of the aneurysm cases. When compared to sonography, both MRI and sonograms provided accurate AP and transverse outer wall measurements, but MRI was superior in determining the presence of renal and/or iliac involvement by the aneurysm. Obviously, sonography remains the better screening mechanism because of cost.

Posttraumatic false aneurysms of the aorta have also come under study by MRI.[25] It was found that the major advantage of MRI over CT scanning was its ability to produce sagittal and coronal images without degradation of spatial resolution. The mediastinal vessels, therefore, can be imaged along their axes. Obviously, such studies would not be done in the acute situation in an unstable patient. However, in the definition of mediastinal masses, MRI appears to have a significant value, since mass lesions are distinctly separated from the blood vessels and bronchi.

In the Cleveland Clinic experience,[21] six patients with documented aortic dissections were examined by MRI, which demonstrated the dissections in all cases and differentiated type A from type B lesions. The coronal and sagittal sections were advantageous in establishing the relationship of the dissection of the three arch vessels and, when cardiac gating was applied, the demonstration of mural thrombus and differentiation of true from false lumen could be accomplished. It was thought that, in five of the six cases, the information obtained by MRI was equal to or surpassed that obtained by CT scanning. In the case of a completely thrombosed dissection, the CT scanning was superior.

In a larger experience from the University of California, the San Francisco School of Medicine,[20] the diagnosis of dissection was clearly made by MRI in the 13 patients with dissection and was excluded in the other patients suspected of having this lesion. This early experience suggested that the MRI could serve as the initial imaging technique in clinically suspected cases of aortic dissection, since the information provided was sufficient to manage many of the cases. In these instances, the MRI obviated the use of contrast media.

At the Massachusetts General Hospital, posterior cerebral territory strokes have been evaluated by MRI.[26] The location of an infarct could be identified in 15 of 16 cases, and in the one case with midbrain subthalmic infarction, motion artifact caused a blurred image. It was concluded that MRI imaging techniques hold great promise in the study of posterior fossa strokes and in differentiating between large- and small-vessel ischemic disease. This, of course, is important in planning therapy for patients with vertebro-basilar insufficiency, since improved surgical techniques allow direct reconstruction of the vertebral system, not only in its first portion but also in bypasses to the third portion of the artery.

In summary, the potential for MRI as a noninvasive screening test for lower extremity vascular disease is evident,[27] but MRI is not a superior imaging instrument at the present time. As stated, in the abdomen and thorax, the limitations of this technique are secondary to a longer acquisition time, which results in respiratory and vascular motion and causes some degradation. Magnetic resonance is in its infancy and, as with CT when it was first introduced in the early 1970s, advances in hardware and software for MRI should rapidly improve the image quality.

While not the subject of this review, it should be noted that positron imaging in ischemic stroke disease is particularly suited to a study of such conditions.[28] This is true because the method has the potential to demonstrate pathophysiologic metabolic changes in brain function and to differentiate viable from nonviable tissue. In early-stage strokes, PET can demonstrate changes that are not initially seen on computed tomography.

COMPUTED TOMOGRAPHY

In contrast to magnetic resonance imaging, CT scanning has found a place in noninvasive evaluation. Since it was introduced to clinical medicine in the early 1970s, sufficient time has passed to make evaluation of this technique accurate. Fur-

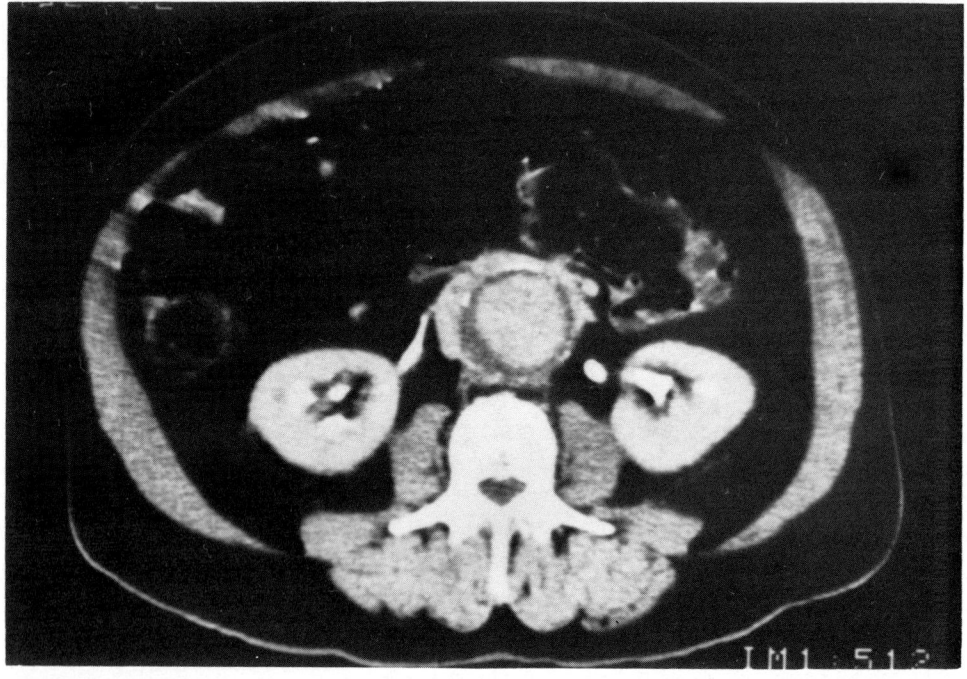

A

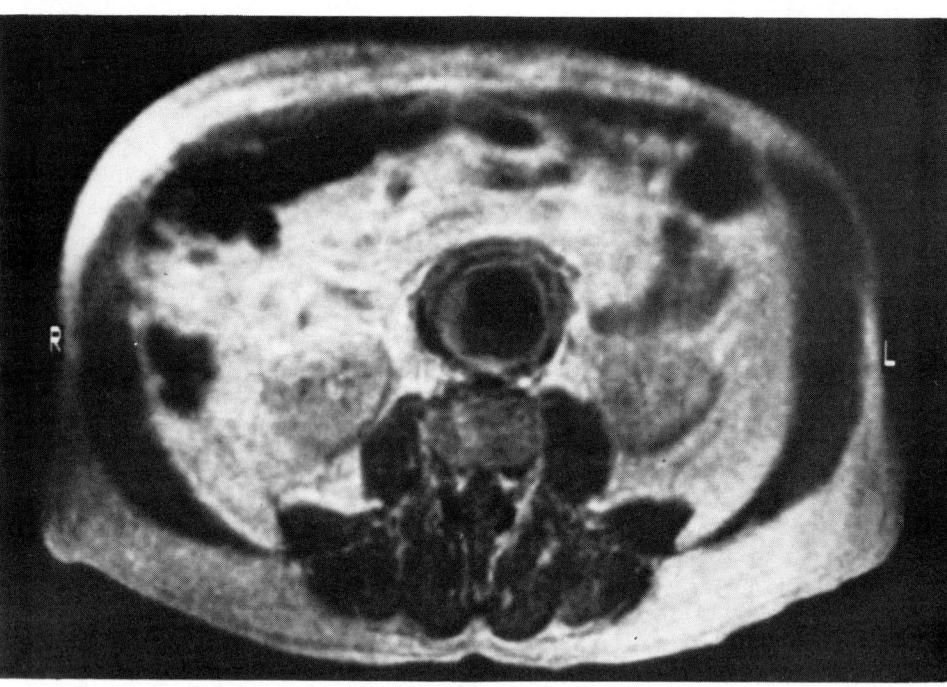

B

Fig. 12-2. (A) This CT scan shows the finding of a so-called inflammatory abdominal aortic aneurysm. Notice the thickness of the hyperlucent tissue anterior to the aneurysm wall, how the ureters are bilaterally attracted to the mass just distal to the renal pelvis, and how they lie in intimate contact with the fibrotic mass on the aneurysm surface. This calls the surgeon's attention to the fact that preoperative ureteral cannulation may allow avoidance of ureteral injury during aneurysm resection. (B) An MRI scan obtained in the same patient demonstrates the aneurysm and the thickened tissue anteriorly, but fails to show the ureteral entrapment.

thermore, the several generations of change in instrumentation have allowed more precision to be applied in imaging portions of the vascular system. The first of the whole-body scanners required an 18-second scan time and made whole-body CT practical, but patient movement, respiration, and normal bowel peristalsis introduced significant image-degrading artifacts, and spatial resolution was poor when compared to current scanners. When rapid scan time was reduced below five seconds, many of the motion artifact problems were resolved. In addition, dynamic scanning allows visualization of transient events, such as arterial opacification and contrast extravasation.

At present, CT scanners are capable of scan times of less than two seconds with excellent spatial and contrast resolution. Thus, CT has become the imaging method of choice for detection of aortic aneurysms, where aortography can be eliminated in many cases.[28-33] Most reports of the use of CT in aortic aneurysm disease describe confirmation of clinical impressions and the fact that sufficient diagnostic information is obtained so that aortography can be eliminated. However, it was found that the CT provides unique information not available by other imaging techniques.[34] In 44 patients with abdominal aortic aneurysms, four were found to have contained retroperitoneal rupture which was not suspected clinically. In addition, two other patients with upper abdominal and back pain and with normal aortograms were shown to have dissection of the thoracic aorta on CT examination. In another patient, a suspected abdominal aortic aneurysm was shown to be a chronic dissecting thoraco-abdominal aneurysm. In another fascinating case, an explanation for weight loss and abdominal mass was provided by the CT, which showed a ruptured superior mesenteric artery aneurysm.

CT provides the best method for making a diagnosis of inflammatory aneurysm of the aorta (Fig. 12-2), and such study alerts the surgeon to possible difficulties to be encountered during the surgical event.[35,36] Although the CT scan has been used to evaluate aorto-iliac occlusive disease, it has been found to be less valuable in that situation.[31] On the other hand, in complex situations such as evaluation of reconstruction complications, the CT provides information additive to that obtained on arteriography. For example, in evaluating patients for the possibility of graft infection, periprosthetic gas has been shown on CT scanning to be a normal finding for as long as 52 days postoperatively,[37] but when the CT scan shows pockets of gas in the thrombus around a graft, this is a distinctive finding of an infected prosthesis[38] (Figs 12-3 and 12-4).

Distinctive features in graft-enteric fistulae have made CT the diagnostic modality of choice in that setting.[29] When compared to indium-labeled white blood cell scans, CT correctly diagnosed the infection in five of five patients studied by showing perigraft fluid collection and/or gas in the graft bed.[39] In three patients in whom groin infection alone was suspected, an extension of this process into the retroperitoneum was displayed on the CT scan. A problem in indium-labeled scanning was that retroperitoneal extension of the infection was not detected and, in patients receiving antibiotics, the indium-labeled cells were not concentrated in the infection.[39]

CT has also been extremely valuable in assessing the postaortic graft patient for anastomotic aneurysm[40] (Fig. 12-5). Therefore, this becomes a useful technique in evaluating the proximal aortic anastomosis in patients with known femoral false aneurysms.

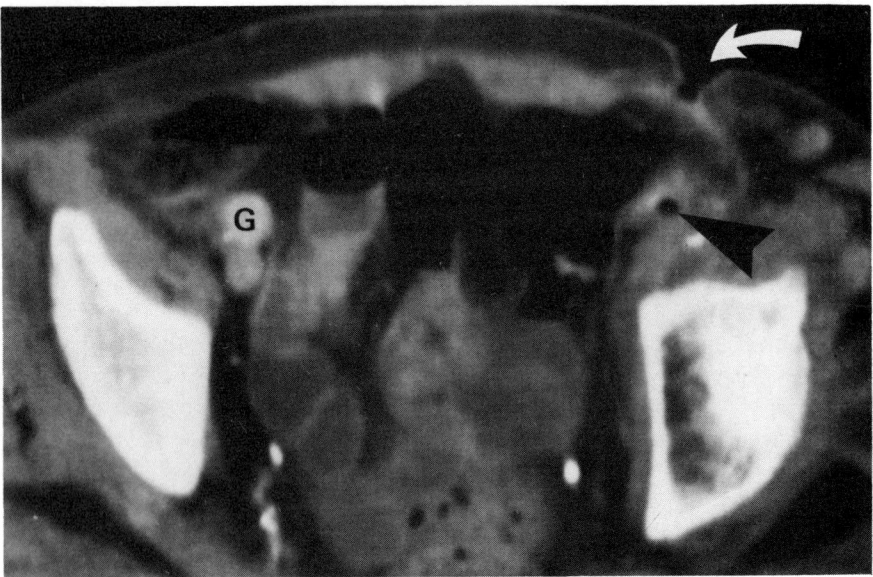

Fig. 12-3. This CT scan was obtained in a patient with a draining left groin wound (arrow). The intragraft air marked by the arrow is pathognomonic of graft infection, while the normal functioning contralateral limb of the graft, marked G, shows no such intragraft or perigraft infection. From Vogelzang RL: The role of CT in reoperative aortic surgery, in Bergan JJ, Yao JST (eds): Reoperative Arterial Surgery. Orlando, Grune & Stratton, 1986, pp 33–58.

Other situations in vascular surgery where the CT has shown itself to be extremely valuable include the detection of jugular venous thrombosis,[41] the evaluation of aorto-coronary bypass patency,[42] in thoraco-abdominal trauma,[43] and in evaluation of retroperitoneal hemorrhage, either spontaneous or as a result of trauma, or following translumbar aortography.[44-46] Computed tomography has even been used in the evaluation of primary lymphedema at the Royal Postgraduate Medical School in London[47] and in the evaluation of the mesentery at Duke University.[48]

In an interesting case in which a mesenteric hematoma was identified by CT, the diagnosis of visceral artery aneurysm was made and successfully treated, suggesting an even greater use for CT in obscure abdominal conditions.[49]

An interesting new use for CT has been the evaluation of cervical carotid plaque.[50] Here, the high-resolution CT scan of the carotid artery is performed with bolus injection and drip infusion of contrast media. Since this technique is relatively noninvasive, it has enormous potential for carotid plaque evaluation where loosened lesions might represent intramural hemorrhage or focal plaque necrosis. Of course, CT angiography has been in use since 1980, and there is no doubt that its applications will increase in the future.[51]

The CT scan has value in evaluating the central nervous system in patients with vascular conditions. The vascular service at the University of Rochester looked at this technique very closely and concluded that the CT scan played a limited role in preoperative evaluation of patients with clear-cut clinical evidence of thromboembolic stroke or transient cerebral ischemia, but that while the CT scan was of no help in selecting patients for elective carotid endarterectomy, it was helpful in planning therapy for patients with acute neurologic problems, whether or not these were caused by extracranial cerebrovascular lesions.[52] Also, in evaluating asymptomatic carotid lesions, it was found by this group that positive CT scans were present in 20% of patients, suggesting that the patient with an asymptomatic carotid lesion and a positive CT scan might no longer be classified as being asymptomatic.

Computerized tomography in our experience at Northwestern University has been extremely valuable in assisting the evaluation of lesions of persistent sciatic artery, intramuscular hemangioma, much as reported from Kuwait,[53] as well as evaluation of hemangiomatous malformations. It is in this last area that CT will have an increasingly important role in planning therapy.

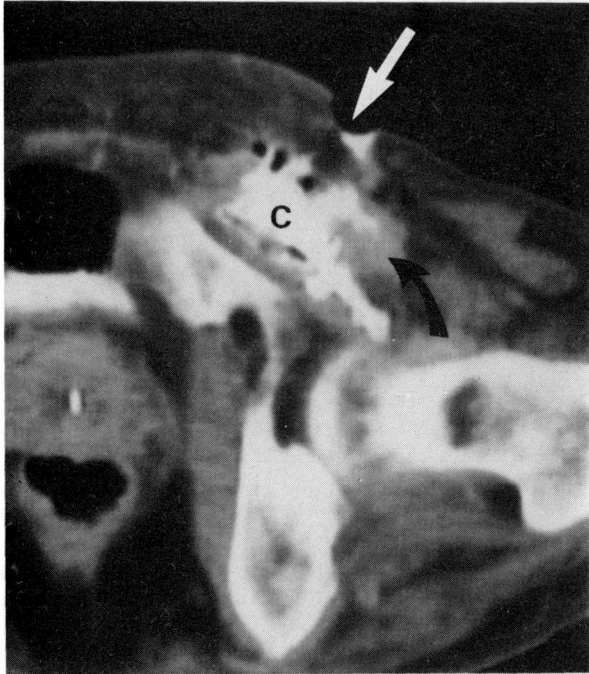

Fig. 12-4. This figure demonstrates the utility of a sinogram and CT together. Water-soluble contrast media has been injected and demonstrates a perigraft fluid collection which is pathognomonic of graft infection. Contrast material is marked by the letter C and the perigraft fluid collection by the curved arrow. From Vogelzang RL: The role of CT in reoperative aortic surgery, in Bergan JJ, Yao JST (eds): Reoperative Arterial Surgery. Orlando, Grune & Stratton, 1986, pp 33–58.

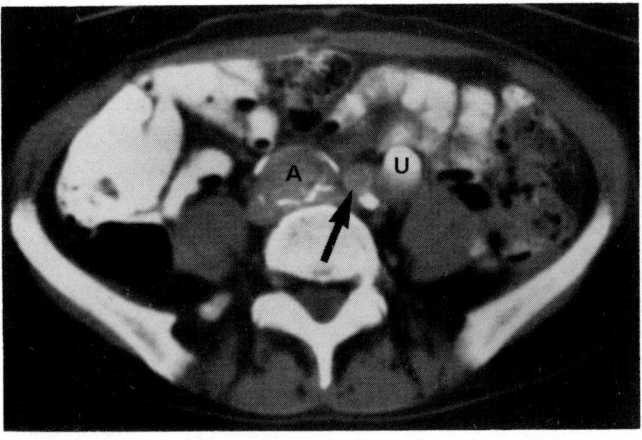

Fig. 12-5. (A and B) These figures showing a CT scan in a patient with a complex problem scheduled for reoperation demonstrate bilateral pseudoaneurysms at the termination of an aorto-biiliac graft. The dilated right ureter, marked U, is seen to terminate in caudad sections. The open arrow shows the incorporation of the ureter into the wall of the left pseudoaneurysm. The right pseudoaneurysm, marked A, and its termination, marked *, also involves the right ureter (solid arrow). These findings alert the surgeon to the need for preoperative ureteral cannulation and aid in the performance of the reoperation. From Vogelzang RL: The role of CT in reoperative aortic surgery, in Bergan JJ, Yao JST (eds): Reoperative Arterial Surgery. Orlando, Grune & Stratton, 1986, pp 33–58.

REFERENCES

1. Bergan JJ, Yao JST: Invited overview: Role of the vascular laboratory. Surgery 88:9–15, 1980
2. Anderson DC, Fischer GG: Impact of digital subtraction angiography on carotid evaluation. Stroke 16:23–28, 1985
3. Roederer GO, Langlois YE, Chan AT, Chikos PM, Thiele BL, Strandness DE Jr: Is siphon disease important in predicting the outcome of carotid endarterectomy? Stroke 14:125, 1983 (Abstr)
4. Earnest F IV, Houser OW, Forbes GS, Kispert DB, Folger WN, Sundt TM Jr: The accuracy and limitations of intravenous digital subtraction angiography in the evaluation of atherosclerotic cerebrovascular disease: Angiographic and surgical correlation. Mayo Clin Proc 58:735–746, 1983
5. Carmody RF, Smith JRL, Seeger JF, Ovitt TW, Capp MP: Intracranial applications of digital intravenous subtraction angiography. Radiology 144:529–534, 1982
6. Modic MT, Weistein MA, Chilcote WA, Pavlicek W, Duchesneau PM, Furlan AJ, Little JR: Digital subtraction angiography of the intracranial vascular system: Comparative study in 55 patients. AJNR 2:527–534, 1981
7. Aaron JO, Hesselink JR, Oot R, Jones RL, Davirs KR, Taveras JM: Complications of intravenous DSA performed for carotid artery disease: A prospective study. Radiology 153:675–678, 1984
8. Reilly LM, Ehrenfeld WK, Stoney RJ: Carotid digital subtraction angiography: Comparative roles of intra-arterial and intravenous imaging. Surgery 96:909–917, 1984
9. Crummy AB, Stieghorst MF, Turski PA, Strother CM, Lieberman RP, Sackett JF, Turnipseed WD, Detmer DE, Mistretta CA: Digital subtraction angiography: Current status and use of intraarterial injection. Radiology 145:303–307, 1982
10. Smith CW, Winfield AC, Price RR, Harding DR, Tucker SW, Witt WS, Hollifield JW: Evaluation of digital venous angiography for the diagnosis of renovascular hypertension. Radiology 144:51–54, 1982
11. Novick AC, Buonocore E, Meaney TF: Digital subtraction angiography for postoperative evaluation of renal arterial reconstruction. J Urol 127:14–17, 1982
12. Pond GD, Osborne RW, Capp MP, Fisher HD, Frost MM, Goldstone J, Malone JM, Nudelman S, Ovitt TW, Roehrig H: Digital subtraction angiography of peripheral vascular bypass procedures. AJR 138:279–281, 1982
13. Shetty PC, Krasicky GA, Sharma RP, Vemuri BR, Burke MM: Mycotic aneurysms in intravenous drug abusers: The utility of intravenous digital subtraction angiography. Radiology 155:319–321, 1985
14. Amundson GM, Wesenberg RL, Mueller DL, Reid RH: Pediatric digital subtraction angiography. Radiology 153:649–654, 1984
15. Goodman PC, Jeffrey RB Jr, Brant-Zawadzki M: Digital subtraction angiography in extremity trauma. Radiology 153:61–64, 1984
16. Hricak H, Amparo EG, Fisher MR, Crooks LE, Higgins CB: Abdominal venous system: Assessment using magnetic resonance imaging. Radiology 156:415–422, 1985
17. Fisher MR, Hricak H, Higgins CB: Magnetic resonance of developmental anomalies. AJR 145:705–710, 1985
18. Amparo EG, Hoddick WK, Hricak H, Sollitto R, Justich E, Filly RA, Higgins CB: Comparison of MR imaging and ultrasonography in the evaluation of abdominal aortic aneurysms. Radiology 154:451, 1985
19. Glazer HS, Gutierrez FT, Levitt RG, Lee JK, Murphy WA: The thoracic aorta studied by magnetic resonance. Radiology 157:149–155, 1985
20. Amparo EG, Higgins CB, Hricak H, Sollitto R: Aortic dissection: Magnetic resonance imaging. Radiology 155:399–406, 1985

21. Geisinger MA, Risius B, O'Donnell JA, Zelch MG, Moodie DS, Graor RA, George CR: Thoracic aortic dissections: Magnetic resonance imaging. Radiology 155:407–412, 1985

22. Baker HL Jr, Berquist TH, Kispert DB, Reese DF, Houser OW, Earnest F IV, Forbes GS: Magnetic resonance imaging in a routine clinical setting. Mayo Clin Proc 60:75–90, 1985

23. Flak B, Li DKB, Ho BYB, Knickerbocker WJ, Fache S, Mayo J, Chung W: Magnetic resonance imaging of aneurysms of the abdominal aorta. AJR 144:991–996, 1985

24. Allgayer B, Rupp N, Reiser M, Lukas HP, Heller HJ, Dörrler J: Das Aortenaneurysm im MR-Tomogramm. Dtsch med Wschr 110:714–718, 1985

25. Moore EH, Webb WR, Verrier ED, Broaddus C, Gamsu G, Amparo E, Higgins CB: MRI of chronic posttraumatic false aneurysms of the thoracic aorta. AJR 143:1195–1196, 1984

26. Kistler JP, Buonanno FS, DeWitt LD, Davis KR, Brady TJ, Fisher CM: Vertebral-basilar posterior cerebral territory stroke: Delineation by proton nuclear magnetic resonance imaging. Stroke 15:417–426, 1984

27. Whitman GJR, Harken AH: Applications of nuclear magnetic resonance to surgical disease: A collective review. J Surg Res 38:187–199, 1985

28. Ackerman RH, Alpert NM, Correia JA, Finklestein S, Davis SM, Kelley RE, Connan GA, D'Alton JG, Taveras JM: Positron imaging in ischemic stroke disease. Ann Neurol 15(Suppl):S126–S130, 1984

29. Vogelzang RL: The role of CT in reoperative aortic surgery, in Bergan JJ, Yao JST (eds): Reoperative Arterial Surgery. Orlando, Grune & Stratton, 1986, pp 33–58

30. Eriksson I, Hemmingsson A, Lindgren PG: Diagnosis of abdominal aortic aneurysms by aortography, computer tomography and ultrasound. Acta Radiol Diagnos 21:209–214, 1980

31. Larsson EM, Albrechtsson U, Christensson JT: Computed tomography versus aortography for preoperative evaluation of abdominal aortic aneurysm. Acta Radiol Diagnos 25:95–100, 1981

32. Anderson PE, Lorentzen JE: Comparison of computed tomography and aortography in abdominal aortic aneurysms. J Comput Assist Tomogr 7:670–673, 1983

33. Gomes MN, Wallace RB: Present status of abdominal aorta imaging by computed tomography. J Cardiovasc Surg 26:1–6, 1985

34. Williams LR, Flinn WR, Yao JST, Vogelzang RL, Roth M, McCarthy WJ III, Bergan JJ: Extended use of computerized tomography in the management of complex aortic problems. J Vasc Surg (in press)

35. Gmelin VE, Burmester E, Valesky A, Weiss HD: So-called inflammatory aneurysm of the abdominal aorta. ROFO 141:56–60, 1984

36. Crawford JL, Stowe CL, Safi HJ, Hallman CH, Crawford ES: Inflammatory aneurysms of the aorta. J Vasc Surg 2:113–124, 1985

37. O'Hara PJ, Borkowski GP, Hertzer NR, O'Donovan PB, Brigham SL, Beven EG: Natural history of periprosthetic air on computerized axial tomographic examination of the abdomen following abdominal aortic aneurysm repair. J Vasc Surg 1:429–433, 1984

38. Haaga JR, Baldwin GN, Reich NE, Beven E, Kramer A, Weinstein A, Havrilla TR, Seidelmann FE, Namba AH, Parrish CM: CT detection of infected synthetic grafts: Preliminary report of a new sign. Am J Roentgenol 131:317–320, 1978

39. Mark AS, McCarthy SM, Moss AA, Price D: Detection of abdominal aortic graft infection: Comparison of CT and indium-labelled white blood cell scans. AJR 144:315–318, 1985

40. Brown OW, Stanson AW, Pairolero PC, Hollier LH: Computerized tomography following abdominal aortic surgery. Surgery 91:716–722, 1982

41. Fishman EK, Pakter RL, Gayler BW, Wheeler PS, Siegelman SS: Jugular venous thrombosis: Diagnosis by computed tomography. J Comput Assist Tomogr 8:963–968, 1984

42. Daniel WG, Döhring W, Lichtlen PR, Stender HS: Non-invasive assessment of aorto-coronary bypass graft patency by computed tomography. Lancet 1:1023–1024, 1980
43. Sherck JP, McCort JJ, Oakes DD: Computed tomography in thoracoabdominal trauma. J Trauma 24:1015–1021, 1984
44. Sagel SS, Siegel MJ, Stanley RJ, Jost RG: Detection of retroperitoneal hemorrhage by computed tomography. Am J Roentgenol 129:403–407, 1977
45. Chuang VP, Fried AM, Chen CO: Computed tomographic evaluation of paraaortic hematoma following translumbar aortography. Radiology 130:711–712, 1979
46. Amendola MA, Tisnado J, Fields WR, Beachley MC, Vines FS, Cho SR, Turner MA, Konerding KF: Evaluation of retroperitoneal hemorrhage by computed tomography before and after translumbar aortography. Radiology 133:401–404, 1979
47. Hadjis NS, Carr DH, Banks L, Pflug JJ: Role of CT in diagnosis of primary lymph-edema of the lower limb. AJR 144:361–364, 1985
48. Silverman PM, Kelvin FM, Korobkin M, Dunnick NR: Computed tomography of the normal mesentery. AJR 143:953–957, 1984
49. Skudder PA Jr, Craver WL: Mesenteric hematoma suggests rupture of visceral artery aneurysm. Arch Surg 119:863, 1984
50. Culebras A, Leson MD, Cacyorin ED, Hodge CJ, Illiya AR: Computed tomographic evaluation of cervical carotid plaque complications. Stroke 16:425–431, 1985
51. Johnson WC, Paley RH, Castronuovo JJ, Gerzof SG, Bush HL Jr, Vincent M, Pugatch RD, Widrich WC, Cho SI, Nabseth DC, Robbins AH: Computed tomographic angi-ography. Am J Surg 141:434–440, 1981
52. Ricotta JJ, Ouriel K, Green RM, DeWeese JA: Use of computerized cerebral tom-ography in selection of patients for elective and urgent carotid endarterectomy. Ann Surg 202:783–787, 1985
53. Christenson JT, Gunterberg B: Intramuscular haemangioma of the extremities: Is com-puterized tomography useful? Br J Surg 72:748–750, 1985

PART III

Arterial Reconstruction

D. E. M. Taylor

13

How May Vascular Grafts Be Modified to Improve Patency?

INTRODUCTION

Despite over 30 years of clinical experience of vascular prostheses, the long-term patency for operations below the groin is still not ideal. A review of a series of papers with long-term follow-up over the past 25 years[1] showed an overall five-year patency rate for femoro-popliteal bypass of only 50% for arterial prostheses, compared to 68% for autologous vein. The poor prosthetic patencies applied to both synthetic and biological materials, despite occasionally exceptional results from individual clinics. The long-term patency rate was even worse for femoro-distal bypass, and there is at present no generally acceptable prosthesis for use in coronary, or similar small artery, surgery. Coronary and cerebrovascular arterial disease each account for about the same incidence of morbidity as, and have a greater mortality than, lower limb occlusive disease. In the case of coronary disease there is competition with the ischaemic lower limb for available autologous vein.

Although manufacturers have tended to concentrate on the improvement of single factors, it should not be forgotten that the causes of graft occlusion and/or failure are multiple: further, there is interaction between the various causative factors. The well known Virchow's triad of aetiological factors in deep venous thrombosis can equally be applied to a consideration of thrombotic occlusion in arterial prostheses. Just as the three factors are interdependent, rather than independent, factors in venous thrombosis, so must their possible interactions be considered in the development of better vascular prostheses, with improved long-term patency.

The occlusive process in a vascular prosthesis depends for its initiation on the aggregation of platelets on the wall, with subsequent progressive thrombus formation. Therefore, any attempt to reduce prosthetic occlusion should logically be based on the prevention of platelet aggregation, rather than on anticoagulation. This is the basis of the use of antiplatelet drugs in such patients. Early attempts at improving prosthetic patency by binding heparin to the prosthesis, however, failed despite the proven efficacy of low-dose heparin in the prophyllaxis against postoperative deep venous thrombosis.

This chapter will review recent advances in the design and construction of vascular prostheses in relation to the aetiological factors in occlusion. The three factors are:

1. stagnation;
2. endothelial damage;
3. increased platelet stickiness.

In terms of improvements in vascular prosthesis, these three factors are addressed in three areas of research and development:

1. reduction in impedance;
2. improved thromboresistance;
3. appropriate cellular lining.

IMPEDANCE

Although stagnation is a major factor in the genesis of any thrombotic process, this aspect has received relatively little attention in the development of vascular prostheses.

In any fluid-filled flow system Ohm's law relationship of

$$\text{Pressure drop} = \text{flow} \times \text{resistance}$$

is approximately correct. However, for pulsatile flow, as in the arterial system, resistance is replaced by impedance. The latter has three components: frictional loss due to viscosity, equivalent to resistance in steady-state flow, turbulent loss due to any flow instability, and nonrecoverable inertial loss due to the pulsatile nature of the flow.[2, 3] The importance of the vessel wall characteristics on pulsile pressure/flow relationships was well summarised by Baird and Abbott in 1976:[4] the stiffer the vessel wall, the less efficient the conversion of pressure drop to flow in a pulsatile system. It has been shown in experimental bypass grafting that whereas in the normal canine aorto-femoral segment nonfrictional losses account for 21% of total pressure energy loss, the nonfrictional loss increases to 80% with an autologous vein bypass, and 81–96% with a synthetic vascular prosthesis bypass.[5]

Clinically the most important cause of low flow through a vascular prosthesis is poor peripheral runoff: this will not be improved by modifications in prosthetic construction and design, but depends on adequate preoperative assessment. Provided peripheral runoff is satisfactory, improvements in vascular prostheses which reduce the impedance to pulsatile flow may help to improve long-term haemodynamic function and patency.

Frictional energy loss is inversely related to the fourth power of the vessel radius, so even small reductions in diameter can have marked effects on pressure drop and flow. If the narrowing is irregular or of short length it can also lead to local turbulence, with further energy loss. The latter is likely to occur where a prosthesis crosses the flexor aspect of a joint, e.g. the knee joint with a femoral-distal bypass, or where there is a long superficial course, as in an axillo-femoral bypass.

These can be associated both with local kinking of the prosthesis on flexion and local narrowing due to external compression. Several manufacturers have tried to minimize these problems by the introduction of prostheses with an external support; synthetic prostheses both of Dacron and of PTFE are available with external support, but follow-up is as yet too short to permit valid assessment of any benefit in terms of patency.[6, 7]

The current generation of synthetic vascular prostheses constructed of either Dacron or PTFE are relatively rigid compared to natural arteries[8, 9] (Fig. 13.1), so that any additional rigidity produced by an external support will have negligible haemodynamic consequences. However, the comparative rigidity of current synthetic vascular prostheses is itself a potential cause of problems; improvement of this aspect constitutes the other main area of advance to improve the low-flow aspect of prosthetic occlusion.

The velocity of transmission of pulsatile pressure and the efficiency of conversion of pressure to flow energy depend on optimal elastic properties of the vessel or prosthetic wall.[10, 11] There is considerable effort being directed to the production of a vascular prosthesis which will have the same compliance after implantation as that of the vessels being replaced or bypassed. Theoretically this would result in reduced nonrecoverable inertial losses on pulsatile flow, with a consequent reduction in pressure drop and increased mean flow. Two approaches to achieve this are being developed, with the production of novel prostheses. First, new

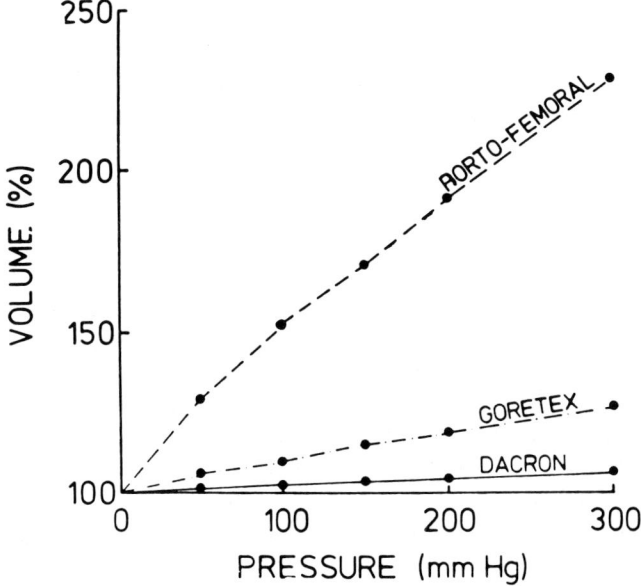

Fig. 13-1. Pressure–volume curves for a natural aorto-femoral arterial segment, a 5 mm i.d. Gore-Tex prosthesis and a 6 mm i.d. DeBakey Dacron prosthesis with the crimp removed. Note the much lower compliance of the synthetic prostheses. Reproduced by permission of the editor of Annals of the Royal College of Surgeons of England.

materials and/or methods of construction can be used to produce a more compliant prosthesis; second, new materials or treatment of materials can be used to minimise the periprosthetic reaction and deposition of fibrous tissue and thrombus after implantation. To assess the magnitude of these two problems, consider the performance of current synthetic prostheses in terms of their circumferential wall elastance. The latter is a measure of the force required per unit length of the vessel or prosthesis to produce a doubling of the diameter. Pulse wave velocity is directly related to the square root of the latter.[11] The circumferential elastance is about 900 N/m for normal femoral artery,[12, 13] compared to about 2600 N/m for a 6-mm i.d. Cooley double velour knitted Dacron prosthesis before implantation and over 3100 N/m for the same prosthesis two hours after implantation.[12] Three months after implantation there is a further slight increase in circumferential elastance to between 3500 and 4000 N/m for Dacron prostheses, but with no further significant increase up to one year after implantation.[1]

Pulse wave velocity is also inversely related to the square root of vessel diameter and, as has been previously stated, viscous resistance is inversely related to the fourth power of the radius. For all types of energy loss the smaller the prosthetic diameter the greater will be the effect of any improvement in long-term compliance—including any reduction in the periprosthetic tissue response.

An improvement in the elastic properties can possibly be achieved by the use of elastomeric polymers. The principle group examined in this respect has been the polyurethanes, both as simple polymers and as block copolymers with other monomers.[14] The work of Annis and his coworkers[15, 16] using electrostatically spun polyurethane has shown considerable promise on animal trials. The latter include follow-up for more than two years. This prosthesis has not yet been able to be introduced for clinical use, but it appears to be ready for a full clinical evaluation. An earlier attempt to introduce an elastomeric prosthesis clinically was not successful. This was a composite of polyurethane and Dacron with a velour construction (CCV–VPI Ltd). The polyurethane used, like many of that polymer family, showed fatigue, with loss of its ability to recover after repeated stressing. This resulted in dilation of the prosthesis with loss of compliance. A further complication was that the materials and method of construction employed led to a marked periprosthetic response, so that much of the inbuilt compliance was lost within a few weeks of implantation and the mechanical properties were similar to those of a Dacron prosthesis.[17] It is apparent from these studies that elastomeric prostheses should be subjected to rigorous long-term in vitro and in vivo studies to assess fully fatigue resistance and chronic biotolerance before being released for clinical use.

A recent experimental approach has been the concept of an elastomeric prosthesis, which is also biodegradable. The planned biodegradation is such that the replacement host tissue itself contains elastin and smooth muscle to give a living conduit with the same mechanical properties as normal arteries.[18] Although this is an attractive prospect, published results to date refer only to subaortic replacement in the rat. The results of long-term animal studies will be required before the likely clinical feasibility of this novel approach can be properly assessed.

Modification of materials and surfaces to minimise periprosthetic response and thus prevent postimplantation stiffening is closely allied to the problems analogous to endothelial damage in the Virchow triad; these will be considered next.

THROMBORESISTANCE

The immediate interaction of the formed elements in the blood with the prosthetic surface is the area of potential improvement which has received the most attention in recent years. The vascular prostheses in current use have an inner surface which is relatively thrombogenic. After implantation of any vascular prosthesis a layer of swept fibrin is deposited on the wall, and it is upon this that any subsequent endothelialisation occurs. Synthetic prostheses tend to show a development of surface endothelium only within a few centimetres of the anastomoses, even after several years. The thickness of the inner fibrin layer will depend not only on the thrombogenicity of the material of construction but also on the velocity and nature of the blood flow over the surface, thus interacting with the impedance factors discussed in the previous section. The converse relationship also applies, for the internal layer deposited will affect both the in-use diameter of the prosthesis (Fig. 13-2) and the wall elastance.[1]

There has in the past been considerable discussion on the importance of porosity and the use of constructions such as velours in improving the nature of the inner lining deposited on a vascular prosthesis. This led to a proliferation of types of Dacron prostheses and conflicting accounts based on clinical experience. Properly controlled comparative studies in animals have demonstrated that porosity and finish of Dacron prostheses have no significant effect on the nature of the inner lining which forms.[1,19] The only consistent differences which have been shown in

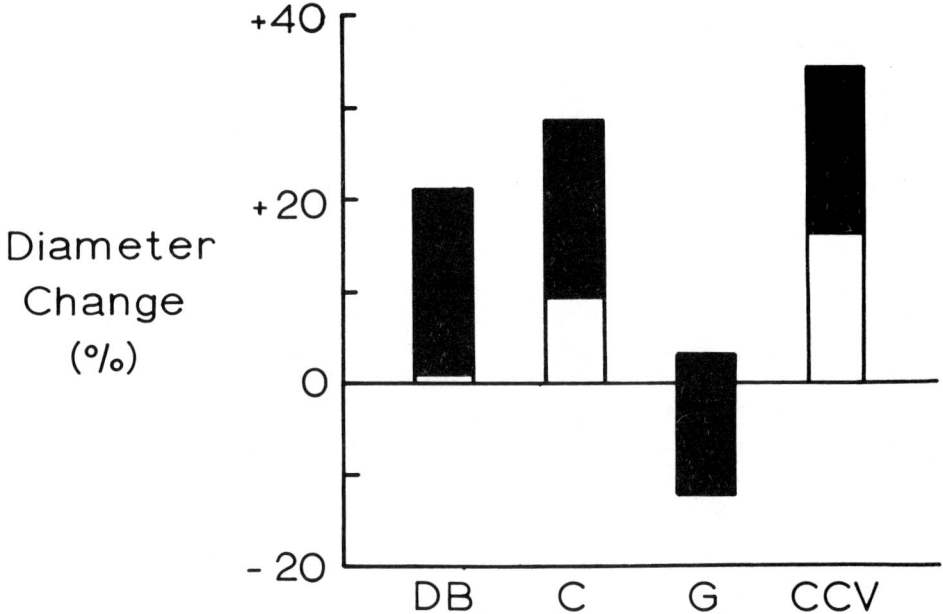

Fig. 13-2. The effect of dilation of the structure and of thrombus deposition on the in-use diameter of various 5 and 6 mm i.d. vascular prostheses. The shaded portion represents the thrombus thickness. DB = DeBakey Dacron (USCI), C = Cooley double velour Dacron (Meadox), G = Gore-Tex, CCV = elastomeric velour (VPI).

Table 13-1
Patency Rates (% mean and range) Reported
in 42 Papers in the Literature from 1978 to
1985 for Different Types of Vascular
Prosthesis in Femoro-popliteal Bypass

Time	Vein	Dacron	PTFE	Biological
2 year	73	75	72	72
	(48–83)	(58–90)	(43–93)	(48–75)
5 year	64	50	64	62
	(55–76)	(28–71)	(38–76)	(52–72)

clinical series relate to the material of construction, with biological and PTFE prostheses having, on average, better long-term patency rates than Dacron prostheses (Table 13-1).

Two new approaches are being developed to improve the surface characteristics of vascular prostheses, so as to reduce thrombogenicity and produce a thinner, more stable and more fully endothelial-covered inner lining. The first method under investigation is to develop new materials or surface treatments of existing materials; the second is to seed endothelial, or similar, cells onto the inner surface of a prosthesis at the time of operation.

The development of new materials or modification of existing materials to reduce thrombogenicity depends on an understanding of the physical and physicochemical properties of healthy endothelium and of platelets. Platelets do not readily adhere to or aggregate on vascular endothelium. If the endothelium is removed to expose the subendothelium, then the platelets migrate, aggregate and adhere to the surface. It is the initial stimulus to adhere to the surface which initiates the complex chemical processes associated with the formation and propagation of a thrombus.

The chemical nature of a surface leaves various charged groups exposed or adsorbed so that there is a net electrical charge on the surface: this is called the surface or zeta potential. A surface potential is present on all cells in the body and also on structural proteins such as collagen. In the case of vascular endothelium, platelets and erythrocytes the surface charge is negative—about -12 to -15 mV. This electrostatic charge is sufficient to repel platelets from each other and from the endothelial surface. Collagen has a net positive surface charge and consequently attracts platelets, causing them to adhere and diminish their negative surface charge, with consequent aggregation and activation.

Surface charge is determined by the balance between hydrophobic and hydrophilic chemical groups, so is related to the wettability of the surface.[20] This can be most easily measured as the water contact angle.[21] It has been accepted in the past that thrombogenicity could best be improved by using hydrophobic materials, such as PTFE. The latter has a water contact angle of 130 degrees, as compared to 68 degrees for Dacron. However, normal endothelium is hydrophilic, and it was calculated that minimum thrombogenicity should be associated with a small water contact angle.[20] This radically different concept of the type of material required for vascular prostheses has been supported by studies on endothelial cell adhesion in vitro[22] and on both periprosthetic cellular response and thrombogenicity in vivo.[1, 17, 23] Work at present in progress in our group indicates that there are two optimal values for water contact angle for maximum biotolerance: a hydrophobic range of more than 110 degrees, in which PTFE falls, and a hydrophylic range of 20–45 degrees, in which new materials are being developed (Fig. 13-3).

The polyurethanes, which were discussed in the previous section, include many hydrophilic materials with a water contact angle within the proposed optimal range. Therefore, in addition to their elastomeric properties, polyurethanes should also exhibit less thrombogenicity. This has been borne out in animal trials.[15,16] As a family of polymers the polyurethanes hold considerable promise in producing better synthetic prostheses.

The surface properties of polymers can be modified by grafting on side-chains of other monomers or polymers: such materials are known as graft copolymers. Many high water content polymers, or hydrogels, possess surface properties which would make them relatively thromboresistant, but they lack the mechanical strength of hydrophobes such as Dacron and PTFE. By producing a graft copolymer of a hydrophilic onto a hydrophobic polymer, a copolymer can be obtained with the surface properties of a hydrogel and the high inherent strength of the base hydrophobic polymer. Work in this field has mainly been concerned with acrylic acid copolymers.[1,17,23] These, like the polyurethanes, show much promise. An acrylic acid/Dacron copolymer vascular prosthesis has been shown in studies of up to one year implantation in the dog, to be associated with a much thinner inner lining (Fig. 13-4) with better compliance, with a slower pulse wave velocity (Fig. 13-5) and less

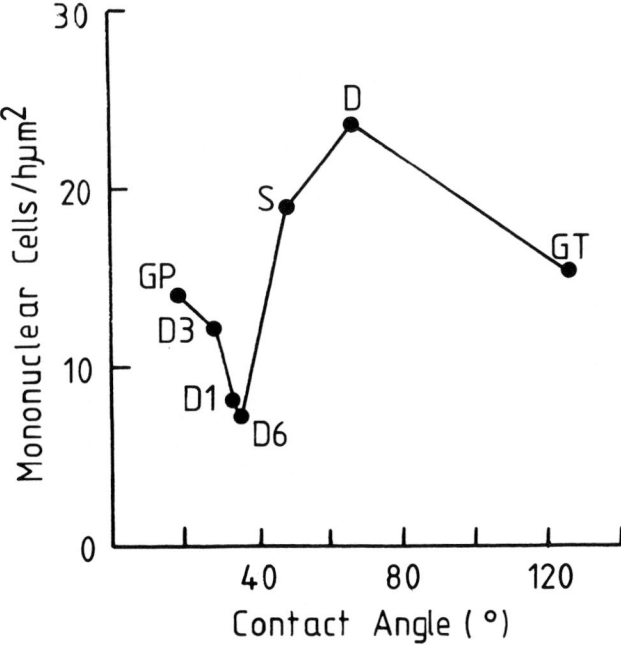

Fig. 13-3. Relation of water contact angle to mononuclear cells in capsule around an implant. GT = Gore-Tex, D = Knitted Dacron, S = Silastic, GP, D3, D1, D6 = novel hydrogels and copolymers. Note minimal reaction troughs for hydrophobe (GT) and hydrophils (D1, D6).

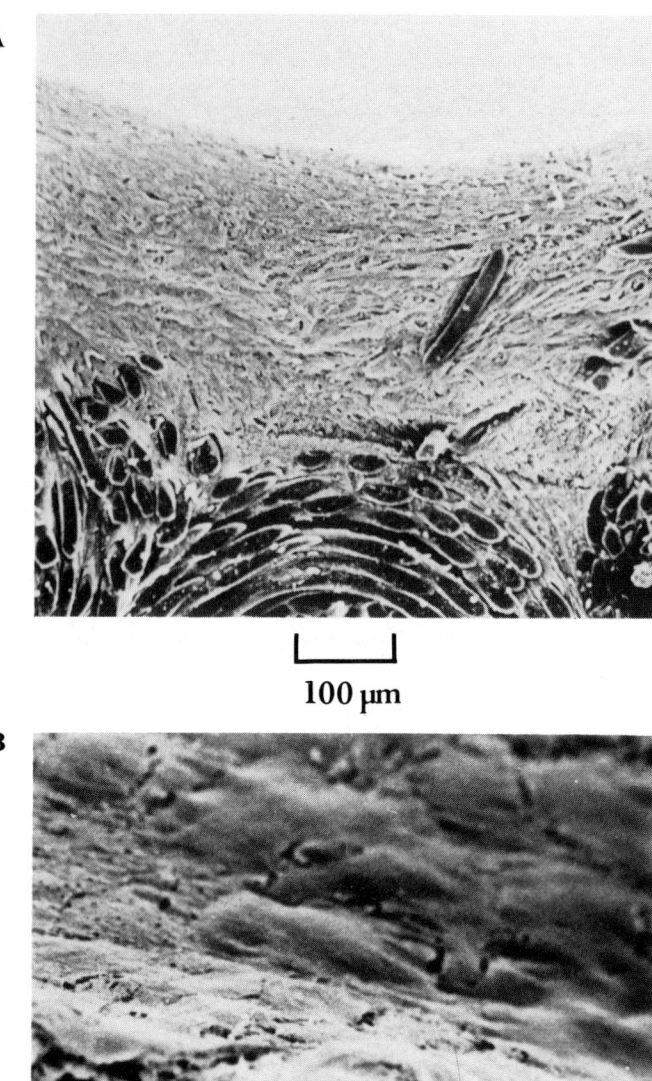

A

100 μm

B

30 μm

Fig. 13-4. SEM pictures of the inner lining of a copolymerised Dacron prosthesis to show (A) a thin layer (< 50 μm) of well-organised thrombus, over which (B) endothelial cells are growing. The prosthesis had been implanted in a dog as a thoracoabdominal aortic bypass for 6/12. Reproduced by permission of RM Miller.

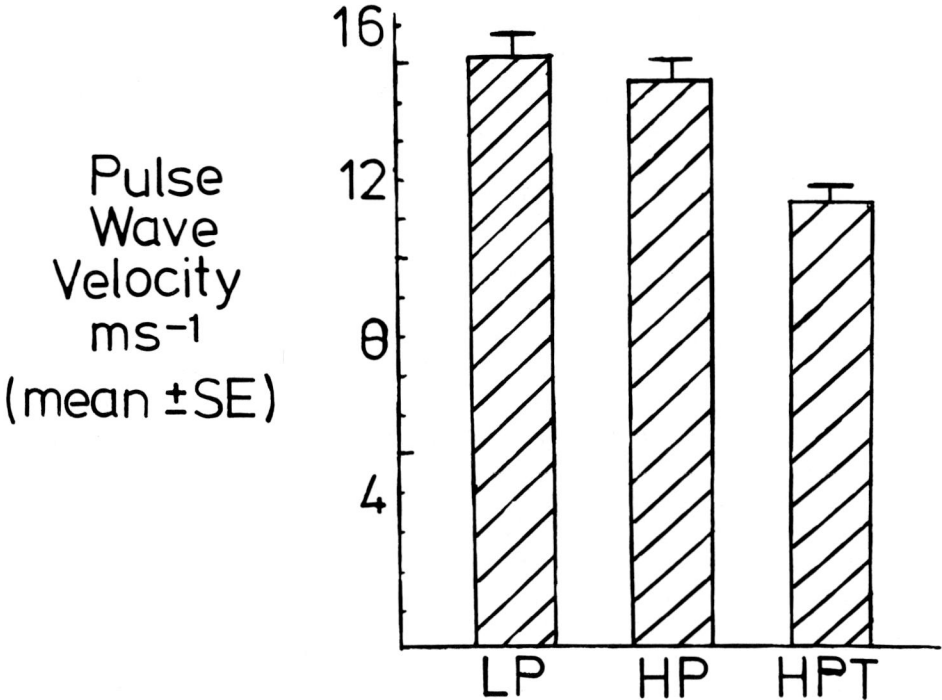

Fig. 13-5. Pulse wave velocity in thoracoabdominal aortic bypass prostheses after 3/12 implantation in the dog. LP = woven Dacron low porosity, HP = high porosity woven Dacron, HPT = acrylic acid graft copolymer of HP. Reproduced by permission of RM Miller.

impedance, and with more complete endothelialisation than a similar unmodified Dacron prosthesis.[1]

As with polyurethane prostheses, the copolymer prostheses are approaching the stage of being submitted to a controlled clinical trial. Their possible place in vascular surgery must also await the results of actual clinical use.

The only well-developed surface modification of an existing synthetic vascular prosthesis is coating a Dacron prosthesis with a protein, or protein-derived, material. The coatings already in clinical use are either collagen or gelatin. Both types of coating transform a porous into a nonporous prosthesis so that preclotting is not required. They also provide a smooth uniform inner surface, encouraging a stable flow close to the surface. The coatings are, however, potentially thrombogenic and in the case of collagen may be recognised by the body as a foreign material. It is too early yet to assess their clinical performance and reports of experimental assessment are sparse; their place in vascular surgery still has to be determined.

The seeding of cells onto the surface of prostheses is an attempt to induce the production on the surface of antiaggregant humoral agents; it will be considered along with the problem of platelet stickiness.

CELLULAR LINING

In the normal vascular system there is an interaction between the platelets and the endothelium with respect to prostaglandin production. The platelet contains thromboxane synthetase, and unless constrained will produce thromboxane A2 from its membrane arachidonic acid. Thromboxane synthesis also occurs in the subendothelial tissue of arteries. The thromboxane produced at these sites is a powerful aggregant of platelets and will initiate thrombosis at the wall of the vessel or prosthesis. The major cycloxygenase pathway for vascular endothelium is for the production of prostaglandin I2, otherwise known as prostacyclin. The latter both inhibits platelet aggregation and activation, and inhibits thromboxane synthesis by the platelet. It is, therefore, highly advantageous for a vascular prosthesis to be lined by vascular endothelium or other cells which synthesise prostacyclin. As has been stated earlier in this chapter, the endothelialisation of present synthetic prosthesis is usually far from complete, even many years after implantation. The inner lining is fibrous connective tissue and a surface of swept fibrin: the term pseudosubintima would be far more apposite for this tissue than the current pseudointima.

Attempts have been made to seed autologous endothelial cells onto synthetic prostheses. This was greatly aided by the development of a single-stage technique.[24] The technique has been further refined, in order to obtain a greater cover with seeded cells, by precoating the prosthesis with fibronectin.[25] Using these methods it has been possible to seed viable endothelial cells onto both Dacron and PTFE,[26] and encouraging results have been obtained with endothelial seeding in experimental animals.[27] Although there are some preliminary results of this method in patients, they are as yet neither in sufficient numbers nor for a sufficient length of time of follow-up for valid assessment.

Another experimental method to achieve the same objective, but more simply, is to place a wrap of autologous vein outside of the prosthesis. It is reported from experiments that there was enhanced endothelialisation of prostheses so treated, with migration of endothelial cells through the interstices of a Dacron prosthesis.[28]

A final modification of the seeding technique is to use not endothelial cells, which may be difficult to harvest or culture, but the more easily obtainable peritoneal mesothelial cells. These also contain prostacyclin synthetase in similar quantities to vascular endothelium. A preliminary experimental report shows that mesothelial cell seeding is as efficacious as endothelial seeding of a Dacron prosthesis.[29]

CONCLUSIONS

This brief review of the factors in and possible solutions of vascular prosthesis occlusion has illustrated that we are dealing with a multifactorial problem which is unlikely to have a unique solution. Improvements in the materials, design and operative treatment of vascular prostheses all offer the possibility of improved long-term patency. Encouraging results from the laboratory, where the prosthesis is being implanted into a normal vasculature, only indicate which novel devices merit a properly controlled clinical trial. The success of any new prosthesis should eventually be decided on an actuarial assessment with a valid follow-up of an adequate number of patients for at least five years.

The various new developments in this paper point the way for clinical evaluation, rather than providing the answers. Despite all the potential advances in vascular prosthesis it is still likely that the major factors in deciding clinical results will be the preclinical assessment of the extent and location of the disease and the adequacy of the peripheral runoff once the prosthesis has been inserted.

REFERENCES

1. Miller RM, Taylor DEM, Ringrose BS: Biotolerant and haemodynamic effects of copolymerisation with acrylic acid on Dacron arterial prostheses. Ann R Coll Surg Engl 68:85, 1986

2. Yellin EL, Liando S, Perkin S, et al: Analysis and interpretation of the normal mitral valve flow curve, in Kalmanson D (ed): The Mitral Valve. Acton, Mass., Publishing Sciences Group, 1976, p 163

3. Taylor DEM, Whamond JS: Computation and modelling of resistive, inertive and turbulent contribution across heart valves. J Physiol 273:24P, 1977

4. Baird RN, Abbot WM: Pulsatile blood flow in arterial grafts. Lancet 2:948, 1976

5. Santiago EJ: Haemodynamic effects of aorto-femoral bypass with various small calibre arterial prostheses in the dog. PhD Thesis, University of London, 1982

6. Stark J, et al: The use of Gore-Tex reinforced with external rings in paediatric cardiac surgery. Ann Thor Surg 39:188, 1985

7. Kennet DA, Sauvage LR, Wood SJ, et al: Comparison of noncrimped, externally supported (EXS) and crimped non-supported Dacron prostheses for axillo-femoral and above-knee femoropopliteal bypass. Surgery 92:931, 1982

8. Santiago EJ, Chatamra K, Taylor DEM: Haemodynamic aspects of lower limb arterial reconstruction using Dacron and Gore-Tex prostheses. Ann R Coll Surg Engl 63:253, 1981

9. Kidson IG: The effect of wall mechanical properties on patency of arterial grafts. Ann R Coll Surg Engl 65:24, 1983

10. McDonald DA: Blood Flow in Arteries. London, Arnold, 1974

11. Taylor DEM, Santiago EJ, Miller RM, et al: Pulse wave velocity in different 5–6 mm i.d. vascular prostheses. Br J Surg, 1986 (in press)

12. Taylor DEM, Santiago EJ: The validity of some methods of estimating circumferential elastance of vascular prostheses. J Biomed Engrs, 1986 (in press)

13. Yamada H: Mechanical properties of circulatory organs and tissues, in Evans FG (ed): Strength of Biological Materials. Baltimore, Williams and Wilkins, 1970, p 106

14. Taylor DEM: Biomaterials in reconstructive surgery, in Bevan PG (ed): Reconstructive Procedures in Surgery. Oxford, Blackwell Scientific Publications, 1982, p 43

15. Annis D, Bornat A, Edwards RO, et al: An elastomeric vascular prosthesis. Trans Am Soc Artif Intern Organs 24:209, 1978

16. Fisher AG, deCossart L, How TW, et al: A small bore Biomer arterial prosthesis: In vivo performance. Life Support Syst 2 (Suppl 1): 340, 1984

17. Whamond JS, Taylor DEM, Fydelor P, et al: Preclinical evaluation of knitted radiation graft copolymer elastomeric vascular prostheses. Life Support Syst 1 (Suppl 1): 443, 1983

18. Gogolewski S, Galleti G: Microporous compliant vascular prosthesis of adjustable rate of degradation. Life Support Syst 2 (Suppl 1): 324, 1984

19. Goldman M, et al: Dacron arterial grafts: The influence of porosity, velour and maturity on thrombogenicity. Surgery 92:947, 1982
20. Sharma CP: Possible contributions of surface energy and interfacial parameters of synthetic polymers to blood compatibility. Biomaterials 2:57, 1981
21. Andrade JD, King RN, Gregonis DE, et al: Surface characterisation of poly(hydroxyethyl methacrylate) and related polymers. 1. Contact angle methods in water. J Polymer Sci 66:312, 1979
22. van Wachem PB, Beugeling T, Feijen J, et al: The interaction of human endothelial cells and biomaterials. Life Support Syst 2 (Suppl 1):98, 1984
23. Fydelor PJ, Ringrose BJ, Taylor DEM, et al: Biotolerance and haemocompatibility of radiation grafted hydrophil/hydrophobe copolymers. Proc Eur Soc Artif Organs 7:72, 1980
24. Herring, M, Garger A, Glover JA: A single staged technique for seeding vascular grafts with autogenous endothelium. Surgery 84:498, 1978
25. Seeger JM, Klingman N: Improved endothelial cell seeding with cultured cells and fibronectin coated grafts. J Surg Res 38:641, 1984
26. Williams SK, Jarrell BE, Friend L, et al: Adult human endothelial cell compatibility with prosthetic graft material. J Surg Res 38:618, 1985
27. Plate G, Hollier LH, Fowl RJ, et al: Endothelial seeding of venous prostheses. Surgery 96:929, 1984
28. Graham LM, Harrell KA, Sell RL, et al: Enhanced endothelialization of Dacron grafts by external vein wrapping. J Surg Res 38:537, 1985
29. Clark JMF, Pittilo RM, Nicholson LJ, et al: Seeding Dacron arterial prostheses with peritoneal mesothelial cells: A preliminary morphological study. Br J Surg 71:492, 1985

Crawford Jamieson

14

What Is the Place of Synthetic Grafts in the Lower Limb?

This chapter will address the clinical and ethical considerations involved in the use of any bypass in the lower limb other than the autogenous saphenous vein. It is generally accepted that autogenous saphenous vein grafts, either reversed or in situ, have significantly better long-term patency and freedom from deleterious side effects than any other bypass below the inguinal ligament, and that these form the gold standard by which the performance of less efficient grafts must be judged.

This gold is not, however, unalloyed. The mean patency of femoro-popliteal saphenous vein bypass grafts at 10 years is not more than 20%,[1] and when inserted to a vessel distal to the popliteal artery the mean patency at one year is not much greater than 50% for reversed vein bypass,[2-4] although there is now uncontrolled evidence which suggests that in situ bypass to the crural vessels fares better than reversed vein bypasses.[5] These are not results of which we, as vascular surgeons, must be particularly proud. They are only made tolerable by the limited life expectancy of our patients.

LIMB SALVAGE AND CRITICAL ISCHAEMIA

The potential benefits of these grafts are fairly obvious. A successful femoro-popliteal or femoro-crural bypass may achieve salvage of a critically ischaemic limb, or lower the level of potential amputation. Patients with critical ischaemia due to atheroma have a mean life expectancy of between three and four years,[6-8] although a few live much longer. It is not, therefore, important to the majority of these patients that the graft should remain patent for a long period, but it is vital that it remain patent for at least a year if it is to be worthwhile, as the majority of patients live longer than that and will still come to amputation if the graft should fail. This point has been hotly disputed, as clearly there would be a much better case for insertion of bypasses of very limited patency if it could be shown that the bypass

VASCULAR SURGERY: ISSUES IN CURRENT PRACTICE
ISBN 0-8089-1839-7

could fail without the limb being lost.[2–5, 9] Most published reports of limb salvage indicate that this is so and that the limb salvage rate exceeds the graft patency figure at all time intervals. Less circulation is required to maintain the nutrition of intact tissue than to heal ulcers and ischaemic sores, so it is conceivable that a graft which remains patent long enough to allow ulcers to heal may then fail and allow the limb to remain intact. This would explain some of the discrepancy between patency rates and limb salvage figures, but I fear that most of the difference is due to inappropriate case selection and the inclusion of patients in these series who were not inevitable candidates for amputation if they had not received a bypass. A prospective study of the British Journal of Surgery's definition of critical ischaemia suggests that it is likely that patients will come to amputation if their grafts fail if they have an ankle blood pressure of < 40 mmHg systolic and rest pain alone, or if they have an ankle blood pressure of < 60 mmHg and ischaemic ulceration or gangrene involving more than a digit. This study has also, however, revealed that many of the patients considered by expert clinicians to be genuine candidates for limb salvage do not meet this definition of critical ischaemia and, in this fraction of the population, the graft may fail without the limb necessarily being lost.[10]

It is important, therefore, for the adequate scientific analysis of these data, that some form of objective classification of critical ischaemia, such as that proposed by the working party of the First International Vascular Symposium and published in the British Journal of Surgery,[11] should be adopted. The apparent discrepancies in patency between various graft materials and the prognoses of these patients might then be greatly reduced. Even if we accept that there is slightly better incidence of limb salvage than graft patency, the difference is probably not greater than 10–15%, so it is essential that a synthetic bypass should remain patent for more than a year, and preferably two years, if it is to be worth using in patients with critical ischaemia.

INTERMITTENT CLAUDICATION

The place of these bypasses in patients with intermittent claudication is less easily defined. Standard teaching has been that they should not be used; in the first generation of vascular surgery Dacron grafts were regularly inserted from the common femoral to the popliteal artery for intermittent claudication alone, but the poor long-term results of this procedure led to disillusionment which made most vascular surgical teachers strongly recommend that patients should not be considered as candidates for synthetic grafts unless they were suffering from critical ischaemia. More recently, however, these tenets have been questioned. Although a superficial femoral artery occlusion is a relatively benign condition and has symptoms which may improve with time, a large proportion of patients remain significantly disabled. They have a limited life expectancy of approximately 8 years[6] and it is sad if their remaining days cannot be free of pain on exercise. A controlled trial has recently shown that the results of PTFE grafts inserted from the common femoral artery to the popliteal artery, particularly above the knee joint,[9] are not much worse than those of the vein and, for that reason, it seems reasonable that, in selected patients with chronic disabling intermittent claudication in whom the vein is unsuitable, one of these grafts should be recommended. A further, smaller, controlled trial has shown, indirectly, that human umbilical vein grafts have as good, if

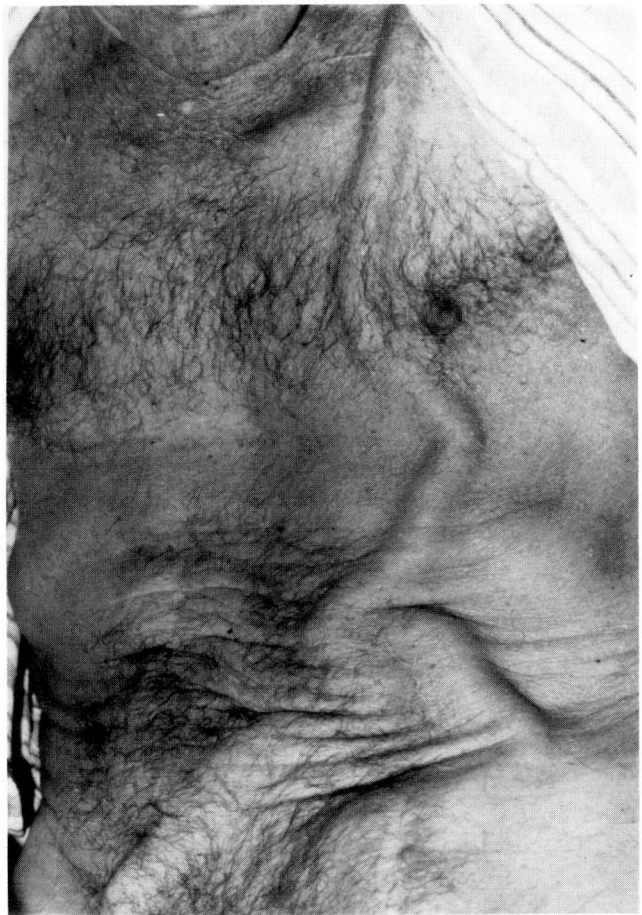

Fig. 14-1. Tortuosity and dilatation of an old knitted
Dacron graft with a false aneurysm in the left groin.

not better, patency rates than PTFE grafts[12] and so it would be reasonable if these
were also employed. Uncontrolled data suggest that knitted, preclotted Dacron
grafts also have comparable patencies.[13, 14] The case exists, therefore, for utilization
of all these materials in claudicants as well as patients requiring limb salvage. In
these patients, however, the long-term patency of the graft becomes of much greater
importance; there is little point in relieving claudication for a year or 18 months,
particularly if this carries any possible additional penalty. The risk of late aneurysmal degeneration of the graft also rises with time in the biograft, though an
aneurysmal graft can usually be replaced.[15]

PENALTIES OF FAILURE

Before it is possible further to evaluate the criteria for insertion of these grafts
the possible penalties of this operation must be carefully considered. Failure of the
graft may cause deterioration in the circulation of the limb, with an increase in

claudication or even amputation. This failure may be due to primary and unexpected thrombosis, sepsis which requires removal of the foreign body, or to the stimulation by the graft of progressive fibromuscular hyperplasia at one or both anastomoses, so that the presence of the graft itself causes deterioration of the arterial tree into which it has been inserted.[16] The first two complications mentioned are obvious, and dreaded by all vascular surgeons. The last, fibromuscular hyperplasia, is less clearly evaluated, but seems to be real and common. If this is the case it has a great bearing upon the site at which one of these grafts should be inserted distally. Were there no risk of causing stenosis and damage to the recipient arterial tree it would be logical to insert the graft into the best artery. If, on the other hand, there is a very real risk of causing further damage to that artery then it would be better if the graft were inserted at the most proximal level, just below the occlusion, so that further occlusion caused by the graft would not have such disastrous consequences, as it would if the graft had been inserted more distally. This applies particularly to grafts for intermittent claudication, and we have recently modified our practice to consider patients for insertion of PTFE or human umbilical vein grafts for intermittent claudication if they have no suitable vein, provided they are fully aware of the risks of the procedure. When these grafts are used they are placed as proximally as possible, in the hope that failure of the graft will not cause circulatory deterioration. This is seldom possible in patients with critical ischaemia as the proximal popliteal segment is frequently highly diseased and we are therefore forced to insert the graft in the distal popliteal artery, or even one of the crural vessels, accepting in these circumstances that failure will almost certainly result in amputation. This would have been inevitable if the operation had not been performed, though the level of amputation might be higher than it would have been if the graft had not been inserted.[17]

RELATIVE CONTRAINDICATIONS TO THE USE OF SYNTHETIC BYPASSES

In addition to these general principles there are certain specific indications in which the insertion of a synthetic graft, if not contraindicated, should be discouraged.

1. When there is a poor chance of its success. In general, the patient with a poor distal runoff, particularly those in whom there is not continuity of the plantar arterial arch,[18] is liable to suffer even worse patency than average. Many studies are in progress at present attempting to evaluate the resistance of the runoff in these patients. Although none has proved to be totally successful their results are encouraging.[19,20] It would be extremely useful if we could decide which patients had the best chance of long-term patency. Clearly grafts should also not be inserted in those patients with compromised proximal arterial trees, in which adequate flowrates cannot be obtained, unless they are simultaneously relieved of this proximal circulatory embarrassment.

2. Synthetic grafts should not be inserted in preference to the use of the autogenous vein, although it has been proposed that, in a patient with a superficial femoral occlusion, an above-knee PTFE graft should be inserted first and the

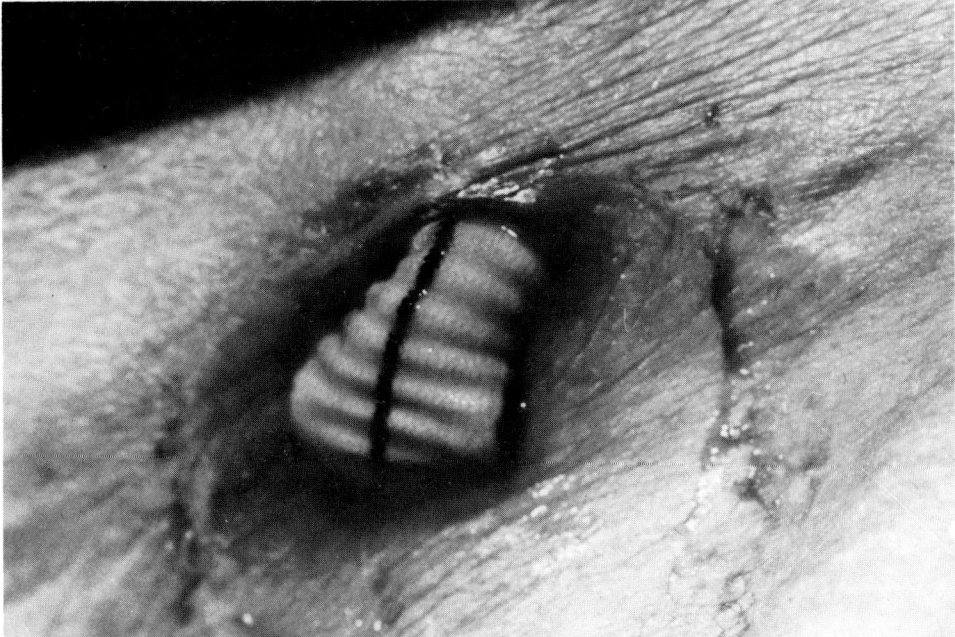

Fig. 14-2. A thrombosed old woven Dacron graft exposed through the skin of the groin.

vein saved either for failure of that graft or for more important bypasses in the future. This philosophy is reasonable if the results of these grafts stand the test of time, the sepsis rate is kept to an acceptable minimum, and they do not cause fibromuscular hyperplasia in the distal vessels.

3. These grafts should not be inserted in the face of flagrant sepsis if any sort of vein bypass is available. Amputation is probably preferable.

4. Previously failed bypass. It is unwise to insert a synthetic bypass in the patient with a bad track record over the insertion of previous bypasses. There is undoubtedly an extraordinary variation between individuals in their receptiveness to these bypasses and the rate at which they undergo unexpected thrombosis and develop distal stenosing fibromuscular hyperplasia. If a patient has already manifested this abnormal response it is unwise to persist with further bypasses, and it may be better to proceed to amputation in critical ischaemia and suggest that the symptoms are tolerated if there is intermittent claudication.

5. Haematological abnormalities. Similarly, it is unwise to operate on a patient with a gross haematological abnormality, such as polycythaemia, thrombocythaemia,[21,22] antithrombin III deficiency, or hyperfibrinogenaemia, if these can be corrected preoperatively.

6. The bed-ridden patient. The place of these bypasses in a nonambulant patient is doubtful. Although he may be spared the psychological trauma of an amputation, the limited patency which they afford is not really acceptable if the patient is not ambulant.

NEW SYNTHETIC BYPASSES

For the reasons outlined at the beginning of this chapter it is extremely difficult to compare bypass materials. Controlled trials are now being published and these, over the next few years, should give us much harder data with which to compare the relative benefits of these prostheses. Surgeons and graft manufacturers continue the search for the "Holy Grail" of an ideal arterial graft, but we are a long way from it. The search has been a rather circular one and the methods by which graft patency may be improved will be discussed in another chapter. Ethical criteria for the release of new vascular prostheses should be improved. It has already become quite clear that, short of a radically different approach in suppression of antigenicity and stabilization of collagen, heterografts, even though stabilized with glutaraldehyde and supported with Dacron, have patency rates which are no better than conventional synthetic tube grafts and suffer from additional hazards related to aneurysm formation.[23,24] I do not believe that any of these grafts should be released, even for

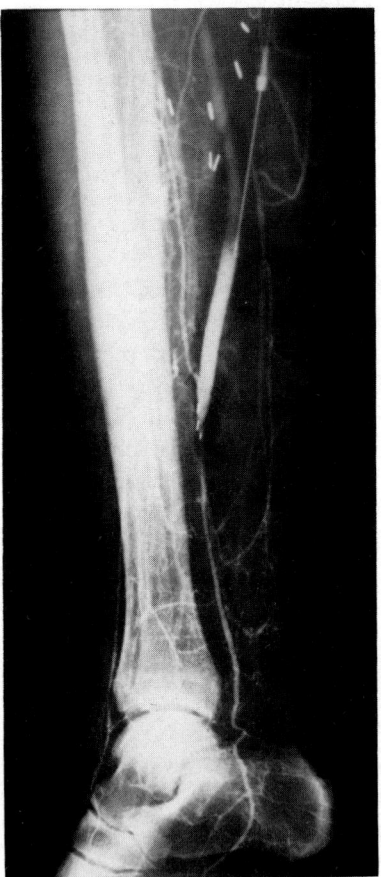

Fig. 14-3. Operative arteriogram of a biograft inserted from the common femoral to posterior tibial artery. This particular graft remains patent four years later.

clinical evaluation, until they have undergone long periods of animal heterograft studies, and subsequent clinical evaluation should be limited to one, or at most two, units for at least *three* years, until they are shown to have a material advantage over cloth grafts (which is highly unlikely). The relative merits of cloth tubes of various sorts are much more subtle and patency figures may be significantly improved by modern endeavours[25-27] such as endothelial seeding techniques and the use of anti-platelet agents. The impregnation of grafts with collagen, although it reduces their porosity and may do away with the need for preclotting, is unlikely, I suspect, to produce major improvements in patency. Collagen is, in itself, slightly thrombo-genic,[28] and this will not improve early patency. In the long term one would expect the collagen graft to be incorporated in a very similar manner to the conventional woven or knitted cloth graft. There is no controlled trial comparing woven with knitted grafts, but anecdotal evidence suggests that knitted grafts below the inguinal ligament have improved patency over woven grafts. There is also no controlled trial comparing Dacron grafts with human umbilical vein grafts or PTFE grafts, and until such a trial is performed we must accept that their results are probably fairly comparable.[13] All these materials produce relatively acceptable patency rates to the upper popliteal artery and, possibly, to the lower popliteal artery, but all of them have unacceptable patency rates to the crural vessels. We have all collected patients who have had a miraculous benefit from one of these grafts in which long-term patency has been achieved, possibly saving the limb for the life of the patient. Against this must be balanced the potentially horrific complications of failure; sepsis, secondary haemorrhage, or conversion to a higher level of amputation with a remnant of infected synthetic graft in the stump.

The controlled trials now in progress will produce some objective evidence of which is the best, or least bad, of the bypasses we have currently available, but even these will not achieve an adequate answer to our dilemma. The primary patency rates of these bypasses may be influenced favourably by adjustments of surgical technique such as composite grafts, patching of the distal anastomosis, or insertion of cuffs of vein at the junction of the anastomosis between the synthetic material and artery. The variety of these techniques, which are finding considerable favour among many surgeons, means that even more trials will be necessary to prove or disprove their value. Similarly, the addition of adjuvant antiplatelet therapy, which has some value in experimental studies in controlling the development of subintimal hyper-plasia,[29, 30] requires careful evaluation. As graft materials appear to vary in the degree to which they promote this fibromuscular hyperplasia[31] separate studies would have to be performed for each of the currently available materials. It will therefore be a long time, if ever, before we know which is the best arterial graft we have available.

OTHER INDICATIONS FOR LOWER LIMB BYPASS

Aneurysms

Aneurysms of the common femoral and popliteal arteries may be successfully replaced using synthetic material rather than vein. Indeed, this may be technically easier, as these patients frequently suffer from arteriomegaly, and end-to-end replacement of the aneurysms may require a conduit of larger diameter than the patient's own saphenous vein. Many patients with aneurysmal disease have extremely good runoff and the flowrate through the reconstruction is therefore high. In these circumstances the patency rates of synthetic bypass are outstanding. In other patients, however, particularly those with popliteal aneurysms, the distal arterial tree has been gradually filling with emboli and the runoff may be very poor. There is no objective evidence in the literature to back this statement, but it would be reasonable in these circumstances to make every effort to utilize a vein rather than synthetic material in their replacement. In my experience it is very unusual in these patients to find a very distal vessel which one could use for a long vein bypass; the distal arterial tree appears to fill sequentially, from the foot upwards, with emboli. For this reason, thrombosis of a popliteal aneurysm may be a disastrous

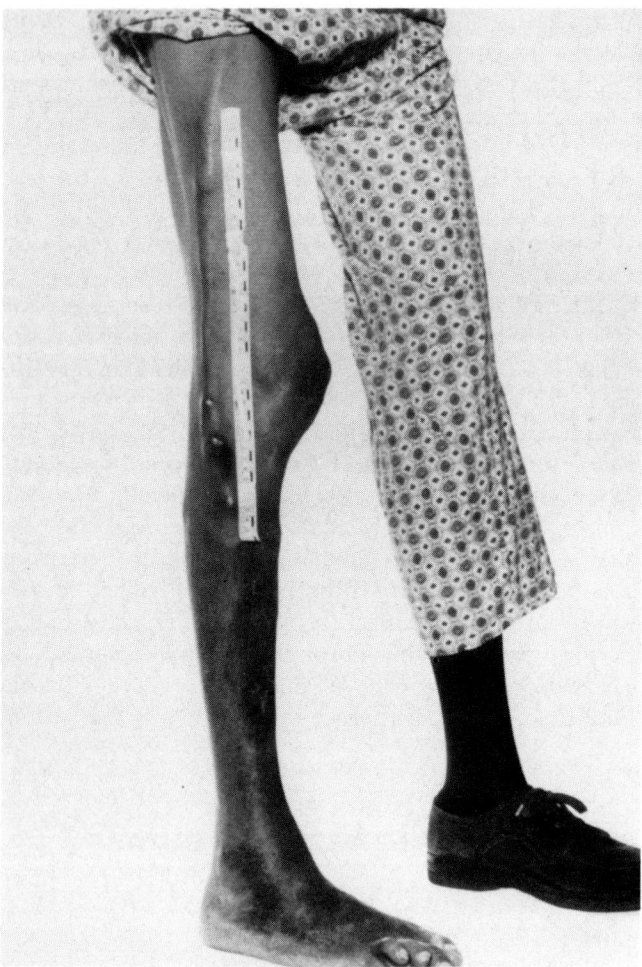

Fig. 14-4A. Aneurysmal degeneration in a biograft two years after insertion from the right common femoral artery to the anterior tibial artery.

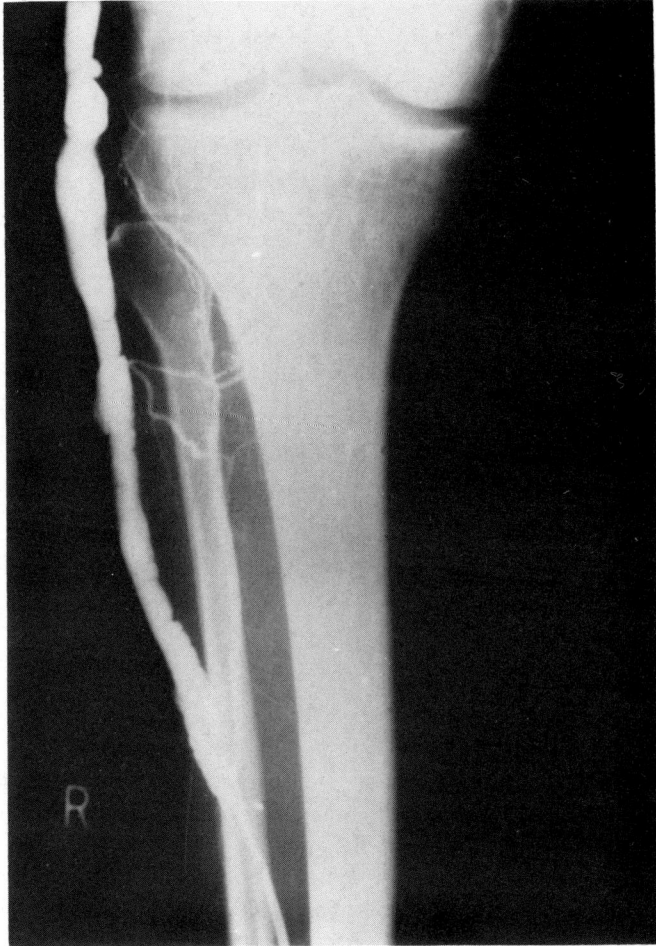

Fig. 14-4B. The angiogram of the aneurysmal graft. The graft was replaced with a similar prosthesis and remains patent 18 months later.

event. The thrombosis tends to occur because of the loss of distal flow and distal thrombectomy is frequently unsatisfactory, as the emboli have been there for some time. In these circumstances adequate runoff cannot be restored and amputation may be inevitable. Vein should be used for any aneurysm distal to the profunda femoris artery when it is available and of adequate calibre as, apart from the possible differences in patency, the use of synthetic material eliminates, to a great extent, the terrors of sepsis.

Trauma

In relatively clean injuries to the vasculature of the lower limb, where there is little or no dead tissue and no contamination, the case may be made for using a synthetic bypass to replace the damaged artery, particularly where there is major

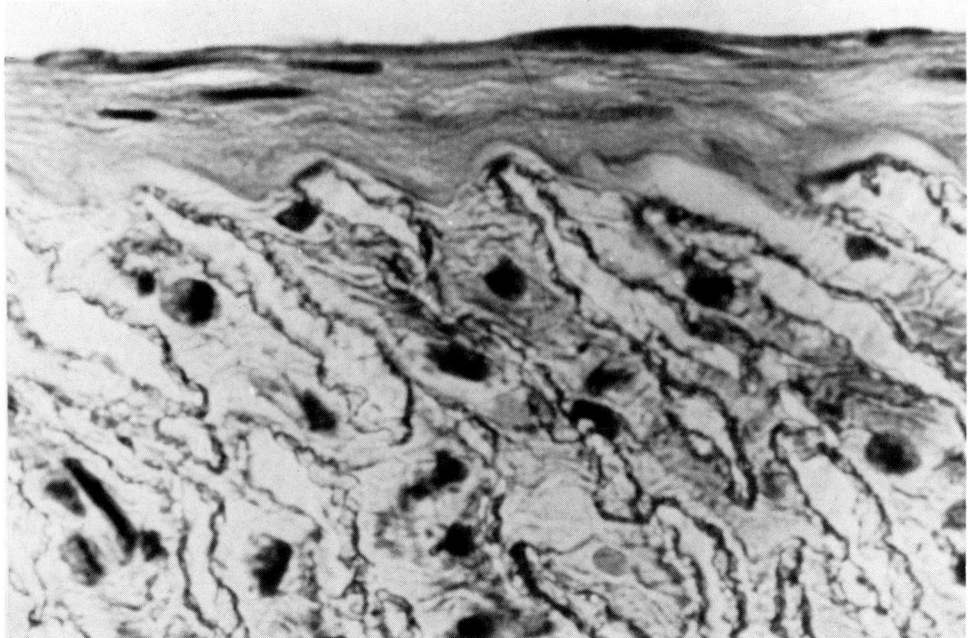

Fig. 14-5. Photomicrograph of an expanded PTFE graft showing well-organized cellularity of its luminal surface.

damage to deep veins and the saphenous vein in that limb should not be removed, to preserve venous collateral. In these circumstances it may be best to harvest the saphenous vein from the other lower limb, to make a composite conduit to replace the damaged deep vein and maintain the saphenous vein in situ in the damaged limb in case the deep venous reconstruction should fail, and to either use a synthetic bypass to replace the artery or, as has been recommended by Wylie, to remove an artery from elsewhere, implant that in the damaged segment, and then use a synthetic bypass in the clean field from which that artery was removed.[32]

CONCLUSION

There may, paradoxically, be a place for the insertion of synthetic bypasses in patients with stable, unremitting intermittent claudication.[33] There is, however, I believe, no place for the insertion of a synthetic bypass in any but a very small number of patients who have critical ischaemia in which a bypass from the distal to popliteal artery is essential, until we can find some method by which we can screen out that very small fraction of the population in whom these grafts will remain patent for more than a year or so. The place of synthetic bypasses to the popliteal artery in critical ischaemia remains to be evaluated. Our practice is now coloured greatly by the prospective study of the definition of critical ischaemia. It is much better to wait and see whether rest pain will be relieved spontaneously or lesions will heal rather than rush precipitously into a bypass which may have highly undesirable consequences. If, however, with the passage of time it is clear that amputation is inevitable the patient has nothing to lose, provided there is a reasonable chance of patency for more than one year, and this depends upon the patient's history and runoff.

REFERENCES

1. DeWeese JA, Rob CG: Autogenous vein graft ten years later. Surgery 82:775–784, 1977
2. Kahn SP, Lindenauer SM, Dent TL, et al: Femorotibial vein bypass. Arch Surg 107:309–312, 1973
3. Nicholas GG, Barker CF, Berkowitz HD, et al: Reconstructive surgery distal to the popliteal trifurcation; effect on the history of arterial occlusive disease. Arch Surg 107:652–656, 1973
4. Szilagyi DE, Elliott JP, Hageman JH, et al: Biologic fate of autologous vein implants as arterial substitutes. Ann Surg 178: 232–248, 1973
5. Leather RP, Shah DM, Karmody AM: Femoropopliteal bypass for limb salvage. Increased patency and utilization of the saphenous vein used in situ. Surgery 196:1000–1008, 1981
6. Boyd MA: The natural course of arteriosclerosis of the lower extremities. Angiology 11:10–15, 1960
7. Little JM: Amputation of the leg—a dull topic revisited. Med J Aust 2:442–451, 1973
8. Kihn RB, Warren R, Beebe GW: The geriatric amputee. Ann Surg 176:305–314, 1972
9. Bergan JJ, Veith FJ, Bernhard VM, et al: Randomization of autogenous vein and poly-tetrafluoroethylene grafts in femoral distal reconstruction. Surgery 92:921–929, 1982
10. Wolfe JHN and the Joint Vascular Research Group: Defining the outcome of critical ischaemia: A one year prospective study. Br J Surg (Abstr) (in press)
11. Report of a working party: The definition of critical ischaemia of a limb. Br J Surg 69(Suppl):2–3, 1982
12. Eickhoff JH, Hansen HJB, Bromme A, et al: A randomized clinical trial of PTFE versus human umbilical vein for femoropopliteal bypass surgery. Br J Surg 70:85–88, 1983
13. Mosley JG, Marston A: A 5 year follow up of Dacron femoropopliteal bypass grafts. Br J Surg 73:24–27, 1986
14. Sauvage LR, Berger K, Davies CC, et al: Composite biosynthetic prosthesis of fibrin and filamentous knitted Dacron for abdominal and lower extremity arterial surgery, in Stanley JC (ed): Biological and Synthetic Prostheses. New York, Grune & Stratton, 1982
15. Layer GT, King RB, Jamieson CW: Early aneurysmal degeneration of human umbilical vein bypass grafts. Br J Surg 71:709–710, 1984
16. DeWeese JA: Anastomotic intimal hyperplasia in vascular grafts, in Sawyer PN, Kadlipp MJ (eds): Vascular Grafts. New York, Appleton Century Crofts, 1978
17. Haimovici H: Failed grafts and level of amputation. J Vasc Surg 2:371–374, 1985
18. O'Mara C, Flinn WR, Bergan JJ: Recognition and surgical management of patent but haemodynamically failed arterial grafts. Arch Surg 193:467–476, 1981
19. Ascer E, Veith FJ, Morin L, et al: Components of vascular outflow resistance and their correlation with graft patency. J Vasc Surg 1:817–828, 1984
20. Parvin SD, Evans DH, Bell PRF: Peripheral resistance measurement in the assessment of severe peripheral arterial disease. Br J Surg 72:751–754, 1985
21. Bouhoutsos J, Morris T, Chavatzas D, Martin P: The influence of haemoglobin and platelet levels on the results of arterial surgery. Br J Surg 61:984–986, 1974
22. Lancet: Familial anti-thrombin III deficiency. Lancet 2:1021–1022, 1983
23. Walden R, L'Italien G, Megerman J: Matched elastic properties and successful arterial grafting. Arch Surg 115:1166–1169, 1980

24. Dale WA, Lewis MR: Further experiences with bovine arterial grafts. Surgery 80:711–716, 1976

25. Herring MB, Dilley R, Gardner AL, et al: Seeding of mechanically derived endothelium on arterial prostheses, in Stanley JC (ed): Biological and Synthetic Vascular Prostheses. New York, Grune & Stratton, 1982

26. Clarke JF, Pittilo RM, Nicholson LJ, et al: Seeding Dacron arterial prostheses with peritoneal mesothelial cells. A preliminary morphological study. Br J Surg 71:492–494, 1984

27. Schmidt SP, Hunter TJ, Falkow Linda, et al: Effects of antiplatelet agents and endothelial cell seeding on small diameter Dacron vascular graft performance in the canine carotid model. J Vasc Surg 2:898–906, 1985

28. Parsonnet V, Tiro AC, Brief DK, et al: The fibrocollagenous tube as a small arterial prosthesis, in Dardick H (ed): Graft Materials in Vascular Surgery. Miami Symposia Specialists, 1978

29. McCann RL, Hagen PO, Fuchs JCA: Aspirin and dipyridamole decrease intimal hyperplasia in experimental vein grafts. Ann Surg 19: 238–243, 1980

30. Harjola PT, Meurala H, Frick MH: Prevention of early reocclusion by dipyridamole and aspirin in arterial reconstructive surgery. J Cardiovasc Surg 22:141–144, 1981

31. Echave V, Koornick AR, Haimov M, et al: Intimal hyperplasia as a complication of the use of polytetrafluoroethylene grafts for femoral popliteal bypass surgery. Surgery 86:791–798, 1979

32. Wylie EJ: Vascular replacement with arterial autografts. Surgery 57:14–21, 1965

33. Sterpetti AV, Schultz RD, Feldhaus RJ, et al: Seven year experience with polytetrafluoroethylene as above knee femoropopliteal bypass graft. J Vasc Surg 2:907–912, 1985

P. R. F. Bell

15

When Are Extra Anatomic Bypasses Indicated?

In general, vascular surgeons prefer to insert bypass grafts in the anatomical position. Sometimes, however, this potentially desirable aim is not possible, usually because the chosen path is not available, is technically too difficult, or the patient is not fit enough to accept what would be a major procedure. Extra anatomic bypasses are usually relatively simpler procedures than the alternative direct operation, and may even be preferable. For these reasons we need to know if extra anatomic bypasses provide better results with fewer complications.

When these techniques were first described they were often intended only as temporary procedures to tide the patient over a difficult situation or to allow an unfit patient to retain a limb until death from some other cause supervened.[1] In modern vascular surgery, therefore, the question of when an extra anatomic bypass is indicated remains difficult to answer, but is best approached by dealing with the different situations in which such bypasses can be placed. Excluding the cerebral circulation and the controversial EC/IC bypass the commonest indications for these procedures are to bypass obstructions in the aortic arch branches, abdominal aorta, or the femoral popliteal trunk. Indications for doing these operations are best discussed with reference to each of these separate areas.

OBSTRUCTION TO BRANCHES OF THE AORTIC ARCH

Occlusion of one of the main arch branches leads to a multiplicity of syndromes depending on the site of obstruction. Occlusion of the origin of the subclavian or innominate artery can, for example, lead to the subclavian steal syndrome and obstruction of the carotid origin can lead to hypoperfusion or embolic states affecting the brain (Fig. 15-1). Such lesions can be dealt with in a number of ways. They can be approached directly by median sternotomy and endarterectomy or bypass of the affected vessel. This approach is entirely acceptable and the results are

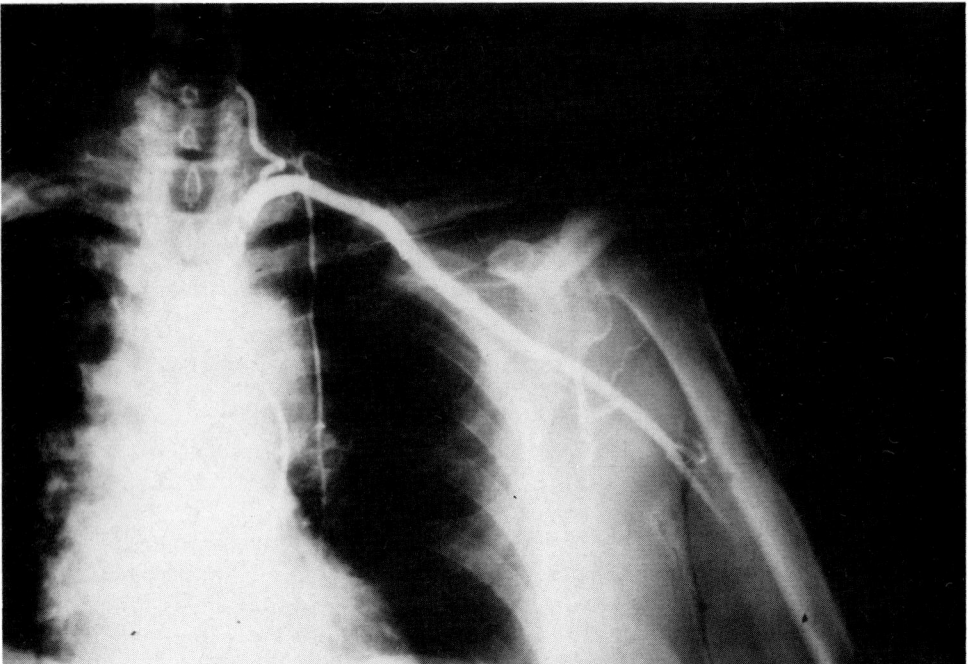

Fig. 15-1. Arteriogram showing severe stenosis of the left subclavian artery.

good.[2, 3] The operation is, however, a major one and in patients who may be suffering from widespread arterial disease and respiratory problems is not always justifiable. For multiple occlusions or stenoses of the arch vessels, particularly if all of them are affected, then a median stenotomy with an extra anatomic bypass from the aortic arch with anastomosis to the various vessels is essential as there is no simple alternative. For unilateral occlusion of the subclavian or carotid origin the options are an axillo-axillary bypass,[4] subclavian bypass,[5] carotid-subclavian bypass,[6] or a direct approach to the aortic arch.[7] These approaches are summarized in Fig. 15-2. The operation decided upon will depend upon the experience of the surgeon, the condition of the patient, and the long-term results with each procedure.

Examining the literature and assessing the results of a number of publications, a definite decision about when an extra anatomic or direct approach should be used is difficult, principally because strictly comparative trials have not been done. Looking at the three areas under discussion, examination of comparative operative mortality, morbidity, and long-term patency, is therefore the best that can be achieved. Mortality rates in experienced hands are low for both procedures, varying from 0 to 2% (Table 15-1). Morbidity in general appears to be slightly higher for the direct approach, but long-term patency is excellent whichever procedure is undertaken[7–11] (Table 15-1).

Where does this then leave us in trying to answer our original question in relation to the aortic arch? It would seem that both operations are safe and produce very good long-term results. The theoretical danger of graft sepsis is small and extra anatomic operations are generally quicker and more straightforward to perform. As a result it would seem reasonable to suggest that the extra anatomic procedures are

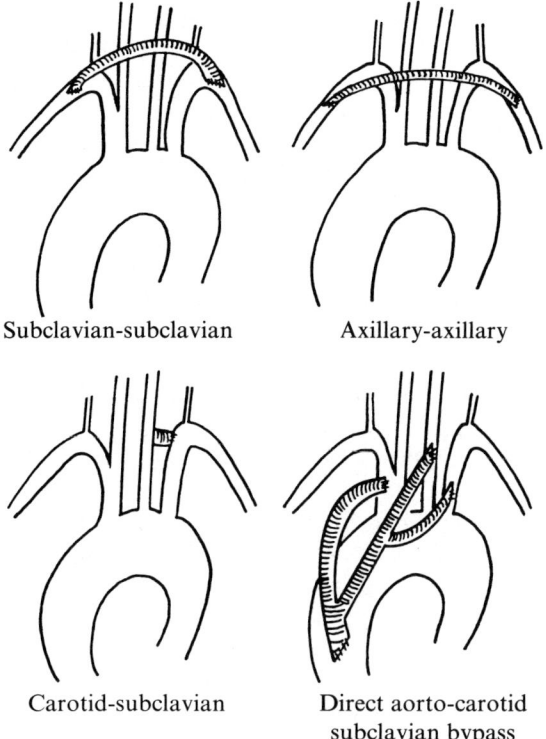

Subclavian-subclavian   Axillary-axillary

Carotid-subclavian   Direct aorto-carotid
                          subclavian bypass

Fig. 15-2. Various anatomic approaches to occlusion of aortic arch branches.

to be preferred in this area. The next question is which operation should be used? In general extra anatomic bypasses do not remove the source of emboli if this is a presenting feature, particularly if transient ischaemic attacks are occurring. In such cases proximal ligation of the artery is advisable in addition to the bypass. Even when this is done, however, certain procedures such as axillary-axillary grafts are not acceptable in patients with cerebrovascular symptoms.[12] Direct anastomosis of the subclavian artery to the common carotid has produced very good results and

Table 15-1
Results of Extra Anatomic Bypass Procedures for
Obstruction of Aortic Arch Branches

Author	Type	Mortality (%)	Morbidity (%)	Patency (%)
Schlosser 1982[7]	EA	0	2	95
	A	2	9	96
Connolly et al 1984[11]	EA	0	2	90
Posner et al 1983[8]	EA	2	3	88
Myers et al 1979[9]	EA	0	—	76
Bentley et al 1982[10]	EA	0	3	80

EA = extra anatomic, A = anatomic, % Patency 1–10 years.

may be the procedure of choice.[13] Our own experience over a 10-year period with these relatively uncommon procedures confirms the view that extra anatomic bypass is the operation of choice in this area. Nine subclavian-subclavian procedures have been performed with no operative mortality, one patient suffered persistent pain in the arm, and graft patency between one and nine years has been 96%. In general Dacron grafts are adequate for the procedure but PTFE is useful, particularly in females where small vessels may have to be used.

PROCEDURES TO CIRCUMVENT OBSTRUCTION OF THE ABDOMINAL AORTA

Although extra anatomic grafts can be used under rare circumstances for problems in the thoracic aorta[14] the main indications relate to obstruction of the abdominal aorta. In this situation where surgery is being performed for severe claudication or limb-threatening ischaemia, the ideal procedure would appear to be some form of direct surgery between the aorta and the femoral vessels which has been shown to be effective with excellent long-term patency.[15] The difficulty arises in older patients where the risks of a transperitoneal operation may be higher. In this situation an extra anatomic bypass procedure between one axillary artery and the femorals is an attractive proposition.[16] The alternative in a patient with a total occlusion is some form of retroperitoneal approach to the aorta. Unfortunately no trial has been performed to compare transperitoneal, retroperitoneal, and axillofemoral grafts in such patients at risk. Some vascular surgeons firmly believe that in view of the good results obtained with a direct transperitoneal approach the matter is not a question of whether the patient is fit but whether the anaesthetist is able to keep the patient in a reasonable condition to take the procedure. Bearing in mind the availability of modern anaesthesia, we have to examine the comparative results of aorto-femoral grafting and axilla-bifemoral procedures in these patients. There is no doubt that transperitoneal bifurcated grafts do well in the long term, with patency rates well over 80% at five years.[15, 17]

This being the case, is the use of an axillo-bifemoral graft to bypass aortic obstruction ever justified? The results of axillo-femoral grafting vary considerably from paper to paper but most authors agree that the outcome for unilateral axillofemoral procedures is relatively poor and these should, if possible, be avoided.[18] There are, however, recent dissenters from this view who claim that an aggressive approach with unilateral grafts paying attention to inflow, outflow, and early unblocking in the event of occlusion can provide comparable results.[19] Axillobifemoral grafts perform better in general with two-year patency rates of 75%,[18] but the results beyond this time do not compare favourably with aorto-femoral grafts.[18-23]

Although mortality from the transperitoneal procedure used to be signficant, modern anaesthesia has largely eliminated the difference.[15] Although extra anatomic grafting in this situation does produce reasonable short-term results (Table 15-2) the operation should probably be limited to patients in whom the risk of laparotomy is held to be excessive. In such situations a decision would be reached between the anaesthetist and the surgeon as to which operation should be performed.

Table 15-2
Results of Uni- and Bilateral Axillo-
Femoral Grafting

Author	Type	% Patency 2 years
Ascer et al 1985[19]	U	71
	B	77
Blaisdell et al 1982[18]	U	50
	B	75
Ward et al 1983[22]	U	67
	B	86
Burrell et al 1982[21]	U	62
	B	73
Bergqvist et al 1984[23]	Mixed	50

U = unilateral, B = bilateral.

A comparison between axillo-bifemoral and retroperitoneal bifurcated grafts[24,25] in our own institution has, however, shown the latter to be inferior, probably because of limited access to the diseased distal aorta, emphasizing that a transperitoneal procedure is the operation of choice. The axillo-bifemoral graft probably comes into its own where an aortic bifurcated graft has to be removed because of infection. Many publications have described its successful use in such a situation.[26-28] Even with this approach, however, there is a significant mortality[29] and it may be that in a case of minor sepsis, particularly where there is a small

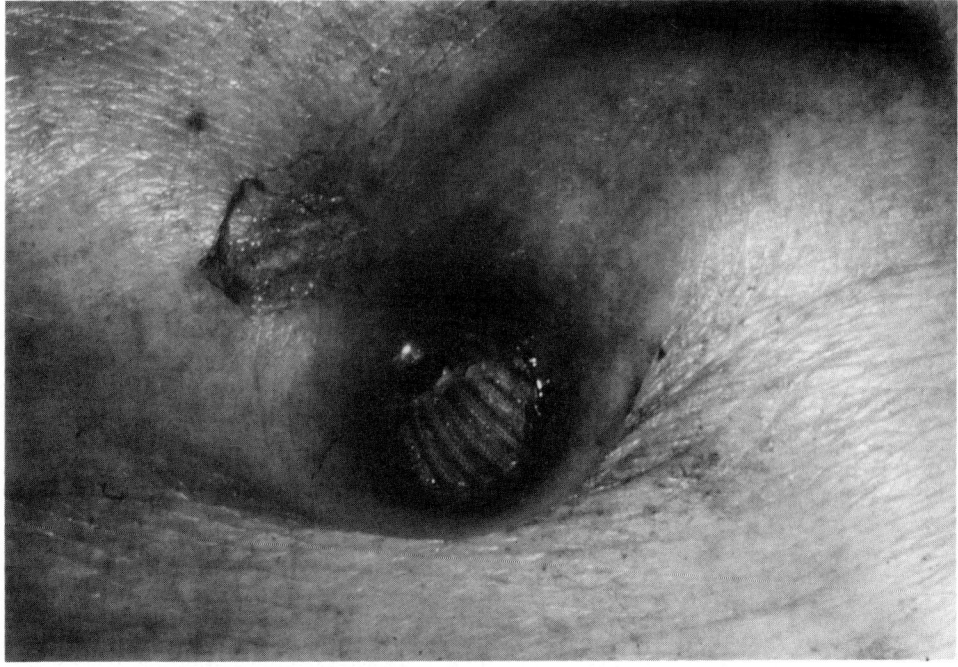

Fig. 15-3. Axillo-femoral graft ulcerating through the skin.

duodenal perforation, local repair will suffice. Where there is major sepsis with pus then the only sensible option is to remove the graft and carry out an axillo-bifemoral procedure. These grafts can, however, cause other problems which include ulceration to the skin (Fig. 15-3), particularly in thin patients, or embolisation with risk to the arm following thrombosis.[30] A steal syndrome with ischaemia to the donor arm rarely occurs in these poor-risk patients. Axillo-unifemoral grafts should probably not be performed, a better option being a cross-over or ilio-femoral graft. Axillo-bifemoral grafts should be limited to poor-risk patients where anaesthesia is a severe risk or where an infected graft has to be removed. In this situation the results of limb salvage in our own institution have been acceptable.[31] A proper trial to compare mortality, morbidity, and the results in comparable patients, however, remains to be done. Unfortunately, the existing results are biased against axillo-bifemoral grafts which tend to be performed in older, poor-risk patients with more advanced disease.

UNILATERAL ILIAC DISEASE

Most patients presenting with arterial symptoms have bilateral disease. A substantial minority do, however, present with unilateral iliac stenosis or occlusion (Fig. 15-4) and a significant number will respond to angioplasty.[32] For the remain-

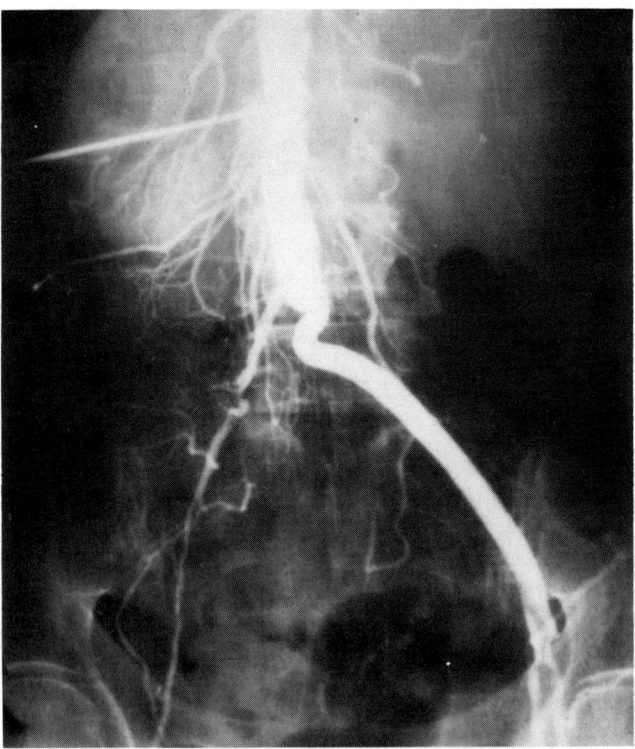

Fig. 15-4. Arteriogram showing a patient with an occluded limb of an aorto-femoral bifurcation shaft suitable for a femoro-femoral cross-over graft.

der, the option lies between an ilio-femoral graft, a unilateral axillo-femoral graft, endarterectomy, or an extra anatomic cross-over femoro-femoral graft. The extra anatomic procedure was popularised in 1962 for the poor-risk patient.[33] The results have been good with five-year patency rates of 60% rising to 90% in patients who successfully stopped smoking.[11,34] The application of this technique to patients with moderate claudication has also produced excellent long-term patency with a low mortality and morbidity.[35-37] The results are therefore very good but two problems remain. The surgeon should be sure to undertake some form of inflow study to make certain that the flow from the donor limb is adequate. In our own institution the papaverine pressure test is used for this purpose, a pressure drop of 20% suggesting an inadequate donor vessel.[38,39] The other problem relates to anxiety about the consequences of graft sepsis, which could be disastrous. For this reason there has been a resurgence of interest in the unilateral retroperitoneal ilio-femoral graft which has many advantages, particularly on the left side, and it remains to be seen if this approach becomes more popular. An extra anatomic graft in unilateral iliac disease is therefore an excellent option even in patients with moderate disease. A comparative study between ilio-femoral grafting and an extra anatomic procedure in such patients needs to be done as the choice still rests between these two excellent alternatives. A theoretical problem with the femoro-femoral graft is ischaemia of the donor limb due to a steal syndrome. Although this occurs to a small degree it is not a serious problem,[36] but might become so if the indications are extended to fitter more active subjects.

EXTRA ANATOMIC PROCEDURES DISTAL TO THE FEMORAL ARTERY

In general, revascularisation of the popliteal or distal tibial, peroneal arteries is by the anatomic route. Examples of extra anatomic grafts include in situ saphenous vein grafting (strictly extra anatomic in one sense but not in another), subcutaneous grafts to the distal vessels, and procedures used to circumvent an infected femoral graft. Of these three examples, the in situ graft is the least controversial. Although the operation was originally described in 1962[40] its popularity waned until recently. Results, particularly when the graft is used to the popliteal and distal tibial arteries, have been excellent[41-43] and it is now the graft of choice in such patients, other materials only being used if it is not available.[44] The alternatives to the in situ graft are PTFE and human umbilical vein. Although good results have been published for PTFE[45] and human umbilical vein,[46] in general the results with such materials for distal procedures are relatively poor.[44] If the umbilical vein is used to vessels below the knee then subcutaneous placement to any of the three lower limb arteries has been described.[47] This route has the advantage that the graft can be easily seen and also allows accurate placement, which is very important with the friable umbilical vein, the position of which cannot be altered once the tunneler has been removed. The route does have disadvantages, however, including ulceration of the graft through the skin with infection, thrombosis, and haemorrhage (Fig. 15-5). For this reason the anatomic route is in general to be preferred.

Finally, in situations where a femoral graft or one limb of a bifurcated graft has become infected removal of the appropriate piece of graft material, closure of the

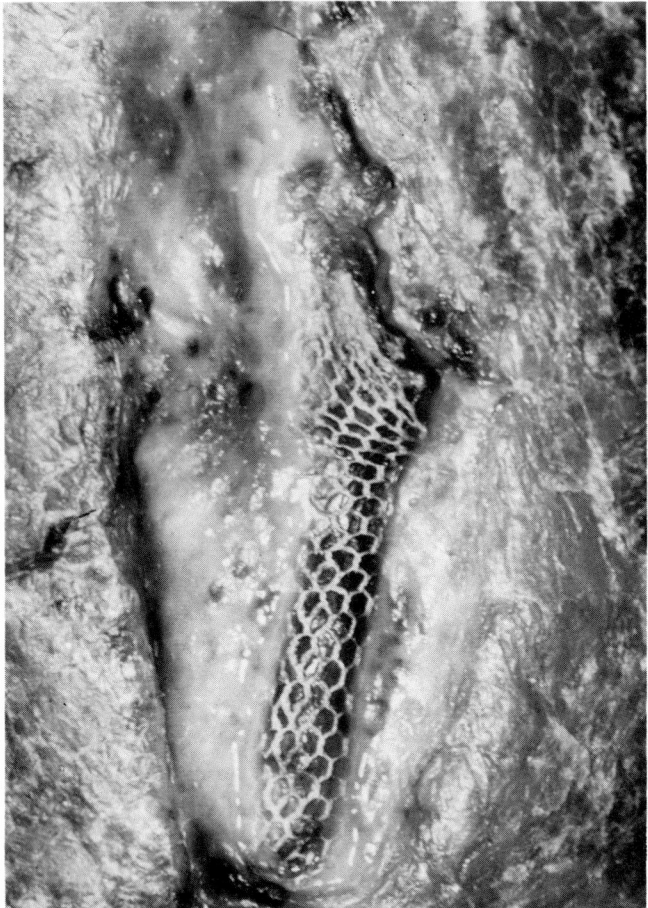

Fig. 15-5. Subcutaneously placed umbilical vein graft ulcerating through the skin.

groin wound, and grafting from the existing graft above the inguinal ligament to the
popliteal artery by the obturator foramen[48,49] (Fig. 15-6), the lateral ilio-popliteal
route,[50] or occasionally by the transperitoneal route using a donor vessel from the
other leg[51] should be considered.

In relation to the three areas discussed we can answer the question originally
posed in the following way. For obstruction of the aortic arch vessels, extra anatomic procedures give good results and should usually be the procedure of choice.
For obstruction of the aorta a transperitoneal bifurcated graft is the procedure of
choice except where there is serious infection or where the patient is held to be unfit
for an appropriate anaesthetic when an axillo-bifemoral graft should be inserted.
For unilateral iliac disease where angioplasty is not applicable, an extra anatomic
cross-over graft gives excellent results but needs to be compared further with the
unilateral ilio-femoral procedure. In the lower limb the "extra anatomic" in situ
graft is the operation of choice for anastomoses below the knee. Other extra anatomic grafts should probably not be used in this location because of the tendency to

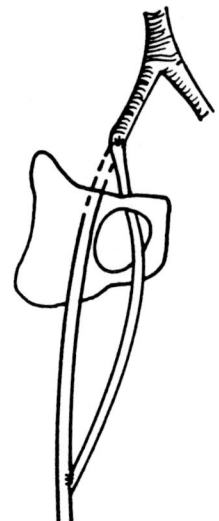

Fig. 15-6. Ilio-popliteal graft utilising the obturator foramen.

ulcerate. Finally, extra anatomic grafts through the obturator foramen to the popliteal artery or the ilio-popliteal route are an excellent method of saving the limb where severe groin sepsis is present.

REFERENCES

1. Blaisdell FW, Hall AD: Axillary-femoral artery bypass for lower limb extremity ischaemia. Surgery 54:563, 1962
2. Lusby RJ, Ehrenfeld WK: The direct approach to the great vessels, in Greenhalgh R (ed): Extra Anatomic and Secondary Arterial Reconstruction. London, Pitman, 1982, p 266
3. Natali J, Kieffer E: Revascularisation of the supra aortic trunks from the thoracic aorta, in Greenhalgh R (ed): Extra Anatomic and Secondary Arterial Reconstruction. London, Pitman, 1982, p 277
4. Myers WO, Lawton BR, Sautter RD: Axillo-axillary bypass graft. JAMA 217:826, 1971
5. Finkelstein NM, Byer A, Russ BF Jr: Subclavian-subclavian bypass for the subclavian steal syndrome. Surgery 71:142, 1972
6. Diethrich EB, Garrett HE, Ameriso J, et al: Occlusive disease of the common carotid and subclavian arteries treated by carotid subclavian bypass. Am J Surg 114:800, 1967
7. Schlosser V: Subclavian steal syndrome correction by transthoracic or extra anatomic repair, in Greenhalgh R (ed): Extra Anatomic and Secondary Arterial Reconstruction. London, Pitman, 1982, p 291
8. Posner M, Riles TS, Ramirez AA, et al: Axillo-axillary bypass for symptomatic stenosis of the subclavian artery. Am J Surg 145:644, 1983
9. Myers WO, Lawton BR, Ray F, et al: Axillo-axillary bypass for subclavian steal syndrome. Arch Surg 114:394, 1979
10. Bentley F, Hollier LH, Batson RC: Axillo-axillary bypass for subclavian and inominate artery revascularisation. Am J Surg 48:70, 1982

11. Connolly JE, Kwaan JH, Brownell D, et al: Newer developments of extra anatomic bypass. SGO 158:415, 1984
12. Wylie EJ, Stoney RJ, Ehrenfeld WK, et al: Manual and Vascular Surgery. New York: Springer-Verlag, 1981, p 1
13. Edwards WH, Mulherin JL: The surgical approach to significant stenosis of vertebral and subclavian arteries. Surgery 87:20, 1980
14. Kieffer E, Natali J: Ascending aorto-abdominal aorto bypass—Technical considerations, indications and report of 15 patients, in Greenhalgh R (ed): Extra Anatomic and Secondary Arterial Reconstruction. London, Pitman, 1982, p 313
15. Brewster DC: Aorto iliac occlusive disease, in Bell PRF, Tilney N (eds): Vascular Surgery. London, Butterworth, 1984, p 78
16. Sauvage LR, Wood SJ: Unilateral axillary bilateral femoral bifurcation graft. A procedure for the poor risk patient with aorto iliac disease. Surgery 60:573, 1966
17. Pierce GE, Turrentine M, Stringfeld S, et al: Evaluation of end to side v end to end proximal anastomosis in aorto bifemoral bypass. Arch Surg 117:1580, 1982
18. Blaisdell FW, Holcroft FW, Ward RE: Axillo femoral and femoro-femoral bypass. History and evolution of technique, in Greenhalgh R (ed): Extra Anatomic and Secondary Arterial Reconstruction. London, Pitman, 1982, p 84
19. Ascer E, Veith FJ, Gupta SK, et al: Comparison of axillo unifemoral and axillo bifemoral bypass operations. Surgery 97:169, 1985
20. Corbett RR, Taylor PR, Chilvers A, et al: Axillo femoral bypass grafts in poor risk patients with critical ischaemia. Ann R Coll Surg Engl 66:170, 1984
21. Burrell MJ, Wheeler JR, Gregory RT, et al: Axillo femoral bypass: A ten year review. Ann Surg 195:796, 1982
22. Ward RE, Holcroft JW, Conti S, et al: New concepts in the use of axillo femoral bypass grafts. Arch Surg 118:573, 1983
23. Bergqvist D, Bergentz SE, Ericsson BF, et al: Extra anatomic vascular reconstruction in patients with aorto iliac arteriosclerosis. Acta Chir Scand 150:205, 1984
24. Rob C: Extra peritoneal approach to the abdominal aorta. Surgery 53:87, 1963
25. Helsby R, Moosa AR: Aorto-iliac reconstruction with special reference to the extra peritoneal approach. Br J Surg 62:596, 1975
26. Baker JD: Axillo profunda bypass for the management of an infected aorto femoral graft. Vasc Surg 17:63, 1983
27. Trout HH, Kozloff L, Giordano JM: Priority of revascularisation in patients with graft enteric fistulas, infected arteries or infected prostheses. Ann Surg 199:669, 1984
28. Casali RE, Tucker WE, Thompson BW, et al: Infected prosthetic grafts. Arch Surg 115:577, 1980
29. Reilly LM, Altman H, Lusby RJ, et al: Late results following surgical management of vascular graft infection. J Vasc Surg 1:36, 1984
30. Hartman AR, Fried KS, Khalil I, et al: Late axillary artery thrombosis in patients with occluded axillary femoral bypass grafts. J Vasc Surg 2:285, 1985
31. Quinton DN, Barrie WW: Extra anatomic grafts for limb salvage. J R Coll Surg Ed 29:158, 1984
32. Harrington DP: Percutaneous transluminal angioplasty—A review, in Bell PRF, Tilney N (eds): Vascular Surgery. London, Butterworth, 1984, p 145
33. Vetto RM: The treatment of unilateral iliac artery obstruction with a transabdominal subcutaneous femero femoral graft. Surgery 52:342, 1962
34. Lamerton A, Nicolaides AN, Kenyon JR, et al: Selection for and long term results of femoro femoral bypass, in Greenhalgh R (ed): Extra Anatomic and Secondary Arterial Reconstruction. London, Pitman, 1982, p 96
35. Brief DK, Brenner BJ, Alpert J, et al: Cross over femoro femoral grafts: Compromise or preference. A reappraisal. Arch Surg 105:889, 1972

36. Harris JP, Flinn WR, Rudo WD, et al: Assessment of donor limb haemodynamics in femoro femoral bypass for claudication. Surgery 90:764, 1981

37. Dick LS, Brief DK, Alpert J, et al: A twelve year experience with femoro femoral cross over grafts. Arch Surg 115:1359, 1980

38. Quin RO, Evans DH, Bell PRF: Haemodynamic assessment of the aorto iliac segment. J Cardiovasc Surg 16:586, 1975

39. Macpherson DS, Evans DH, Bell PRF: Common femoral artery Doppler waveforms: A comparison of three methods of objective analysis with direct pressure measurement. Br J Surg 71:46, 1984

40. Hall KV: The great saphenous vein used "in situ" as an arterial shunt after exterpation of the vein valves. Surgery 51:492, 1962

41. Leather RP, Karmody AM: In situ saphenous vein for arterial bypass, in Stanley JC (ed): Biologic and Synthetic Vascular Prostheses. New York, Grune & Stratton, 1982, p 351

42. Leather RP, Shah DM, Karmody AM: Femoropopliteal arterial bypass for limb salvage. Increased patency and utilisation of the saphenous vein used in situ. Surgery 190:1000, 1981

43. Hall KV, Rostad H: In situ vein bypass in the treatment of femoro popliteal atherosclerotic disease. A ten year study. Am J Surg 136:158, 1978

44. Bell PRF: Are distal vascular procedures worthwhile? Br J Surg 72:335, 1985

45. Gupta SK, Veith FJ: Three year experience with expanded polytetrafluoroethylene arterial grafts for limb salvage. Am J Surg 140:214, 1980

46. Dardik H: In Bell PRF, Tilney N (eds): Vascular Surgery. London, Butterworths, 1984, p 108

47. Dardik H, Ibrahim IM, Sussman B, et al: Indications and critical factors for the success of lower extremity bypass in the subcutaneous position, in Greenhalgh R (ed): Extra Anatomic and Secondary Arterial Reconstruction. London, Pitman, 1982, p 368

48. Van-Det RJ, Brands LC: The obturator foramen bypass: An alternative procedure in iliofemoral artery revascularisation. Surgery 89:543, 1981

49. Erath HG, Gale SS, Smith BM, et al: Obturator foramen grafts—The preferable alternative route. Am J Surg 48:65, 1982

50. Trout HH, Smith CA: Lateral iliopopliteal arterial bypass as an alternative to obturator bypass. Am J Surg 48:63, 1982

51. Taylor RSF, Massouth F: The transperitoneal graft. An alternative for femoro femoral bypass, in Greenhalgh R (ed): Extra Anatomic and Secondary Arterial Reconstruction. London, Pitman, 1982, p 237

Allan D. Callow

16

The "Tissue Culture" Arterial Graft—How Soon?

The desire to develop a biologic arterial graft made up entirely of living tissues of the same cell lines and with close to identical functions as the human artery is prompted by the increasing realization that a satisfactory small-caliber substitute is not available. The high initial patency rate seen in large vessels such as the aorta has not been duplicated in a more critical small-vessel location, such as below the knee. The five-year patency rate of the reversed autogenous saphenous vein is approximately 50% in the femoro-popliteal position, and less than half of that when a synthetic tube is utilized in the same location.[1,2] Even the much shorter reversed saphenous vein in the aorto-coronary position undergoes thrombosis at the rate of 20–25% during the first year, and as much as 2–4% per year thereafter. At 10 years, approximately 50% of these grafts have failed.[3]

Contemporary reconstructive arterial surgery is based upon the use of biologically inert, nonresorbable, synthetic polymer tubes introduced by Blakemore and Voorhees in 1952, who noted that synthetic fabric tubes implanted in the canine aorta for up to 153 days became covered by a glistening intima-like coat.[4] Ignoring the complex anatomic and physiologic characteristics of the artery and with no experimental efforts to study and duplicate them, innovative surgeons sought and found fabrics which could serve as a blood conduit, conceptually at least, the simplest function of the human artery.

The ability to transport blood, limited to a narrow range of hemodynamic variables, is the only quality the synthetic arterial conduit shares with the normal, live human artery. They remain a foreign body for life, as evidenced by their failure in the human to develop an endothelial lining and to maintain a biologically stable, anastomotic zone which remains free of stenosing cellular proliferation (Fig. 16-1).

"No material so far developed is completely passive to blood when implanted within the vasculature."[5] From what are possibly the most extensive investigations of the reactions of synthetic materials implanted in the human arterial tree, Anderson suggests that the first event when blood contacts the graft is the adsorption of several proteins, fibrinogen, albumin, gamma globulin, and fibronectin on the

VASCULAR SURGERY: ISSUES IN CURRENT PRACTICE
ISBN 0-8089-1839-7

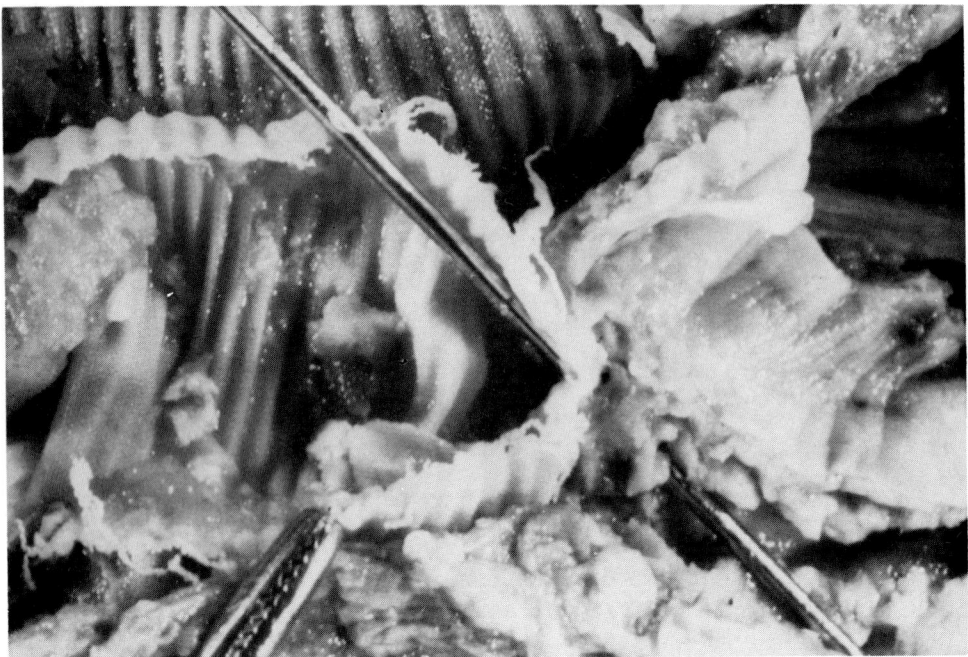

Fig. 16-1. Crimped Dacron aortic bifurcation graft recovered at operation, showing fragments of avulsed and discontinuous "neointima" hyperplasia.

surface of the polymer,[6] followed by platelet adhesion, and then "pavementing" of leukocytes.[7] Platelet activation and release of the granules may be accompanied by activation of the coagulation system and fibrin formation. Because blood does not control the entire reaction, a great deal of investigative effort has been expended upon various modifications of the graft. Nevertheless, the fundamental defects in fabric tubes have not been corrected by modifications in surface characteristics, and textile composition and fabrication, despite claims to the contrary. In the critical small-vessel location, all grafts in current use are essentially equal in terms of clinical applications and limitations.

Because of the role of platelets in activation of the coagulation process, numerous investigations with antiplatelet agents have been reported. Increased vein graft patency in the aorto-coronary position was reported by Chesebro,[8] but a similar regimen in the hands of others did not.[9, 10] Whether the discrepancy is due to hypercoagulation and platelet activation during the critical perioperative period in some but not all patients, as suggested by McDaniel and coworkers,[11] is unknown, but no clear-cut beneficial effect on either short- or long-term patency rates of antiplatelet drugs has been consistently noted.[12–17] In the canine carotid experimental model, Sharp and his coworkers reported significantly better mean patencies of endothelial seeded double-velour Dacron grafts in antiplatelet medicated dogs than in endothelial cell seeded grafts from nonmedicated dogs.[18, 19] Despite occasional reports of success, the use of antiplatelet agents in small-caliber prostheses in the clinical setting has not improved long-term patency rates.

The major cause of intermediate and late graft failure appears to be the development of a hyperplastic response at the anastomotic line. Modified fibroblasts, modified endothelial cells, and smooth muscle cells have been identified within the thickened "pseudointima."[20–22] Even in the vein graft in the rabbit model, endothelial cells continue to proliferate for up to 12 weeks, and because of the accumulation of smooth muscle cells and extracellular matrix, the wall continues to thicken.[23] Thus, not only is the synthetic graft unsatisfactory in low-flow, high-resistance situations, but so is the autogenous vein with its relatively intact intima (Fig. 16-2).

Endothelial cells have become available for the seeding of synthetic prostheses as a result of the huge growth of tissue culture technology in the past decade. Uncertain results of these experimental efforts with seeded grafts have been reported in terms of improved short- and long-term patency rates.[24, 25] Some of the experiments were of poor experimental design and the results of others reflected in the bias of the investigator.[18, 19, 26–29] Not only has there been no clear-cut evidence of improved long-term patency but insofar as the human endothelial cell is concerned, no incontrovertible data have been provided confirming actual growth of the endothelial cell within the graft despite positive findings on tissue culture ware. Despite the experience with the canine model, there is no evidence that the human endothelial cell continues to grow, to replicate, to replace dead or dying cells, and to perform all the functions the endothelial cell does perform in its normal milieu. However, inasmuch as these functions occur predominantly in the microenvironment of the microvasculature rather than in large elastic and muscular arteries, their absence in the seeded graft may not matter. All that may be required is that the endothelial cell retain its nonthrombogenic monolayer and aid in suppression of smooth muscle cell proliferation and anastomotic hyperplasia.

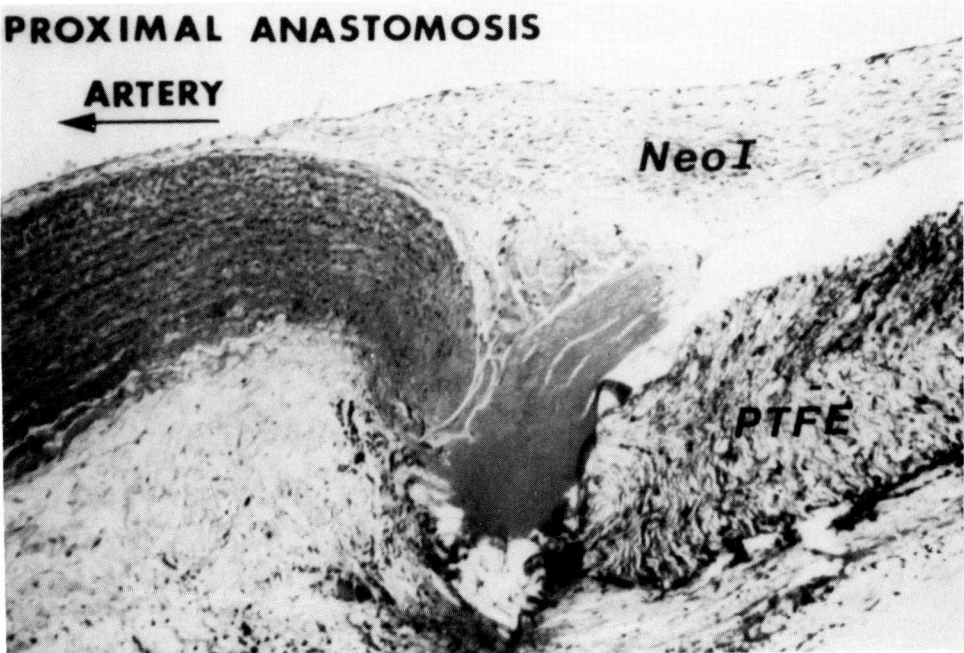

Fig. 16-2. ePTFE graft removed one month after implantation showing the host artery to the left, the ePTFE graft to the right, and a neointimal proliferating response extending from the normal artery across the anastomotic line on the surface of the ePTFE graft.

The observation that platelets continue to demonstrate their most intensive adhesion reaction in the area of the host–graft junction for long after implantation[30,31] focused attention upon the hyperplastic reaction seen at the anastomosis (Fig. 16-3).[32–34] Compliance mismatch of graft and artery[35] and the rheology of flow through anastomoses came under close experimental scrutiny.[36]

In a baboon model, Clowes and coworkers[37] noted that endothelium and smooth muscle cells, presumably derived from the cut end of adjacent artery, formed a new intima and migrated together along the luminal surface of an ePTFE graft.[23] In animals with a less porous graft, for example, 30 μm PTFE, healing was accomplished by the slow ingrowth of endothelium and smooth muscle cells from the cut edges of adjacent arteries. These cell types were identified by morphologic analysis only. In more porous grafts, for example, 60 μm PTFE, the process of new intima formation took place along the entire length of the graft by ingrowth through the graft wall of capillaries containing endothelial and smooth muscle cells. Whether these events occur in the human is unknown. Although it seemed evident that the smooth muscle cell was the principal connective tissue cell in the intima of these grafts, questions remain as to their origin, their method of proliferation, and the regulation of their accumulation. The authors conclude that: (1) endothelium upon the graft does not stop proliferating even when it has reached the confluent state; (2) chronic endothelial proliferation implies chronic endothelial injury; (3) graft "intima" is formed by the proliferation of the smooth muscle cell; and (4) smooth muscle cells proliferate acutely and chronically underneath the endothelial layer and not only in regions lacking endothelium.

Although it is known that platelets contain several smooth muscle cell mito-

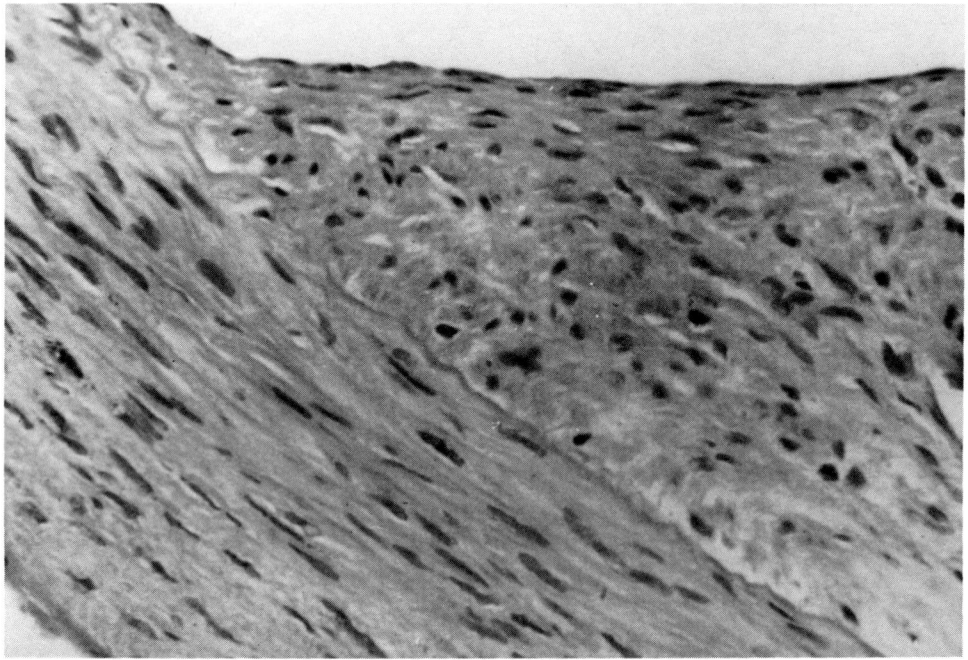

Fig. 16-3. Hyperplastic response. Courtesy of Dr Peter Madras.

gens, suggesting that smooth muscle proliferation in the injured artery is regulated by platelet products, most of the smooth muscle cell proliferation in vascular grafts occurs in endothelialized regions where platelet adherence accumulation is not evident.[38] Platelets do, however, accumulate in neighboring denuded regions.[39] Endothelial cells in vitro produce several smooth muscle cell mitogens and one of these appears to be identical to the platelet-derived growth factor.[40,42] In addition, under limited circumstances, smooth muscle cells appear to make PDGF.[43] This secretion is further stimulated if the endothelial cells are also in some fashion injured or otherwise stimulated. It is a short step from these observations to the speculation that the endothelial cells at the artery–graft junction may be subjected to chronic repetitive injury and repair, and this may be accompanied by continued smooth muscle cell proliferation despite the absence of platelets. If this experimental observation in the baboon can be confirmed, e.g., that smooth muscle cell proliferation occurs despite EC coverage, and in the absence of platelets, the erratic, unpredictable influence of antiplatelet agents to influence favorably long-term graft patency becomes more understandable. In addition, smooth muscle cell proliferative activity may well vary from one individual to another, as, for example, in the patient with increased plasma LDL[3] and other risk factors such as continued cigarette smoking.[44]

If this chronic endothelial proliferation is indeed secondary to chronic endothelial injury, the solution to the problem of zonal anastomotic hyperplasia may not come, as is now anticipated by some investigators, from simple endothelial cell seeding of synthetic grafts. Whether pharmacologic agents can be developed to suppress this smooth muscle proliferation, whether more rapid endothelialization of the seeded synthetic prosthesis can be induced, whether polymers with more "blood congenial" surfaces can be fabricated, and whether more effective chemical inhibitors of smooth muscle cell mitogens can be isolated are unanswered questions and worthy of investigation. For the present, however, all of these endeavors, some of which have been used in concert, have failed to alter the poor performance of small-caliber arterial substitutes, and the long overdue study of the arterial wall at the cellular and molecular level must begin. A biologic graft composed of all the elements of the normal arterial wall becomes an attractive challenge. The current "synthetic era" may yield to the biologic as the concept of a graft raised from tissue culture is tested.

The important anatomical and physiologic characteristics of the artery include its ability:

1. to serve as an efficient and unremitting conduit;
2. to exist in a state of active tension to assist in the regional distribution of blood;
3. to maintain an endothelium which inhibits clotting when intact but initiates it when injured;
4. to possess an elastic lamina for the storage of kinetic systolic energy;
5. to supply nutrients via vasa vasora in elastic arteries and via a process of selected permeability and diffusion across the endothelium and small muscular arteries; and
6. to exist in a microenvironment containing from time to time a host of evanescent substances of direct and indirect activity acting upon the cell membrane, and other wall and blood-borne elements.

The arterial wall is a biologically complex structure. It consists of the endothelial cell and its basement membrane, the extracellular matrix, the smooth muscle cell, and the adventitia with its many components.

The intima is a single layer of squamous endothelial cells lining the vascular wall, resting on a thin basal lamina of approximately 80 nm thickness, and a subendothelial layer composed of collagenous bundles, elastic fibrils, smooth muscle cells, and perhaps some fibroblasts.

Prevention of platelet aggregation and thrombus formation are critically dependent upon the integrity of the endothelial monolayer. Exposure of the surface underlying the endothelial cell is a very potent stimulus for thrombosis. The endothelial monolayer also serves as a permeability barrier or transport system for withholding or moving components of blood from and to the media.

The media is made up of smooth muscle cells, a varied number of elastic sheets or laminae, bundles of collagenous fibrils, and in large arteries such as the human aorta, 40–60 fenestrated elastic lamina which gradually decrease toward the periphery into smaller arteries. A network of delicate elastic fibrils interconnects the elastic lamina thus providing an elaborate elastic framework of great resilience and strength. Small arteries have only a limited number of smooth muscle cells, and in capillaries the wall consists of endothelial cells and basal lamina only.

The smooth muscle cell is the principal connective tissue cell of the arterial wall. It synthesizes collagen, elastic fibers, and proteoglycans. Unlike the fibroblast, which forms concentric whorls of cells, the smooth muscle cell forms a series of hills and valleys which may pile upon one another to form as many as 10–15 layers.

The adventitia, or external wrap of the vascular wall, varies in thickness with the type and location of the blood vessel. It provides stability to the wall, attaches the blood vessel to its surrounding tissues, and serves as a conduit to carry nutrients to the smooth muscle cells of the media.

Probably the first attempt to develop a viable arterial graft was made by Gross and his associates in the 1940s from arteries aseptically removed from healthy human subjects dying of trauma. Stored at 4°C in a balanced salt solution of 10% human serum, fibroblastic proliferation in tissue culture retained some evidence of viability for as long as 37 days after harvesting, at which time these supposedly viable cells began to disintegrate and disappear. Early expectations[45] were not confirmed by clinical trials.[46]

A second attempt to develop a viable biologic graft, this from the tissues of the host, consisted of the insertion of a silicone polymer rod, or mandril, in the subcutaneous fat of the thigh, which by six weeks was surrounded by a collagenous tube. At a second operation, the mandril was removed, and the ends of the tube connected to the femoral and popliteal arteries. Although associated with early success, extensive aneurysmal dilatation led to its abandonment. Still other sporadic efforts have consisted of attempts to develop a fibrous collagenous tube around an implanted bioresorbable graft.[47] A bioresorbable tube of 95% polyurethane–5% poly-L-lactic acid implanted into the rat abdominal aorta was associated with formation of an antithrombogenic neointima, elastic laminae, and a supporting neoadventitia. Regeneration of a neoarterial wall of sufficient strength, compliance, and thromboresistance to function as a small-caliber arterial substitute was claimed. The fibrohistiocytic tissue organization of the disintegrating scaffold resembled a foreign body reaction. Macrophages formed multinucleated giant cells, possibly an ominous portent for good long-term results.[48]

Because of a better understanding of the mechanisms of intermediate and long-term graft failure, of the response to injury of the arterial wall, and because of the great advances in tissue culture science, it now appears reasonable to attempt to develop an arterial graft, consisting of the primary endothelial and smooth muscle cells grown from tissue culture upon a supporting scaffold of a biopolymer matrix with a predictable rate of degradation and resorption. This approach, departing from present technology based on synthetic fabrics, rejects the precept that arterial prostheses must be biologically inert, and assumes the contrary view that for long-term success with small-caliber grafts, the ideal substitute must be biologically active. This concept presupposes that such a vascular substitute will maintain an intact, self-renewing, thromboresistant endothelial lining, that its cells will synthesize appropriate extracellular matrix components, that its compliance and elasticity will duplicate the native vessel, and that it will maintain its total biological and mechanical integrity in vivo.

Human vascular EC and SMC can now be grown routinely in tissue culture and maintain many of their complex cell functions. The introduction of "artificial skin" in 1981 by Burke and coworkers opened the way for the use of biopolymer matrices to replace normal human tissue while preserving normal tissue biology.[49, 50]

Resorbable biopolymer matrices suitable for vascular cell support and growth are available. Some can orient cells in vitro and in vivo can assume characteristics of the native tissue. Their fabrication into a tubular conformation requires attention, particularly with respect to the behavior of cells accustomed to a flat surface. Methods for creating tubes composed of collagen and collagen–GAG complexes have already been described.[51] Such biopolymers fabricated into tubes must be evaluated in vitro for tensile strength, suturability, protein adsorption, leukocyte migration and attachment, complement and platelet activation, and a host of other possibilities. A candidate matrix may be available by the coprecipitation of collagen and the GAG chondroitin 6-sulfate.[51] Several methods for covalently cross-linking these coprecipitates into insoluble materials have been described as well as separate techniques for fabrication into seamless tubes.[51] The tensile strength of these tubes approaches 400 lb/in^2, a value which has been shown to be adequate for both secure suture holding and resistance to fatigue caused by physiologic blood pressure.[51] The strength of this material and its rate of degradation by collagenase appear to be dependent on its GAG content.[52] Whether vascular smooth muscle, which is known to produce a collagenase in vitro, is capable of remodelling and slowly resorbing such a biopolymer matrix[53] remains to be seen, as well as whether or not the extracellular matrix normally produced by SMC and EC in vivo can be controlled at a satisfactory replacement rate.

Preliminary studies in our laboratory have demonstrated the feasibility of the collagen gel matrix coculture system.[54] These experiments demonstrated: (1) that stable collagen matrix gels can be seeded with smooth muscle cells, (2) that a surface layer of endothelial cells can be established and maintained in a viable state with stable morphology, and (3) that morphologic techniques can be developed to examine these preparations, which later could be adapted for immunohistochemical studies. These cocultures were maintained for time periods from 24 hours to 5 days. Morphologic evaluation consisted of light, phase contrast, scanning electron, and transmission electron microscopy. The studies revealed a confluent monolayer of normal-appearance endothelium on the surface of these gels. Smooth muscle morphology was equally good. No basement membrane-like structure, however, has been identified at the EC–gel interface at the 24-hour period, although no specific immunohistochemical studies have been completed (Figs 16-4 to 16-13).

That the problem is a large one is obvious from a consideration of the many specific, delicately balanced, closely interrelated functions assumed by the components of the arterial wall. The most important of these is the selective permeability of the endothelium and its capability to inhibit thrombosis, the viscoelasticity of the medial smooth muscle and collagen fibers, the influence of the extracellular matrix on growth and metabolism of the cellular elements, and the apparent self-reparative capability of all of these elements.[38, 55]

The endothelial cell synthesizes components of the extracellular matrix: fibronectin,[52] type IV collagen,[56] laminin,[57] and probably others. Cultures of EC layered over SMC accumulate an extracellular matrix similar to that of the normal arterial wall.[58] The chemical composition and physical properties of this matrix appear to be controlled by the interaction between these two cell types (Merriless and Scott[59]). ECs interact directly with SMC by secreting both growth-inhibiting[60] and growth-stimulating substances.[61] The vascular smooth muscle cell also synthesizes components of the extracellular matrix, specifically collagen types I and III, procollagen,[62] elastin, microfibrillar proteins, and glycosaminoglycans.[63] By means of this framework, vascular wall structural integrity is maintained (Fig. 16-14).

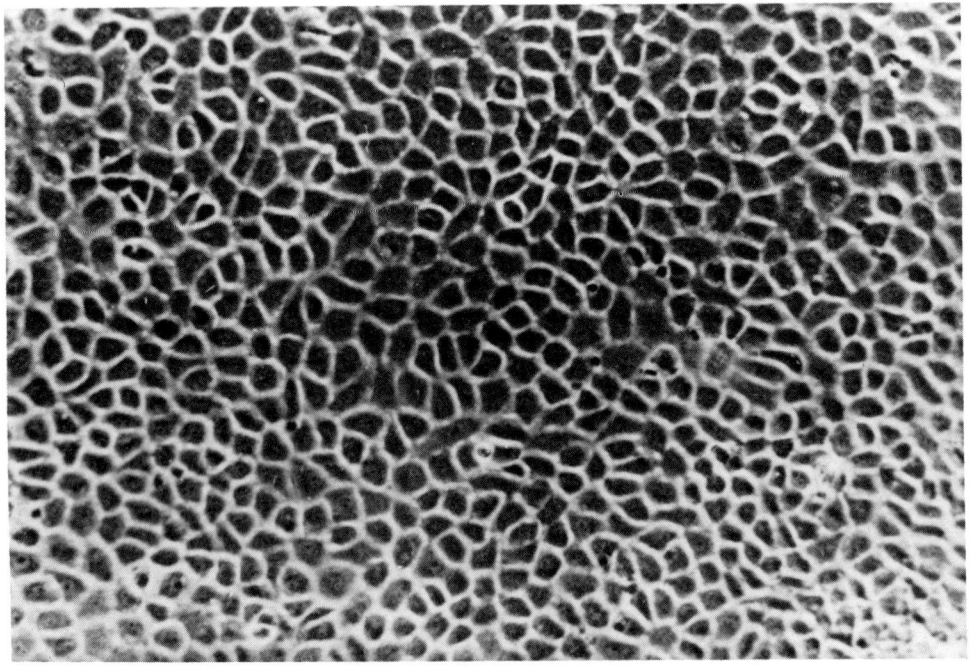

Fig. 16-4.   Bovine aorta EC in culture. Phase contrast. 300 ×.

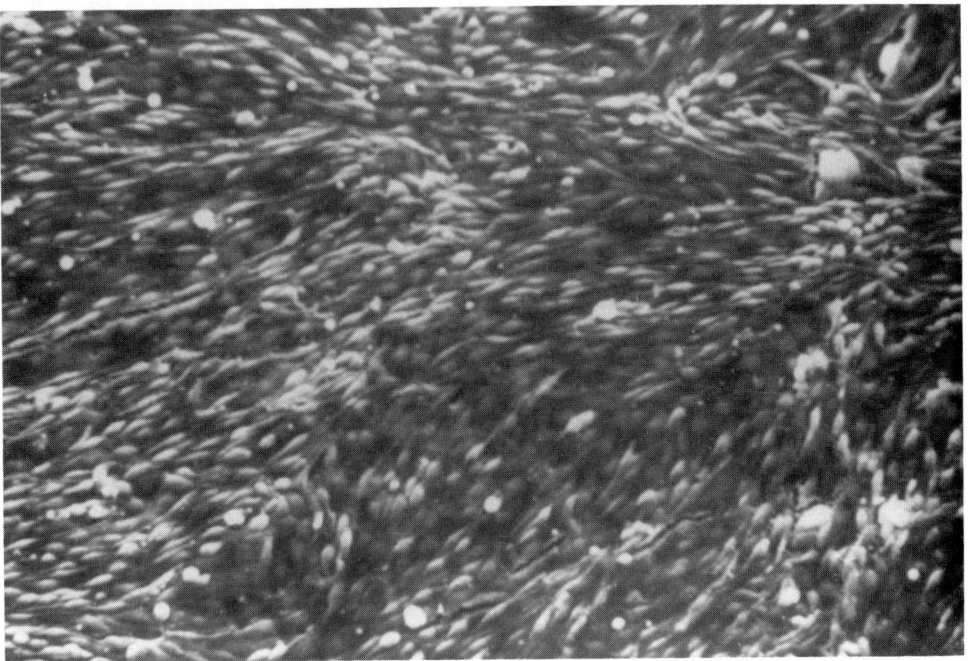

Fig. 16-5. A confluent monolayer of bovine endothelial cells on top of a smooth muscle cell impregnated collagen gel. These cells were seeded at 1.05×10^5 cells/cm². Note the more polar share and linear arrangement of the cells. $200\times$.

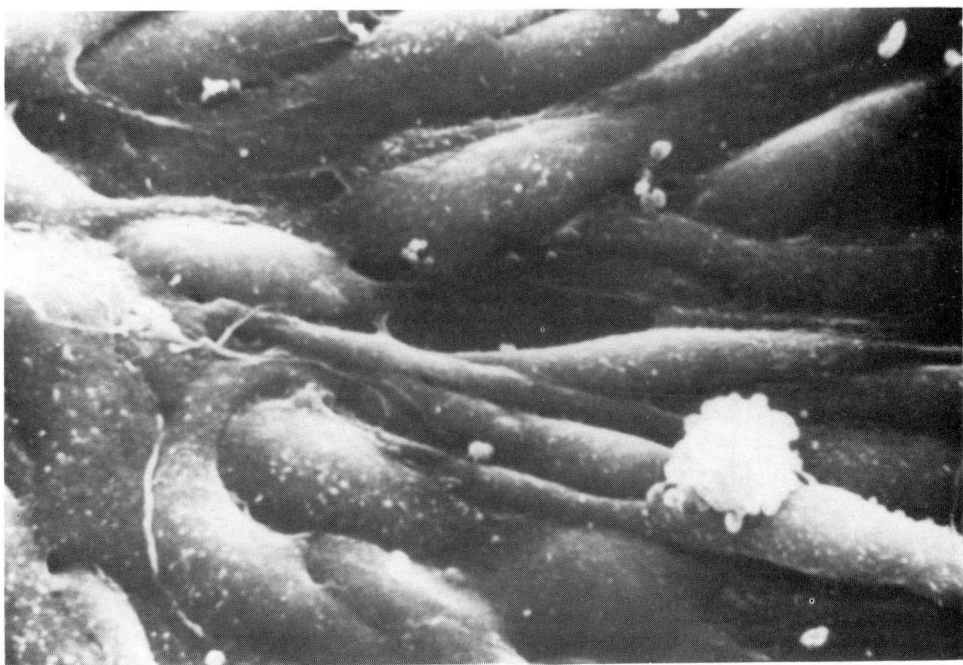

Fig. 16-6. The endothelium seeded surface of a smooth muscle cell impregnated collagen gel. This gel had been seeded with 1×10^5 bovine smooth muscle cells/ml and the surface had been seeded with 1.05×10^5 bovine endothelial cells/cm². The gel was fixed 48 hours after seeding. $1900\times$.

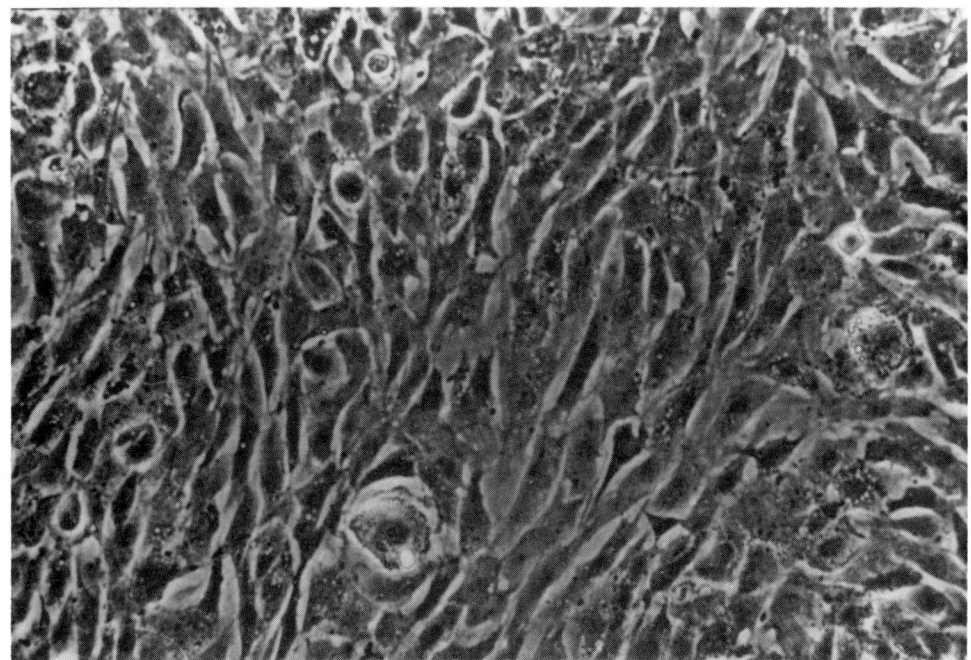

Fig. 16-7. Bovine aorta SMCs in culture. Phase contrast. 300×.

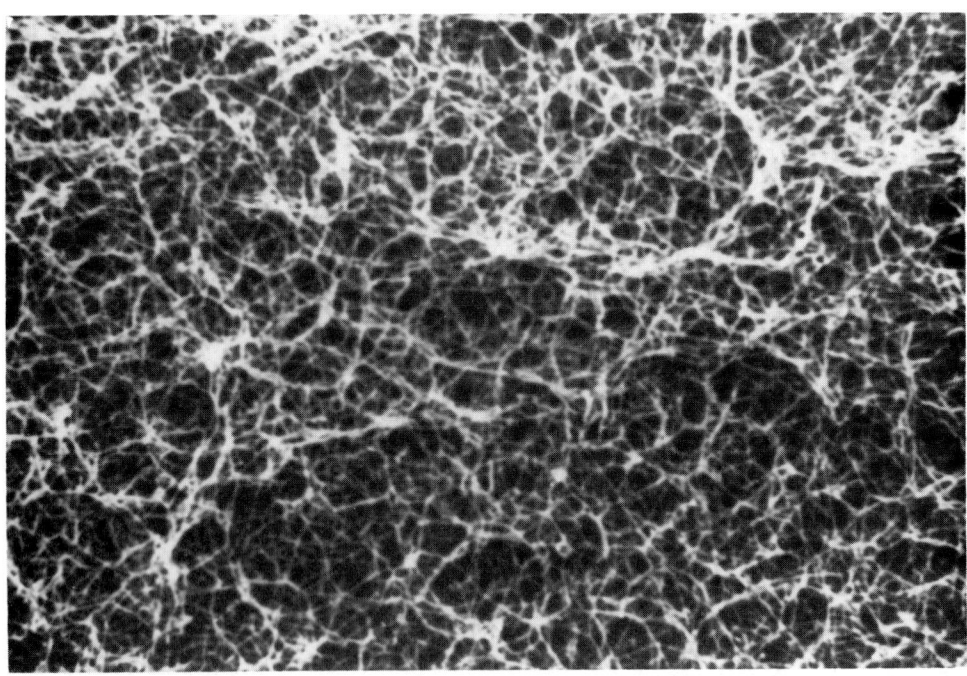

Fig. 16-8. A section of the bottom of a collagen gel where no cells were present. The gel had been fixed and critical point dried. The gel is made from bovine dermal collagen. 200×.

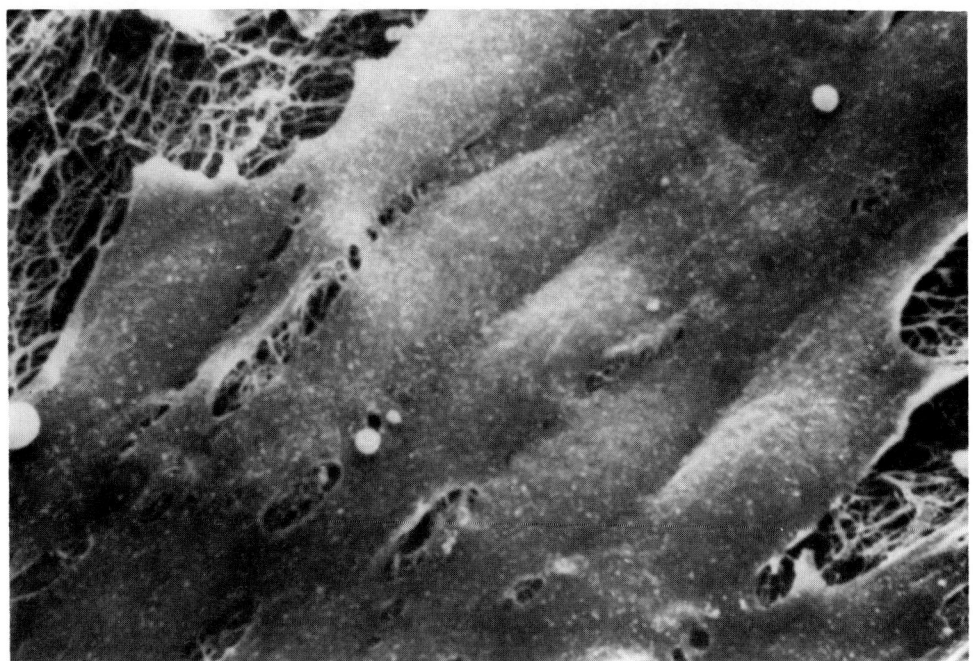

Fig. 16-9. Bovine smooth muscle cells on the bottom surface of a collagen gel seeded with these cells at 1×10^5/cm. 2000 ×.

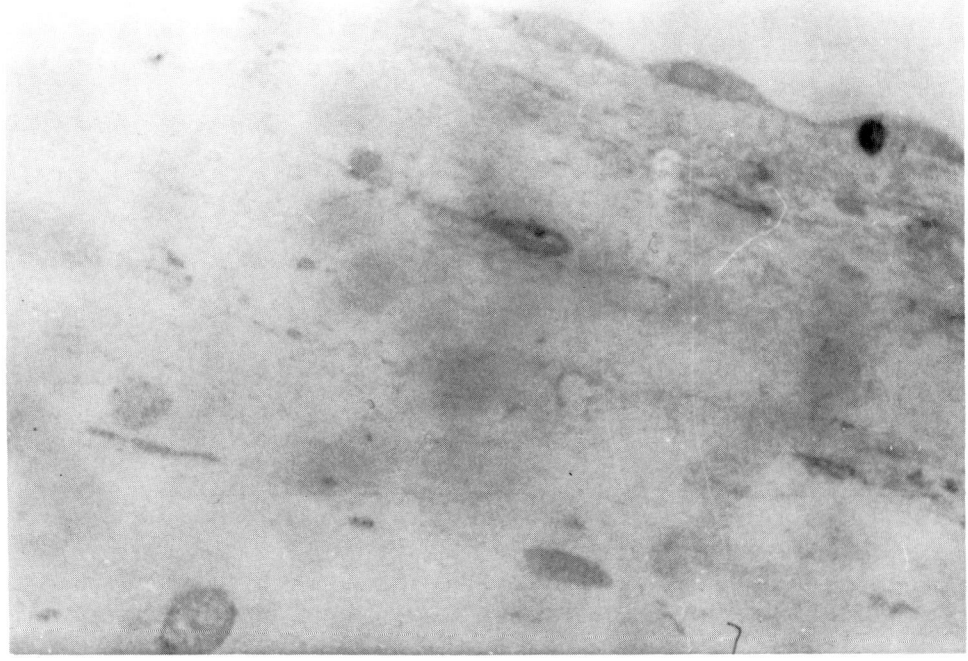

Fig. 16-10. A cross section of a collagen gel containing SMC (1×10^5/ml) and a surface seeded with EC at 1.05×10^5 cells/cm^2. The ECs were confluent and can be seen to be in contact with each other. SMCs and collagen fibers are visible within the gel. Trichrome stain of an epoxy embedded thick section. 750 ×.

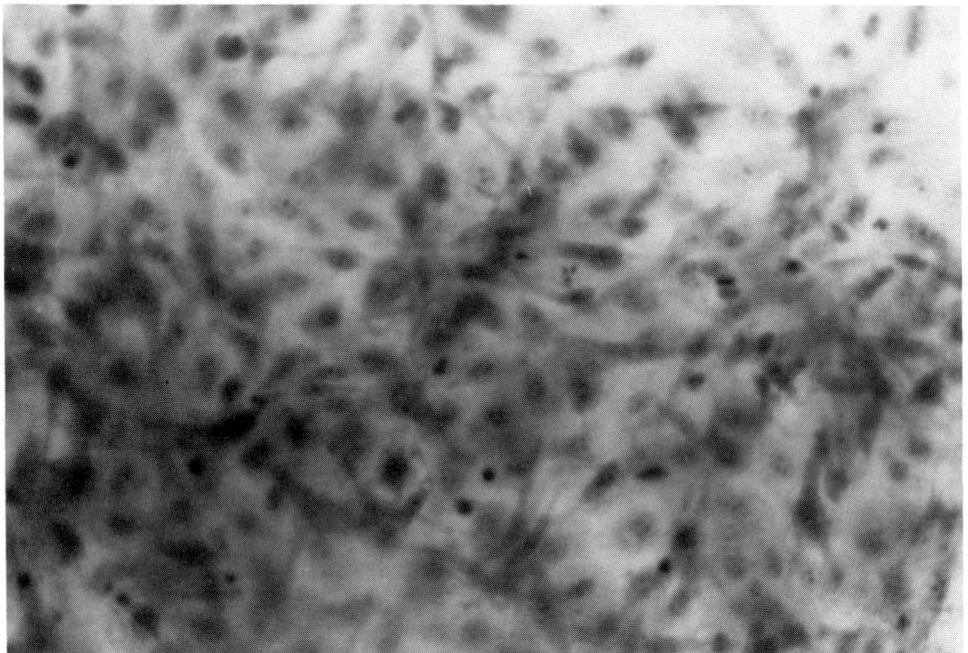

Fig. 16-11. A toluidine blue stained whole-mount section from an SMC containing collagen gel that had EC seeded onto the surface. The plane of focus is on the top surface of the gel where more polygonal, lightly stained EC can be observed. 300 × .

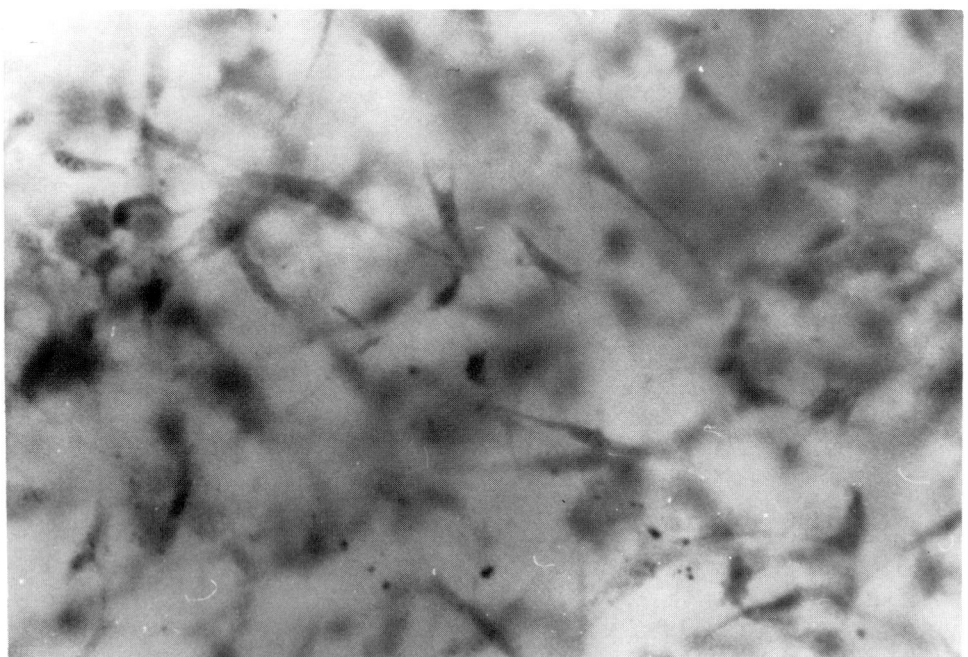

Fig. 16-12. The same gel as in Fig. 16-11 only here the plane of focus is deeper in the gel and the more polar and more darkly stained SMCs can be seen.

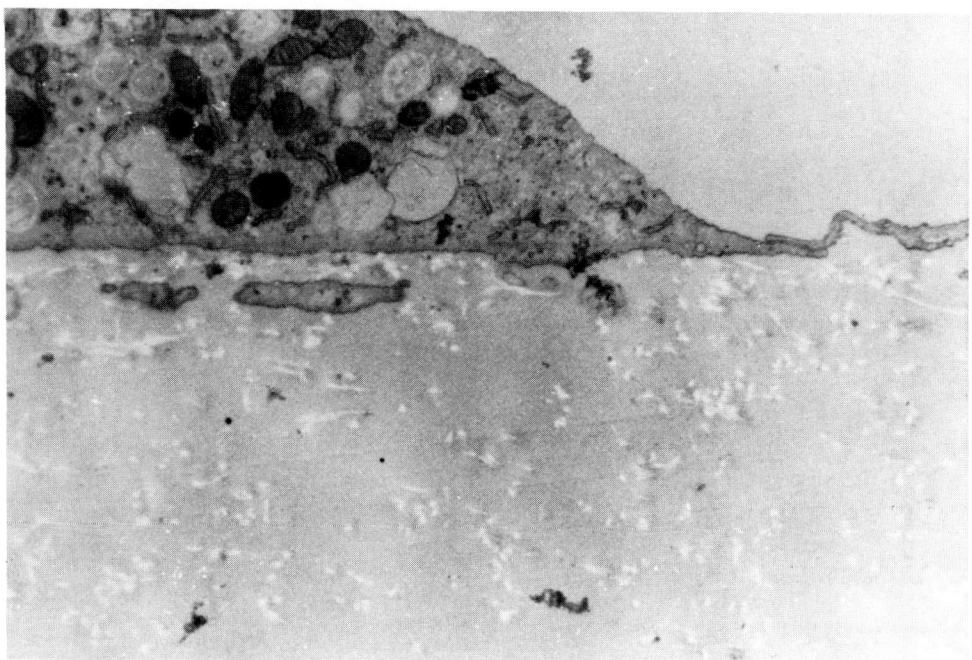

Fig. 16-13. EC on the surface of an SMC containing collagen gel. Note the junction where two ECs are joined to the right of the EC body. Collagen fibrils and a portion of an SMC are seen within the gel below the EC layer. 9500 × .

LUMINAL SURFACE

PROCOAGULANT:	INDUCIBLE IMMUNE FUNCTIONS:	ENZYMES:	ANTICOAGULANT:
Tissue factor vWf	Class II HLA determinants Interleukin-1 production	ACE I & II Nucleotidases Histamine Bradykinin	Prostacyclin Thrombomodulin t-PA Heparin-like molecules

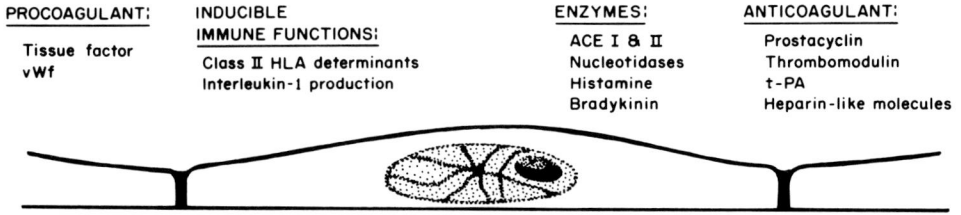

ABLUMINAL SURFACE

BIOSYNTHESIS OF EXTRACELLULAR MATRIX:	ELABORATION OF VASODILATORS:	GROWTH STIMULATORS:	GROWTH INHIBITORS:
Collagens Fibronectin Laminin Glycosaminoglycans	Prostacyclin "Endothelial-dependent Relaxation Factor"	C-sis product Interleukin-1	Heparin-like molecules

Fig. 16-14. Vascular endothelial cell.

Resolution of these problems requires attention to the following questions:

1. What is the orientation of the EC and SMC within these matrices?
2. Does the smooth muscle cell engender contraction of the matrix gels, and, if so, what is its extent and time course, and can it be controlled? Will the SM overgrow and engulf the EC? Can this tendency be controlled?
3. Does the EC seeded on these matrices secrete substances for the synthesis of the basement membrane and extracellular matrix components and in the appropriate location? Does the composition of the collagen matrix influence the type and amount of extracellular structural products secreted by EC? Does the presence of the smooth muscle cell influence the type and amount of these products?
4. Does a synthesis of the normal components of the extracellular matrix provided by the smooth muscle cell occur under these circumstances? Is this function of the SMC affected by the overlying layer of EC?
5. Is the thromboresistant property of the endothelial layer maintained in this coculture system or is it adversely affected by the composition of the collagen gel?
6. What is the tensile strength of these temporary exogenous collagen matrices? How durable are they? How durable should they be? How does the introduction of GAGs or other variations in the collagen type affect this strength? Can a balance be developed between resorption of the degradation of the collagen gel–GAGs supporting scaffold and the formation of a replacement structure by the SMC?

It should be apparent from this consideration that the construction of a tissue culture arterial substitute is one of enormous magnitude and enormous need. It requires the collaboration of many investigators in many disciplines. From the theoretical point of view, it appears to be a task capable of achievement given sufficient time, dedication of personnel, and availability of resources. Justification is validated by the need.

"It is surprising that given the availability of all necessary ingredients, e.g. endothelial monolayers and main components of basement membranes, that no one has reported an attempt to reconstitute in vitro . . . a capillary wall with its proper basement membrane and its continuous endothelium."[64]

REFERENCES

1. Reichle FA, Martinson MW, Rankin KP: Infrapopliteal arterial reconstruction in the severely ischemic lower extremity. Ann Surg 191:59, 1980
2. Ricco JB, Flinn WR, McDaniel MD, et al: Objective analysis of factors contributing to failure of tibial bypass grafts. World J Surg 7:347, 1983
3. Campeau L, Enjalbert M, Lesperance J, et al: The relation of risk factors to the development of atherosclerosis in saphenous vein bypass grafts and the progression of disease in the native circulation. N Engl J Med 311:1329, 1984
4. Voorhees AB, Jaretski A, Blakemore AH: The use of tubes constructed from Vinyon "N" cloth in bridging arterial defects. Ann Surg 135:332, 1952

5. Anderson JM, Kottke-Marchant K: Platelet interactions with biomaterials and artificial devices. CRC Critical Reviews in Biocompatibility 1:111, 1985
6. Brash JL: Protein interactions with artificial surfaces, in Salzman EW (ed): Interaction of the Blood with Natural and Artificial Surfaces. New York, Marcel Dekker Inc, 1981, pp 37
7. Mason RG, Kim SW, Andrade JD, Hakim RM: Blood surface interactions. Trans Am Soc Artif Intern Organs 26:603, 1980
8. Chesebro JH, Clements IP, Fuster V, et al: A platelet-inhibitor drug trial in coronary-artery bypass operations. N Engl J Med 307:73, 1982
9. Pantely GA, Goodnight SH Jr, Rahimtoola SH, et al: Failure of antiplatelet and anti-coagulant therapy to improve patency of grafts after coronary-artery bypass. A controlled, randomized study. N Engl J Med 301:962, 1979
10. McEnany MT, Salzman EW, Mundth ED, et al: The effect of antithrombotic therapy on patency rates of saphenous vein coronary bypass grafts. J Thorac Cardiovasc Surg 83:81, 1982
11. McDaniel MD, Pearce WH, Yao JST, et al: Sequential changes in coagulation and platelet function following femorotibial bypass. J Vasc Surg 1:261, 1984
12. Mackey WC, Connolly RJ, Callow AD, et al: Aspirin decreases platelet uptake on Dacron vascular grafts in baboons. Ann Surg 200:93, 1984
13. Green RM, Roesersheimer LR, DeWeese JA: Effects of aspirin and dipyridamole on expanded polytetrafluoroethylene graft patency. Surgery 92:1016, 1982
14. Gloviczki P, Hollier LH, Dewanjee MK, et al: Quantitative evaluation of ibuprofen treatment on thrombogenicity of expanded polytetrafluoroethylene vascular grafts. Surgery 95:160, 1983
15. Chesebro JH, Fuster V, Eleveback LR, et al: Effect of dipyridamole and aspirin on late vein-graft patency after coronary bypass operations. N Engl J Med 310:209, 1984
16. Kohler TR, Kaufman JL, Kacoyanis G, et al: Effect of aspirin and dipyridamole on the patency of lower extremity bypass grafts. Surgery 96:462, 1984
17. McCready RA, Price MA, Kryscio RJ, Hyde GL, Mattingly SS, Griffen WO: Failure of antiplatelet therapy with ibuprofen (Motrin) to prevent neointimal fibrous hyperplasia. J Vasc Surg 2:205, 1985
18. Schmidt SP, Hunter TJ, Hirko M, et al: Small-diameter prostheses: Two designs of PTFE and endothelial cell-seeded and nonseeded Dacron. J Vasc Surg 2:292, 1985
19. Schmidt SP, Hunter TJ, Falkow LJ, Evancho MM, Sharp WV: Effects of antiplatelet agents in combination with endothelial cell seeding on small-diameter Dacron vascular graft performance in the canine carotid artery model. J Vasc Surg 2:898, 1985
20. Herring M, Baughman S, Glover J, et al: Endothelial seeding of Dacron and PTFE grafts. The cellular events of healing. Surgery 96:745, 1984
21. Kern WH, Dermer GB, Lindesmith GG: The intimal proliferation in aortocoronary saphenous vein grafts: Light and electron microscopic studies. Am Heart J 84:771, 1972
22. Vlodaver Z, Edwards JE: Pathologic changes in aortic-coronary arterial saphenous vein grafts. Circulation 44:719, 1971
23. Clowes AW, Adams MC: Smooth muscle cell proliferation and arterial graft failure, in Bergan JJ, Yao JST (eds): Reoperative Arterial Surgery. Orlando, Florida, Grune & Stratton, 1986, p 3
24. Herring MB, Dilley R, Jersild RA, Boxer L, Gardner A, Glover J: Seeding arterial prostheses with vascular endothelium. Ann Surg 190: 84, 1979
25. Stanley JC, Burkel WE, Ford JW, et al: Enhanced patency of small diameter externally supported Dacron iliofemoral grafts seeded with endothelial cells. Surgery 92:994, 1982
26. Gembarowicz R, Connolly R, Callow AD, et al: Effect of PGI2 on the interaction of platelets with small-caliber Dacron grafts. Surg Forum 33:466, 1982
27. Ramberg K, Keough EM, Callow AD, et al: Indium-111 labeled platelet imaging of endothelial cell seeded small caliber synthetic grafts in the baboon. ASAIO 8:95, 1985

28. Harker LA, Slichter SJ, Sauvage LR: Platelet consumption by arterial prostheses: The effects of endothelialization and pharmacologic inhibition of platelet function. Ann Surg 186:594, 1977

29. Callow AD, Connolly R, O'Donnell TF, et al: Platelet-arterial synthetic graft interaction and its modification. Arch Surg 117:1447, 1982

30. Dewanjee MK, Pumphrey CW, Murphy KP, et al: Evaluation of platelet-inhibitor drugs in a canine bilateral femoral graft implant model. Trans Am Soc Artif Intern Organs 28:504, 1982

31. Goldman M, Norcott HC, Hawker RJ, Drolc Z, McCollum CN: Platelet accumulation of mature Dacron grafts in man. Br J Surg 69:S38, 1982

32. Pomposelli F, Schoen F, Cohen R, O'Leary D, Johnson WR, Madras PN: Conformational stress and anastomotic hyperplasia. J Vasc Surg 1:525, 1984

33. Madras PN, Ward CA, Johnson WR, Singh PI: Anastomotic hyperplasia. Surgery 90:922, 1981

34. Abbott WM, Cambria RP: Control of physical characteristics (elasticity and compliance) of vascular grafts, in Stanley JC (ed): Biologic and Synthetic Vascular Prostheses. New York, Grune & Stratton, 1982, p 189

35. Hasson JE, Megerman J, Abbott WM: Increased compliance near vascular anastomoses. J Vasc Surg 2:419, 1985

36. LoGerfo FW, Quist WC, Nowak MD: Downstream anastomotic hyperplasia: A mechanism of failure in Dacron arterial grafts. Ann Surg 197:497, 1983

37. Clowes AW, Gown AM, Hanson SR, Reidy MA: Mechanisms of arterial graft failure. 1. Role of cellular proliferation in early healing of PTFE prostheses. AJP 118:43, 1985

38. Ross R, Glomset JA: The pathogenesis of atherosclerosis. N Engl J Med 295:369, 420, 1976

39. Reidy MA, Schwartz SM: Endothelial injury and regeneration. IV. Endotoxin: A non-denuding injury to aortic endothelium. Lab Invest 48:25, 1983

40. Gajdusek CM, DiCorleto P, Ross R, et al: An endothelial cell derived growth factor. J Cell Biol 85:467, 1980

41. Fox PL, DiCorleto P: Regulation of production of platelet-derived growth factor-like protein by cultured bovine aortic endothelial cells. J Cell Physiol 121:298, 1984

42. Barrett TB, Gajdusek SM, McDougall JK, et al: Expression of the sis gene by endothelial cells in culture and in vivo. Proc Natl Acad Sci USA 1:6772, 1984

43. Seifert RA, Schwartz SM, Bowen-Pope DF: Developmentally regulated production of platelet-derived growth factor-like molecules. Nature 311:699, 1984

44. Greenhalgh RM, Laing SP, Cole PV, et al: Effect of risk factors on the outcome of arterial reconstruction, in Greenhalgh RM (ed): Smoking and Arterial Disease. Bath, England, Pitman Press, 1981, pp 187

45. Gross RE, Bill AH, Pierce EC: Methods for preservation and transplantation of arterial grafts: Observations on arterial grafts in dogs: Report of transplantation of preserved arterial grafts in nine human cases. Surg Gynecol Obstet 88:689, 1949

46. Gross RE, Hurwitt ES, Bill AH, et al: Preliminary observations on the use of human arterial grafts in the treatment of certain cardiovascular defects. N Engl J Med 239:578, 1948

47. van der Lei B, Bartels HL, Nieuwenhuis P, Wildevuur CRH: Microporous, compliant, biodegradable vascular grafts for the regeneration of the arterial wall in rat abdominal aorta. Surgery 98:955, 1985

48. Anderson JM, Miller KM: Biomaterial biocompatibility and the macrophage. Biomaterials 5:5, 1984

49. Yannas IV, Burke JF, Orgill DP, Skrabut EM: Wound tissue can utilize a polymeric template to synthesize a functional extension of skin. Science 215:174, 1982

50. Burke JF, Yannas IV, Quinby WC, Bondoc CC, Jung WK: Successful use of a physio-

logically acceptable artificial skin in treatment of extensive burn injury. Ann Surg 194:413, 1981

51. Yannas IV, Forbes JM, Stein JA, Salzman EW: Tube fabrication from collagen/glycosaminoglycan dispersions. Fourth Annual Progress Report for NIH Contract NIH-N01-HV-4-2969-4; 6/78

52. Jaffee EA, Mosher DF: Synthesis of fibronectin by cultured human endothelial cells. J Exp Med 147:1779, 1978

53. Delvos U, Gajdusek C, Sage H, Harker LA, Schwartz SM: Interactions of vascular wall cells with collagen gels. Lab Invest 46:61, 1981

54. Callow AD, et al: Creation of a small caliber arterial prosthesis. NIH Proposal 1 RO1 HL32790, submitted 1 Nov 1983

55. Burton AC: Relation of structure to function of the tissues of the wall of blood vessels. Physiol Rev 34:619, 1954

56. Jaffee EA, Minick CR, Adelman B, Becker CG, Nachman R: Synthesis of basement membrane collagen by cultured human endothelial cells. J Exp Med 144:209, 1976

57. Foidart JM, Bere EW, Yaar M, et al: Distribution and immunoelectron microscopic localization of laminin, a noncollagenous basement membrane glycoprotein. Lab Invest 42:336, 1980

58. Jones PA: Construction of an artificial blood vessel wall from cultured endothelial and smooth muscle cells. Proc Natl Acad Sci USA 76:1882, 1979

59. Merrilees MJ, Scott L: Interaction of aortic endothelial and smooth muscle cells in culture. Atherosclerosis 39:147, 1981

60. Karnovsky MJ: Endothelial-vascular smooth muscle cell interactions. Rous-Whipple Award Lecture. Am J Pathol 105:200, 1981

61. DiCorleto PE, Bowen-Pope DF: Cultured endothelial cells produce a platelet-derived growth factor-like protein. Proc Natl Acad Sci 80:1919, 1983

62. Burke JM, Balian G, Ross R, Bornstein P: Synthesis of types I and II procollagen and collagen by monkey aortic smooth muscle cells in vitro. Biochem 16:3243, 1977

63. Muir LW, Bornstein P, Ross R: A presumptive subunit of elastic fiber microfibrils secreted by arterial smooth muscle cells in culture. Eur J Biochem 64:105, 1976

64. Palade GE: Annals of the New York Academy of Sciences, 1982

Robert B. Rutherford,
Anita Patt,
and David A. Kumpe

17

The Current Role of Percutaneous Transluminal Angioplasty

INTRODUCTION

Percutaneous transluminal angioplasty (PTA) is no longer "the new kid on the block." Though technical refinements continue, percutaneous transluminal dilation with the Gruntzig balloon has had an opportunity to show what it is capable of achieving and settle into its rightful place in management of arterial occlusive disease. Initially, the criteria upon which successful outcome was reported varied tremendously, leaving the readers confused by the contrast between the enthusiastic claims of interventional radiologists and critical appraisals by vascular surgeons. Now reporting practices for PTA are more uniform and sizable, carefully evaluated long-term experiences have emerged, allowing the ultimate role of angioplasty to be projected. This report will analyze such experiences, including the authors' own, in relation to a number of specific considerations which, in combination, should allow proper definition of the current role of transluminal angioplasty.

The discussion will begin by balancing risk, in terms of technical failure and serious complications, against benefit, in terms of frequency, degree, and duration of improvement. Comparison with the results of surgical alternatives will focus on significant differences in patient selection and lesions treated. The effect of patient selection, criteria for success or failure, operator skill, lesion morphology and location, diabetes, and other risk factors on the reported outcome of PTA will be elaborated upon. The major emphasis in this report will be on transluminal angioplasty as a primary mode of treatment for arteriosclerosis obliterans, though some consideration will also be given to its role as an adjunct to arterial reconstruction, in preserving graft patency, and its use in combination with thrombolytic therapy in the management of arterial occlusions.

VASCULAR SURGERY: ISSUES IN CURRENT PRACTICE
ISBN 0-8089-1839-7

RISKS AND COMPLICATIONS

The primary justifications for PTA are its relatively low risk and cost, both monetarily and in terms of morbidity and mortality, compared to arterial reconstruction. In general, it does not produce as good a hemodynamic result, nor is it as durable as arterial bypass, but it infrequently results in the deterioration of the patient's prior clinical status, can be repeated if stenosis recurs, avoids severing autonomic nerves, and does not interfere with subsequent vascular reconstructions.[1] Furthermore, PTA is done under local anesthesia and the patient is discharged one day after the procedure unless a complication occurs.[2] Several centers now perform PTA as an outpatient procedure.

The list of PTA complications is long but most are of minor consequence, do not require surgical intervention, and can be minimized by experience and judgment.[3] Total complications in some high-risk series may be as high as 30–50%,[4, 5] but usually range between 4 and 22%.[2, 6–12] Those complications requiring surgical intervention rarely exceed 5%.[2, 13] The incidence of complications appears to be higher in patients in whom the PTA was unsuccessful[14] and the radiologist inexperienced.[2] In our series as many complications occurred in the first 15 as in the subsequent 95 dilatations. Zeitler and coworkers showed a progressive drop in the complication rate over three time periods from 14 to 4% and, of those requiring surgical intervention, from 2.3 to 0.45%.[15] Deaths following PTA are extremely rare, although a one-month mortality of 3% was reported in one series of high-risk patients.[5] The majority of deaths are only indirectly related to the procedure and occur in such high-risk patients as those suffering from severe diffuse atherosclerotic disease.

Complications can occur at both the puncture site and the dilatation site. The majority of complications occurring at the catheter introduction site consist of small or large hematomas. Less frequently reported are spasm, thrombosis, false aneurysms, and arterio-venous fistulas. At the dilatation site the formation of a contained false passage is most common; however, intimal dissection, intimal flaps, thrombosis, arterial perforation, balloon rupture, and distal embolization are reported. The latter are of clinical significance in less than 1% of cases, even though microembolization occurs more commonly during femoro-popliteal dilatation. Microembolization of no clinical consequence was seen in 8% of our first 50 femoro-popliteal lesions.[16] Splitting of the atheroma results in the dislodgement of superficial plaque elements or thrombi which are carried distally and, in the majority of cases, are thought to undergo lysis and absorption. Occasionally, particularly in patients with poor runoff, this embolization may put a patient's limb at risk and require surgical intervention, especially if the artery is freshly thrombosed.[17] The incidence of embolization of any type is much lower for iliac than for femoro-popliteal dilatations.

A list of complications and their incidences in various series is shown in Table 17-1.

"Technical failure" should be considered under complications, particularly since it is so often excluded in projecting success rates against time. The site of dilation, as well as the severity of the lesion, correlate with success of the initial dilation. Failures are more common in segments with severe long stenosis, occlusions, and in femoro-popliteal lesions. Failure may be caused by inability to

Table 17-1

Complications of Percutaneous Transluminal Angioplasty (%)

Complications	Kumpe and Jones[16]	Glover and coworkers[4]	Knight and Knight and coworkers[13]	Sinning, Dixon, and Pinkerton[12]	Campbell and coworkers[17]	Johnstone and Colapinto[29]	Jones and coworkers[8]	Krepel and coworkers[26]
A. *Puncture site*								
Hematoma	3.8	5.5	22.0	18.0	15.0	6.5		1.8
Thrombosis			5.0				1.2	
False aneurysm	1.5						0.3	
Arterio-venous fistula								
Arterial perforation with dye extravasation			10.0		5.0			
Arterial spasm								0.6
B. *Dilation site*								
Contained false passage	4.5							
Intimal dissection		4.5					1.2	
Intimal flaps								
Thrombosis		6.4	5.5	4.5				1.2
Balloon rupture or failure	4.5	3.7						
Embolization	3.3	2.8	1.0	9.0	5.0	1.8		2.4
C. *Other*	7.0	2.8					2.4	
Overall complication rate	25.1	26.0	43.5	32.0	20.0	9.0	5.0	6.0
D. *Complications requiring surgical intervention*	5.5	5.0	13.0		5.0	0.8	0.8	1.2
E. *Technical failure*	8.1	22.0	13.0	4.0	23.0	7.0	7.0	16.0
F. *Mortality (up to 1 month)*	0	0	0	9.0	0	1.0	2.0	0

cannulate the artery, inability to advance the guide wire, through the lesion, failure of the diseased segment to dilate adequately, and dissection or thrombosis of the dilated segments.

The technical failure rate is not always reported[12, 23] and in one series repeated dilations were considered to be part of the initial transluminal angioplasty procedure.[5] Most series report an overall technical failure rate close to 15% (11.5–20%) with iliac dilatations having a higher success rate than distal dilatations.[1, 4, 5, 8, 9, 13, 14, 17] The failure rate for proximal lesions ranges from 4 (in our series) to 17% and the rate for distal lesions from 15 to 20% (our series 17.5%).[4, 8]

Delayed complications other than recurrent stenosis are extremely rare. It is not an uncommon observation, when recurrences are arteriogrammed, that the site of stenosis is distal or proximal to the dilation site. Of the first seven patients in our series having repeated arteriography for deterioration, six had new areas of stenosis either adjacent to or remote from the dilated areas.[16] This suggests that there are some deleterious local effects produced by dilations, probably from catheter-induced local trauma.[18] The restenosis rate is influenced by systemic risk factors, such as smoking, diabetes, hyperlipidema, and hypertension, and local factors such as the number plus length of lesions, the extent of the disease, and the adequacy of outflow vessels.[19] The mechanisms of restenosis are still under investigation but some studies suggest aggressive dilation resulting in plaque rupture, medial disruption, and subendothelial collagen exposure may cause extensive platelet deposition and subsequent accelerated atherosclerosis and restenosis, especially in the presence of hyperlipidemia.[20–22] In addition, areas of medial rupture and intimal dissection may propagate into adjacent nondilated areas. Flow irregularities are not uncommon and further predispose to restenosis and long-term failure.[19]

HEMODYNAMIC RESPONSE TO TRANSLUMINAL ANGIOPLASTY

It is obvious that dilation of an occlusive lesion does not always produce a wide-open lumen. When dilation fails to enlarge the lumen to a point where the lesion no longer constitutes a critical stenosis and thus does not eliminate the pressure gradient across that segment, it is considered a technical failure. This occurred in 4.7% of our series and was greater for distal than proximal dilations. Even if dilation significantly reduces the gradient, it may not produce sufficient overall hemodynamic improvement to relieve the patient's symptoms. This is particularly true for proximal dilations done in the face of distal disease where, in our series, 25% failed to improve the ankle–brachial index (ABI) by a significant degree. Other studies concur with a 26–28% failure to increase the ABI.[1, 7, 9] However, it should be pointed out that this also occurs to the same degree with aorto-bifemoral bypass done in the face of superficial femoral occlusive disease.

The degree by which transluminal angioplasty falls short of producing an equivalent hemodynamic response to arterial reconstruction or bypass is hard to gauge, primarily because they are rarely performed on the same or equivalent lesions. Transluminal angioplasty tends to be performed at either clinical extreme of the disease spectrum and not on the same anatomically extensive and usually completely occlusive lesions subjected to bypass. Tables 17-2 and 17-3 illustrate this

Table 17-2
Aorto-bifemoral Bypass versus Transluminal
Angioplasty for Iliac Occlusive Disease:
Comparison of Pre- and Post-TBI and ABI Indices

	Aorto-bifemoral Bypass	Transluminal Angioplasty (Iliac Lesion)
n =	57	59
Pre-TBI	0.70 ± 0.15	0.70 ± 0.18
Post-TBI	1.15 ± 0.19	0.99 ± 0.19
Diff-TBI	0.45 ± 0.22	0.29 ± 0.14
Pre-ABI	0.48 ± 0.19	0.60 ± 0.17
Post-ABI	0.86 ± 0.23	0.86 ± 0.23
Diff-ABI	0.38 ± 0.27	0.28 ± 0.28
Pre-TBI–ABI	0.22	0.10
Post-TBI–ABI	0.29	0.13

point. In Table 17-2, iliac dilations are compared with aorto-femoral bypass. Serendipitiously the mean preoperative thigh–brachial indices are equal in both groups, suggesting equal degrees of severity of the proximal disease, but the mean ankle–brachial indices are significantly lower in the bypass group, indicating a higher proportion of patients with associated occlusive lesions. The posttreatment thigh–brachial index is significantly higher in the bypass group, indicating greater luminal improvement, and the ankle–brachial indices are no longer lower but equal, indicating this greater improvement has compensated for the greater distal disease. From Table 17-3 it can be seen that, similarly, the ankle–brachial indices are increased to a greater degree by femoro-popliteal bypass than by dilation of femoro-popliteal lesions, more than compensating for the greater severity of occlusive disease.

Noninvasive limb pressure movements can not only successfully gauge the hemodynamic response to dilation but have prognostic significance, for we, as well as others,[1,7,9,14,16,23] have found that the late rate of failure or deterioration is considerably higher in those with lesser degrees of hemodynamic improvement. It has been pointed out that the hemodynamic response, as measured by the ankle–brachial index, does not always correlate with the angiographic appearance.[5,8,24] Many have felt that complete anatomical correction, as judged by radiographic appearance, is unnecessary[24] and that there is no relationship between the presence

Table 17-3
Comparison of Femoro-popliteal Bypass and
Transluminal Angioplasty for Femoro-popliteal Lesions:
Pre- and Post-ABIs

	Femoro-popliteal Bypass	Transluminal Angioplasty of Femoro-popliteal Lesions
n =	32	36
Pre-ABI	0.42 ± 0.28	0.57 ± 0.24
Post-ABI	0.85 ± 0.25	0.82 ± 0.28
Diff-ABI	0.43 ± 0.27	0.24 ± 0.26

of lumen contour irregularities or dissection channels with the final hemodynamic or clinical result.[5,19,21] Figure 17-1 shows the results of Charoenkul, Tey, and Ahmed,[25] comparing two-year clinical outcome with initial hemodynamic measurements versus radiographic appearance. Contrary to this general impression, however, one study[26] has actually suggested that good postdilatation morphology carried a better long-term prognosis.

There are several explanations offered for this lack of correlation between clinical success and radiographic appearance in addition to the known difficulty of judging luminal size by two-dimensional angiographic views. First, a minor luminal change in the stenotic lesion, e.g., an increase from 40 to 60%, may render it no longer hemodynamically significant. Second, delayed improvement can be due to relief of associated vasospasm or lysis of a distal emboli. Third, opening up of collaterals around residual distal occlusive lesions has also been credited for delayed improvement. However, the most interesting cause is the phenomenon of "remod-

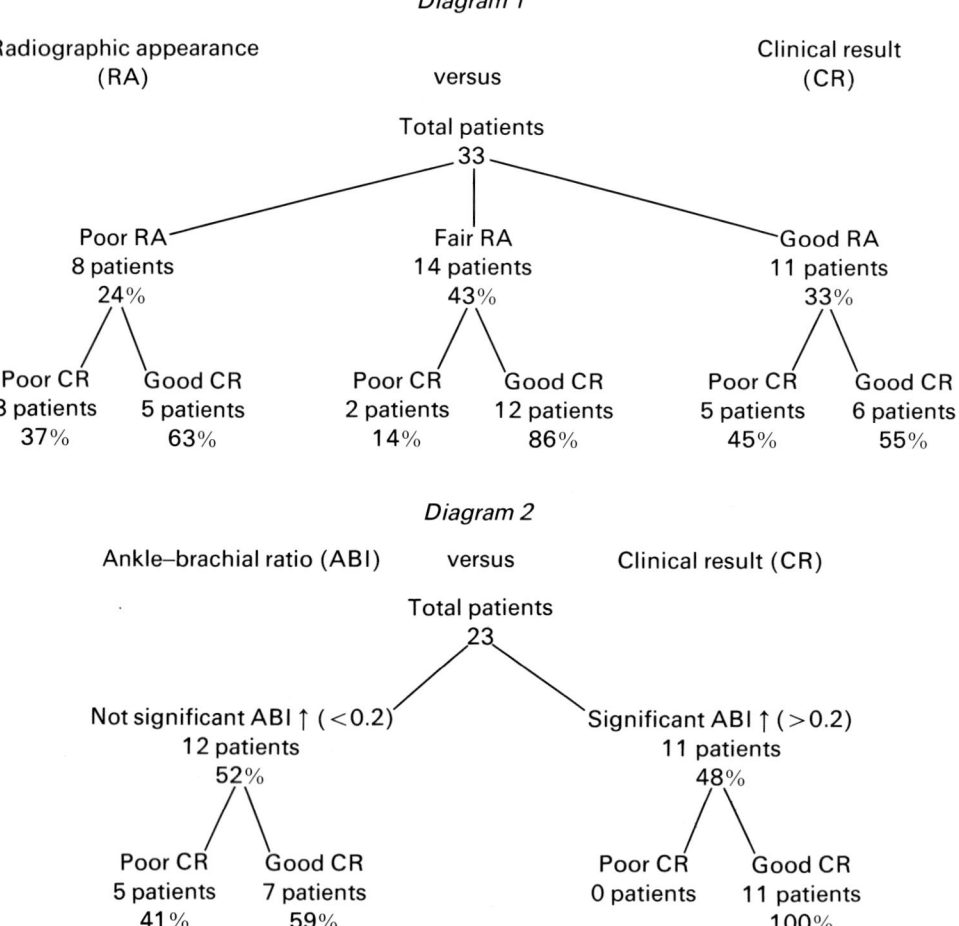

Fig. 17-1. Diagram 1 compares the postdilation radiographic appearance to the two-year clinical outcome. Diagram 2 compares the postdilation ABI increase to the two-year clinical outcome. Adapted from Charoenkul V, Tey PH, Ahmed A: Hemodynamic improvement after percutaneous transluminal angioplasty. Mount Sinai J Med 49:468–471, 1982.

eling." This relates to the characteristic morphologic changes produced by transluminal angioplasty. It was formerly thought that dilation was achieved by compression of deformable plaque, but it is now well appreciated that there is usually both a longitudinal tear along the length of the plaque and a dissection or shearing of the plaque from the underlying media and adventitia produced by the expansion of the inflating balloon. Sometimes the hinged flap of plaque thus created is immediately pinned down by blood flow and soon adheres to the outer lumen. At other times, it remains suspended in midstream and clots may even form in the crevice behind it. Ultimately this "remodels" and the lumen becomes bigger, often much larger and smoother than the narrow irregular lumen visualized by angiography immediately after dilation.

Regardless of cause, the observation of delayed improvement is clinically important in that several days should be allowed before judging the end-result of transluminal angioplasty, and, therefore, it is wise to wait before proceeding with further therapy, particularly when contemplating a distal reconstruction following a proximal dilation.

FREQUENCY, DEGREE, AND DURATION OF BENEFIT

Outcome Criteria

Though the risks are minimal, the benefits of PTA require careful analysis as well in order to define its role. Judging an outcome as "successful" requires objective and uniform criteria. Uniform reporting practices for PTA have not been adopted and the criteria upon which successful outcome is claimed vary considerably. Continued relief of symptoms in claudicators or avoidance of amputation in those deemed to be in a "limb salvage" situation might seem reasonable enough criteria, but their correlation with actual patency of the treated arterial segment is as poor for PTA as it is for the arterial bypass, and possibly poorer because angioplasty does not always restore normal luminal dimensions in the first place. Obviously, monitoring patients by serial angiography is not practical. However, they can be evaluated by noninvasive vascular studies. Many authors require an ankle–brachial index increase of close to 0.10, if not a 0.15 increase in lieu of angiography, as proof of patency.[24, 25] Others have required this degree of ABI increase plus categorical improvement in clinical status (e.g., a change from rest pain or threatened tissue loss to claudication, or from claudication to asymptomatic) as criteria for success. A similar approach has been adopted by the Committee on Reporting Standards of the SVS/ISCVS, and, while this should help in the future, this review of past PTA reports will require additional qualification if an accurate perspective is to result.

There is a further problem in relying on ankle pressures (or plethysmography in diabetics) to evaluate the initial success of proximal dilations carried out in the face of distal occlusive disease (typically superficial femoral artery occlusion). Lack of improvement in the ankle–brachial index can occur in spite of significantly improved dimensions and flow through the dilated iliac segment, if the distal disease is severe enough. This has caused some to report on the fallibility of noninvasive testing in this setting,[27] while others have considered that if the ankle pressure is not improved and the patient's distal circulation remains impaired, the PTA has failed

Table 17-4
Comparison of Success Rate of Iliac PTAs as
Evaluated by Different Criteria (three-year follow-up)

	All† (%)	Initial Successes (%)
Elevation of TBI > 0.10 over baseline	77	89
Sustained elevation of TBI*	74	79
Elevation of ABI > 0.10 over baseline	64	68
Sustained elevation of ABI*	54	58
Significant symptomatic improvement	52	54

* Counts deterioration only with treadmill testing also.
† All with VDL follow-up.

in achieving its goal, even if this is an error in judgment rather than technique. The authors and others have dealt with this dilemma by using elevation of the thigh–brachial index as a "patency marker" for proximal dilations, but still requiring categorical symptomatic improvement for ultimate consideration as a "success." In contrast, van Andel and coworkers[28] have credited those with subjective improvement and a palpable femoral pulse with continued patency after iliac dilation. At the other extreme, Johnston and Colapinto require categorical improvement in clinical status plus improvement in the ankle–brachial index.[29]

In the same vein it should be noted that many authors do not count technical failures into their projections of cumulative patency; in fact some also eliminate not only technical failures but all dilations thrombosing within two weeks.[28] Others freely admit to discounting technical failures in such calculations, in order to evaluate the primary patency of successful dilatations, but some do not even document the frequency of such technical failures.[15, 27] Table 17-4 shows the effect of these varying criteria for success on the results of iliac dilations when applied to a single (the authors') series. As can be seen, depending on the criteria for success and whether or not one includes technical failures, one can report three-year success rates between 89 and 52%. Similarly, with our distal dilations, the same varying criteria produced a range in reported success of from 63 to 27%. Finally, some reports consider restenoses as continuing success if they have been successfully redilated. This approach obviously obscures the true rate of deterioration or failure of the primary dilatation, but may be of value in determining the ultimate value of serial dilations to maintain arterial patency.

Case Selection

Another major consideration in gauging the success of transluminal angioplasty is the manner in which cases are selected for such intervention. The percentage of patients submitting themselves to an institution for treatment who undergo transluminal angioplasty is usually not mentioned. However, in those reports where it is documented, it varies from 10 to 56%, reflecting wide variations in case selection. Some institutions use very liberal indications for PTA, reasoning that it is now safe and rarely makes matters worse.[1] Others are screened through vascular surgeons and angiographers who may still feel that the procedure is palliative and should be restricted to poor-risk candidates in a limb salvage situation. Others feel that transluminal angioplasty at least should not be performed on any claudicating patient who would not otherwise be an acceptable candidate for arterial reconstruction, since the complications of angioplasty may force operation. At the other extreme, some radiologists primarily restrict PTA to those in whom the morphology of the lesion is very favorable, such as a superficial femoral occlusion less than 2 cm in length[23, 26] or an iliac stenosis less than 3 cm.[23] More will be said of this in the subsequent discussion which focuses on factors influencing outcome.

Factors Potentially Affecting Outcome (and, Ultimately, Case Selection)

Location of Lesion

The dilation site probably has a greater effect on outcome than any "anatomic" consideration, i.e., the morphologic characteristics of the lesion. As a generalization, it can be said that PTA results worsen as one goes distally into smaller caliber arteries, so much so that most authors separate the results of proximal (ilio-femoral) and distal (femoro-popliteal) dilations, just as is done in surgical bypass series. The results of isolated peroneal or tibial dilations are probably worse still, but thus far too few have been done to make any statistically significant comparison. Profunda and hypogastric stenoses are also infrequently reported and cannot be readily monitored by segmental pressures or plethysmography.

Even within larger arterial segments, the location of the lesion may affect the outcome. For example, distal femoro-popliteal lesions, i.e., those located at the level of the adductor canal, have been reported to do better than more proximal superficial femoral lesions in one series.[26] External iliac–common femoral stenoses, in the authors' and others'[29] experience, do worse than common iliac stenoses, although other series do not find that this makes a significance difference.[30] Table 17-5 shows the three-year success rate for dilations in our series, showing the steady trend of worsening results as one goes distally.

Degree of Occlusion

In general, worse initial results have been obtained for occlusions than for stenoses, but this deserves qualification. Occlusions tend to be longer as clots often propagate proximally to the next major collateral takeoff. Also, the dimensions of

Table 17-5
PTA Outcome Related to Site of Lesion (% of total)

	Early Failure			Late Outcome*		
	Technical	Hemo-dynamic	Total	Failed	Deteri-orated	Sustained Success
Common iliac	0	0	0	12.5	21.5	89.5
External iliac–common femoral	6.7	6.7	13.5	5.7	16.7	70.0
Superficial femoral	13.0	0	13.0	43.0	59.0	28.0
Popliteal	30.0	20.0	50.0	0	0	50.0

* Three-year follow-up.

the underlying stenotic lesions are obscured and possibly the dilation is not as well applied. Early results with iliac occlusions, and particularly the risk of significant distal embolization, almost eliminated these lesions from consideration for PTA. Therefore, proximal dilations in most series consist almost exclusively of iliac stenoses. This may change, however, as the preliminary use of intraarterial thrombolysis, using urokinase or streptokinase prior to transluminal angioplasty, is now being applied more frequently with encouraging preliminary results.[3, 31] Occasionally, localized distal aortic stenoses have been dilated with multiple and single large balloons. At the superficial femoral level, short occlusions (≤ 10 cm) as well as stenoses are dilated. In our series the long-term results for the two were not significantly different, possibly because of the more extensive nature of the stenoses subjected to dilation. In Krepel's series it also did not make a difference, but in two other series there was a 10–20% difference in the late outcome in favor of stenoses over occlusions.[30, 32]

Length of Lesion

In most experiences results worsened with increasing length of the occlusive lesion to be dilated. For example, at the femoro-popliteal level, Krepel and coworkers report continuing improvement at five years *after technically successful dilation* of 89% of occlusions less than 3 cm in length versus 26% for those over 3 cm, and 77% for stenoses less than 2 cm versus 54% for those greater than 2 cm.[26]

Extent of Disease

The extent of the occlusive disease focuses on the disease adjacent to the dilated segment. However, the length of the dilated segment and the extent of disease commonly go together and, therefore, there is cross-correlation. In the previously mentioned series from Holland, an 83% five-year success rate was reported for initially successful femoro-popliteal dilations in which the lesion was discrete, as opposed to 62% for diffusely involved segments.[26] In the same series, stenoses with an eccentric lumen had a 77% five-year success rate versus 69% for concentric stenoses. Another variable that indirectly reflects the same basic characteristic as length of lesion or extent of disease is the need to dilate multiple rather than single occlusive lesions in a given arterial segment. In the authors' experience single discrete stenoses gave a 91% three-year patency versus 56% when two or more iliac lesions required dilating.

Calcification

Calcification in the occlusive lesion does not appear, in itself, to adversely affect long-term outcome. In fact, in our series such lesions tended to do better after successful dilation, for example, 89% versus 78% at the iliac, and 59% versus 42% at the femoro-popliteal level (not statistically significant).

Runoff

Patients who have more extensive disease also tend to have occlusive lesions in the outflow tract beyond the arterial segment that has been dilated. This "poor runoff" appears to affect the durability of the dilation just as it does with arterial bypass or reconstruction. The difficulty comes in judging, by arteriogram, when the runoff is "poor" enough to adversely effect outcome. This may explain why some reports show no effect and others show a significant difference related to runoff.[20, 24, 26, 30] One series reported major differences in their results of iliac dilation based on the presence or absence of poor runoff. They reported an 89% versus 74% difference in initial success and a 50% versus 25% difference in late outcome, the higher figures applying to those cases without significant distal occlusive disease.[11] In the authors' series, the difference between iliac dilations done with an open runoff versus those with superficial femoral occlusion was not statistically significant (92% versus 83% respectively). For femoro-popliteal dilations the recent report from Eindoven, Holland, reported 77% versus 59% five-year success rates for good and poor runoff cases respectively.[26] Another series[6] showed results that steadily dropped off for femoro-popliteal dilations as the number of patent infrapopliteal vessels decreased from 3 (75%) to 2 (63%) to 1 (43%).

Diabetes

Diabetes appears to correlate with worse results following transluminal angioplasty if one only looks at overall results. However, this is because of the characteristically different distribution of lesions in the diabetics, i.e., they have proportionately fewer proximal iliac lesions which of course have the more favorable outcome. In our series and others,[9] there was no difference at either level for diabetics versus nondiabetics, but in one series, where no difference was found for proximal dilations, diabetics had only a 53% success rate with femoro-popliteal dilations versus 85% for nondiabetics.[30] However, if there is an effect of diabetes, it probably relates to the frequent presence of infrapopliteal occlusive lesions which produce poor runoff.

Durability and Late Patency Rates

As can be seen from the foregoing discussion, quoted patency rates following transluminal angioplasty should not be simply accepted at face value. Overall patency is obviously affected by the distribution and severity of occlusive lesions represented in the experience. At the very least, proximal and distal dilations should be reported separately, as is the case for aorto-iliac versus femoro-popliteal grafts. Even then one should determine whether technical errors and early failures have been excluded, redilations counted as continued successes, and whether or not the criteria for patency are "hard" or "soft." Finally, the cases or lesions selected for dilation obviously greatly influence both the initial and long-term success rate. All the aforementioned variables are responsible for the widely different estimates of continued success reported in the literature. Table 17-6 demonstrates the effect of individual variables on the authors' two-year patency rate for proximal and distal PTAs; Table 17-7 demonstrates the variation in the two-year results for proximal and distal dilations reported in the literature, keeping in mind the possible variations in patient population and criteria that each reference may represent.

With these considerable reservations, let us examine long-term results. There arc three reported experiences using life table analysis of balloon dilatations besides the authors' which reach out past the five-year level; most articles in the literature report one-, two-, and three-year success rates. One of the best documented long-term reports comes from van Andel and coworkers in Eindoven, Holland.[26, 28] They report impressive five-year success rates of over 70% for femoro-popliteal dilations

Table 17-6

Effect of Individual Variables on Two-year
Patency Rate of Proximal and Distal TLAs

	Iliac (%)	Femoral/ Popliteal (%)	All (%)
I. Lesion site	87.5	40	
II. Length of lesion			
> 2 cm stenosis		54	
< 2 cm stenosis		77	
III. Single lesions	91.0	45	75
IV. Multiple lesions	56.0	30	42
V. Good runoff	92.0	65	
VI. Poor runoff	83.0	44	
VII. Calcification	89.0	59	79
VII. Noncalcification	78.0	42	62
IX. Diabetic	57.0		
X. Nondiabetic	64.0		

and 90% for iliac lesions. However, again it should be pointed out that these results have been achieved by selecting a high proportion of favorable lesions (e.g., most lesions were less than 3 cm in length), by eliminating a 5–16% technical failure rate, and by judging patency in iliac dilations by palpable groin pulse and symptomatic improvement rather than noninvasive testing, although arm–ankle indices were used to evaluate femoro-popliteal results. Gallino and coworkers,[34] using arm–ankle pressure differences to evaluate all patients, found five-year patencies of 83% for iliac lesions and 58% for femoro-popliteal lesions. Technical failures were *not* excluded in their series.

Table 17-7

Variation in Two-year Results for Proximal and
Distal Dilations

(a) Results of Iliac Angioplasty

Principal Investigator	No. of Patients	Initial Success Rate (%)	Five-year Patency
Gruntzig (1977)[33]	36	92	85
Gallino (1984)[34]	134	95	83
van Andel (1985)[28]	194	96	90

(b) Results of Femoro-popliteal Angioplasty

Principal Investigator	No. of Patients	Initial Success Rate (%)	Five-year Patency
Gruntzig (1977)[33]	122	84	68
Gallino (1984)[34]	251	87	58
Krepel (1985)[26]	164	84	70

The authors have separately analyzed those transluminal angioplasties which had gone *at least* five years beyond the date of initial dilation. At least a 0.10 increase in the appropriate distal segmental limb pressure or normalization of that pressure was required as a criteria for patency. The five-year patency rate for 66 proximal dilations was 74%; at seven years, 58% (this excludes a 4% technical failure rate). However, distal dilations had only a 23% primary patency at five years (this excludes a technical failure rate of 17.5%). However, it should be pointed out that in the early years of our experience which are represented in these figures, it was not our practice to treat short isolated femoro-popliteal stenoses since these patients have minimal symptoms and are well managed conservatively. Patients treated were commonly bad-risk patients with jeopardized limbs and diffuse ather- omatous lesions, often requiring long segment dilation or recanalization and dila- tation at multiple sites in an attempt to tide the patients over. Arteries kept open with repeat dilatation (secondary patency) were also excluded. Even with this, there was a 56% relief of symptoms and/or preservation of limb at three years in initially successful cases. In our series of iliac dilatations we also found a significant symp- tomatic deterioration due to progression of distal disease in the presence of a patent iliac segment. At 36 months 89% of patients had improvement of the resting thigh– brachial index, while 68% of patients had an improved resting ankle–brachial index.

Recurrence Rate

In those with primarily favorable lesions mostly performed for claudication, the extended benefit reaches 90%. The recurrence rate even for relatively favorable lesions was 27.5% for femoro-popliteal lesions and 7% for iliac lesions in the Dutch series, whereas, in the Indiana experience, almost half the dilations recurred within six months.[4] Our experience has been intermediate between these two reports; 18% of iliac dilations failed during a mean follow-up of one year and 37.5% of femoro- popliteal dilations failed or deteriorated within a mean follow-up of nine and a half months. On the other side, only 2 of 11 femoro-popliteal dilations that were patent failed after one year and only 7 out of 44 iliac dilations failed between 2 and 5 years (16%).

It is also important to recognize that the consequences of failure of PTA are not severe. Recurrent stenosis at the dilatation site or new stenosis in the same arterial segment usually returns the patient to clinical baseline. Kalman and Johnston[1] reported that, of 223 eventual failures among 631 angioplasties, 85% returned to their baseline state, 5.5% were still better off, and 9.5% were clinically worse than before PTA. The 12 amputations in this series were due to advanced atheromatous disease and in no instance were attributed to failure of the PTA. Among those patients undergoing subsequent reconstructive surgery, a failed PTA had little effect on the type and outcome of the operation, although vascular reconstruction was often technically more demanding because of fibrosis at the puncture site and peri- vascular inflammatory response at the dilatation site.

SUMMARY

The current role of angioplasty will be reviewed differently by different clini- cians for biases persist. It is the authors' view, or bias if you will, that transluminal angioplasty has claimed an important role in the current management of arteriosclerosis obliterans. That role has emerged in sufficient clarity that the procedure is no longer competitive with, but rather is complementary to, arterial reconstructive surgery. It tends to be applied at the extremes of the clinical spectrum, where either arterial surgery cannot be justified (in the claudicator with a discrete stenosis) or cannot be tolerated (because of extreme operative risk in a patient with limb-threatening ischemia). An extensive experience with the latter type of case has been reported by Lu and Zarins with very acceptable morbidities and limb salvage.[5, 7] However, since transluminal angioplasty has a high technical success rate and is most durable in rather discrete occlusive lesions, it is best applied to lesions with very favorable morphology, whereas arterial reconstruction is applied to that distinct majority of cases with diffuse, extensive, or multiple in-series occlusive lesions. Since these are the more common lesions, even in our institution, where transluminal angioplasty is fairly liberally applied, PTA accounts for the sole primary treatment only in about 25% of the total cases, the remainder being managed by arterial reconstruction. Transluminal angioplasty is also being increasingly applied as an adjunct to arterial surgery to simplify arterial reconstruction or to salvage them should graft stenoses be detected.

There is a significant cost incentive to use PTA in the minority of patients where it is applicable. Two studies of initial costs of PTA compared with reconstructive vascular surgery found that the costs of iliac PTA were 18 and 30% those of aorto-femoral bypass, while femoro-popliteal PTA costs were 22 and 34% those of femoro-popliteal bypass.[35, 36] The Johns Hopkins study excluded professional fees. In both studies the principle cost benefit came from reduced length of hospitalization. Doubilet and Abrams[37] estimated the effects of using PTA as the initial modality in treating varying percentages of patients with aorto-iliac and femoro-popliteal occlusive disease, with surgery used to treat the remainder and all of the angioplasty failures. If 40% of patients with peripheral vascular disease were treated initially with angioplasty, they estimated an annual saving of 352 lives, 5006 additional limbs patent, and $99.8 million saved. If 20% were so treated, their figures indicated 176 lives saved, 2053 additional limbs patent, and $49.9 million saved.

To be more specific, transluminal angioplasty is the treatment of choice in good-risk patients for discrete (less than 5 cm) stenoses or, in the superficial femoral artery, occlusions of the same magnitude. Those patients with isolated lesions of this magnitude will invariably be claudicators and surgery can rarely be justified because of its small but significant risk when viewed against the generally benign prognosis for claudicators. In contrast, PTA can be applied to active, young, and disabled claudicators with discrete lesions because of its negligible risk in experienced hands.

Long stenoses of occlusive lesions, or multiple short stenoses in the same segment, or a single critical stenosis in a diffusely involved irregular segment are all best treated by arterial reconstruction, presuming the balance between operative risk and the threat of limb loss or restriction in essential activities justifies such intervention. PTA should be used in these instances only when surgery is contraindicated, in order to gain a relatively short-term benefit. Total iliac occlusion runs a significant risk of embolization when treated with transluminal angioplasty, even if preliminarily treated with thrombolytic drugs. The role of preliminary treatment with infraarterial fibrinolytic drugs followed by PTA to treat iliac occlusion remains to be defined.[3, 31]

If a discrete iliac stenosis exists on the side opposite to an extensive or totally occluded contralateral iliac artery or an ipsilateral superficial femoral lesion, it is appropriate to dilate it several days prior to proceeding with a femoro-femoral or femoro-popliteal bypass respectively.

Only a very limited experience with concomitant intraoperative dilation of stenoses proximal or distal to a reconstruction, using a Fogarty Chin catheter, has been reported at this writing. Therefore, secure recommendations cannot be made for this practice, but it makes more sense to the authors to dilate intraoperatively discrete SFA stenoses at the end of an aorto-bifemoral bypass than to dilate an iliac lesion intraoperatively before proceeding with femoro-popliteal bypass. Reliable inflow is essential; improved runoff is desirable.

Stenoses developing adjacent to a bypass graft and recurrent stenoses in a previously dilated segment can be detected by serial follow-up using noninvasive testing. Balloon angioplasty of such lesions is appropriate and can add significantly to the cumulative patency rate of such grafts and arteries.[38]

Finally, in categorically poor-risk patients with limb-threatening ischemia, it is often appropriate to apply transluminal angioplasty, with or without the aid of intraarterial infusions of thrombolytic drugs, to avoid inevitable amputation.

REFERENCES

1. Kalman PG, Johnston KW: Outcome of a failed percutaneous transluminal dilation. SGO 161:43–46, 1985
2. ACP: Percutaneous transluminal angioplasty. Ann Int Med 99:864–869, 1983
3. Auster M, Kadir S, Mitchell SE, et al: Iliac artery occlusion: Management with intra-thrombus streptokinase infusion and angioplasty. Radiology 153:385–388, 1984
4. Glover JL, Bendick PJ, Dilley RS, et al: Balloon catheter dilation for limb salvage. Arch Surg 118:557–560, 1983
5. Rush DS, Gervertz BL, Lu CT, et al: Limb salvage in poor risk patients using transluminal angioplasty. Arch Surg 118:1209–1212, 1983
6. Graor RA, Young JR, McCandless M, et al: Percutaneous transluminal angioplasty: Preview of iliac and femoral dilations at the Cleveland Clinic. Cleveland Clinic Quarterly 51:149–154, 1984
7. Lu CT, Zarins CK, Yang CF, Turcotte JK: Percutaneous transluminal angioplasty for limb salvage. Radiology 142:337–341, 1982
8. Jones BA, Maggisono R, Robbe C. et al: Transluminal angioplasty: Results in high risk patients with advanced peripheral vascular disease. Canadian J Surg 28:150–152, 1985
9. Johnston KE, Colapinto RF, Baird RJ: Transluminal dilation: An alternative? Arch Surg 117:1604–1609, 1982
10. Engel A, Adler OB, Rosenberger A: Percutaneous transluminal angioplasty of the iliac and lower limb vessels: One year's experience. IS J Med Sci 18:921–926, 1982
11. Cumberland DC: Percutaneous transluminal angioplasty: A review. Clinical Radiology 34:25–38, 1983
12. Sinning MA, Dixon GD, Pinkerton JA: Percutaneous transluminal angioplasty. J Kansas Med Soc 1983:331–334, 1983
13. Knight RW, Kennoy GJ, Lewis EE, Johnston GG: Percutaneous transluminal angioplasty: Results and surgical implications. Am J Surg 147:578–582, 1984
14. Glover JL, Bendick PJ, Dilley RS, et al: Efficacy of balloon catheter dilatation for lower extremity atherosclerosis. Surgery 91:560–565, 1982
15. Zeitler E, Richter EI, Roth F, Schoop W: Results of percutaneous transluminal angioplasty. Radiology 146:57–60, 1983

16. Kumpe DA, Jones DN: Percutaneous transluminal angioplasty—Radiological viewpoint. Vasc Diag and Therapy 3:19–35, 1982

17. Campbell WB, Jeans WD, Cole SEA, Baird RN: Percutaneous transluminal angioplasty for lower limb ischemia. Br J Surg 70:736–739, 1983

18. Gallino A, Mahler F, Probst P: Progression to total occlusion of lower limb artery stenoses selected for percutaneous transluminal angioplasty. Lancet 1983:59–60, 1983

19. Zarins CK, Lu CT, Gevertz BL, Lyon RT, Rush DS, Alagor S: Arterial disruption and remodeling following balloon dilatation. Surgery 92:1086–1095, 1982

20. Zollikofer CL, Salmonowitz E, Sibley R, et al: Transluminal angioplasty evaluated by electron microscopy. Radiology 153:369–374, 1984

21. Pope CF, Ezekowitz MD, Smith EO, et al: Detection of platelet deposition at the site of peripheral balloon angioplasty using indium-111 platelet scintography. Am J Cardiol 55:495–497, 1985

22. Faxon DP, Sanborn TA, Weber VJ, et al: Restenosis following transluminal angioplasty in experimental atherosclerosis. Arteriosclerosis 4:189–195, 1984

23. Katzen BJ: Percutaneous transluminal angioplasty for arterial disease of the lower extremities. AJR 142:23–25, 1984

24. Kaufman SZ, Barth KH, Kadir S, et al: Hemodynamic measurements in the evaluation and follow-up of transluminal angioplasty of the iliac and femoral arteries. Radiology 142:329–336, 1982

25. Charoenkul V, Tey PH, Ahmed A: Hemodynamic improvement after percutaneous transluminal angioplasty. Mount Sinai J Med 49:468–471, 1982

26. Krepel VM, van Andel GJ, van Erp WFM, Breslau PJ: Percutaneous transluminal angioplasty of the femoropopliteal artery: Initial and long term results. Radiology 156:325–328, 1985

27. Samson RH, Sprayregen S, Veith FJ, et al: Inadequacy of the noninvasive hemodynamic evaluation of percutaneous transluminal angioplasty. Am J Surg 147:212–215, 1984

28. van Andel GJ, van Erp WFM, Krepel VM, Breslau PJ: Percutaneous transluminal dilatation of the iliac artery: Long term results. Radiology 156:321–323, 1985

29. Johnston KE, Colapinto RF: Peripheral arterial transluminal dilatation: early results. Canadian J Surg 25:532–534, 1982

30. Lally ME, Johnston KW, Andrews D: Percutaneous transluminal dilation of peripheral arteries: An analysis of factors predicting early success. J Vasc Surg 1:704–709, 1984

31. Pilla TJ, Peterson GJ, Tantana S, et al: Percutaneous recanalization of iliac artery occlusions: An alternative to surgery in the high risk patient. AJR 143:313–316, 1984

32. Council on Scientific Affairs: Percutaneous transluminal angioplasty. JAMA 251:764–768, 1984

33. Schneider E, Gruntzig A, Bollinger A: Long term patency rates after percutaneous transluminal angioplasty for iliac and femoropopliteal obstructions, in Dotter CT, et al (eds): Percutaneous Transluminal Angioplasty. Berlin, Springer-Verlag, 1983, pp 175–180

34. Gallino A, Mahler F, Probst P, Nachbur B: Percutaneous transluminal angioplasty of the arteries of the lower limbs: A five year follow-up. Circulation 70:619–623, 1984

35. Freiman DB, Freiman MP, Spence RA, et al: Economic impact of transluminal angioplasty. Angiology 36:772–777, 1985

36. Kinnison ML, White RI, Bowers WP, Dunlap ED: Cost incentives for peripheral angioplasty. AJR 1241–1244, 1985

37. Doubilet P, Abrams HL: The cost of underutilization. Percutaneous transluminal angioplasty for peripheral vascular disease. NEJM 310:95–102, 1984

38. Howell HS, Ingram CH, Parham AR: Transluminal angioplasty of the iliac artery combined with femorofemoral bypass. Southern Med J 76:49–51, 1983

Richard H. Dean

18
What is New in Renal Revascularization?

Optimal methods for diagnostic evaluation and management of renovascular disease and renovascular hypertension continue to be controversial, with proponents of conflicting viewpoints espousing the superiority of their respective bias based on results of selected experiences with various modes of evaluation and treatment. Unfortunately, most recommendations are defended by data collected in an uncontrolled fashion based on preselected populations, and rarely are derived from scientifically sound comparisons of respective modalities of evaluation or therapy. Nevertheless, issues currently obtaining most attention in renal revascularization include the role of revascularization for salvage of function in the azotemic patient, the use of visceral vessels as donors for renal artery bypass, the relative role of percutaneous transluminal angioplasty (PTA) and surgery, and the value of "prophylactic" renal revascularization in the absence of renovascular hypertension or impaired renal function.

REVASCULARIZATION FOR RENAL SALVAGE

The 1962 report by Morris, DeBakey, and Cooley[1] underscored the potential value of renal revascularization in the management of patients with impaired renal function. In that study they described the salutary effect of revascularization on both hypertension and renal function in eight azotemic patients with either severe bilateral renal artery occlusions or unilateral occlusive disease and absence of the contralateral kidney. Novick and coworkers[2] similarly found a beneficial functional response to renal revascularization when bilateral lesions were corrected in azotemic patients. These previous observations have been mimicked in our experience only by severely azotemic patients (serum creatinine ≥ 3.0 mg/dl) with correctable bilateral disease; these patients demonstrated a significant improvement in serum creatinine after revascularization (Fig. 18-1).[3]

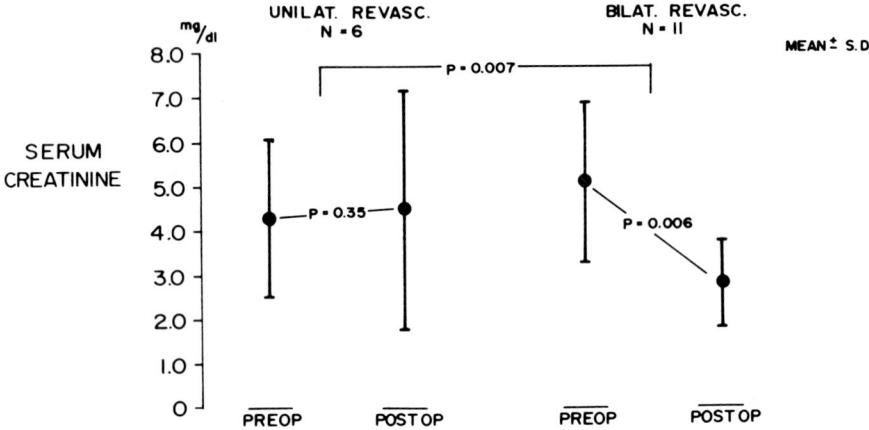

Fig. 18-1. Effect of revascularization of a unilateral lesion compared to bilateral lesions on serum creatinine.

There is a theoretic possibility that a unilateral lesion may develop which, while protecting the distal renal parenchyma from nephrosclerosis, produces severe hypertension that destroys the "unprotected kidney" and causes severe azotemia. In this frequently hypothesized situation, unilateral revascularization of the "protected kidney" would be expected to produce a significant benefit in overall excretory function. Such a presentation is rare, however, and has only occurred once in our experience. In all other instances, overall renal function has not benefited. In the group of six patients with a preoperative serum creatinine greater than or equal to 3.0 mg/dl, there was an insignificant increase in serum creatinine after such unilateral reconstructions. With these findings we believe that such unilateral reconstructions in severely azotemic patients should be undertaken only for purposes of blood pressure control. In this circumstance, there is potential that better blood pressure control might decrease the rate of progressive bilateral arteriolar nephrosclerosis.

A more common clinical controversy surrounds the management of patients who present with hypertension secondary to renal artery occlusive disease in whom the ischemic kidney has little or no residual excretory function but overall excretory function is not severely impaired. Many physicians believe that such kidneys predominantly have end-stage nephrosclerosis and that they have little potential for salvage. Indeed, if retrieval of function is unlikely, then either continued control by drug therapy or primary nephrectomy would be superior. Clearly the aggressive attitude adopted in our center toward the potential value of revascularization for retrieval of function and our desire to identify the lower limits of retrievability led to revascularization of some kidneys in which no functional response was achieved. In such patients, primary nephrectomy would have been simpler and equally beneficial in blood pressure control. Nevertheless, this aggressive approach has provided a spectrum of responses from which the value of potential preoperative predictors of response can be examined. In this regard, data received from split renal function studies, isotope renography, and renal length measurement merit special comment.

Split renal function studies (SRFS) have been employed in our center for over 24 years to supplement renal vein renin assays in the diagnosis of renovascular hypertension as well as to define parameters of excretory function in the involved kidney. Through this long experience, the methodology of their performance and their interpretation have been well standardized.[4] Since the physiologic response of the normal kidney is to increase the tubular reabsorption of water during periods of decreased perfusion, the presence of urinary hyperconcentration of nonreabsorbable solutes such as creatinine is an indication that both a physiologically important renovascular lesion is present and that there are significant numbers of intact nephron units present within the ischemic kidney. This later premise becomes particularly important in the patient with a poorly functioning kidney. In this circumstance, the presence of hyperconcentration should reflect the presence of a potentially retrievable function. This hypothesis was examined in the current study. However, the absence of urine flow from the affected kidney does not allow useful calculation of hyperconcentration. In such circumstances this parameter has no value as a predictor of functional response.

Isotopic studies of renal function have been modified several times over the past several years in our center. The current study combines the determination of glomerular filtration rate by ^{99m}Tc-DPTA with a calculation of relative functioning mass from each kidney using ^{99m}Tc-DMSA. The derived value of the individual kidney or split GFR has primarily been used to provide a noninvasive means of determining changes in renal function during serial observations. The finding that a statistically significant negative correlation exists between the preoperative split GFR and the change in creatinine clearance from the affected kidney is particularly exciting, for it suggests that a noninvasive means of functional assessment and prediction of retrieval of function may be possible. This premise is strengthened by the finding that patients with a split GFR less than or equal to 20 ml/min from the affected side had a statistically significantly greater response than patients with a higher preoperative split GFR.

Results of renal length analyses show that a negative linear relationship may exist between the preoperative length and the change in length following an operation. Many physicians have adopted a lower limit of renal length below which they suggest that there is no value of revascularization. Although our data include revascularization of only two kidneys with lengths less than or equal to 8.0 cm, regression analysis suggests that when other parameters predict the presence of retrievable renal function in a kidney with a correctable lesion that short renal length alone is not a valuable negative predictor of response. In contrast, one might expect the greatest percentage improvement in length in such kidneys. Nevertheless, the premise that renal length improvement can be equated to improvement in renal function is speculative. The demonstrated interrelationships between preoperative renal length, changes in renal length following revascularization, and changes in functional parameters as identified in this study, however, suggest that such a relationship may exist.

Adequate angiographic evaluation of the renal vasculature is imperative for accurate selection of patients for revascularization. Successful retrieval of function by revascularization implies that macroscopic occlusive disease has been either bypassed or removed at operation. None of the examined preoperative parameters would be expected to have pertinence when significant branch and intrarenal segmental vessel occlusions are present. Therefore, a preoperative demonstration of disease-free distal vessels is required before retrieval of function or benefit in blood pressure control can be anticipated. Most kidneys in which the distal vessel can not be visualized on preoperative angiography have severe distal disease. Nevertheless, if preoperative functional assessment provides data which suggest the presence of retrievable renal function, then exploration of the nonvisualized distal vessel and revascularization when a disease-free distal vessel is found is appropriate in selected cases. Otherwise, primary nephrectomy is more appropriate for treatment of such patients.

Although Zinman and Libertino have found preoperative renal biopsy to be of value as a predictor of functional retrieval in patients managed in their center,[5] we have not found it worthwhile. Having identified diffuse hyalinization of glomerulae in specimens obtained by open biopsy from selected sections of kidneys with adequate renal function and in kidneys which had marked improvement in excretory function, we abandoned the technique in the remote past as misleading and potentially hazardous.

RENAL ARTERY BYPASS FROM VISCERAL ARTERIES

Renewed enthusiasm for the use of visceral artery branches as donor vessels for renal artery bypass has received renewed publicity in the recent literature. Donor sites for such alternate methods of renal revascularization include the hepatic artery,[6-8] splenic artery,[9,10] gastroduodenal artery,[11] and mesenteric arteries.[12] Experience with use of these alternate donor vessels, however, varies widely among centers with wide experience with the surgical management of RVH. Dominant among the reasons for such disparity in frequency of use are the perceived indications for their preferential use.

Although a rare reason for using these techniques, they are extremely valuable in the treatment of aortic graft infections where no infrarenal stump is available for closure after graft removal. In this circumstance, transfer of the site of renal perfusion to the splenic and hepatic arteries allows the juxtarenal aorta to be securely closed without compromise of renal perfusion.

A more commonly employed reason for use of visceral donor vessels for renal revascularization is a desire to not molest the aorta in a variety of situations. Included among the publicized reasons are the presence of a diffusely atherosclerotic aorta, previous aortic dissection, aortic aneurysms, or other instances which would lead to simultaneous aortic replacement in order to facilitate the performance of an aorto-renal bypass. Implicit in the choice for use of such alternate methods is a desire to limit the magnitude of the operative procedure, to reduce the risk of combined aortic and renal reconstruction, and to minimize the cost in morbidity of the more complicated dissection in an area of previous intervention. Certainly, total experiences with combined aortic and renal artery surgery carry higher operative mortality rates than when the procedure is limited to renal artery surgery alone. This apparently appropriate logic, however, compares two different populations undergoing operation and the risk of operation in these different populations. This point is exemplified in our experience with renal artery surgery in over 700 patients. Although renal revascularization alone has had an attendant 0.8% operative mortality rate and combined simultaneous aortic and renal artery surgery has had a 12% operative mortality rate, the risk in the latter combined procedure group primarily has been related to the preoperative status of the patient and can be predicted. In a review of our experience with such combined procedures, the operative risk clearly could be stratified and was negligible in the majority of patients.[13] In the subgroup of patients at high risk, another nonaortic procedure was not a clinically realistic alternative. Further, this experience was developed with the philosophy that aorto-renal bypass alone should be performed if there was no clinically justifiable reason for aortic replacement. In other words, the aorta was not replaced simply to facilitate aorto-renal bypass. Therefore, in conditions of diffuse atherosclerosis, mild subrenal ectasia of the aorta, and in the face of previous aortic dissections, aorto-renal bypass or another direct renal artery procedure alone was performed. In these circumstances, alternate donor sources for renal artery bypass were not used, and no untoward consequences of this more standard approach ensued. Considering the success of this approach, which currently includes a 98% technical success rate of aorto-renal bypass and an operative mortality rate in a predominantly atherosclerotic patient population of less than 1%, I believe the nonaortic donor vessel techniques must be shown to have at least an equal success before a liberal use of such procedures in the population in question is justifiable. In this regard, in the 1984 review of the Cleveland Clinic[14] experience with spleno-renal bypass in 69 patients, there were four operative deaths (6%) and an additional 6% who were failures of intervention. Therefore, I continue to believe that such alternate methods of renal revascularization are a valuable adjunct to our surgical armamentarium but that their use should be limited primarily to management of patients in whom the aorta truly is not a viable donor site. Using this philosophy, we have not required the use of such a technique in over 450 cases.

In any event, when such visceral vessels must be used, one must accurately assess the entire donor vessel for clinically silent occlusive disease. Since the orifice of the celiac axis is a common site for asymptomatic stenosis, lateral aortography and selective visceral angiography is necessary for assurance that the chosen vessel is free of significant occlusive disease.

THE ROLE OF PERCUTANEOUS TRANSLUMINAL ANGIOPLASTY

The introduction of the alternative interventional modality percutaneous transluminal angioplasty (PTLA) by Grüntzig in 1978[15] has led to a new era in the management of hypertensive patients with renal artery stenosis. Early reports of the results of this technique showed that stenotic renal arteries frequently could be dilated successfully with immediate improvement in levels of hypertension in patients with RVH. Following these reports and attendant widespread publicity, euphoric acceptance of the technique in many centers has ensued prior to the availability of any follow-up data on its safety, success, and durability compared with operation in similar groups of patients. Like results with operative management, experience with PTLA in a given center may vary; however, in centers experienced with its use, immediate results of PTLA serve as a comparison to address relevant unanswered questions regarding the relative merit of this modality.

In comparing published results of PTLA[16–22] to experience with operation, the risk of death from either modality should be negligible. Immediate technical success gauged by postoperative angiography has demonstrated that 97% of renal revascularization procedures have been technically successful in our center. PTLA has been feasible in over 90% of attempted cases in these centers. Similar to the variability of operative results in respective hospitals, patient selection and the actual technique of PTLA are important factors in describing its safety and success. Although atheromatous embolism, irretrievable renal artery trauma, renal failure, and other major complications have resulted from inappropriate patient selection for PTLA and improper technique, these risks are low ($< 10\%$) in centers experienced with its use and are comparable to the cumulative risks of similar complications in our experience with operative management.

Immediate results of successful PTLA in regard to amelioration of hypertension are difficult to compare with our experience with operation. Most reports suggest that at least 90% of patients will have improved hypertension at one month after PTLA.[16–22] In our center 96% of patients have had significant benefit in hypertension at six months after operation. Since early results of renal revascularization from any method traditionally have been based on the six-month postoperative status, and less than 30% of reported patients treated by PTLA have been followed up for even this period, comparison is impossible from currently available data. Nevertheless, in a recent report by Tegtmeyer, Kofler, and Ayers,[16] a cure rate at 1–52 months after PTLA was reported to be 44% in 80 patients. These data are not broken down into patients with atherosclerotic lesions and those with fibro-dysplastic lesions. The authors do state that 11 of 23 patients (48%) with fibro-muscular dysplasia were cured. In contrast, 73% of patients with FMD have been rendered normotensive without medication in a recent report of our operative experience.

Finally, since the value of either operation or PTLA is related to the ability to provide lasting relief of renal ischemia and long-term reduction of hypertension-related cardiovascular risk factors, durability of revascularization should be a central ingredient. Our review of follow-up angiography obtained 1–23 years after operation in 198 patients has demonstrated a 5% incidence of progressive fibrotic stenosis of the reconstruction during follow-up. Since each of these changes became apparent by 12–18 months after operation, comparison of the one-year durability of operation (95%) to that seen after PTLA seems appropriate. Unfortunately, minimal follow-up angiographic data are available in reports on patients treated by PTLA. To date, less than 10% of patients included in such reports have one-year follow-up angiographic data. Within the limitations imposed by the lack of follow-up data, however, there appears to be some discrepancy among the centers performing PTLA in regard to the frequency of restenosis after successful dilatation. In addition, the type of lesion (atherosclerosis versus fibromuscular dysplasia) also appears to be important in regard to the probability of restenosis after PTLA. Follow-up over this short period suggests that the dilatation by PTLA of the medial dysplasia type of fibromuscular dysplasia appears to be maintained. In contrast, restenosis of atherosclerotic lesions appears to be frequent. The actual rate of restenosis and frequency are unknown, but published reports suggest that 10–100% of atherosclerotic lesions treated by PTLA will recur to their original severity within a year.[16-22]

In the review of Grim and coworkers,[22] all patients with angiographic follow-up had developed restenosis by one year. In the recent review by Tegtmeyer, Kofler, and Ayers,[16] restenosis occurred in 10% of the patients, yet they summarized the results in five other large series in which the reported recurrence rate was 19–30%.[17-21] Again, these results are not segregated into the respective types of lesions, and few of the patients in any of the series have been restudied. Nevertheless, factors potentially increasing the rate of failure of PTLA due both to failure of successful dilatation and to recurrence of the lesion are calcification in the lesion, lesions situated at the orifice of the renal artery, and residual narrowing of the PTLA of more than 30%. Although PTLA of fibromuscular dysplastic lesions of the "chain-of-beads" variety (medical dysplasia) appears to be maintained during follow-up, similar permanency of PTLA of unifocal lesions has not been demonstrated. Nonetheless, we have seen and operatively managed several patients, both children and adults, with unifocal lesions—congenital and acquired—who did not respond to PTLA. In addition, the lower incidence of cure after PTLA of fibromuscular dysplastic lesions when compared with operation is probably related to the presence of lesions not seen angiographically and thereby not dilated. Certainly, this is a uniform observation at operation, where involvement of the vessel is always more extensive than that appreciated angiographically.

Although the considerations reviewed in the foregoing paragraphs have not been resolved, a common practice in many centers at this time is to proceed with PTLA whenever a significant renovascular lesion is demonstrated in the hypertensive patient who is undergoing angiographic evaluation. The logic for this attitude is that PTLA is both diagnostic and therapeutic and that no functional assessment or proof of a causal relationship between the renovascular lesion and the hypertension is required prior to intervention. When only 50% of such lesions are, in fact, the source of hypertension, this logic suggests without proof that untoward effects are so uncommon as to make them of no concern. Further, this also suggests that there may be salutary effects on incidental lesions by preventing their progression to produce RVH or to deteriorate renal function. Certainly, if such were the case, the relative risks and costs of management of all patients in this manner might be lower than the combined risks and costs of diagnostic studies and subsequent interventional therapies.

Since none of these questions has been addressed in a scientific manner, one is left with a personal bias based on personal experience and available literature to describe the current role of PTLA as a means of renal revascularization. Clearly, when results are summarized, operative management is somewhat superior, yet results in subgroup populations are clearly divergent. PTLA clearly has an associated high rate of either inadequate dilatation or rapid recurrence when orificial and bilateral lesions are managed. Similarly, congenital lesions and unifocal lesions as well as multiple-branch lesions are more successfully managed by operation. In contrast, the patient with a totally nonorificial atherosclerotic lesion and the patient who is at an unacceptable high risk for operation are best managed by PTLA. In these groups, operation can legitimately be the therapeutic alternative when success with PTLA is not achieved.

PROPHYLACTIC RENAL REVASCULARIZATION

Following reports of a progressive loss of renal function during nonoperative follow-up of patients with renal artery stenosis and RVH, there has been increased enthusiasm for empiric intervention, either by operation or PTLA, regardless of the results of functional studies or in the absence of such studies performed to define the clinical relevance of the renovascular lesion. The justification for such an aggressive approach toward the value of intervention is that this empiric or "prophylactic" revascularization will prevent subsequent loss of renal function. Although such logic appears potentially sound, two factors impact on its utility. First, such reasoning implies that one can predict which lesion will cause progressive loss of renal function. Serial follow-up data collected in our center suggests that 41% of patients treated medically who had initially positive functional studies, i.e., presumptive proof of the presence of a hemodynamically significant lesion, will have significant reduction in some parameter of renal function during follow-up.[23] There has been no definition of the characteristics predictive of such subsequent deterioration, however. Further, if the lesion has no functional or hemodynamic significance, there are no data available which define the rate of loss of renal function. Intuitively, one would surmise that the frequency of deterioration in such patients would be significantly less than in those patients seen later in their course when the lesion has progressed to functional significance and is, thereby, the source of RVH.

Second, there is no published data comparing the incidence of deterioration of renal function after intervention. Implicit in empiric or "prophylactic" revascularization is the premise that such deterioration is less frequent when revascularization is attempted. Although we currently are evaluating this comparative frequency in a prospective randomized trial of operative management and drug therapy for RVH, this trial is incomplete and no other data are available. Therefore, we continue to believe that renal revascularization should be performed for the management of RVH and hope that this has a favorable effect on preventing loss of renal function as well as retrieval of lost function. Nevertheless, we believe functional proof should be required when appropriate and that there is no justification for attempted revascularization without such foundations.

REFERENCES

1. Morris GC Jr, DeBakey ME, Cooley DA: Surgical treatment of renal failure of renovascular origin. JAMA 182:113–116, 1962
2. Novick AC, Pohl MA, Schreiber M, et al: Revascularization for preservation of renal function in patients with atherosclerotic renovascular disease. J Urol 129:907–911, 1983
3. Dean RH, Englund R, Dupont WD, et al: Retrieval of renal function by revascularization: Study of preoperative outcome predictors. Ann Surg 202:367–375, 1985
4. Dean RH, Rhamy RK: Split renal function studies in renovascular hypertension, in Ernst CB, Fry WJ, Stanley JC (eds): Renovascular Hypertension. Philadelphia, WB Saunders, 1984, pp 135–145
5. Zinman L, Libertino JA: Revascularization of the chronic totally occluded renal artery with restoration of renal function. J Urol 118:517–521, 1977
6. Libertino JA, Zinman L: Hepatorenal bypass in the management of renovascular hypertension. J Urol 115:369–372, 1976

7. Novick AC, Palleschi J, Straffon RA, Beven EG: Experimental and clinical hepatorenal bypass as a means of revascularization of the right renal artery. Surg Gynecol Obstet 148:557–561, 1979

8. Chibaro EA, Libertino JA, Novick AC: Use of hepatic circulation for revascularization. Ann Surg 199:406–411, 1984

9. Novick AC, Banowsky LH, Stewart BH, Straffon RA: Splenorenal bypass in the treatment of stenosis of the renal artery. Surg Gynecol Obstet 144:891–898, 1977

10. Brewster DC, Darling RC: Splenorenal arterial anastomosis for renovascular hypertension. Ann Surg 189:353–358, 1979

11. Libertino JA, Lagneau P: A new method of revascularization of the right renal artery by the gastroduodenal artery. Surg Gynecol Obstet 156:221–223, 1983

12. Khauli RB, Novick AC, Coseriu GV, Beven E, Hertzer NR: The superior mesenterorenal bypass in patients with infrarenal aortic occlusion. J Urol 133:188, 1985

13. Dean RH, Keyser JE III, Dupont WD, Nadeau JH, Meacham PW: Aortic and renal vascular disease: Factors affecting the value of combined procedures. Ann Surg 200:336–344, 1984

14. Khauli RB, Novick AC, Ziegelbaum M: Splenorenal bypass in the treatment of renal artery stenosis: Experience with sixty-nine cases. J Vasc Surg 2:547–551, 1985

15. Grüntzig A, Vetter W, Meier B, et al: Treatment of renovascular hypertension with transluminal dilatation of a renal artery stenosis. Lancet 1:801, 1978

16. Tegtmeyer CJ, Kofler TJ, Ayers CA: Renal angioplasty: Current status. AJR 142:17, 1984

17. Colapinto RF, Stronell RD, Harries-Jones EP, et al: Percutaneous transluminal dilatation of the renal artery: Follow-up studies on renovascular hypertension. AJR 139:727, 1982

18. Katzen BT, Chang J, Knox WG: Percutaneous transluminal angioplasty with the Grüntzig balloon catheter: A review of 70 cases. Arch Surg 114:1389, 1979

19. Puijlaert CBAJ, Boomsma JHB, Ruijs JHJ, et al: Transluminal renal artery dilatation in hypertension: Technique, results and complications in 60 cases. Urol Radiol 2:201, 1981

20. Schwarten DE: Percutaneous transluminal renal angioplasty. Urol Radiol 2:193, 1981

21. Sos TA, Saddekni S, Sniderman KW, et al: Renal artery angioplasty: Technique and early results. Urol Radiol 3:223, 1982

22. Grim CE, Weinberger MH, Yune HY, et al: Balloon dilatation as a treatment of hypertension due to renal artery stenosis: Preliminary results in 25 patients. Proceedings of the First SCOR-Hypertension Conference, Cornell Medical Center, New York City, March 7–8, 1980, pp 125–129

23. Dean RH, Kieffer RW, Smith BM, et al: Renovascular hypertension: Anatomic and renal function changes during drug therapy. Arch Surg 116:1408–1415, 1981

Peter J. Morris
and John A. Murie

19

Vascular Complications after Renal Transplantation

INTRODUCTION

Vascular complications after renal transplantation are of considerable importance as they may lead to the loss of the transplanted kidney and even to loss of life. They may involve both the arterial and the venous systems. Arterial complications may be related to the graft itself, such as transplant renal artery thrombosis, or stenosis of the renal artery of the graft or secondary haemorrhage. General arterial complications also occur due principally to cardiac or peripheral atheromatous disease. Venous problems may also be related to the graft itself, such as renal vein thrombosis, or may be more distant, such as deep vein thrombosis in the lower limbs with or without pulmonary embolism. Each of these subgroups will be discussed in turn.

LOCAL ARTERIAL COMPLICATIONS

Transplant Renal Artery Thrombosis

This is fortunately a rare complication in experienced units, for it will almost certainly result in loss of the graft, even if recognised early and treated appropriately. In Oxford it has occurred twice in 540 (0.4%) transplant operations, one of which was a technically difficult third-transplant procedure. Renal artery thrombosis is generally due to technical error producing twisting or kinking of the vessel when the kidney is placed in its extraperitoneal pouch, and careful assessment of the artery is required at this stage of the operation.

This complication should be suspected in any patient who suddenly becomes anuric within 48 hours of surgery. Rapid confirmation of arterial occlusion may be obtained by isotope scanning of the kidney, but the problem is of such urgency that it may be more appropriate if the diagnosis is strongly suspected to return the patient immediately to the operating room for exploration. If the blood supply is not reconstituted by thrombectomy or revision of the anastomosis within 90 minutes, warm ischaemic damage will almost certainly cause irreversible damage to the graft. It is apparent that the likelihood of rescuing a graft when renal artery thrombosis has occurred is remote.

Thrombosis may also affect accessory renal arteries, occlusion of which may not be attended by any major problems provided that only a small segment of kidney is vascularised by such an accessory artery. On the other hand, hypertension may result, requiring medical and even surgical intervention. In the case of a lower polar accessory artery, which usually provides a blood supply to the ureter, its occlusion may predispose to urine leak in the early days after transplantation, or ureteric stenosis at a later stage.

Transplant Renal Artery Stenosis

This complication is not uncommon, and although it has been found after seven (1.3%) out of 540 transplant operations in Oxford, a much higher incidence was reported following routine angiography in a small series of patients with hypertension after renal transplantation.[1] There are two types. In the first, vessel narrowing occurs at the site of the anastomosis in an end-to-end anastomosis of the renal artery to the internal iliac artery, and in the second it occurs more distally in the renal artery, usually between 5 and 20 mm from an end-to-end or end-to-side anastomosis (Fig. 19-1).

The first type is generally a short stenosis which may be atheromatous in nature. It is technical in origin caused either by a poorly constructed anastomosis or by reaction to the suture material. A fall in incidence of this complication has occurred in tandem with increased utilisation of nonreactive suture material such as Prolene, in preference to silk, and anastomotic line stenosis is now rarely seen.

The second type is more common and accounts for all those in the Oxford series. It is usually more diffuse than the anastomotic type and may extend from near the anastomosis itself up to the first branch artery of the graft. The affected vessel is surrounded by a dense fibrosis and although the exact aetiology of post-anastomotic stenosis is not known, it probably has little in common with atheromatous disease. It has been suggested that angulation in the renal artery may cause turbulent flow which predisposes to vessel wall changes or that arterial trauma at the time of organ perfusion is responsible.[2] The most likely explanation is that the stenosis results from a fibrotic response of the periadventitial tissue to the generalised homograft reaction.[3]

The diagnosis of transplant renal artery stenosis may be difficult on clinical grounds as the principal features of hypertension and decreased renal function occur commonly in transplant recipients from other causes. The appearance of a bruit over the kidney, especially when difficulty in control of hypertension is encountered, is a serious sign, for it is rare not to hear a bruit in the presence of a functional stenosis. Antihypertensives such as captopril or enalopril which act as competitive inhibitors of angiotensin I converting enzyme may compromise renal function in patients with renal artery stenosis and so provide a useful diagnostic clue.[4] Final elucidation, however, depends on angiography. Digital subtraction angiography has

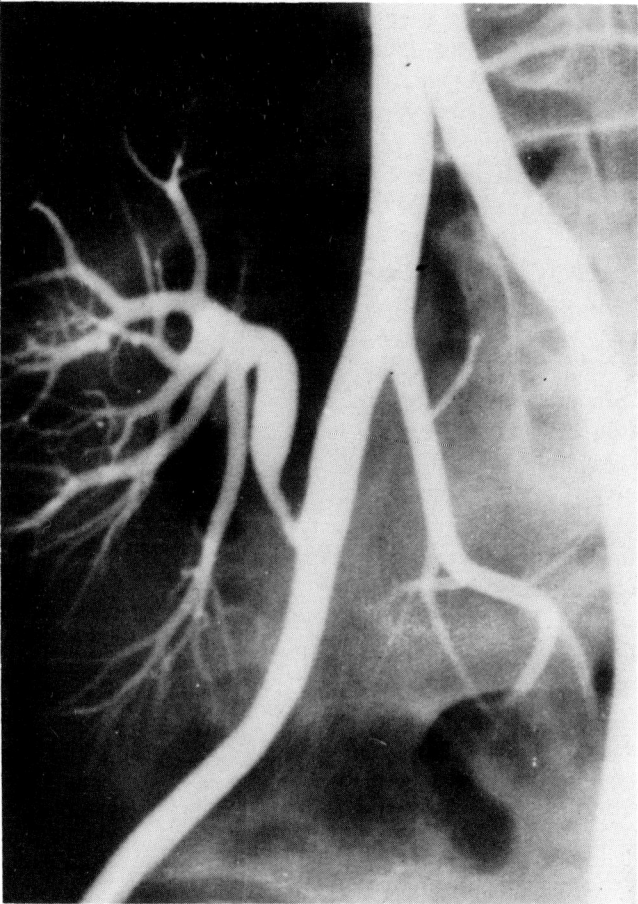

Fig. 19-1. Transplant renal angiogram showing a post-anastomotic stenosis of the renal artery.

been applied in this situation but has yet to be shown to be sufficiently accurate compared to conventional techniques. Other forms of noninvasive vascular assessment are not generally applicable, principally because of the variation in anatomical disposition of vessels encountered in the area of the transplant. The significance of a renal artery stenosis may be determined sometimes by venous sampling, demonstrating a high plasma renin activity in the renal vein effluent, or by a renal biopsy excluding severe chronic rejection as a cause of hypertension and deteriorating renal function.

Once the diagnosis is clear, if hypertension is difficult to control or if renal function is compromised, an attempt to correct the stenosis should be made. Operative correction is difficult and should only be undertaken by those experienced in both transplant and vascular surgery. The approach may be made through the old transplant incision, but a new longitudinal abdominal incision is generally preferable. In either case the peritoneal cavity is entered and the iliac and renal vessels are identified intraperitoneally. The overlying peritoneum is incised and the iliac arteries and renal artery dissected out. The stenosis is identified and one of a variety of techniques used for its correction. Assessment of blood flow through the renal artery before and after correction using an electromagnetic flowmeter is useful.

Twenty operations in 18 patients have been performed by one of the authors (PJM) for transplant renal artery stenosis in Melbourne and Oxford over the past 18 years. All patients had severe preoperative hypertension and all but one had reduced renal function. The average age was 34 years (range 16–45 years) and the stenoses were diagnosed at a mean of 21 months after transplantation (range 2–72 months). In 10 cases the transplant anastomosis was end-to-side between the renal artery and external iliac artery and in eight was end-to-end between the renal artery and internal iliac artery. All diagnoses were made using conventional angiography and recent biopsies were available to exclude significant changes of rejection in the kidneys. Surgery was usually performed by a transperitoneal route and in all cases dissection was difficult due to the fibrosis surrounding the vessels.

The most frequent technique used in 20 operations was to divide the internal iliac artery and anastomose it end-to-end or end-to-side with the renal artery distal to the stenosis (eight cases). Alternatively, especially when the internal iliac vessel had been used to revascularise the kidney at the time of transplantation, a vein graft was used. This ran from the external iliac (five cases) or the common iliac (one case) or the internal iliac artery (one case) to the renal artery distal to the stenosis. Other less commonly used techniques were to divide the renal artery distal to the stenosis and reimplant it in the external iliac artery (two cases), to endarterectomise the renal artery with vein patch closure of the arteriotomy (one case), or to use an angioplasty balloon catheter to dilate the stenosis (one case). In one case, reconstruction was not feasible and a transplant nephrectomy was performed. Thus reconstruction was technically impossible in only one out of 20 (5%) cases.

Excluding the nephrectomy, 18 out of 19 (95%) procedures resulted in an improvement in hypertension. Only the operative balloon catheter angioplasty failed in this respect. Excluding both the nephrectomy and the single patient with good preoperative renal function, 16 out of 18 (89%) operations resulted in a significant improvement in renal function. The balloon catheter angioplasty and one other reconstruction failed to improve renal function.

Although percutaneous transluminal angioplasty (PTA)[5] has been very successful in treating atheromatous stenosis at various sites including the native renal artery, its use in the treatment of transplant renal artery stenosis has been attended by mixed results. The overall reported success rate of PTA for this condition is not better than 50%.[3,6] Complications such as renal artery thrombosis and graft loss have been reported. The inferior results in transplant renal artery stenosis may be due to a pathological process different from atheroma causing the lesion. In Oxford, three attempts at PTA for transplant renal artery stenosis have been made and although the technique has not been responsible for graft loss, in no case was it possible to negotiate the balloon catheter into the stenosis itself.

Secondary Haemorrhage

This is an uncommon but potentially life-threatening complication due to infection of the anastomosis. The source of sepsis may be contamination from the graft itself before storage. Now that the administration of prophylactic antibiotics at the time of transplantation has become routine practice, this complication is much less frequently encountered. Transplant nephrectomy is usually necessary if the graft is in situ, but the complication may also occur after graft nephrectomy. Usually it is necessary to ligate the internal iliac artery proximally in the case of an end-to-end anastomosis or the external iliac artery above and below the anastomosis in the case of an end-to-side anastomosis. In the latter operation, immediate reconstruction of the arterial supply to the lower limb is generally not required.[7]

GENERAL ARTERIAL COMPLICATIONS

Data from the European Dialysis and Transplant Association Registry show that more than half of all deaths among patients receiving renal replacement therapy are from vascular disease.[8] The principal causes of death are myocardial infarction and cerebrovascular accident and there is little evidence that renal transplantation reduces the incidence of death from generalised arterial disease from that found in patients treated either by haemodialysis or by continuous ambulatory peritoneal dialysis. It is certain when survival is related to the cause of renal failure that, whatever the mode of treatment, patients with either hypertension or diabetes mellitus as the primary diagnoses fare worse than those with other primary pathologies.[9] Cardiovascular mortality in patients after renal transplantation may be due to any of the well-defined risk factors for the general population, either singly or in combination. In those with renal disease, however, two factors are of special importance, namely hypertension and hyperlipidaemia.

Although uraemia itself may be associated with hypertension, elevated blood pressure remains a problem all too often in those with functioning renal transplants. Despite improvement in renal function after grafting, there must be new causes for raised blood pressure. Bachy has shown that 30% of patients are hypertensive one month after transplantation and 65% are hypertensive between six months and three years. Although the incidence tends to fall in later years, 40% remain long-term hypertensives.[10] Kirkman has also noted that hypertension is the commonest complication in long-term survivors after transplantation, affecting no less than 46% of patients with a functioning graft.[11]

The mechanism of hypertension in renal transplant patients is well reviewed by Raine and Ledingham.[12] Whatever the cause, there is little to suggest that the problem is less severe after grafting than on dialysis. Although some reports show no greater prevalence of hypertension posttransplant,[10] others have suggested that those with renal failure may be even more prone to blood pressure elevation when treated by transplantation than by haemodialysis.[13] The causes of hypertension in the patient with a renal transplant include rejection, the influence of diseased native kidneys, transplant renal artery stenosis, steroid therapy, and cyclosporin therapy. Hypertension is more common in those receiving cadaver grafts than in recipients of kidneys from living related donors.[14]

Hypertension is usual but not invariable in acute rejection and is due to increase in plasma renin activity[15] and fluid retention. In chronic rejection a direct relationship exists with hypertension. Kirkman has shown that 72% of long-term survivors with chronic rejection are also hypertensive.[11] Conversely, many transplant recipients with elevated blood pressure have normal renal function.

Although disease of the native kidneys may produce hyperreninaemia and blood pressure elevation which can be corrected by pretransplant nephrectomy in individual patients, Kirkman found no correlation between the prevalence of hypertension and the frequency of prior nephrectomy in 217 transplanted patients.[11] The problem of transplant renal artery stenosis was discussed in the previous section and although the Oxford incidence is low, others have reported an incidence as high as 16%.[16] Variation in the criteria for recognition accounts for the variation in incidence, but it must be appreciated that the association of renal artery stenosis and hypertension is not always causal.

Steroid immunosuppressive therapy predisposes to hypertension[15] and conversion to alternate-day therapy[17] or low-dose regimens[18] are less hazardous in this respect. Steroids may not, however, be a primary cause of blood pressure elevation since in some series no difference in steroid dose was found between normotensive and hypertensive patients.[10] In the European Multicentre Trial comparing cyclosporin with azathioprine and prednisolone as immunosuppressive regimens, mean arterial pressure was similar and in the normotensive range in both groups.[19] However, in the Oxford randomised trial of short-term use of cyclosporin for three months followed by conversion to azathioprine and prednisolone, there was a marked improvement in hypertension after conversion.[20]

Drug therapy for posttransplant hypertension is reviewed elsewhere.[12] If this is not successful, nephrectomy of the native kidneys may be curative, especially if they are shown to be the source of raised plasma renin activity.[21] Renal artery embolisation is an alternative and has resulted in significant reduction in mean blood pressure in eight out of 12 patients so treated in Oxford, with no serious morbidity.[22]

Although the most profound effect of arterial disease is death from myocardial infarction or stroke, nonfatal arterial occlusive disease may also be more common in renal transplant recipients, not only than in the normal population but also than in those treated by dialysis.[23] Peripheral arterial disease in transplant recipients may cause not only limb ischaemia but also loss of the graft due to occlusion of the iliac artery on the side of the transplanted organ. This has accounted for the loss of two out of 540 kidneys transplanted in Oxford.[7]

It has long been recognised that uraemic patients commonly have type IV hyperlipidaemia with marked hypertriglyceridaemia.[24] Cholesterol levels in the uraemic patient tend to be normal or below normal. After transplantation, although the type IV abnormality may persist, patients may also develop type IIa or IIb hyperlipidaemia with cholesterol as well as triglyceride elevation. Curtis has shown that both cholesterol and triglycerides were elevated on a 15 mg per day maintenance dose of prednisolone but fell to normal after a 30 mg per alternate day regimen was started.[25] An inverse relationship exists between very low-density lipoprotein (VLDL) and high-density lipoprotein (HDL) cholesterol. VLDL cholesterol is elevated in transplant recipients[26] and HDL cholesterol is low, a feature known to be associated with ischaemic heart disease.[27] Although HDL can be measured as a risk factor there is no evidence that raising its concentration by dietary or drug therapy will reduce the risk of atheroma in transplant patients. Nevertheless, it seems reasonable to correct hyperlipidaemia by simple calorie restriction.[28]

Despite the undoubted lipid changes which occur in the posttransplant patient, it must be remembered that it is hypertension which is the major risk factor and its control is essential. Everything possible must be done in transplant recipients to slow the progression of atherosclerosis; this includes stopping smoking, which itself doubles the risk of generalised arterial disease for any other given set of risk factors.[29]

LOCAL VENOUS COMPLICATIONS

Although renal vein thrombosis may be seen in grafts removed after irreversible rejection has occurred, as a primary event it is a rare complication after transplantation. It may be due to technical factors causing kinking or twisting of the vein[30] and it has been suggested that postoperative swelling of the kidney due to rejection, acute tubular necrosis, or ureteric obstruction might cause compression of the renal vein itself.[31] It is also recognised that ilio-femoral deep vein thrombosis may occur on the side of the transplant with extension of the thrombosis into the renal vein.[32] Deep venous thrombosis is discussed in the next section.

Despite all of these possibilities, after 540 transplants in Oxford renal venous thrombosis causing loss of the graft has occurred on only three occasions (0.6%) and was in no case obviously due to any of the above factors. All thromboses occurred within two weeks of transplantation. Two patients were receiving triple therapy (cyclosporine, azathioprine, and prenisolone) as immunosuppression and one was receiving azathioprine and steroid at the time of the thrombosis. The diagnosis may be suspected on clinical grounds after the onset of sudden pain and graft swelling. If the kidney is functioning, haematuria and proteinurea are usually observed and isotope scanning shows no perfusion in the graft. Preoperative confirmation of the diagnosis requires direct or pertrochanteric venography[33] but immediate surgical exploration may be more appropriate, although thrombectomy resulting in graft salvage is rare.

Merion has reported seven instances of transplant renal vein thrombosis, six of which occurred in patients receiving cyclosporin.[34] As in the Oxford series, however, the numbers were too small to detect a true association between the occurrence of renal vein thrombosis and the use of cyclosporin.

GENERAL VENOUS COMPLICATIONS

Venous thrombosis in transplant patients, as in the general population, affects principally the veins of the lower limbs and pelvis. It is not an uncommon source of morbidity and the European Dialysis and Transplant Association report of 1983 shows a mortality of no less than 4.4% after renal transplantation attributable to pulmonary embolism.[8]

The causes of deep venous thrombosis and/or pulmonary embolism are no different in transplant recipients than in others undergoing major surgery. In addition, it has been suggested that the presence of a kidney near the pelvic veins may cause thrombosis by compression, especially if the graft swells during periods of rejection.[31] It is interesting, however, that Bergquist has demonstrated that the presence of the kidney does not influence venous emptying from the lower limb[35] and in the Oxford series deep venous thrombosis has not been significantly more common on the transplanted side. The principal factors governing risk of deep venous thrombosis and/or pulmonary embolism in transplant patients are age (Fig. 19-2), surgery including the transplant operation itself, and incidents requiring periods of bedrest. Bergquist has also incriminated diabetes mellitus as a risk factor.[35] It is not clear to what extent particular immunosuppressive agents are associated with venous thrombosis but cyclosporine has been implicated by others.[36] In the Oxford series, however, no patient developed either deep venous thrombosis or pulmonary embolism while receiving this drug alone, whereas immunosuppression involving steroid therapy was a universal feature in those with these diagnoses.

Diagnosis of deep venous thrombosis may be made on clinical grounds. In the first month after transplantation, however, leg swelling on the same side as the kidney may be due to lymphatic obstruction by a lymphocele. This may confuse the issue, especially as deep venous thrombosis may also arise secondary to a lymphocele, a finding in three out of 35 lymphoceles diagnosed in Oxford. Although isotope studies and ultrasonography may be used to diagnose deep venous thrombosis objectively, it has been our policy to submit all clinically suspected gases to venography. Patients with suspected pulmonary embolism are routinely assessed by

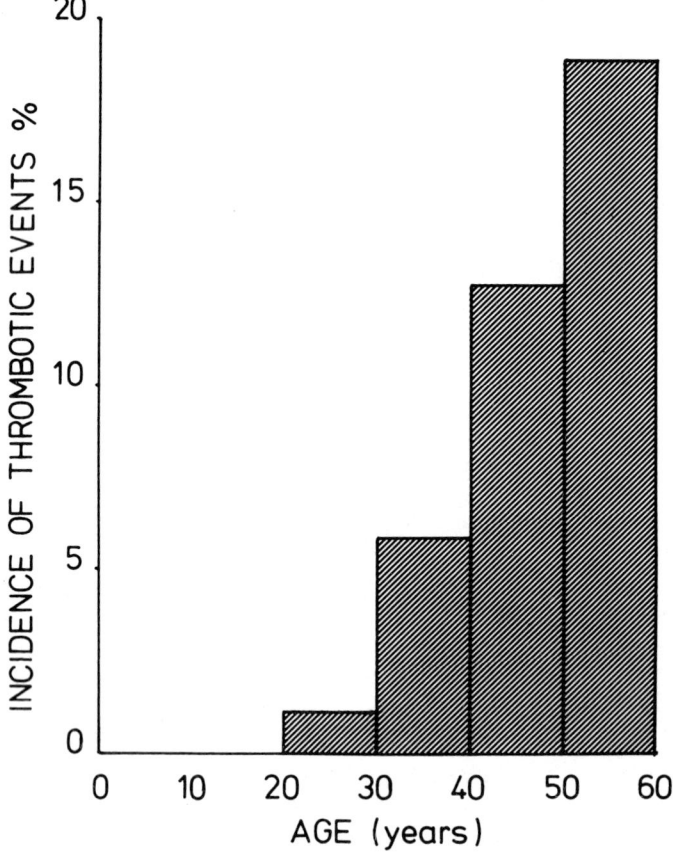

Fig. 19-2. Incidence of thrombotic events (deep venous thrombosis and/or pulmonary embolism) for various age groups of renal transplant patients.

ventilation/perfusion isotope scanning. Using such criteria, 40 thrombotic events (25 DVT, 11 DVT and pulmonary embolism, and 4 pulmonary embolism without clinical evidence of DVT) were recognised after 480 adult renal transplants, an incidence of 8.3% in Oxford.

The timing of the thrombotic event is interesting for although 20% occurred within one month of the transplantation operation itself, the remaining occurred later. The median time of thrombosis for these later presentations was at four months after transplantation and they were generally associated with periods of enforced bedrest or further surgery. It is worthy of note that those suffering a late thrombosis had increased their haemoglobin concentration from a mean of 8.5 g/dl at the time of transplantation to a mean of 11.9 g/dl at the time of thrombosis. No rise in platelet concentration was found. While a similar rise in haemoglobin concentration was found in patients with functioning grafts but without thrombosis, there is little doubt that the correction of anaemia which occurs after a successful kidney transplant plays a major role in increasing susceptibility to venous thrombosis.

In Oxford, patients with thrombosis in the popliteal or more proximal veins or who have a pulmonary embolism are treated actively by full anticoagulation with heparin for seven days followed by warfarin therapy for at least three months. In two patients regular venesection has been required for control of polycythemia. In general, almost all cases of deep venous thrombosis are satisfactorily managed by this policy and no kidney has been lost due to extension of thrombosis into the renal vein. Similarly, pulmonary embolism which does not result in sudden death can be expected to respond well to this regimen.

While the therapeutic use of anticoagulation is well recognised, its role in prophylaxis in renal transplant patients is less certain. The low risk of thrombosis in the first month after the transplant operation itself is due to a coagulation defect associated with anaemia and uraemia. Chemical prophylaxis is not warranted at this time although antiembolism stockings, early ambulation, or other mechanical forms of prevention are probably worthwhile. On the other hand, patients with a functioning graft which has corrected the anaemia and uraemia, especially if they are over 40 years old, seem particularly at risk of deep venous thrombosis and pulmonary embolism when confronted with incidents such as further surgery or infection which require prolonged bedrest. It is wise to offer chemical prophylaxis to such patients and our current policy is to give 5000 units of subcutaneous heparin every eight hours until normal ambulation is resumed.

CONCLUSIONS

The vascular complications seen in the renal transplant patient are diverse. Those affecting principally the transplant renal artery or vein may threaten the viability of the graft itself and occasionally even the life of the patient. Those with more generalised effects on the arterial or venous systems can pose a major threat to the patient's life and atheroma is an especially insidious but major problem in the transplant recipient. Those who care for transplant patients must guard against such complications as far as is possible in the light of our present knowledge. It must be remembered that these complications may present at any time after successful renal transplantation.

REFERENCES

1. Morris PJ, Yadav R, Kincaid-Smith P, et al: Renal artery stenosis in renal transplantation. Med J Aust 1:1255, 1971
2. Lacombe M: Surgical techniques, in Hamburger J, et al (eds): Renal Transplantation: Theory and Practice, 2 ed. Baltimore, Williams and Wilkins, 1981, p 301
3. Belzer FO, Glass N, Sollinger H: Technical complications after renal transplantation, in Morris PJ (ed): Kidney Transplantation, 2 ed. London, Grune and Stratton, 1984, p 407
4. Curtis JJ, Luke RG, Whelchel JD, Diethelm AG, Jones P, Dustan HP: Inhibition of angiotensin-converting enzyme in renal transplant recipients with hypertension. New Engl J Med 308:377, 1983
5. Gruntzig A, Velter W, Meier B, Kuhlmann U, Lutoff U, Siegenthaler W: Treatment of renovascular hypertension with percutaneous transluminal dilatation of renal artery stenosis. Lancet 1:801, 1978
6. Grossman RA, Dafoe DC, Shoenfeld RB, et al: Percutaneous transluminal angioplasty treatment of renal transplant artery stenosis. Transplantation 34:339, 1982
7. Chiverton SG, Murie JA, Allen RD, Morris PJ: Renal transplant nephrectomy: A ten year experience. Surg Gynecol Obstet (in press)
8. European Dialysis and Transplant Association Registry: 1983
9. Vollmer WM, Wahl PW, Blagg CR: Survival with dialysis and transplantation in patients with end-stage renal disease. New Engl J Med 308:1553, 1983
10. Bachy C, Alexandre GPJ, de Strihou CY: Hypertension after renal transplantation. Br Med J 2:1287, 1976
11. Kirkman RL, Strom TB, Weir MR, Tilney NL: Late mortality and morbidity in recipients of long-term renal allografts. Transplantation 34:347, 1982
12. Raine AEG, Ledingham JGG: Cardiovascular complications after renal transplantation, in Morris PJ (ed): Kidney Transplantation, 2 ed. London, Grune and Stratton, 1984, p 469
13. Ibels LS, Stewart JH, Mahoney JF, Neal FC, Sheil AGR: Occlusive arterial disease in uraemic and haemodialysis patients and renal transplant recipients. Quart J Med 46:197, 1977
14. Jacquot C, Idatte JM, Bedrossian J, Weiss Y, Safar M, Bariety J: Long-term blood pressure changes in renal homotransplantation. Arch Intern Med 138:233, 1978
15. Poportzer MM, Pinnggera W, Katz FH, et al: Variations in arterial blood pressure after kidney transplantation. Circulation 47:1297, 1973
16. Faenza A, Spolaore R, Poggioli G, Selleri S, Roversi R, Gozzetti G: Renal artery stenosis after renal transplantation. Kidney Int 23(Suppl 14):S54, 1983
17. Siegal RR, Luke RG, Hellesbusch AA: Reduction of toxicity of corticosteroid therapy after renal transplantation. Am J Med 53:159, 1972
18. Morris PJ, Chan L, French ME, Ting A: Low dose oral prednisolone in renal transplantation. Lancet 1:525, 1982
19. European Multicentre Trial: Cyclosporine as a sole immunosuppressive agent in recipients of kidney allografts from cadaver donors. Lancet 2:57, 1982
20. Chapman JR, Morris PJ: Cyclosporin nephrotoxicity and the consequences of conversion to azathioprine. Transplant Proc 17(Suppl 4):254, 1985
21. Curtis JJ, Lucas BA, Kotchen TA, Luke RG: Surgical therapy for persistent hypertension after renal transplantation. Transplantation 31:125, 1981
22. Thompson JF, Fletcher EWL, Chalmers DHK, Wood RFM, Morris PJ: Bilateral renal embolization for the control of hypertension in transplant recipients. Br J Surg 70:681, 1983
23. Ibels LS, Stewart JH, Mahoney JF, Shiel AGR: Deaths from occlusive arterial disease in renal allograft recipients. Br Med J 3:552, 1974

24. Bagdade JD, Porte D, Bierman EL: Hypertriglyceridaemia. A metabolic consequence of chronic renal failure. New Engl J Med 279:181, 1968

25. Curtis JJ, Galla JH, Woodford SY, Lucas BA, Luke RG: Effect of alternate day prednisolone on plasma lipids in renal transplant recipients. Kidney Int 22:42, 1982

26. Gokal R, Mann JI, Moore RA, Morris PJ: Hyperlipidaemia following renal transplantation. Quart J Med 48:507, 1979

27. Kindler J, Sieberth HG, Hahn R, Glockner WM, Vlaho M, Pelzer R: Does atherosclerosis caused by dialysis limit this treatment? Proc Eur Dial Transplant Assoc 19:168, 1982

28. Chan MK, Varghese Z, Moorhead JF: Lipid abnormalities in uraemia, dialysis and transplantation. Kidney Int 19:625, 1981

29. Kannel WB: Update of the role of cigarette smoking in coronary artery disease. Am Heart J 101:319, 1981

30. D'Apuzzo V, Bretscher D, Oetliker O, et al: Renal vein thrombosis in kidney allografts. Lancet 2:975, 1973

31. Sorenson BL, Nissen TH, Nissen HM: Silent iliac compression syndrome as a cause of renal vein thrombosis after transplantation. Scand J Urol Nephrol 6(Suppl 15):75, 1973

32. Arruda JAL, Gutierrez LF, Jonasson O, Pillay VKG, Kurtzman NA: Renal vein thrombosis in kidney allografts. Lancet 2:585, 1973

33. Smellie WAB, Vinik M, Freed TA, Hume DM: Pertrochanteric venography in the study of human renal transplant recipients. Surg Gynecol Obstet 126:777, 1968

34. Merion RM, Calne RY: Allograft renal vein thrombosis. Transplant Proc 17:1746, 1985

35. Bergquist D, Bergentz SD, Bornmyr S, Husberg B, Konrad P, Ljungner H: Deep vein thrombosis after renal transplantation: A prospective analysis of frequency and risk factors. Eur Surg Res 17:69, 1985

36. Vanrenterghem Y, Roels L, Lerut T, et al: Thrombotic complications and haemostatic changes in cyclosporin treated cadaveric kidney allograft recipients. Lancet 1:99, 1985

Anthony M. Imparato

20

How Much Can the Risk of Stroke be Influenced by Surgery?

INTRODUCTION

It seems clear and is generally accepted that ischemic strokes are due mainly to extracranial occlusive arterial lesions which involve the carotid bifurcations most often and the vertebral origins second in incidence.[1] The aim of surgical procedures is to decrease the long-term risk of stroke by eliminating threatening extracranial lesions without producing additional neurologic deficits by the surgical maneuvers. That this can be achieved was first demonstrated by the results of the Joint Study of Extracranial Arterial Occlusion, a prospective randomized study in progress from 1959 to 1972. All patients with neurologic events which might have been construed as having been due to ischemia including profound strokes with altered consciousness were subjected to four-vessel angiographic study visualizing the extracranial circulation from its origin at the aortic arch, and the intracranial circulation as well. All lesions which produced 30% or more narrowing of surgically accessible arteries were subjected to surgical correction by endarterectomy for the carotid bifurcations and by a variety of procedures for other lesions.[2] Since the carotid bifurcation has received the major attention because of its predominant incidence, this discussion will be limited to it.

This study revealed that the two groups with the most advanced carotid lesions, namely those with bilateral carotid stenosis and those with stenosis opposite occlusion subjected to surgical intervention, enjoyed a lowered stroke rate during 48 months of follow-up compared to randomized comparable nonsurgical patients, provided that only the survivors of surgical intervention who had suffered no intraoperative strokes were compared to the nonrandomized surgical group.[3] Late strokes unrelated to the surgical procedure nevertheless occurred in late follow-up in the operated group.

Two issues were clearly defined thereby which can be posed as questions, namely: (1) What are the preventable mechanisms of intra- or perioperative strokes? (2) What are the circumstances of late strokes?

PERIOPERATIVE STROKES

The most vulnerable period in the surgical management of patients with carotid lesions is during the operative procedure. Great emphasis has been placed upon the susceptibility of the brain to ischemic infarction during the period of carotid clamping. There is a voluminous bibliography attesting to the superiority of one technique of management over another with differences of opinion regarding whether or not the brain should be monitored, whether one monitoring technique or another is more sensitive and what protective measures should be taken to insure that ischemic damage will not occur. Each advocate of a technique then reports a perioperative stroke rate with the prevailing opinion being that if the stroke rate in any series is less than 3% the technique is a satisfactory one (Table 20-1). There is very little reliable data to analyze the strokes as to mechanisms, in large measure because of the difficulty of differentiating cerebral damage due to embolization as opposed to that occurring from clamping ischemia in patients who, in the main, are operated upon under general anesthesia. It therefore becomes impossible to evaluate the value in preventing strokes from cerebral ischemia resulting from carotid clamping, of various monitoring techniques such as continual electroencephalographic monitoring,[4] internal carotid pressure,[5] regional cerebral blood flow,[6] or even some of the earlier monitoring methods such as jugular venous oxygen saturations.[7] As much can be said for protective measures including carotid shunts to bypass carotid

Table 20-1

Incidence of Perioperative Stroke Related to Monitoring and Utilization of Shunt

Series	Technique	Number of Patients	Incidence of Stroke (%)
Haynes et al (1979)	Routine shunt	276	4.0
Nunn (1975)	Routine shunt	234	4.7
Thompson (1979)	Routine shunt	516	2.1
Callow et al (1978)[4]	EEG-selective shunt	399	3.5
Sundt et al (1977)[6]	EEG-selective shunt	474	4.4
Hays et al (1972)[5]	Stump pressure selective shunt	200	3.0
Moore et al (1973)	Stump pressure selective shunt	107	4.7
Rich et al (1975)	Regional-selective shunt	209	5.7
Imparato et al (1980)	Regional-selective shunt	933	2.5
Whitney et al (1980)[9]	No shunt	1197	3.5
Baker et al (1977)	No shunt	304	5.3

Modified from Arch Surg 117:1076, 1982.

clamps during the period of carotid arteriotomy,[8] of general anesthesia,[9] or even of the older techniques of inducing hypercarbia,[10] arterial hypertension, or the administration of carbonic anhydrase inhibitors.

Our own experience since 1962 has been in operating upon carotid arteries in conscious patients with either local infiltration anesthesia or more recently cervical block with minimal preanesthetic sedation testing various monitoring techniques and suggested protective measures against the neurologic condition of the patient.[11] More recently, routine immediate postoperative oculoplethysmography has also been performed. All newly occurring neurologic events and newly appearing abnormalities of oculoplethysmography have led to investigation of the cause through immediate exploration of operated arteries with reopening of the endarterectomy sites if the internal carotid artery was no longer pulsatile, by the performance of intraoperative angiography if the internal carotid artery after the exploration was still pulsatile, and by the performance of CT scans of the brain.[12]

The combination of operating in conscious patients and the aggressive exploration of all postoperative neurologic events, whether major or minor, has helped to place the problem of perioperative stroke, monitoring techniques, and protective devices in perspective.

Incidence of Intolerance of Carotid Clamping and Perioperative Strokes[11]

Although the overall incidence of intolerance to carotid clamping in our experience was 7.6% and the overal incidence of perioperative strokes was 2.5%, both varied markedly in different subgroups, permitting the identification of risk factors associated with carotid clamping as well as for susceptibility to stroke.

Carotid Clamping Intolerance (Table 20-2)

In conscious patients intolerance to carotid clamping is quickly recognized since within 8–45 sec of application of a clamp to occlude the internal carotid artery there results the development of contralateral weakness followed quickly by loss of consciousness, recovery occurring within 1–2 minutes of removal of clamps. On occasion, merely clamping the common carotid artery produces the same results. Of those undergoing operations upon a stenotic carotid artery opposite total occlusion 27% develop such ischemic symptoms and signs, while in the presence of bilateral flow impeding stenoses ischemia develops only 10% of the time. On occasion patients with unilateral carotid lesions also develop cerebral ischemia. Shunting was performed in those intolerant to carotid clamping, but the shunts were placed in the common carotid artery first since most of those who failed to tolerate the clamping of the internal carotid artery tolerated clamping of the common carotid artery, provided the internal and external arteries remained in communication. In eight patients insertion of the common carotid end of the shunt required extensive dissection of the more proximal portion of the common carotid artery to clear the shunt of atheromatous debris or to relieve stenosis in the mid and more proximal portions of the common carotid arteries.

Clamping intolerance could be reversed in three-quarters of the patients by artificial elevation of the blood pressure to above 180 mmHg, but this was associated with an increased incidence of acute myocardial infarction and has been dis-

Table 20-2

Relationship of Major Risk Factors
Affecting Perioperative Stroke Rates to
Clamping Ischemia

	Clamp Intolerance (%)
Contralateral carotid	
Less than 70%	5.4
70–99%	4.2
Totally occluded	27.2
Neurologic status	
No CVA	7.4
CVA	8.3
Contralateral stenosis and neurologic status	
No CVA	
Less than 70% stenosis	5.5
70–99% stenosis	3.8
Total occlusion	28.4
CVA	
Less than 70% stenosis	5.2
70–99% stenosis	6.1
Total occlusion	25.0

Modified from Arch Surg 117:1075, 1982.

continued. Attempts to induce hypocarbia by inhalation of carbon dioxide–oxygen mixtures or by the administration of carbonic anhydrase inhibitors did not convert intolerance to carotid clamping to tolerance. A review of preoperative angiographic studies has shown that intolerance to carotid clamping may be related to the phenomenon of carotid predominance in that the artery which supplies more than its own hemispheric vessels is the one which will, when clamped, be associated with cerebral ischemia. Failure to visualize a posterior communicating artery also identifies those susceptible to clamping ischemia.[12] These observations, however, do not permit identification of all those who are susceptible to carotid clamping ischemia since there are instances in which there is a balanced carotid circulation and cerebral clamping ischemia occurs in spite of careful blood pressure control.

Perioperative Stroke Incidence

The incidence of perioperative strokes varies greatly from 0.6% for patients who are neurologically intact who tolerate carotid clamping to 9.9% for patients who have contralateral carotid occlusion requiring shunts because of intolerance to carotid clamping and who also have a neurologic deficit remaining from a previous stroke. Table 20-3 relates the details of the three major risk factors encountered for perioperative strokes, namely the status of the contralateral artery, the preoperative neurologic condition of the patient, and the tolerance to carotid clamping, indicating the specific risks of each and the results of combining risk factors.

Causes of Stroke

Table 20-4 lists the causes of perioperative strokes and indicates that there is no single mechanism for their occurrence. Although the factor which has received major attention, namely clamping ischemia, is a potential in a significant number of

Table 20-3

Incidence of Clamping Intolerance to Other Risk
Factors of Contralateral Carotid Stenosis and
Neurological Status and Its Effect on Perioperative
Stroke Rates

	Perioperative Stroke (%)
No CVA	
Tolerated clamping	1.6
Less than 70% stenosis (contralateral)	1.7
70–99% stenosis (contralateral)	0.6
Total occlusion (contralateral)	5.3
Did not tolerate clamping	5.9
CVA	
Tolerated clamping	2.7
Less than 70% stenosis (contralateral)	2.8
70–99% stenosis (contralateral)	28.0
Total occlusion (contralateral)	14.0
Did not tolerate clamping	20.0

Modified from Arch Surg 117:1076, 1982.

Table 20-4

Analysis of Perioperative Strokes

Technical problems	
Narrowed outflow	2
Intimal flap	1
Shunt displaced	1
Attempted opening of total occluded internal carotid	1
Clamp injury	1
Bland clot	2
Total	35%
Embolic	
Prior to clamping internal carotid	2
Source other than carotid	2
From operative site postoperatively	1
Total	22%
Intracerebral hemorrhage	17%
Other	
Stroke from contralateral carotid	1
Stroke in evolution progressed	1
Myocardial infarct with shunt in place	1
Bradycardia	1
Total	17%
Unknown	8.7%

Modified from Arch Surg 117:1076, 1982.

patients it can be reduced to an incidence of approximately one-half of 1% by selective shunting in patients who exhibit clamping ischemia under local anesthesia. Of equal importance are technical misadventures which result in thrombosis at the site of the endarterectomy, which incidentally apparently occurs far more often than is expected from the incidence of perioperative stroke when searched for by routine immediate postoperative duplex scanning or by oculoplethymography. Of similar importance is embolization from the site of operation and intracerebral hemorrhage occurring between the first and fifth postoperative days, rarely as late as the ninth in patients who have no detectable evidence of having suffered a cerebral infarct but who have had relief of tight carotid stenosis. In a fifth group the precise mechanism of stroke could not be determined.

In approximately an additional 5% of patients signs of cerebral ischemia occurred after the initial clamping tolerance had been established and while the endarterectomy was being performed. Most often this occurred in relation to a drop in arterial pressure which might be as little as 20–30 mmHg and restoration of blood pressure with vasopressors restored neurologic integrity. In three patients restoration was not possible because of there having occurred an acute myocardial infarct in one and an uncontrollable cardiac arrhythmia in another, in both of whom insertion of the shunt did not reverse the cerebral ischemia. In a third patient displacement of the shunt resulted in significant blood loss with hypotension on the table, stroke, and finally death.

PREVENTION OF PERIOPERATIVE STROKES

Of major significance, then, in the answer to the question "How much can the risk of stroke be influenced by surgery?" is the fact that one must deal with the prevention of perioperative strokes as the first and foremost factor to be considered. Cerebral protection during the surgical management is an all-out effort aimed at preventing or dealing with clamping ischemia upon its recognition, upon the avoidance of technical errors which lead to thrombosis at the operative site, to the prevention of embolization to intracranial vessels, to the prevention of intracerebral hemorrhage, to the protection of the heart to avoid myocardial infarction and cardiac arrhythmias, and to the prevention of intracerebral hemorrhage.

Selection of Patients

Patients who have suffered acute and massive strokes with altered states of consciousness are extremely poor candidates for carotid arterial operations since the mortality rate following surgical intervention when compared to similar patients medically treated is doubled.[13] In our experience those with totally occluded internal carotid arteries or with marked stenoses who have evidence of recent cerebral infarction appear to be at higher risk of suffering intracerebral hemorrhages if operated upon within four weeks of the acute episode. Those with lesser degrees of stenosis which are not producing marked flow gradients perhaps are not at increased risk.

Management to Prevent Cerebral Embolization

Embolization from the operative site is guarded against in a number of ways. Antiplatelet therapy which is begun in the preoperative period is continued through the operative procedure and heparin is administered prior to carotid clamping. The endarterectomy site is liberally irrigated with heparin solution to prevent the formation of thrombus at the operative site during closure of the arteriotomy which can occur, even with seemingly adequate heparinization, from blood which may leak into the operative site through the vasa vasorum. The internal carotid artery is clamped prior to clamping the common carotid and a stereotyped flushing maneuver is employed for each of the three major vessels prior to restoration of flow to the internal carotid. Care is taken to apply vascular clamps to the common carotid artery well below the bifurcation, usually at the level of the omohyoid muscle, a level which is usually though not always free of friable atherosclerotic plaque. Careful attention is paid to the preoperative angiographic study to detect such sites of involvement.

Management to Prevent Clamp Ischemia

Although clamping ischemia is usually often downgraded as a cause of perioperative stroke in the conscious patient it is recognizable in different subgroups occurring at different rates and can be documented to result in severe neurologic deficits when it exceeds a period as short as four minutes. Those at high risk for exhibiting clamping ischemia are those with stenosis opposite occlusion, those who exhibit a predominant carotid artery when that artery must be clamped, those who have nonvisualization of posterior communicating arteries, and those with neurologic deficits from prior strokes, especially if there is a contralateral flow-impeding stenosis. In those who have such risk factors it would seem prudent to either shunt routinely or to monitor either the conscious patient or to employ a direct monitoring technique—be it continuous electroencephalographic monitoring which may result in a higher than necessary incidence of shunting or the elaborate and not universally available regional blood flow studies. Retrograde internal carotid back pressure has given false negative and false positive correlations with the effect upon consciousness and can be expected to fail to detect regional cerebral blood flow deficits which appear to be a major manifestation of clamping ischemia. At present there appears to be no entirely reliable technique for protecting the brain from clamping ischemia short of with a well-functioning shunt. Because of the difficulty sometimes encountered in placing the shunt in the common carotid artery and because the majority of patients intolerant to carotid clamping exhibit ischemia only when the internal is clamped, tolerating clamping of the common alone quite well, the sequence of shunt placement should be placement in the common carotid artery first while the internal and external are open to each other. This will minimize the period of clamping ischemia.

Avoidance of technical errors which can occur during carotid artery endarterectomy relate to the performance of blind endarterectomy in the internal carotid artery, such that the cutoff point is not visualized, and to failure to recognize acute kinking of the internal carotid artery which may become accentuated after endarterectomy and lead to acute thrombosis and failure to remove significant plaque in the common carotid across which clamps might be placed. Most technical errors can be avoided by achieving wide exposure through longitudinal incisions placed anterior to the sternocleidomastoid muscle, identifying the omohyoid muscle as the lower extent of the dissection and the digastric muscle as the upper extent of the dissection. In most patients exposure of the internal carotid artery can be obtained by mobilization of the XII nerve dividing the sternocleidomastoid artery and the sometimes numerous veins which obscure the upper portion of the hypoglossal nerve. In approximately 5% of patients the digastric muscle is also divided to permit adequate exposure of the internal carotid artery and the descending branch of the XII nerve may be divided. This avoids the need to place retractors on the hypoglossal nerve. Rarely is division of the styloid process required. The arteriotomy is longitudinal and extends to beyond the uppermost extent of the internal carotid plaque and well below the bulb in the common carotid to a site where the common carotid intima is neither markedly thickened nor friable. If such intima is encountered the incision is extended downward to as far as the head of the clavicle if necessary, the omohyoid muscle is divided, and additional endarterectomy is performed. Closure of the vessel is most easily performed with an autologous saphenous vein roof patch. If marked redundancy of the internal carotid is present it is corrected, employing a plication technique.

General Measures

Postoperatively, careful control of blood pressure is achieved. Elevation of blood pressures above 180 mmHg and depressions below 120 mmHg are treated to achieve stability between 120 and 180 mmHg. Heparin is not continued postoperatively but antiplatelet agents are. All neurologic deficits, major and minor, are immediately investigated as previously described. Those which occur following the day of operation, if not associated with evidence of flow impairment detectable either by duplex scanning of the operative site or by oculoplethysmography, are investigated by angiography in the angiographic suite. Serious irregularities at the site of operation are treated surgically.

Neurologic deficits not explained either by rethrombosis of the vessel or by finding a site of embolization, whether or not associated with hemorrhage, are also investigated by CT scanning of the brain to detect intracerebral hemorrhage. If associated with a rapidly deteriorating neurologic condition, evaluation by the neurosurgical staff is performed to determine the advisability of craniotomy with evacuation of hematoma.

Unanswered Questions

Unanswered questions regarding operative management have to do with the most reliable technique for monitoring the response to carotid clamping. At present it would appear that the most precise technique is monitoring the conscious patient.

Another unanswered question deals with whether or not routine intraoperative postendarterectomy angiography should be performed in all patients. It is likely that some form of imaging is required to detect sites of clamp trauma, of asymptomatic rethromboses, which may be of considerable importance in late follow-ups.

LATE STROKES

The question of whether late strokes can be prevented by surgical intervention upon the carotid artery is equally hotly contested.[14] It is clear that there is no single model which when studied will answer the question. It is complicated by the fact that the true incidence of stroke in any population group is an unknown, that strokes appear to spontaneously be decreasing in incidence, and that the risk of recognizable ischemic stroke appears to be markedly different in different population subgroups characterized by their clinical status and the distribution of lesions in the extracranial circulation. It is perhaps informative to examine the effects of surgical intervention in these specific subgroups. It is also informative to examine narrative data to help place the problem in perspective. As has already been stated in the introduction, it became clear during the early phases of the Joint Study of Extracranial Arterial Occlusion that carotid surgery could only be effective if employed prophylactically before serious brain damage had occurred. Rarely were major neurologic deficits dramatically reversed by operative intervention. Occasionally dramatic results were obtained at the cost of a very high operative complication rate. Operations upon patients with acute strokes and altered consciousness were attendant with a 40% mortality, whereas the randomized non-surgical group had only a 20% mortality. Nevertheless, in a few of these there was a dramatic and almost instantaneous improvement upon disobliteration of either totally occluded or markedly stenotic internal carotid arteries.[15] It was also apparent from the Joint Study that surgical interventions were most effective in those with the most advanced lesions in the extracranial circulation in whom the surgical risk was greatest, and it has already been discussed how critical is the need to perform the surgical procedures with exceedingly low complication rates which then renders surgical management effective. Our own report on the effects of operation upon stenotic carotid arteries opposite total occlusion illustrates the manner in which this can be accomplished.[16]

The follow-up data in patients with bilateral lesions underscores the fact that these patients are afflicted with what often proves to be progressive arterial degeneration. Three groups of patients undergoing operations with bilateral lesions were compared. The first had operations performed upon the symptomatic side only, the second upon hemodynamically significant stenosis opposite total occlusion, and the third prophylactic contralateral endarterectomy after relief of the symptomatic side if certain criteria were satisfied. These were that the symptomatic artery exhibited either intraplaque hemorrhage, intraplaque atheromatous debris, ulceration of the luminal surface, or thrombus deposition at sites of stenosis, and the asymptomatic contralateral side had a clearly defined 50% stenosis. The five-year stroke rate in those with bilateral operations was approximately one-quarter of that in those who had undergone unilateral operations or who had had endarterectomy of a stenotic carotid artery opposite total occlusion.[17] This perhaps illustrates the importance of recognizing that the pathologic changes at the carotid bifurcation have certain characteristics which place the patient at risk of stroke.

What of patients with transient symptoms—patients with the transient ischemic cerebral episodes and amaurosis fugax? The risk of stroke is variously estimated at 30–50 percent within five years. In this group operative risks tend to be low and although a universally accepted prospective randomized study impeccably performed and analyzed by statistical techniques which are universally accepted does not exist the reports from many groups indicate that surgical intervention favorably influences the late stroke rate.

For some time the presence of neck bruit was considered an identifying characteristic of patients at risk of stroke. This led to a frequently quoted study by Thompson and coworkers[18] in which a prospective nonrandomized study compared 132 patients treated surgically with 138 patients followed nonsurgically. Those who had prophylactic carotid endarterectomies had a significantly lower incidence of transient cerebral episodes as well as strokes. The nonoperated patients had a 27% incidence of transient cerebral episodes and a 17% stroke rate while the operated patients had a 4.5% incidence of TIA and a 2.3% incidence of stroke. This was in spite of the fact that it has been shown that bruits identify a significant number of patients who do not have treatable involvement of the carotid bifurcation.

When the identification of the patients at risk from carotid lesions is refined by determining their effects on flow then there are a number of reports which indicate that positive oculoplethysmography, an identifying characteristic of hemodynamically significant lesions, further emphasizes the effectiveness of prophylactic carotid operation. In the report by Busutil and coworkers[19] the incidence of stroke was 1.9% in the operated group compared to 16% in the nonoperated group. Virtually all of the strokes which occurred in the nonoperated group occurred from the side of the positive OPG.

In an attempt to further relate the pathologic characteristics of the carotid lesion to the stroke risk Moore[19] compared the stroke rate in nonrandomized sets of patients with nonstenotic ulcerations in whom operation was performed. A stroke rate of 12.5% per year was noted for those with advanced carotid bifurcation changes compared to 1.47% per year for the operated group.

The pathologic studies of the author and his colleagues[20, 21] have emphasized the importance of the changes at the carotid bifurcation which appear to correlate with symptoms. Intramural hemorrhage and its consequences appear to identify the process which beyond mere fibrous proliferation at the carotid bifurcation causes the patient to be at risk of stroke. Indeed, in approximately one-half of the patients operated upon for asymptomatic carotid lesions in whom the degree of stenosis is considered to be hemodynamically significant either from the angiographic study or from the noninvasive studies, evidence of prior embolization is found at operation and consists of deep pits, of obviously recent ulcerations in which portions of the arterial wall have literally disappeared from the carotid bifurcation, sites of either intramural hemorrhage producing marked stenosis or intramural atheromatous debris producing stenosis. It is reasonably clear that the carotid bifurcation is subject to proliferative changes in virtually all of us. It is equally clear that strokes occur when the pathologic changes at the carotid bifurcation progress beyond the stage of mere fibrous proliferation and that these progressive changes occur secondary to intramural hemorrhage and consist of embolization of portions of the arterial wall, of embolization of portions of the intramural hemorrhage, and of the atheromatous debris which appears to result from the intramural hemorrhage and from thrombosis of the internal carotid artery secondary to marked stenosis and ulceration. Surgical intervention should be directed at correcting these lesions with secondary changes or with the potential for secondary change.

How then can one identify such dangerous plaques? Patients with transient ischemic attacks are identifiable as a group in whom recurrent embolization is occurring. Patients with advanced lesions opposite symptomatic lesions can similarly be identified. Patients who are totally asymptomatic but have advanced lesions recognizable by the fact that flow impeding stenosis has occurred, implying that the dangerous secondary changes in the artery have already occurred, are also recognizable as a group at high risk for stroke. In each of these groups it can be demonstrated that performing the surgical procedures with a sufficiently low mortality and morbidity will influence favorably the late stroke rates. It seems equally clear that those who have suffered profound damage to the brain with altered consciousness can neither be restored neurologically by surgical intervention nor be salvaged except at exorbitant risk. The totally occluded internal carotid artery can rarely be disobliterated and a great disappointment has been that the extracranial–intracranial bypass procedure does not decrease late stroke rates.

Unanswered questions relate to whether prophylactic intervention is indicated in patients undergoing surgical procedures unrelated to their cerebrovascular circulation. Here, perhaps, the data from hemodynamic studies is of value, but nevertheless the incidence of stroke secondary to noncardiac operations is quite low. It is not clear whether the patients with acute neurologic deficits who are either at risk of repeated embolization or who are suffering from flow impairment of hemodynamically significant lesions can be operated upon safely with a sufficiently low complication rate to favorably alter their long-term prognosis.

CONCLUSION

The conclusion that can be drawn in spite of the rather heated debate to the contrary is that removal of either severely ulcerated or hemodynamically significant lesions from the carotid bifurcation in patients with or without symptoms if performed with a sufficiently low complication rate will favorably alter the long-term prognosis for stroke.

REFERENCES

1. Hass WK, Fields WS, North RR, Kricheff II, Chase NE, Bauer RB: Joint Study of Extracranial Arterial Occlusion. II. Arteriography, techniques, sites and complications. JAMA 203(11):159–166, 1968
2. Fields WS, et al: Joint Study of Extracranial Arterial Occlusion as a cause of stroke. I. Organization of study and survey of patient population. JAMA 203:955, 1968
3. Fields WS, Maslenikov V, Meyer JS, Hass WK, Remington RD, Macdonald M: Joint Study of Extracranial Arterial Occlusion. V. Progress report of prognosis following surgery or nonsurgical treatment for transient cerebral ischemic attacks and cervical carotid artery lesions. JAMA 211(12):1993–2003, 1970
4. Callow AD, Matsumoto G, Baker G, et al: Protection of the high risk endarterectomy patient by continuous electroencephalography. J Cardiovasc Surg 19:55, 1978
5. Hays RJ, Levinson SA, Wylie EJ: Intraoperative measurement of carotid backpressure as a guide to the operative management for carotid endarterectomy. Surgery 72:953, 1972
6. Sundt TM Jr, Hauser OW, Sharbrough FW: Carotid endarterectomy results, complications and monitoring techniques. Adv Neurol 16:97, 1977

7. Larson CP Jr, Ehrenfeld WK, Wade JG, Wylie EJ: Jugular venous oxygen saturation as an index of adequacy of cerebral oxygenation. Surgery 62:31, 1967
8. Thompson JE, Talkington CM: Carotid endarterectomy. Ann Surg 184:1–15, 1976
9. Whitney DG, Kahn EM, Estes JW: Carotid artery surgery without an indwelling temporary shunt. Arch Surg 115:1393, 1980
10. Ehrenfeld WK, Hamilton FN, Larson CP Jr, et al: Effect of CO_2 and systemic hypertension on downstream cerebral arterial pressure during carotid endarterectomy. Surgery 67:87, 1970
11. Imparato AM, Ramirez A, Riles TS, et al: Cerebral protection in carotid surgery. Arch Surg 117:1073, 1982
12. Imparato AM: The "major" and "minor" carotid artery in arterial reconstructions. Current concepts of cerebrovascular disease. Stroke IX:15–19, 1974
13. Blaisdell WF, Clauss RH, Galbraith JG, Imparato AM, Wylie EJ: Joint study of extracranial arterial occlusion. IV. A review of surgical considerations. JAMA 209(12):1889–1895, 1969
14. Barnett HJM, Plum F, Walton JN: Carotid endarterectomy—An expression of concern. Stroke 15:941, 1984
15. Meyer FB, Sundt TM Jr, Piepgras DG, et al: Emergency carotid endarterectomy for patients with acute carotid occlusion and profound neurological deficits. Ann Surg 203:82, 1985
16. Riles TS, Imparato AM, Kopelman I: Carotid artery stenosis with contralateral internal carotid occlusion: Long-term results in fifty-four patients. Surgery 87(4):363–368, 1980
17. Riles TS, Imparato AM, Mintzer R: Comparison of results of bilateral and unilateral carotid endarterectomy five years after surgery. Surgery 91(3):258–262, 1982
18. Thompson JE, Patman RD, Talkington M: Asymptomatic carotid bruit: Long-term outcome of patients having endarterectomy compared with unoperated controls. Ann Surg 188:308–316, 1978
19. Busutil RW, Baker JD, Davidson RK, et al: Carotid artery stenosis—Hemodynamic significance and clinical course. JAMA 245:1438–1441, 1981
20. Imparato AM, Riles TS, Gorstein F: The carotid bifurcation plaque: Pathologic findings associated with cerebral ischemia. Stroke 10(3):238–245, 1979
21. Imparato AM, Riles TS, et al: The importance of hemorrhage in the relationship between gross morphologic characteristics and cerebral symptoms in 376 carotid artery plaques. Ann Surg 197:197–203, 1983

C. William Cole
and Wesley S. Moore

21

The Natural History of Lesions of the Carotid Artery

The importance of atherosclerotic lesions in the extracranial carotid artery as potential causes of ischemic stroke has been recognized for more than a century,[1] but widespread awareness of its clinical importance was kindled by the first reports of successful surgical management.[2,3] Despite the long familiarity with this lesion, the management of patients with extracranial carotid artery occlusive disease remains one of the most controversial subjects of present-day medical practice. There are several reasons for this, principally because the literature on stroke and stroke-related syndromes has many inconsistencies related to the classification of patients, and the numbers of patients in the reported series are generally too small for firm conclusions to be drawn. Comparisons between such studies are hazardous at best, and usually result in confusing the issues rather than clarifying them. Nevertheless, significant facts regarding the natural history of carotid artery occlusive disease have been established, upon which rational investigation and treatment of patients should be based.

This chapter focuses on the natural history of extracranial carotid artery occlusive disease with emphasis on the significance of symptomatic lesions as precursors of stroke and the growing evidence that treatment of critical but asymptomatic lesions may prevent its occurrence.

PATHOGENESIS OF CEREBRAL ISCHEMIA DUE TO CAROTID ARTERY LESIONS

There is general agreement that an ischemic insult to the brain as a result of carotid artery lesions is due to a reduction in blood flow in the carotid territory, either by narrowing of the vessel to flow-limiting proportions or by embolic material released from the diseased artery which produces the same effect in the smaller vessels in the distal cerebral circulation. Either mechanism may be

VASCULAR SURGERY: ISSUES IN CURRENT PRACTICE
ISBN 0-8089-1839-7

responsible in an individual patient, but the majority of cerebral events due to these lesions are embolic. Stenotic lesions must reduce the diameter of the vessel by more than 75% before significant reduction in flow occurs[4] and collateral circulation via the circle of Willis usually provides adequate perfusion unless other flow-limiting lesions are present. Besides their flow-limiting effects, stenotic lesions may cause enough turbulence to initiate platelet and platelet–fibrin aggregates to form which then embolize into the distal circulation. Obviously, progressive stenosis will ultimately lead to complete occlusion and thrombosis of the vessel with catastrophic results in some, but not all, patients. Frequently symptoms caused by emboli released from a preocclusive lesion will be relieved once the internal carotid artery is completely occluded. In some patients, emboli may be released even when the vessel is occluded, either from the terminal end of the thrombus into the distal circulation, or from the proximal end into the collateral circulation via the external carotid.[5, 6]

Nonstenotic, ulcerative lesions may form a nidus for platelet and thrombus deposition with subsequent embolization,[7–10] or hemorrhage may occur into an atherosclerotic plaque, producing further stenosis and possibly releasing emboli from exposed thrombus. Ulcerated atherosclerotic plaques may also release cholesterol crystals directly into the cerebral circulation and if they come to lodge in the vessels of the retina may be observed with an ophthalmoscope.[11]

Patients who experience neurologic symptoms from causes unrelated to atherosclerotic lesions affecting the bifurcation of the carotid artery must be distinguished, and excluded whenever possible, from consideration for carotid endarterectomy. These include emboli emanating from the heart or its valves, atherosclerosis or inflammatory processes affecting the arch of the aorta and its branches (Takayasu's disease, syphilis, polyarteritis nodosa, systemic lupus erythematousus, giant cell arteritis, granulomatous angiitis, sarcoid angiitis, fibromuscular dysplasia) or from hematologic disorders such as polycythemia. These disorders are responsible for the minority of cases,[12] however, and can usually be identified when present.

RISK FACTORS

Atherosclerosis affecting the carotid arteries is a local manifestation of a generalized process and the risk factors associated with it are generally the same as those associated with other clinical manifestations of atherosclerosis. They include age, cigarette smoking, hypertension, diabetes, and a strong family history of related disorders. The factors which have the most influence on both survival and recurrence following ischemic cerebral events, the majority of which are due to carotid artery lesions, are concomitent coronary artery disease and hypertension.[13, 14] These factors should be included as part of any study design so that accurate comparisons can be made between reports.

COMPLETED STROKE

Stroke is a leading cause of death and disability, exceeded in importance only by heart disease and cancer.[15] In the population study of Rochester, Minnesota, reported from the Mayo Clinic, stroke affected from 276.8 per 100,000 population in the age group 55–65, to 1786.4 per 100,000 population for the age group over 75. Men had an incidence of cerebral infarction 1.5 times that of women of comparable age.[16] Mortality from the initial stroke was 38%, 10% from a subsequent stroke, and 18% from heart disease. When all causes of stroke were included the recurrence rate was 35% among survivors of the initial attack, 10% within the first year and 20% within five years. Similar rates were observed in a population study of the city of Goulburn, Australia, reported by Wallace.[17] The overall incidence of stroke was 330 per 100,000 population per year. Mortality from the initial event was 37% with a recurrence rate of 35%.

A high recurrence rate among survivors of completed stroke was also noted by Sacco and coworkers[18] in their review of the Framingham population. They noted that the recurrent attack frequently occurred in the same anatomic region, which is a characteristic feature of experimentally induced cerebral occlusion by emboli from the carotid artery. In a model employing metal beads released from a focal point into the carotid territory circulation the beads repeatedly followed the same path and lined up one behind the other in the same cortical vessel.[19]

The natural history of carotid artery atheromata is to increase in thickness, progressively narrowing the lumen of the vessel. In a series of carotid artery atheromatous lesions followed angiographically, Javid and coworkers[20] noted only 38% to remain stable in size while the remaining 62% increased in size and effect on the lumen of the artery. In a large proportion of the lesions under study (34%) the progression was rapid—25% per year.

The role of the carotid endarterectomy in preventing patients who have suffered a stroke from having another stroke is unclear, but evidence is accumulating that this is the case. Thompson, Austin, and Patman[21] were the first to suggest that carotid endarterectomy decreased the mortality and lowered the incidence of recurrent stroke. This study was uncontrolled and the stroke group included patients with waxing and waning signs as well as patients with mild, fixed deficits that may have favorably influenced their conclusions. However, in a nonrandomized study, but one which did include a control group of patients treated medically, McCullough and coworkers[22] reported new neurologic deficits in only two of 59 patients treated surgically, compared to 12 in their control group. There were no stroke-related deaths in the group treated surgically and three in the group treated medically. Survival was unaffected by the surgical procedure, but stroke-free survival was clearly improved. Without randomization the parallel group was not entirely comparable, as Bernstein pointed out in the discussion of this paper, and the inclusion of patients with mild, fixed deficits in the stroke group may have played a significant part in determining their favorable results. Prior stroke increases the risk for patients undergoing carotid endarterectomy and outweighs other risk factors to a large degree. Bardin and coworkers[23] noted the risk of stroke associated with carotid endarterectomy to double in patients who had experienced a previous stroke. In their experience with 456 consecutive carotid endarterectomies the incidence of perioperative stroke in patients who were free from prior stroke was 2.1% but occurred in 3.9% in patients who had experienced a prior stroke. Operative mortality in their group was 0.9% overall, but was 3.1% in the stroke group. On balance, the available data seem to suggest that the natural history of completed stroke may be favorably altered by surgical treatment only in carefully selected patients with fixed, mild to moderate neurologic deficits, but more data from randomized, controlled studies are clearly needed.

Patients experiencing crescendo transient ischemic attacks, attacks abruptly increasing in frequency to at least several per day, or stroke-in-evolution, are in imminent danger of progressing to a completed stroke. Similarly, patients who have suffered small strokes, but are not presently progressing, represent a group of patients at risk of developing another more dense stroke. There are few reports in the literature which focus on this small, but distinct, clinical spectrum. The available data suggest that progression to completed stroke in the first case or recurrent stroke in the second, can be prevented by prompt surgical treatment when a responsible carotid artery lesion is identified. Goldstone and Moore[24, 25] reported on 26 patients with crescendo transient ischemic attacks (hemispheric or monocular) or stroke-in-evolution, with carotid occlusive lesions managed by emergency endarterectomy with complete resolution of symptoms. The authors of this study emphasize that their patients did not have fixed deficits, but were neurologically unstable. Even when signs of a completed stroke are present, but are mild and stable, it may be a greater risk to wait four to six weeks before carrying out an indicated carotid endarterectomy than to perform the procedure expeditiously. In the interval a second, more severe, stroke may occur. A group of 28 such patients with clinically small, fixed neurologic deficits who were considered to have carotid territory at risk of further ischemic events has been reported by Whittemore and coworkers[26] from the Brigham and Women's Hospital, Boston. They successfully carried out carotid endarterectomy an average of 11 days after the ischemic event and reported two new neurologic events over the course of two years of follow-up: one fatal stroke and one transient deficit. Unfortunately, there was no control group in this study to show the efficacy of the procedure.

Computerized axial tomography (CT) may be helpful in distinguishing which patients might be suitable for earlier correction of carotid lesions than the minimal four to six weeks frequently recommended.[27] Ricotta and coworkers[28] found CT to be of limited or no use in elective carotid artery surgery, but in 27 patients with acute neurologic changes were able to achieve a successful outcome by urgent endarterectomy (within 10 days of presentation) in 15 out of 17 when preoperative CT was normal versus 5 out of 10 when CT demonstrated an area of infarction. These studies represent important attempts to identify patients at highest risk of cerebral infarction due to carotid occlusive disease and to apply earlier surgical treatment to prevent progression to stroke or a recurrent, possibly more dense, stroke. The results stand in stark contrast to those from reports of similar treatment of patients with dense strokes who have an operative mortality rate ranging from 40 to 50%.[29, 30]

There have been no randomized clinical trials of emergency anticoagulation for patients with stroke-in-evolution or patients with mild fixed neurologic deficits.

TRANSIENT ISCHEMIC ATTACKS

A large population of patients experience warning neurological signs in the carotid territory manifested as a transient, focal deficit before stroke actually occurs. A clear understanding of what a transient ischemic attack (TIA) is (and is not) is crucial to accurate classification of patients and for interpretation of the relevant medical literature. TIA is best defined as "an acute loss of focal, cerebral or ocular function with symptoms lasting less than 24 hours and which, after adequate investigation, is presumed to be due to embolic or thrombotic vascular disease."[31] Studies which do not use strict criteria for case selection cloud rather than clarify an already complex issue.

Significance of TIA

The significance of TIA on the risk of subsequent stroke has been well demonstrated in the Rochester, Minnesota, study in which 33 strokes were observed in a group of patients who had experienced a TIA compared with two that were expected from that number of patients based on the experience of the whole population.[32] The incidence of stroke in 118 patients from the same series who experienced TIA, followed without treatment, was 23% at one year after the initial attack, 37% after three years, and 45% after five years of follow-up. As an approximate rule of thumb, based upon the available data, Wiebers and Whisnant estimate the expected rate of stroke for patients experiencing TIA to be 7% per year over the first five years after the initial attack. Stated another way, one-third of patients with TIA will have a stroke within five years.[33] The importance of these observations to the management of such patients is clear in the light of the joint study of extracranial arterial occlusion,[34] which has documented that 75% of patients with cerebrovascular ischemia have a surgically accessible lesion.

ASYMPTOMATIC CAROTID LESIONS

Perhaps the most controversial subject related to extracranial cerebrovascular disease is the management of patients with asymptomatic lesions. Despite a vast literature on the subject, there are many conflicting reports resulting in differing, yet firmly held, opinions, usually based on relatively few concrete data. Here, especially, the numbers of patients necessary in a study to establish the case for, or against, a particular therapy are prohibitive, unless subgroups of patients are carefully selected and studied with appropriate parallel controls.[35] In the main, the presence of a cervical bruit has a rather benign influence on the majority of patients. This has been confirmed by the paucity of untoward cerebral ischemic events observed in patients with cervical bruits undergoing general surgical procedures[36] as well as aorto-coronary bypass grafting.[37] The widespread prevalence of cervical bruits in the general population accounts for the benign course of the majority of these patients. The significance of a cervical bruit only becomes apparent when the lesion causing it has been further categorized. In selected populations, particularly in those with generalized vascular disease, the presence of a cervical bruit should alert the physician to the possibility of a significant carotid lesion.[38] More severe stenosis is associated with an increased risk of stroke as well as of myocardial infarction. The most convincing evidence of this correlation has been published by Moore and coworkers.[39] In this study, 303 consecutive patients underwent noninvasive assessment of their carotid arteries for whom the follow-up data for more than five years was available in 90% of cases. Half the deaths were due to myocardial infarction, the risk of which was doubled in patients with carotid stenosis >50%. The overall incidence of stroke was 13.5%. A strong correlation was demonstrated between the incidence of stroke and severity of disease; no stenosis (10%), 0–49% stenosis (11%), and >50% stenosis (19%). In their second analysis,[40] carotid stenosis >50% predicted a 15% stroke incidence at two years compared to a 3% incidence with 1–49% stenosis. Five-year cumulative stroke incidence was 9% with 0% stenosis, 14% with 1–49% stenosis, and 21% with stenosis >50%. Both hypertension and age increased cardiac mortality in patients with carotid stenosis >50%. Patients >70 years old with carotid stenosis >50% had a 37% incidence of stroke. The beneficial effects of carotid endarterectomy was most apparent in the group of patients with the most severe disease. Surgery reduced the five-year stroke rate from 21 to 8%, mitigated the effects of age and hypertension, and improved survival.

In a study by Roederer and coworkers[41] of nonoperated carotid arteries opposite an endarterectomy in 134 patients, followed by noninvasive methods, 12.6% showed progression of the disease, 7.4% to a diameter greater than 50% over the four years of the study. Disease progression was more rapid in patients under 65 years of age. Again, there was a strong relationship between the development of symptoms and stenoses greater than 80%. The generalized nature of atherosclerosis and its propensity to affect vessels on both sides of the body in a symmetrical pattern suggests that patients found to have a significant lesion in one carotid artery will eventually develop a similar lesion in the contralateral vessel. Therefore, patients with carotid artery disease should have periodic reexamination of the contralateral vessel in an effort to identify patients at risk of developing further significant carotid lesions. Hertzer and Arison,[42] reporting from the Cleveland Clinic, noted that contralateral hemispheric strokes occurred in 36% of patients with uncorrected contralateral stenosis compared with 8% of those who had elective bilateral reconstruction. Only 10% of strokes occurred ipsilateral to previously endarterectomized carotid arteries. This figure is similar to reports of recurrent carotid artery stenosis after endarterectomy (see below).

Noninvasive tests have become an invaluable tool in distinguishing patients at greatest risk of developing cerebral ischemic events and, therefore, those who stand to benefit most from carotid endarterectomy.[43,44] Busuttil and coworkers,[43] for example, found the risk of cerebral ischemic events to be 2.2% (2 out of 90) in patients with nonhemodynamically significant carotid stenosis, while patients with hemodynamically significant stenosis had a 16.2% risk of stroke compared to 1.9% risk of stroke in similar patients who underwent carotid endarterectomy. Chambers and Norris,[45] in a report ironically titled the case *against* surgery for asymptomatic carotid stenosis, found that TIA or stroke occurred at more than twice the rate in asymptomatic patients with carotid stenosis >75% than in patients whose lesions were <75% stenotic.

Increasingly, it is possible with noninvasive studies to identify patients whose stenotic carotid artery lesions are most likely to cause a stroke. Low morbidity and mortality rates for angiography and carotid surgery can be achieved in specialized units, but this may not be the case in all centers. Noninvasive methods may be helpful in reducing the risks of angiography, including the inevitable delay entailed in obtaining the study, particularly in high-risk patients.

Asymptomatic nonstenotic, ulcerative lesions

Unfortunately, noninvasive methods do not consistently distinguish patients with ulcerative plaques, and angiography is usually necessary for this purpose. The physician must recognize this limitation of noninvasive methods and carry out angiography in all patients when ulcerative lesions are suspected. The natural history of these lesions is comparable to that of patients with TIA.[9,10] Ulcerations of the carotid artery have been classified according to their dimensions as measured on the cut films after arteriography. Medium-sized ulcers are associated with an annual stroke rate of 4.5% while large, complex ones pose a stroke risk of 7.5% per year.[10] The natural history of patients who have undergone surgical correction for these lesions is unknown since no long-term follow-up studies have been carried out; nor have randomized prospective trials comparing surgical versus medical management been reported. Based upon the favorable outlook for patients treated with carotid endarterectomy for TIA and the very large numbers of patients that would be necessary to carry out appropriate comparative studies, carotid endarterectomy is currently recommended for patients who are not otherwise in a high-risk category for surgery.

RECURRENT CAROTID ARTERY STENOSIS

Carotid artery stenosis recurs in approximately 10% of patients following endarterectomy.[46,47] Women have a higher recurrence rate than matched male subjects. Thomas and coworkers[48] reported an overall recurrence rate of 15%: 25% in women, 9% in men. A similar preponderance of women in the group with recurrent carotid artery stenosis after endarterectomy was noted by Clagett and coworkers.[49] Many recurrences occur within the first year after surgery, but no apparent factors apart from sex were found to explain this difference. It has been suggested that differences in platelet function between men and women might account for the difference in recurrence rates since the vessel usually has intimal hyperplasia as the root cause of the recurrence, which may be mediated by platelets.[50]

ESTABLISHED INTERNAL CAROTID ARTERY OCCLUSION

Occasionally occlusion of the common carotid and/or the internal carotid artery may be associated with symptoms of cerebral ischemia. Thrombectomy of an occluded common carotid artery can be performed to reestablish patency to the external carotid artery and, on occasion, to the internal carotid artery.[51,52] However, thrombectomy of an occluded internal carotid artery may be associated with further cerebral damage due to hemorrhage. Extracranial-intracranial bypass has been recommended to alleviate symptoms of cerebral ischemia in the presence of an occluded internal carotid and a patent external carotid artery. However, the true benefit of this procedure remains in considerable doubt following an internal randomized trial.[53]

The external carotid artery may provide an important source of collateral flow in the presence of an occluded internal carotid artery. A cul-de-sac formed by the proximal oriface of the internal carotid artery may release fragments of thrombus that can embolize to the cerebral circulation or eye via the open external carotid artery.[6, 54] This phenomenon may progress to cerebral or retinal infarction and can be prevented by angioplasty of the external carotid artery in which the stump of the internal carotid artery is removed. Endarterectomy of the external carotid artery may also be required to maximize flow through this important collateral.[55] The literature is rather sparse in reporting series of patients whose symptoms are due to external carotid disease, but the references cited here outline its importance as a potentially treatable lesion.

REFERENCES

1. Gunning AJ, Pickering GW, Robb-Smith AHT, Russell RR: Mural thrombosis of the internal carotid artery and subsequent embolism. Q J Med 33:155–195, 1964
2. Carrea R, Molins M, Murphy G: Surgical treatment of spontaneous thrombosis of the internal carotid artery in the neck. Carotid-carotideal anastomosis. Report of a case. Acta Neurol Latinoamer 1:71–78, 1955
3. Eastcott HHG, Pickering GW, Rob C: Reconstruction of internal carotid artery in a patient with intermittent attacks of hemiplegia. Lancet 2:994–996, 1954
4. Brice JG, Dowsett DJ, Lowe RD: The effect of constriction on carotid blood flow and pressure gradient. Lancet 1:84–85, 1964
5. McIntyre KE, Ely RL III, Malone JM, Bernhard VM, Goldstone J: External carotid artery reconstruction: Its role in the treatment of cerebral ischemia. Am J Surg 150:58–64, 1985
6. Barnett HJM, Peerless SJ, Kaufmann JCE: "Stump" on internal carotid artery—A source for further cerebral embolic ischemia. Stroke 9:448–456, 1978
7. Moore WS, Hall AD: Ulcerated atheroma of the carotid artery. A cause of transient cerebral ischemia. Am J Surg 116:237–242, 1968
8. Dixon S, Pais O, Raviola C, Gomes A, Machleder HI, Baker JD, Busuttil RW, Barker WF, Moore WS: Natural history of nonstenotic, asymptomatic ulcerative lesions of the carotid artery. Arch Surg 117:1493–1498, 1982
9. Moore WS, Hall AD: Importance of emboli from carotid bifurcation in pathogenesis of cerebral ischemic attacks. Arch Surg 101:708–716, 1970
10. Moore WS, Boren CB, Malone JM, et al: Natural history of nonstenotic asymptomatic ulcerative lesions of the carotid artery. Arch Surg 113:1352–1359, 1978
11. Hollenhorst RW: Vascular status of patients who have cholesterol emboli in the retina. Am J Ophthalmol 61:1159–1165, 1966
12. Millikan CH: The pathogenesis of transient focal cerebral ischemia. Circulation 32:438–450, 1965
13. Sacco RL, Wolf PA, Kannel WB, McNamara PM. Survival and recurrence following stroke. The Framingham study. Stroke 13:290–295, 1982
14. Hertzer NR, Arison R: Cumulative stroke and survival ten years after carotid endarterectomy. J Vasc Surg 2:661–668, 1985
15. Silverberg E: Cancer statistics, 1984. Ca-A Cancer Journal for Clinicians 34:8–10, 1984
16. Matsumoto N, Whisnant JP, Kurland LT, Okazaki H: Natural history of stroke in Rochester, Minnesota, 1955 through 1969. Stroke 4:20–29, 1973
17. Wallace DC: A study of the natural history of cerebral vascular disease. Med J Aust 1:90–93, 1967
18. Sacco RL, Wolf PA, Kannel WB, McNamara PM: Survival and recurrence following stroke in the Framingham study. Stroke 13:290–295, 1982

19. Millikan CH, reported by Moore WS: Pathogenic mechanisms of cerebral dysfunction in vascular disease, in Rutherford Robert B (ed): Vascular surgery. Philadelphia, WB Saunders Co, 1984, p 1214

20. Javid H, Ostermiller WE, Hengesh JW, Dye WS, Hunter JA, Najafi H, Julian OC: Natural history of carotid bifurcation atheroma. Surgery 67:80–86, 1970

21. Thompson JE, Austin DJ, Patman RD: Carotid endarterectomy for cerebrovascular insufficiency: Long-term results in 592 patients followed up to thirteen years. Ann Surg 172:663–679, 1970

22. McCullough JL, Mentzer RM Jr, Harman PK, Kaiser DL, H DrP, Kron IL, Crosby IK: Carotid endarterectomy after a completed stroke: Reduction in long-term neurologic deterioration. J Vasc Surg 2:7–14, 1985

23. Bardin JA, Bernstein EF, Humber PB, Collins GM, Dilley RB, Devin JB, Stuart SH: Is carotid endarterectomy beneficial in prevention of recurrent stroke? Arch Surg 117:1401–1407, 1982

24. Goldstone J, Moore WS: A new look at emergency carotid artery operations for the treatment of cerebrovascular insufficiency. Stroke 9:599–602, 1978

25. Goldstone J, Moore WS: Emergency carotid artery surgery in neurologically unstable patients. Arch Surg 111:1284–1291, 1976

26. Whittemore AD, Ruby ST, Couch NP, Mannick JA: Early carotid endarterectomy in patients with small, fixed neurologic deficits. J Vasc Surg 1:795–799, 1984

27. Dosick SM, Whalen RC, Gale SS, Brown OW: Carotid endarterectomy in the stroke patient: Computerized axial tomography to determine timing. J Vasc Surg 2:214–219, 1985

28. Ricotta JJ, Ouriel K, Green RM, DeWeese JA: Use of computerized cerebral tomography in selection of patients for elective and urgent carotid endarterectomy. Ann Surg 202:783–787, 1985

29. Wylie EJ, Hein MF, Adams JE: Intracranial hemorrhage following surgical revascularization for treatment of acute strokes. J Neurosurg 21:212–215, 1964

30. Blaisdell WF, et al: Joint study of extracranial arterial occlusion. JAMA 209:1889–1895, 1969

31. Warlow C, Morris PJ (eds): Transient Ischemic Attacks. New York, Marcel Dekker, 1982, p ix

32. Whisnant JP, Matsumoto N, Elveback LR: Transient cerebral ischemic attacks in a community: Rochester, Minnesota, 1955 through 1969. Mayo Clin Proc 48:194–198, 1973

33. Wiebers DO, Whisnant JP: Epidemiology, in Warlow C, Morris PJ (eds): Transient Ischemic Attacks. New York, Marcel Dekker, 1983, p 8

34. Fields WS, Lemak NA: Joint study of extracranial arterial occlusion as a cause of stroke—I. Organization of study and survey of patient population. JAMA 203:955–960, 1968

35. Taylor DW, Sackett DL, Haynes RB: Sample size for randomized trials in stroke prevention. How many patients do we need? Stroke 15:968–971, 1984

36. Ropper ASH, Wechsler LR, Wilson L: Carotid bruit and the risk of stroke in elective surgery. N Engl J Med 307:1388–1401, 1982

37. Furlan AJ, Craciun AR: Risk of stroke during coronary artery bypass graft surgery in patients with internal carotid artery disease documented by angiography. Stroke 16:797–799, 1985

38. Sutton KC, Dai WS, Kuller LH: Asymptomatic carotid artery bruits in a population of elderly adults with isolated systolic hypertension. Stroke 16:781–784, 1985

39. Moore DJ, Sheehan MP, Kolm P, Russell JB, Sumner DS: Are strokes predictable with noninvasive methods? A five-year follow-up of 303 unoperated patients. J Vasc Surg 2:654–660, 1985

40. Moore DJ, Miles RD, Gooley NA, Sumner DS: Noninvasive assessment of stroke risk in asymptomatic and nonhemispheric patients with suspected carotid disease. Ann Surg 202:491–504, 1985

41. Roederer GO, Langlois YE, Jager KA, Primozich JF, Beach KW, Phillips DJ, Strandness DE Jr: The natural history of carotid arterial disease in asymptomatic patients with cervical bruits. Stroke 15:605–613, 1984

42. Hertzer NR, Arison R: Cumulative stroke and survival ten years after carotid endarterectomy. J Vasc Surg 2:661–668, 1985

43. Busuttil RW, Baker JD, Davidson RK, Machleder HI: Carotid artery stenosis— Hemodynamic significance and clinical course. JAMA 245:1438–1441, 1981

44. Kartchner MM, McRae LP: Noninvasive evaluation and management of the asymptomatic carotid bruit. Surgery 82:840–847, 1977

45. Chambers BR, Norris JW: The case against surgery for asymptomatic carotid stenosis. Stroke 15:964–967, 1984

46. Baker WH, Hayes AC, PA-C, Mahler Debbie, Littooy FN: Durability of carotid endarterectomy. Surgery 94:112–115, 1983

47. Salvian A, Baker JD, Machleder HI, Busuttil RW, Barker WF, Moore WS: Cause and noninvasive detection of restenosis after carotid endarterectomy. Am J Surg 146:29–34, 1983

48. Thomas M, Otis SM, Rush M, Zyroff J, Dilley RB, Bernstein EF: Recurrent carotid artery stenosis following endarterectomy. Ann Surg 200:74–79, 1984

49. Clagett GP, Rich NM, McDonald PT, Salander JM, Youkey JR, Olson DW, Hutton JE Jr: Etiologic factors for recurrent carotid artery stenosis. Surgery 93:313–318, 1983

50. Ross R, Glomset J, Kariya B, Harker L: A platelet-dependent serum factor that stimulates the proliferation of arterial smooth muscle cells in vitro. Proc Natl Acad Sci USA 71:1207–1210, 1974

51. Rushton RW Jr, Kukora JS: Surgical management of the occluded carotid artery. Surgery 96:845–853, 1984

52. Moore WS, Blaisdell FW, Hall AD: Retrograde thrombectomy for chronic occlusion of the common carotid artery. Arch Surg 95:664–673, 1967

53. Barnett HJM, et al: Failure of extracranial-intracranial arterial bypass to reduce the risk of ischemic stroke. N Engl J Med 313:1191–1200, 1985

54. Lamberth WC: External carotid endarterectomy: Indications, operative technique, and results. Surgery 93:57–63, 1983

55. Connolly JE, Stemmer EA: Endarterectomy of the external carotid artery. Arch Surg 106:799–802, 1973

PART IV

Special Problems

William K. Ehrenfeld
and Steven P. Okuhn

22

Can We Reduce the Mortality of Abdominal Aortic Aneurysms?

The perioperative mortality associated with abdominal aortic reconstructive surgery has been variously reported between 0.9 and 15%, averaging 7% in a review of eight large series.[1-8] Not surprisingly, the majority of deaths were cardiac related with from 48 to 100% of the mortality rate in these patients ascribed to cardiac events (Table 22-1). Other less common factors directly responsible for perioperative mortality included exsanguinating hemorrhage (either intra- or postoperative), aortic declamping shock, visceral infarction, embolization or thrombosis of the distal vasculature, renal failure, graft infection, cerebrovascular accident, and pulmonary insufficiency. This chapter will review the techniques employed at the University of California, San Francisco, to reduce the operative mortality of abdominal aortic *aneurysm* surgery.

Table 22-1
Variation in Perioperative Mortality for
Abdominal Aortic Aneurysm

Series	Mortality/Total Events/Patients	Mortality Due to Cardiac Events
Szilagi et al (1966)[5]	59/401	48
Hicks et al (1975)[3]	19/225	53
Thompson et al (1975)[6]	6/108	83
Young et al (1975)[8]	7/144	100
Mulcare et al (1978)[4]	14/140	79
Whittmore et al (1980)[7]	1/100	100
Crawford et al (1981)[1]	41/860	54
Hertzer (1983)[2]	22/523	64

VASCULAR SURGERY: ISSUES IN CURRENT PRACTICE
ISBN 0-8089-1839-7

It has been clearly demonstrated that perioperative mortality is greatly elevated with emergent aneurysmectomy, and the following discussion will be limited to elective aneurysm surgery. It should, however, be mentioned that to minimize the high operative mortality associated with a ruptured abdominal aneurysm, urgent operation is advised if the aneurysm is symptomatic or semi-urgently if there is documented substantial recent enlargement. All aneurysms greater than 6 cm should be electively repaired if the patient can tolerate operation. In very good-risk patients repair of smaller aortic aneurysms is also justified in the light of their reported 20% risk of rupture.[9]

PERIOPERATIVE EVALUATION AND MANAGEMENT

The presence of an abdominal aortic aneurysm is usually detected by physical examination and confirmed by plain film of the abdomen or by B-mode ultrasonography. While arteriography is not a mandatory part of the preoperative evaluation, this study should be selectively employed to: (1) determine the extent of the aneurysm when renal, visceral, or thoracic involvement is suspected; (2) assess the distal circulation when peripheral vascular disease is present. With this information the surgeon can more safely plan the operative approach (transabdominal versus thoraco-retroperitoneal) and will be forewarned about abnormal anatomic findings (e.g., horseshoe kidney, multiple renal arteries) and deal appropriately with distal occlusive disease.

The remainder of the preoperative evaluation is devoted to detection of risk factors that warrant special perioperative attention. A careful history and physical examination, routine laboratory studies including a complete blood count, urinalysis, renal and electrolyte panel, EKG, and chest X-ray are performed on all patients. Then, based on clues from these data, further evaluation to lower risk is performed. For example, in patients with suspected pulmonary insufficiency, pulmonary function studies and arterial blood gases are obtained. Then the obvious steps of cessation of smoking, aggressive pulmonary toilet, and patient education regarding intubation and postoperative care are taken. Some patients will also require further intervention including preoperative intravenous bronchodilators to lessen their pulmonary risk to acceptable levels.

A similar risk-minimization approach is undertaken with regard to coronary artery disease, almost ubiquitous in this patient population. While cardiac events are the leading cause of death following repair of abdominal aortic aneurysms, this does not justify coronary angiography with prophylactic bypass of significant lesions in all of these patients. Instead, careful cardiac evaluation including the routine workup already described is first performed. Those patients with suspected coronary artery disease by history, physical exam, or abnormal EKG, would then undergo some form of stress testing, either exercise–thallium or dipyridamole–thallium imaging. Because exercise–thallium scintigraphy is a more specific indicator of myocardial ischemia than multigated radionuclide scanning, the former approach is preferred. Additionally, because it is often difficult to obtain adequate stress testing in these vascular patients, dipyridamole-induced coronary vasodilation when combined with thallium scanning provides results comparable to exercise–thallium scans alone.[10] Patients without thallium redistribution may safely undergo aneurysm resection, while those who show evidence of redistribution are then considered for coronary angiography. Those patients of acceptable risk who have demonstrably significant coronary artery disease should undergo aorto-coronary bypass prior to aneurysmectomy. Some patients, because of globally poor left ventricular function or unreconstructable coronary artery disease, will of necessity undergo aneurysm resection alone with accompanying aggressive cardiac management. This might include control of hypertension and optimization of fluid status and cardiac indices by preoperative insertion of a Swan–Ganz catheter and pharmacologic treatment with combinations of intravenous dopamine, dobutamine, nitroprusside, and nitroglycerine.

All patients are intravenously hydrated, beginning the evening prior to aneurysmectomy, to prevent rapid swings in the blood pressure associated with anesthetic induction and the surgical repair. Since skin flora are often related to graft infection, preparation of the skin before the operation is important. Whenever possible, the patient should bathe with an antibacterial soap for a day or two preoperatively. Mechanical cleansing of the bowel facilitates surgical exposure and may also be worthwhile in preventing infection if the bowel is accidentally entered. Even though almost all surgeons administer antibiotics prophylactically for arterial reconstructions, such usage had been highly controversial until about five years ago. A recent prospective double-blind randomized trial has now clearly demonstrated the efficacy of cefazolin in reducing wound and prosthesis infections in vascular reconstructions, and thus the use of prophylactic antibiotics in vascular cases can now be advocated on more than just an empiric basis.[11] For optimal efficacy, the antibiotics should be administered preoperatively and supplemental doses given at the appropriate intervals during a long procedure.

Anesthetic Management

On the morning of surgery, patients are given all of their usual cardiac medications and, once in the operating room, a conventional electrocardiographic system is attached. A radial arterial catheter is inserted and central venous access is obtained. The majority of patients have Swan–Ganz catheters inserted; however, in the better-risk aneurysm patient, central venous monitoring may be sufficient. All patients are anesthetized with either a halogenated anesthetic or fentanyl, paralyzed, and mechanically ventilated. The myocardial depressant actions of the halogenated inhalation anesthetics make these agents less desirable in higher cardiac risk patients.

As has been discussed, myocardial ischemia remains the most common cause of perioperative mortality in abdominal aortic aneurysm patients, despite the availability of aggressive intraoperative cardiac monitoring and therapy. It has been shown that the standard surface electrocardiogram can miss the presence of subendocardial ischemia and will occasionally miss transmural myocardial ischemia.[12] Two-dimensional transesophageal echocardiography (2D-TEE), a new and minimally invasive cardiac monitoring technique, accurately identifies intraoperative segmental wall motion abnormalities (SWMAs), a highly sensitive and specific marker of myocardial ischemia. Smith has recently demonstrated that intraoperative

Table 22-2

Changes Occurring with Clamping at the
Supraceliac (SC), Suprarenal (SR), and Infrarenal
(IR) Aortic Levels

	SC(%)	SR(%)	IR(%)
MAP[†]	54	5*	2*
PCWP[‡]	38	10*	0
EDA	28	2*	9*
ESA	69	10*	11*
EF	−38	−10*	−3*
With wall motion abnormalities	92	33	0
New MIs	8	0	0

* Statistically different from the SC group at the $p < 0.05$ level.
† Mean atrial pressure (MAP).
‡ Pulmonary capillary wedge pressure (PCWP).

SWMAs are detected by 2D-TEE four times more frequently than ST segment changes on the ECG.[13] Additionally, those patients having new persistent SWMAs (present at skin closure) are more likely to have a myocardial infarction (MI) than those with transient SWMA (resolving by skin closure). No patients without new SWMA suffered a myocardial infarction in this study. When 2D-TEE was used to compare myocardial function in patients undergoing supraceliac, suprarenal-infraceliac, or infrarenal aortic occlusion, differences were observed which were not detectable by conventional hemodynamic monitors.[14]

Occlusion at the supraceliac (SC) level caused significantly greater increases in left ventricular end-systolic (ESA) and end-diastolic areas (EDA), decreases in ejection fraction (EF), and more frequent SWMAs. Occlusion at the suprarenal (SR)-infraceliac level caused similar but smaller changes, and occlusion at the infrarenal (IR) level caused only minimal cardiovascular effects (Table 22-2).

2D-TEE is easy to use and of proven safety with no observed complications in over 700 applications at the University of California, San Francisco. Once the endotracheal tube is in place, a 9 mm gastroscope tipped with a 3.5 mHz phased-array transducer is positioned in the esophagus. The transducer is connected to an ultrasonograph to provide real-time, short-axis, cross-sectional views of the left ventricle at the level of the papillary muscles (Figs 22-1 to 22-3).

Armed with this monitor, the anesthesiologist can optimize volume status and myocardial function during the aneurysmectomy. This optimization becomes critically important when the heart is subjected to the increased afterload associated with aortic cross-clamping and then again to prevent declamping shock when the cross-clamp is removed (Figs 22-4 and 22-5). Myocardial performance throughout the procedure can be closely monitored and therapeutic intervention based on interpretation of 2D-TEE findings is made in the hope of reducing myocardial morbidity and mortality. We have recently looked at the role of 2D-TEE on the outcome in cerebrovascular reconstructions and found a lower myocardial complication rate among patients who were studied with 2D-TEE versus risk-matched controls.[15]

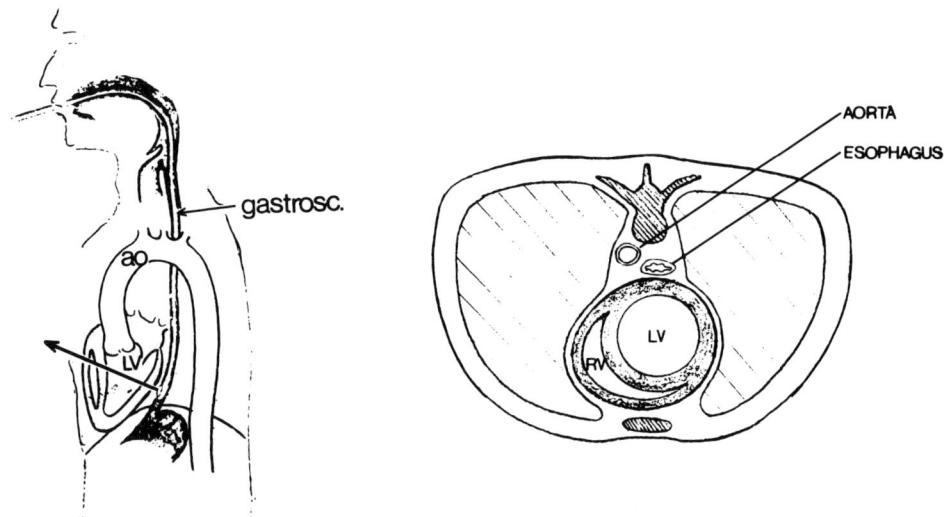

Fig. 22-1. (Left) An illustration of a 2D-TEE tipped gastroscope positioned in the distal esophagus. (Right) A cross-sectional view of the patient at the level of the papillary muscles (arrow) schematically demonstrating the view obtained with 2D-TEE.

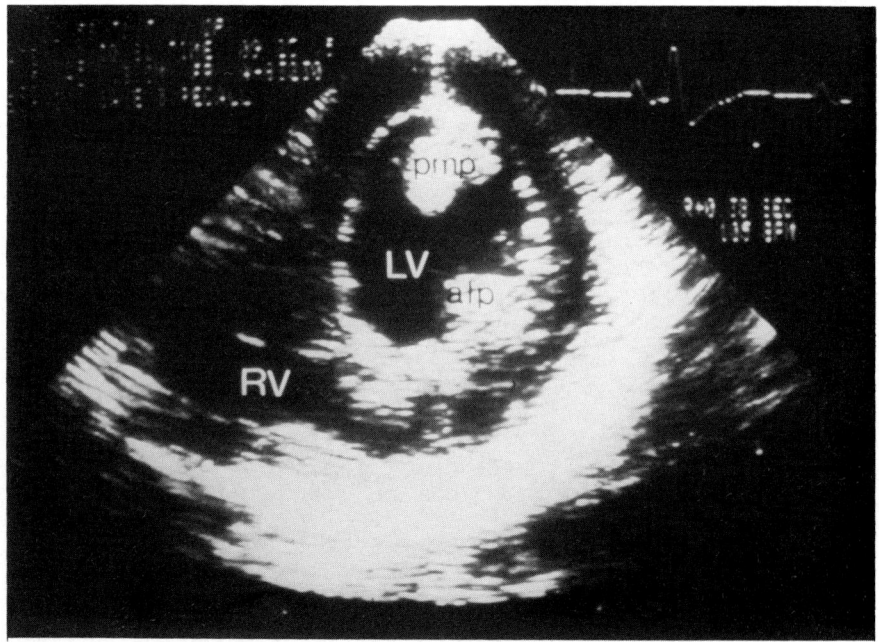

Fig. 22-2. A 2D-TEE image of the heart at the level depicted in Fig. 22-1. RV = right ventricle, pmp = posteromedial papillary muscle, LV = left ventricle, alp = anterolateral papillary muscle.

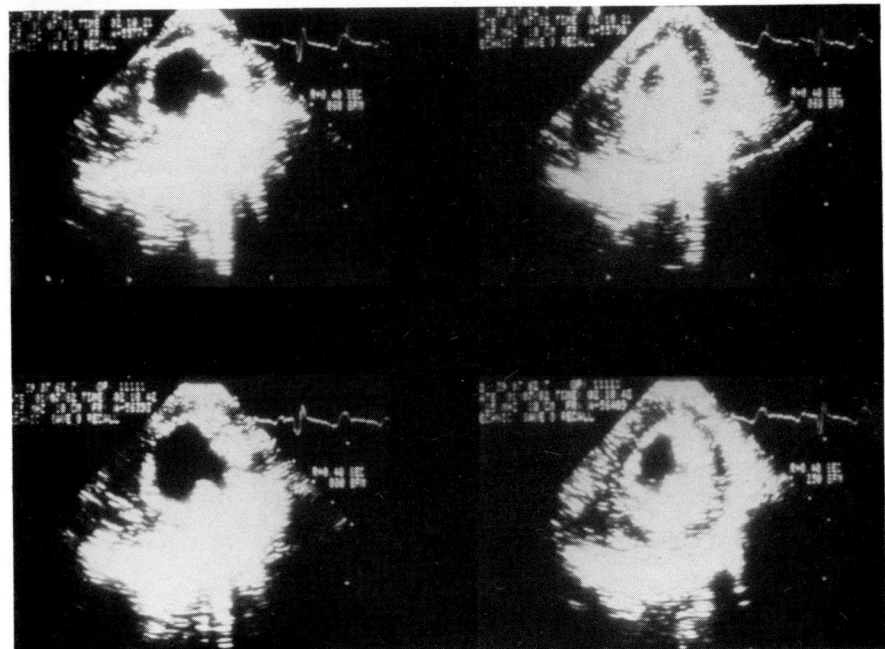

Fig. 22-3. 2D-TEE images demonstrating the effect of aortic cross-clamping in the setting of hypovolemia. (Top left) End diastole, decreased volume. (Top right) End systole, decreased volume. (Bottom left) End diastole, cross-clamp placed. (Bottom right) End systole, cross-clamp placed. Note that the combination of cross-clamping with hypovolemia yields a near-normal 2D-TEE image of the LV.

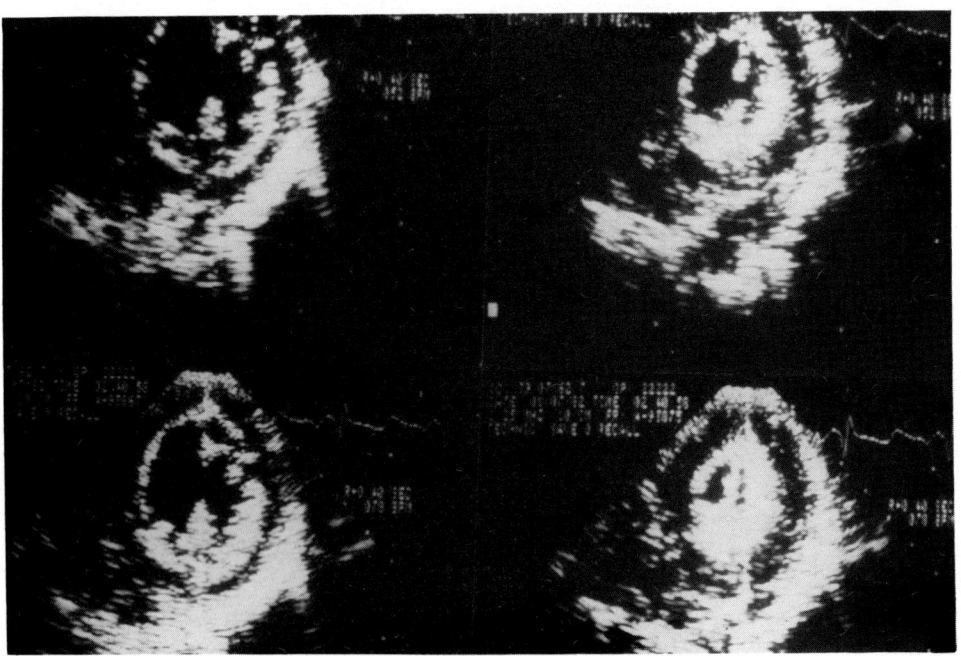

Fig. 22-4. 2D-TEE images demonstrating the effect of unclamping on a volume-loaded heart. (Top left) End diastole, volume-loaded, cross-clamp in place. (Top right) End systole, volume-loaded, cross-clamp in place. Note the near-normal appearance of the LV. (Bottom left) End diastole, hypovolemia, clamp-off. (Bottom right) End systole, hypovolemia, clamp-off.

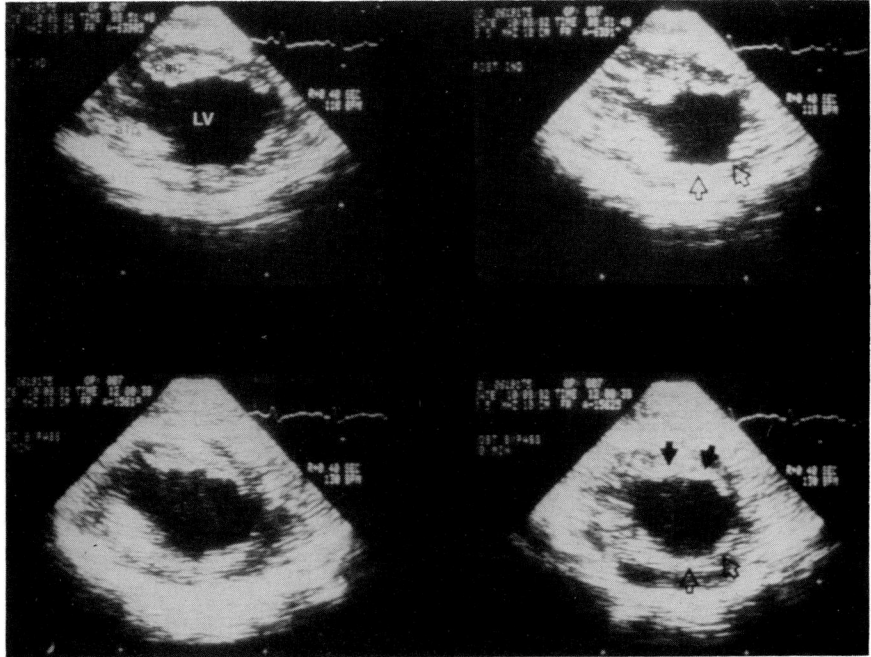

Fig. 22-5. 2D-TEE demonstration of new segmental wall motion abnormalities (SWMAs) in the presence of preexisting SWMA. (Top left) End diastole. (Top right) End systole, anterior ventricular SWMA (clear arrows). (Bottom left) End diastole, later in the procedure. (Bottom right) End systole, new posterior ventricular SWMA (black arrows) as well as preexisting anterior ventricular SWMA.

Along with continuous cardiac monitoring, the anesthesiologist follows arterial blood gases and urine output throughout the procedure. Fluids are aggressively given to replace the substantial evaporative and third-space losses associated with aneurysmectomy. If urine output falls below the accepted minimum of 0.5 cm^3/(kg h), additional fluids are administered. Low urine output in the face of adequate filling pressures and reasonable myocardial function as evidenced by either cardiac index and/or 2D-TEE requires the use of diuretics. If low-output myocardial failure is the cause of oliguria, then pharmacologic support is instituted in the form of ionotropic agents and afterload reduction.

The other significant advance in anesthetic/fluid management involves the more liberal use of intraoperative autotransfusion in abdominal aortic aneurysm surgery. The detrimental effects of severe anemia on the heart, brain, and kidneys are obvious, and this technique has helped reduce the incidence of myocardial ischemia, stroke, and renal failure at this institution. Even more importantly, homologous blood transfusion requirements drop significantly with autotransfusion, decreasing the risk of blood-borne infections including hepatitis and AIDS.

Operative Management

Once endotracheal anesthesia has been administered and appropriate monitors placed, attention is then directed toward the conduct of the aneurysm resection. With regard to risk minimization the first major consideration is infection. Intraoperative prophylaxis against the grave consequences of prosthetic graft infection consists of efforts to reduce the number of microorganisms reaching the wound via the operative team, the operating room environment, and the patient. The most important feature affecting the operating room milieu is the level of human activity, and traffic in and out of the room should therefore be minimized.

The least expensive and easiest compound to use for preparing the operative skin site is 1% iodine in 70% ethyl alcohol (tincture of iodine). Other agents such as povidone-iodine, other iodophores, hexachlorophene, chlorhexidine gluconate, and benzalkonium are also satisfactory. Even after disinfection, however, the anatomy of the skin makes it impossible to maintain sterility. For this reason, the skin edges are lined with antibiotic soaked sponges, and plastic surgical adhesive drapes are used to prevent the prosthetic graft from contacting the skin.

Laparotomy is most expeditiously accomplished through a full-length midline incision from the xyphoid process to the symphysis pubis.[16] A transverse abdominal incision to provide access to the aorta either transperitoneally or retroperitoneally is often adequate and lessens postoperative incisional pain. Although exposure via this transverse incision may be limited if an unanticipated problem is encountered, this incision should be used for patients with poor pulmonary function.

The small intestines are placed in a plastic bag and brought out onto the abdominal wall to the right of the incision. Maintenance of gastrointestinal tract integrity is of obvious importance in preventing prosthetic graft infection. If accidental enterotomy is made while exposing the aorta during an elective aneurysmectomy, the bowel and laparotomy wounds should be closed and the procedure deferred for one to two weeks. Additionally, since the risks associated with infectious complications are so high, elective surgical procedures on the gastrointestinal or urinary tract should not be performed concomitantly with aneurysm resection.

The posterior peritoneal incision is made longitudinally on the dome of the aneurysm to the right of the vascular arcade supplying the left colon. The incision is extended to the left renal vein superiorly, and inferiorly it swings to the right over the anterior surface of the right common iliac artery. In this way, the medially oriented pelvic branches of the IMA are avoided, providing protection against subsequent colon devascularization. The anterior two-thirds of the aneurysm is then unroofed, separating it from the duodenum on the right to the depth of the inferior vena cava. Should this normal dissection plane between the aorta and the duodenum be absent, as seen with inflammatory aneurysms, then the bowel is left attached to the aneurysm wall to prevent possible enterotomy. An underlying principle of aneurysm exposure is gentle dissection of the patient from the aneurysm to minimize the risk of distal embolization.

Control of both external iliac and hypogastric arteries is obtained prior to control of the proximal aorta. Special care should be exercised when mobilizing these vessels at the aortic bifurcation to avoid troublesome hemorrhage associated with caval or iliac vein laceration at this level. Where one dissects the aorta proximally depends on the aneurysm neck and the presence of luminal disease (thrombus or atheroma). The arteriogram and careful palpation guide the surgeon in this regard and, if necessary, suprarenal or supraceliac cross-clamping is utilized. Generally, circumferential exposure of the aneurysm is easiest at the neck because of its anterior displacement. If this becomes difficult to accomplish without a high probability of perforating the aorta or dislodging friable intima, then the posterior wall of the aorta is left undivided and the posterior anastomosis is sewn with deep sutures that doubly penetrate the full thickness of the aortic wall.

Except for the very elderly patient or the rare case where a bleeding diathesis is encountered, the appropriate size *knitted* graft is then chosen and preclotted with blood obtained by puncture of the vena cava. The patient is then systemically anticoagulated with from 3000 to 4000 units of heparin. Because of the complications associated with protamine sulfate, reversal of heparin is not routinely performed.

After communication with the anesthesiologist, the distal clamps are applied. Distal clamping is performed first to allow more gradual increase in afterload and to eliminate the possibility of embolic material dislodging with application of the more proximal clamp. In the usual situation there is a short cuff of nonaneurysmal aorta distal to the renal arteries. The proximal aortic clamp is applied as closely as possible to the renal artery origins without impinging on their orifices. Occasionally, the aneurysm will involve only a more distal segment of the infrarenal aorta. It is important to recognize that aortic dilation at a higher level will develop in time and aortic transection should still be performed at the customary level immediately distal to the renal arteries.

A bulldog clamp is placed on the IMA after dissecting this vessel at least 1 cm from the aneurysm wall. This is important to insure preservation of the major branches of this vessel. The aneurysm is opened longitudinally and the contained thrombus is removed manually. If necessary, a thromboendarterectomy of the aorta is performed to facilitate identification and suture closure of back-bleeding lumbar vessels. Small figure-of-eight transfixion sutures will firmly seal each bleeding orifice.

The aortic cuff is then prepared either by partial endarterectomy or, more commonly, simple removal of loose material by vigorous flushing. Close, deeply placed sutures at the proximal anastomosis adequately bind the less loosely attached intimal fragments that remain. Bifurcation grafts are preferred to prevent the possibility of distal anastomosis thrombosis or disruption because of aneurysmal disease in the distal aortic segment. The common iliac artery is the usual site for distal end-to-end anastomosis. If these vessels are unacceptable because of aneurysmal or occlusive disease, then variations in performing the distal anastomosis become necessary to insure outflow via at least one hypogastric artery. This is important to provide a source of collateral blood supply to the descending and sigmoid colon. Hypogastric preservation also minimizes the consequences of distal embolization by allowing another avenue for flushing and opening the graft than the external iliac arteries.

Adequacy of blood flow to the left colon is insured if vigorous pulsatile back-bleeding from the IMA stump can be demonstrated. If this back-bleeding is inadequate and a large and patent IMA was noted on preoperative aortography, then reimplantation of the IMA should be performed. Reimplantation is also necessary whenever there is evidence of left colon ischemia. It is important to note, however, that when safeguards are taken to preserve the vascular supply to the colon, adequate collaterals are almost invariably present largely via the hypogastric arteries.

A final flush through the unsutured opposite iliac arm of the graft is then performed. This momentary release of the aortic clamp removes clotted blood and debris that may have accumulated in the graft. After allowing adequate preparation by the anesthesiologist, the anastomosed graft limb is flushed, first into the hypogastric artery and then into the external iliac artery. If properly managed, declamping hypotension should be minimal (10–20 mmHg) and lasts only 1–2 minutes. Following completion of the opposite iliac anastomosis a similar staged release of the distal clamps is performed. The redundant aneurysm wall is sutured around the graft to close the retroperitoneal dead space and interpose a thick layer of viable tissue between the graft and duodenum. The posterior peritoneum is then approximated with a lock-suture to prevent telescoping of the duodenum. This two-layer retroperitonealization of the graft is performed in the hope of minimizing the late risk of aorto-enteric fistula.

The patients are observed overnight in the intensive care unit and generally remain intubated until they are fully awake with reasonable arterial blood gases. Fluids are vigorously replaced to maintain adequate urine output and cardiac function, as discussed earlier. Antibiotics are continued until all catheters are removed and patients are generally discharged after one week to 10 days of hospitalization.

REFERENCES

1. Crawford ES, Saleh SA, Babb JW III, et al: Infrarenal abdominal aortic aneurysm. Factors influencing survival after operation performed over a 25-year period. Ann Surg 193:699, 1981
2. Hertzer NR: Myocardial ischemia. Surgery 93:97, 1983
3. Hicks GL, Eastland MW, DeWeese JA, et al: Survival improvement following aneurysm resection. Ann Surg 181:863, 1975
4. Mulcare RJ, Royster TS, Lynn RA, et al: Long-term results of operative therapy for aortoiliac disease. Arch Surg 113:601, 1978
5. Szilagyi DE, Smith RF, DeRusso FJ, et al: Contribution of abdominal aortic aneurysmectomy to prolongation of life. Ann Surg 164:678, 1966
6. Thompson JE, Hollier LH, Patman RD, et al: Surgical management of abdominal arotic aneurysms: Factors influencing mortality and morbidity—A 20-year experience. Ann Surg 181:654, 1975
7. Wittemore AD, Clowes AW, Hechtman HB, et al: Aortic aneurysm repair. Reduced operative mortality associated with maintenance of optimal cardiac performance. Ann Surg 192:414, 1980
8. Young AE, Sandberg GW, Couch NP: The reduction of mortality of abdominal aortic aneurysm resection. Am J Surg 134:585, 1975
9. Darling RC, Messina ER, Morrison G, et al: Autopsy study of unoperated abdominal aortic aneurysms: The case for early resection. Circulation 56 (Suppl 2):11, 1977
10. Boucher CA, Brewster DC, Darling RC, et al: Determination of cardiac risk by dipyridamole–thallium imaging before peripheral vascular surgery. NEJM 312:389, 1985
11. Wilson SE, Van Wagenen P, Passaro E Jr: Arterial infection, in Ravitch MM, Steichen FM (eds): Current Problems in Surgery. Chicago, Year Book Medical Publishers, 1978
12. Barnard RJ, Buckberg GD, Duncan HW: Limitations of the standard transthoracic electrocardiogram in detecting subendocardial ischemia. Am Heart J 99:476, 1980
13. Smith JS, Cahalan MK, Benefiel DJ, et al: Intraoperative detection of myocardial ischemia in high-risk patients: Electrocardiography versus two-dimensional transesophageal echocardiography. Circulation 72:1015, 1985
14. Roizen MF, Beaupre PN, Alpert RA, et al: Monitoring with two-dimensional transesophageal echocardiography. J Vasc Surg 1:300, 1984
15. Okuhn SP, Benefiel DJ, Ehrenfeld WK, et al: Unpublished data
16. Wylie EJ, Stoney RJ, Ehrenfeld WK: Manual of Vascular Surgery, vol I. New York, Springer-Verlag, 1980

T. Coddington, J. Waller,
A. Drew, Claire Martin,
C. N. McCollum, and R. M. Greenhalgh

23

How Can We Improve Amputation Practices?

Improvements in amputation practices can be made in three main areas: (1) reduction in the number of major amputations performed, (2) in the performance of a good surgical amputation stump, and (3) by providing a rapid limb-fitting service. There is very little doubt that the number of major amputations can be reduced when severely ischaemic limbs are managed by vascular specialists. In the first section we shall discuss the amputation rates recorded in a district general hospital and compare them with our results in a specialist vascular service. In the second section we shall stress the importance of a good amputation stump in reducing the period of rehabilitation and the discomfort of the patient. Finally, we consider the steps which might be taken to reduce the time between major amputation and the provision of the final prosthetic limb.

AMPUTATION FOR PERIPHERAL ARTERIAL DISEASE: COMPARISON BETWEEN OUR EXPERIENCE AND THAT OF A DISTRICT GENERAL HOSPITAL

Haynes and Middleton reported the experience of a general surgeon with a special interest in vascular surgery working in a large district general hospital and assisted by annually rotating general surgical registrars.[1] The authors welcomed comparison with specialist vascular units such as ours which has two full-time consultant surgical staff, a highly trained junior staff, and the facilities of a University Department of Surgery. Haynes and Middleton's patients were treated in a large district general hospital with 1200 beds on an ordinary general surgical service. Frequently the patients came from geriatric wards and the level of amputation was determined on clinical grounds. The authors note that ". . . in some cases peripheral angiography had previously been performed which will determine whether or not the integrity of the limb could be maintained. Emphasis was placed on achieving

VASCULAR SURGERY: ISSUES IN CURRENT PRACTICE
ISBN 0-8089-1839-7

primary healing and therefore few of the more sophisticated and complicated procedures such as Gritti–Stokes and below knee amputations were attempted."

During the 11-year period from January 1969 to December 1979, 290 amputations for vascular insufficiency of the lower limb were performed on 286 patients at the East Birmingham Hospital. Of the patients 70% were male and 30% female. Thirty-six (12.6%) of the patients were diabetic. The mean age of the amputees was 70.2 years. The indication for operation was ischaemic rest pain (174) and gangrene (116).

These authors report that the commonest site of amputation by far was mid-thigh amputation (224 patients—77.2%). Gritti–Stokes (34—11.7%) and below-knee amputation (32—11.1%) were clearly performed far less commonly. Primary healing was achieved in 202 (75.9%) of the 226 early survivors. A total of 73 amputees (25.5%) died during the period of hospital admission (28.6% for mid-thigh amputation). These authors draw attention to the absence of any specialist rehabilitation unit for the care and supervision of amputees in the early weeks after operation: "In our own District General Hospital these facilities are not available." Patients were sent home and from home they were referred to the Artificial Limb and Appliance Centre for rehabilitation. The limb-fitting doctors did not see the patient's stump till this stage; communication between them and the surgical team was minimal.

The importance of this paper is to draw attention to what must be the pattern for a number of general surgical units throughout the country. A general surgical registrar will stay with a consultant surgeon with a vascular interest for a period of 12 months. Frequently the safest treatment is a major amputation either below knee or, more frequently, above knee. A comparison of the management of comparable patients in a specialist vascular unit in the same country is striking.

AMPUTATION FOR PERIPHERAL ARTERIAL DISEASE IN OUR SPECIALIST VASCULAR SERVICE

In the Vascular Surgical Service at Charing Cross Hospital there are two whole-time vascular surgeons, one with a senior registrar and the other with a registrar and other junior staff. A 24-hour Vascular Surgical Service is provided with approximately 50% of the patients referred from outside of the region. This involves the patients in some travelling to the hospital and some are tertiary referrals from other consultant surgeons who do not have such a marked vascular interest. Over the past five years, approximately 140 patients per year with severe ischaemia have been referred to this service. In the first instance, the patients are seen and assessed clinically and then evaluated with noninvasive Doppler ultrasound tests. These are performed during the outpatient consultation and made available to the clinician for a decision. All patients with potentially reversible ischaemic rest pain and early minor gangrene receive complete arteriography and thorough assessment and consideration of arterial reconstruction. The cardiac status of the patients is assessed by ECG and evaluation of ventricular ejection fraction. The carotid vessels are assessed by duplex scanning to estimate the risk of potential stroke. Within 2–3 days of presentation to hospital, patients with ischaemic rest pain or pregangrene are operated upon by a reconstructive arterial procedure. A major amputation is very rarely considered as a primary procedure.

From Table 23-1 it can be seen that between 11 and 23 major amputations were performed each year in the six years from 1980 to 1985 inclusive, an average of 15 major amputations per year. In other words, of the patients referred with pregangrene or early gangrene only approximately 11% (15 of 140) per year came to major amputation either above knee or below knee and the rest had limb salvage from the benefit of arterial reconstructive procedures. In Table 6-1 the deaths which occurred after amputation can also be seen. From this we see that only 16 deaths occurred in a follow-up of up to five years from a total of 89 major amputations.

During the same period of time, minor amputation in association with limb salvage was performed far more frequently: in 1980, 23 times; in 1981, 22 times; in 1982, 35 times; in 1983, 22 times; in 1984, 23 times; and 1985, 24 times. These were either amputation of digits or, at most, transmetatarsal amputation.

An implied comparison between these services as we have done is in many ways not legitimate. Patients in one group are in Birmingham and in the other group are in London. The years chosen are not the same and the severity of arterial disease in each group cannot be accurately compared. However, the age range and male–female ratio are very similar and it is likely that both groups had end-stage arterial disease. The severity of arterial disease in the East Birmingham Hospital would not have been available because frequently arteriography was not performed. At least some comparisons are legitimate. The Vascular Surgical Service specialist group have investigated all patients fully and shown that a relatively small fraction come to amputation. These facilities are not available at the present time in many parts of the United Kingdom and the comparison draws attention to the need for Vascular Surgical Services across the country. This would involve strategic replacement of consultant surgeons by general surgeons with a vascular interest, to work in

Table 23-1
Charing Cross Hospital: Major Amputations—Primary and Post Reconstruction

Year	Total	Age Range	Male–Female Ratio	Above Knee	Below Knee	Through Knee	Deaths
1980	11	60–80	6 : 5	3	8	0	1 AK 1980
							1 BK 1980
1981	11	59–79	4 : 7	5	6	0	1 BK 1981
							1 BK 1983
1982	23	53–88	12 : 11	6	15	2	1 BK 1983
							1 BK 1985
							1 AK 1983
1983	11	48–87	8 : 3	3	8	0	1 BK 1983
							1 BK 1984
							1 AK 1985
1984	20	59–80	16 : 4	5	15	0	1 BK 1984
			4 : 1				2 BK 1985
							1 AK 1984
							1 AK 1986
1985	13	55–79	10 : 3	3	9	1	Nil
Mean	15	48–88		4.1	10.2	0.5	

pairs in one district hospital such that this speciality is possibly withdrawn from an adjacent district hospital. Instead, in the other hospital a speciality such as urology could be offered. Facilites for proper investigations should be made available, including proper noninvasive investigation with a technician and adequate angiography, so that arterial reconstructive surgery can be offered where appropriate. This could lead to a dramatic reduction in the number of major amputations and above-knee amputation would become a very rare event.

From Table 23-1 it can be seen that above-knee amputation would be performed on average four times per year in a practice in which 140 patients are referred with severe lower limb ischaemia in a 12-month period—an incidence of 2.9%. By comparison, an ever-increasing number of minor amputations would be performed in association with such Vascular Surgical Services. The services of an orthotist would increase to provide footwear after partial amputation as the need for above-knee and below-knee prostheses reduces. If these recommendations were implemented the revenue consequences to the country would be enormous. By increasing the limb salvage rate by setting up Vascular Surgical Services, fewer support services would be required as more patients would be able to take care of themselves at home. Fewer ambulance journeys for limb fittings would be required as well as actually fewer artificial limbs being made. On occasions, patients would need to travel further from their home for specialist expertise than at present, but this they would surely gladly do if they knew the issues.

PERFORMANCE OF THE SERVICEABLE AMPUTATION

It has been extremely beneficial to work together with the visiting team of limb-fitting doctor, prosthetist, orthotist, and physiotherapist. Surgeons are not always aware of the difficulties the prosthetist has with certain amputation stumps and proper communication is a vital ingredient. This team regards the below-knee amputation as the best major amputation at the present time and strive to conserve the knee joint at all cost.

Once attempted limb salvage fails to enable amputation to occur at the transmetatarsal level, the next desirable amputation level is the below-knee amputation position. If this is not possible neither the through-knee nor the Gritti–Stokes amputations are recommended, but rather the patient is thought to have a better mobility with a mid-thigh amputation with myoplastic flaps. If the knee joint is not conserved then the weight of the patient is taken mainly on the ischial tuberosity and this applies both to the through-knee and Gritti–Stokes as well as mid-thigh amputations.

Conservation of the knee joint is considered to be of prime importance and the long posterior flap Burgess below-knee amputation method is preferred (Fig. 23-1).[2] The Burgess below-knee amputation greatly improves the chances of primary healing. The blood supply is carried in the muscles to the skin edges and muscles and skin are cut together and not separated so as not to disturb the vital blood supply. This has led to a very much better primary healing rate. It is important to avoid leaving unsightly "dog ears" at the corner and in Fig. 23-1 the best shape of Burgess amputation is demonstrated. This shape is ideal for the prosthesis. More recently, the skew flap amputation (Fig. 23-2) has been described by Kingsley

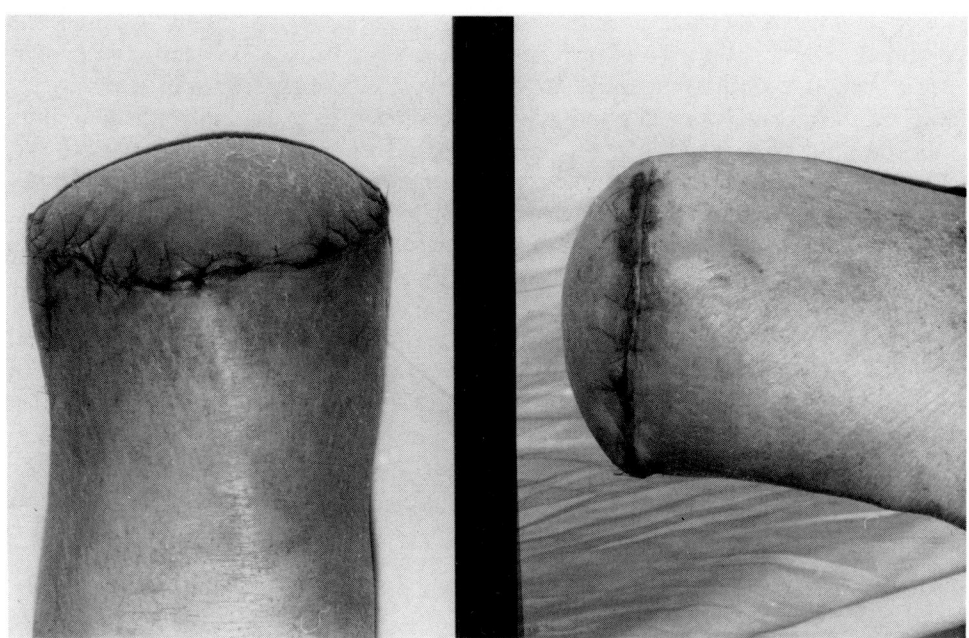

Fig. 23-1. The Burgess below-knee amputation demonstrating the avoidance of "dog-ears".

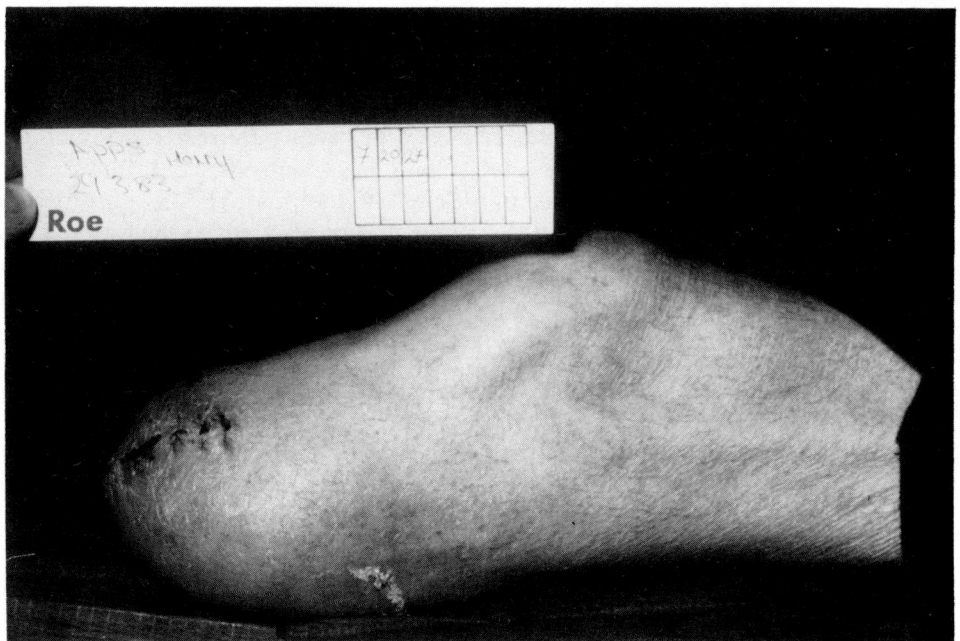

Fig. 23-2. The skew flap amputation stump as described by Kingsley Robinson.

Robinson and good results have been reported.[3] Using this technique it is sometimes possible to achieve a below-knee amputation where a Burgess amputation
would not be possible. The reason for this is that the long posterior flap of the
Burgess amputation is cut quite far down the back of the calf and if disease has
reached this area, a skew flap may be possible whereas a long posterior flap amputation would not.

The through-knee amputation has largely gone out of favour but it does have a
place in a very sick patient, allowing a soft tissue amputation without the need to
cut bone. The benefit of this procedure is that it requires a small dissection through
soft tissue and the procedure can be performed under light anaesthesia or even
strong analgesia. The through-knee amputation is at present reserved by our group
for this sort of patient. It is not considered to be an ideal amputation for rehabilitation as the prosthetic limb has many drawbacks.

In the postoperative period, the wound is left sealed for about a week and we
avoid firm amputation bandaging intended to "shape" the stump. We are more
concerned with achieving primary healing at this stage and specifically avoid any
firm bandaging which might reduce blood supply to the wound edges. The sutures
are left in between 14 and 21 days but rehabilitation of the patient begins at once
after amputation.

ARTIFICIAL LIMBS AT THE DISTRICT HOSPITAL

The weekly visit of the artificial limb and appliances team to the district hospital is to be highly recommended. As has been recorded above, it is beneficial for the
surgeon, prosthetist, orthotist, and limb-fitting doctor to work together to discuss
amputation levels. This visiting team is also of value to the specialist physiotherapist
on the rehabilitation of the amputee which should begin immediately before surgery.
This is the reverse of the system mentioned by Haynes and Middleton. Over the
past six years our team has visited patients together in the wards at the hospital and
usually managed to cast and provide a prosthesis for use within three-weeks. This
involves a visit of the limb-fitting doctor, prosthetist, or orthotist to the district
hospital once per week in a single half-day session. This totally cuts out the need for
the patient to travel to the Artificial Limb and Appliance Centre except for follow-
up visits for maintenance purposes at a future stage. This system also demands that
a workshop is available.

Equally, we would not favour the setting up of specialist amputation units
across the country. Vascular disease accounts for about 80% of major amputations
and it would be a retrograde step to encourage referring doctors to send ischaemic
limbs direct for amputation. Limb salvage must be the prime issue. Nor should
patients be shipped off for amputation when limb salvage fails. Not only is this
dreadful for patient morale, leading to slower and therefore more costly rehabilitation, but time is lost and inpatient bed occupancy would increase. As soon as an
amputation is unavoidable, it is best that it should be performed quickly, but where
possible after the visiting team has seen the patient. Immediately after the prosthesis
has been supplied the patient receives approximately one more week of rehabilitation before discharge home independently with the artificial limb. This system is

clearly much more desirable than that which occurs as described by Haynes and Middleton in a large number of district general hospitals in the United Kingdom.

Before 1980, when the system of casting and supplying artificial limbs at our hospital began, we had a choice. Either we could send patients home in a wheelchair as soon as the wound was healed, without any rehabilitation at all and without the prosthesis, or else we could keep the patients in hospital for a period of 10-12 weeks while the limb was cast, with the patient attending a limb-fitting centre on three occasions. Clearly, use of a hospital bed for 10–12 weeks is quite inappropriate and unnecessarily costly and quite the wrong use of an acute surgical bed. It is equally wrong not to commence rehabilitation of a patient and not to commence the learning process to walk before the patient is discharged home, as this is not only bad for the patient but also expensive on social support services.

IMPROVEMENTS IN AMPUTATION PRACTICES

In summary, improvements in amputation practices can only be achieved by grouping together surgeons so that two vascular surgeons can offer a 24-hour Vascular Surgical Service with proper facilities for investigation and correction of severe ischaemia of the limbs to avoid an unnecessarily high amputation rate. Saving of revenue consequences have been discussed in this respect. Such an expert group would also work more closely with the prosthetist, limb-fitting doctor, and orthotist, and encourage the prosthetist to take more clinical responsibility and work as part of the clinical team. The travelling prosthetist would benefit the patient by determining optimal amputation levels with the surgeon. With such a Vascular Surgical Service, the prosthetist would come to the patient rather than the patient to the prosthetist. This could lead to the need for an increasing number of prosthetists in the country and an increase in clinical awareness of the prosthetists. This would be no bad thing. This need for increasing responsibility in prosthetists may require

Table 23-2
Charing Cross Hospital: Rehabilitation
Time after Major Amputation

	Total Prosthesis Supplied	Surgery to Prosthesis Supply
1980	11	11 in 3 weeks
1981	8	8 in 3 weeks
1982	15	10 in 3 weeks
		5 in 4 weeks
1983	8	3 in 3 weeks
		5 in 4 weeks
1984	17	5 in 3 weeks
		8 in 4 weeks
		3 in 5 weeks
1985	10	2 in 3 weeks
		3 in 4 weeks
		1 in 5 weeks
		1 in 6 weeks

that they undergo further training and undoubtedly as a group they would seek more financial reward. The financial savings involved in reducing the journeys of patients on at least three occasions from their home or from the hospital to an artificial limb centre would in part go towards paying for the increased expenditure of prosthetists.

With this system, fewer major amputations would be performed, and then at the best level. The prosthesis would be supplied at the district hospital within a minimum period of time and rehabilitation would commence during the three-week period of hospitalisation after amputation and before discharge. Very shortly after that date, the patient with the prosthesis would walk out of hospital and further expensive ambulance travelling time and home services would be avoided. The system would not only be better for the patient but would be cheaper for the country to provide.

REFERENCES

1. Haynes IG, Middleton MD: Amputation for peripheral vascular disease: Experience of a district general hospital. Ann R Coll Surg Engl 63:342–343, 1981
2. Burgess EM, Romano RL, Zettl JH: The management of lower extremity amputations. Prosthetic and Sensory Aids Service, US Veterans Administration 11 TR:10–16, 1969
3. Robinson KP, Hoile R, Coddington T: Skew flap myoplastic below knee amputation: A preliminary report. Br J Surg 69(9), September 1982

Ronald J. Stoney
and Linda M. Reilly

24

How Should We Treat Infected Grafts?

The introduction of prosthetic vascular grafts three decades ago has resolved most of the reconstructive challenges for the vascular surgeon, while at the same time introducing a unique set of problems—graft complications. The most serious of these is the prosthetic graft infection, and the most commonly involved graft is an aortic prosthesis originally inserted to replace an aneurysm or bypass an obstructive lesion. The threat to life and limb of the infected aortic graft and its treatment are higher than for any other vascular surgical lesion. Because of its infrequent occurrence, few surgeons have enough experience with its management to become familiar with the complex and innovative surgical techniques required to provide alternative routes for limb revascularization and complete removal of the infected prosthesis itself. The expertise in employing these principles dictates a satisfactory and durable outcome for the threatened patient. This chapter will review two decades of experience with aortic graft infection at the University of California, San Francisco, emphasizing the types of infection, diagnostic techniques, operative strategy, and the management of late complications associated with successful initial treatment.

DEFINITIONS

A prosthetic graft is infected when there is successful colonization of the host tissue which incorporates the prosthesis. This usually occurs late after implantation (28 months mean) and varies with the source and type of organisms (Gram negative, enteric organisms—33 months; Gram positive, skin organisms—25 months). Usually, the infection is *diffuse* at the time of clinical presentation and diagnosis, and the entire graft must be removed and an alternate route for revascularization of the limbs must be established. On rare occasions, the infection is *limited* to one graft segment, usually as a result of a late re-do groin operation to restore graft patency or repair a noninfected false aneurysm. The delayed appearance of infection may include pain, redness, or sinus drainage following such an operation, and this may signify a localized graft limb infection. Treatment of this entity can proceed with retention of the aortic portion of the graft and the contralateral limb which greatly simplifies the management for such a patient.

DIAGNOSIS

The successful management of a patient who harbors an infected aortic prosthetic graft is total removal of the infected graft itself and limb revascularization using either remote prosthetic bypass or in situ autogenous reconstruction. This is a formidable task for patient and surgeon alike and one must be certain of the diagnosis before embarking on such treatment. Aortic graft infection is the most *unpopular* diagnosis in vascular surgery, yet delay through unproductive, conservative treatment only complicates the problem for the patient and its ultimate solution for the vascular surgeon.

Aortic graft infections arise from either an enteric erosion fistula between the retroperitoneal graft and overlying bowel (usually duodenum or proximal jejunum) or skin organisms, most likely from the groin. Characteristically, gastrointestinal bleeding is reported to herald the former, while sinus drainage or false aneurysm are features of the latter. Unfortunately, these classic reported features are not that common, and subtle symptoms and signs must be sought whenever this diagnosis is a possibility. Gastrointestinal bleeding occurred in only two-thirds of our patients proven to have a prosthetic-enteric fistula as the source of the graft infection and it was massive, life-threatening bleeding in only 5% of patients. Endoscopy is definitive if an experienced endoscopist reaches the site of fistulization, but the presence of another bleeding source, gastritis, does not rule out an associated prosthetic-enteric fistula.

Evidence of a groin infection involving a graft limb is variable. Pain, erythema, tenderness, and mass are sometimes present, though a skin sinus, when present, is classic. Systemic manifestations include malaise, back pain, fever, and weight loss, usually with an elevated sedimentation rate as the only laboratory abnormality.

The retroperitoneal portion of an aortic prosthesis is the most challenging to assess for possible infection. CT scans and MRI are the most specific imaging methods we have found, while indium white blood cell scans and ultrasound are less specific. When clinical suspicion for graft infection warrants a diagnosis, exploration of the graft will detect incorporation of the graft, excluding graft infection or peri-graft purulent fluid which establishes the diagnosis, when all other diagnostic tests are negative.

OPERATIVE STRATEGY

In order to plan the method of limb revascularization which is essential for the optimal management of a patient with an aortic graft infection, a current aortogram with runoff views of the arteries in the legs is required. This will reveal the site and configuration of the graft anastomoses, and the patent and occluded native circulation. This information will assist in planning the revascularization method as well as the technique of prosthetic graft removal and the sequence and timing of both.

AORTO-ILIAC GRAFT INFECTION

The usual indication for an intraabdominal retroperitoneal aorto-iliac graft is the replacement of an aortic aneurysm. The involved native aorta and iliac segment is essentially absent after graft replacement whereas the distal arteries of the extremities are usually patent and preformed collateral pathways are absent. There is no possibility of groin contamination in such a graft replacement.

STAGED REMOTE PROSTHETIC BYPASS AND GRAFT REMOVAL

The simplest and safest operative strategy in this situation is the creation of a remote prosthetic bypass (right axillo–right common femoral) and a cross femoral (right femoral–left femoral) through clean incisions which are then closed and sealed. A transabdominal removal of the infected graft with two-layer tension-free closure of the aortic stump, repair of the intestinal fistula if present, and wide debridement of the retroperitoneal graft bed are completed. Depending on the condition of the patient, these two procedures can be performed sequentially under the same anesthetic, or staged (two or three day interval between the first and second stage). Only the rare situation of life-threatening gastrointestinal bleeding from a prosthetic fistula located at the level of the proximal aortic anastomosis requires that the transabdominal procedure precede the extremity revascularization. In this setting, the surgeon is concerned only with controlling life-threatening bleeding, and it may be safer and simpler to control the aorta above the site of the fistula, separate the bowel, and reinforce or re-graft the proximal anastomosis. The bowel can then be repaired leisurely and the abdomen closed. After recovery and hemodynamic stability, the patient can undergo the procedure as originally described, namely a prosthetic remote axillo-bifemoral bypass, followed by the transabdominal graft removal and aortic stump closure.

This strategy is recommended rather than initial emergent transabdominal graft removal, closure of the aortic stump and bowel repair, followed by immediate extraanatomic limb revascularization for two reasons:

1. The prolonged period of limb ischemia is associated with major ischemic sequela in many patients.
2. The remote prosthetic bypass is frequently contaminated with the same organisms responsible for the graft infecting low, despite efforts to isolate and separate the initial (contaminated) and the subsequent (clean) procedures.

AORTO-FEMORAL GRAFT INFECTION

The usual indication for an aorto-femoral graft is limb ischemia caused by aorto-iliac occlusive disease. The involved native arterial segments are present. There is likely to be coexisting occlusive disease in the arteries of the thighs and preformed, well-functioning collateral circulations are usually present. The presence of prosthetic graft limbs in the groins makes both groins contaminated or infected; hence they are both avoided when planning remote prosthetic limb revascularization.

The simplest and safest method of remote prosthetic limb revascularization is a right axillo–mid-superficial femoral (if patient) or distal profunda femoris artery bypass. This is performed through clean incisions which are then closed and sealed. If the segment superficial femoral artery is occluded, a 15–20 cm segment is removed, opened using an oscillating loop endarterectomy stripper, and temporarily stored for later use as an autogenous cross-femoral bypass. The two original groin incisions (contaminated) are reopened and the graft femoral anastomoses mobilized. The right graft limb is ligated near the inguinal ligament and the distal segment excised together with the femoral anastomotic suture line. The autograft is then anastomosed end-to-end or end-to-side to the femoral artery which is perfused retrograde from the functioning remote prosthetic bypass. The autograft is placed through a subcutaneous, suprapubic tunnel and anastomosed to the left femoral artery after detachment of the left femoral graft limb as previously described. The anastomoses are performed with fine monofilament suture. The wounds are debrided and the deep layers approximated leaving subcutaneous tissue and skin open for packing with Povidone-soaked gauze sponges. When patent superficial femoral arteries preclude their use as autografts, the greater saphenous vein is harvested and used as the autogenous cross-femoral graft.

At a second operation three to five days later, the infected aortic graft (now thrombosed) is mobilized at its proximal anastomosis to the aorta. If the end of the graft is attached end-to-side to a patent aorta, following removal of the graft and anastomotic suture line, a local aortic endarterectomy and autogenous patch aortoplasty is used to restore flow in the native aorta. This avoids division of the aorta and aortic stump closure with its potential for later dehiscence. The patch of autogenous artery can usually be obtained from a convenient site on one of the occluded iliac arteries. If the graft is attached end-to-end to the divided infrarenal aorta, temporary suprarenal aortic control facilitates accurate and complete excision and debridement of the native infrarenal aortic cuff above the level of the original anastomosis. A precise two-layer (horizontal mattress inner layer and over-and-over running outer layer) tension-free monofilament closure can be accomplished within the ischemic tolerance of the kidneys. The now completely detached infected aorto-femoral graft is withdrawn from its retroperitoneal tunnels and the retroperitoneum is irrigated with antibiotic solution. The retroperitoneum is reapproximated in the posterior midline, and the abdominal fascia is closed with monofilament sutures. The skin and subcutaneous tissues are left open to allow healing by secondary intention. Drains, aortic stump reinforcement, and omementum transposition are not employed.

IN SITU AUTOGENOUS AORTO-FEMORAL RECONSTRUCTION

An alternative one-stage approach exists in the rare patient with an aorto-femoral graft infection whose native bypassed aorto-iliac segments are either patent or, if occluded, have abundant collateral circulation to provide a viable limb without the aorto-femoral graft. The patient can undergo a transabdominal and femoral exposure and mobilization of the infected graft and the bypassed native arteries. If these are patent, and existing collateral adequate, following graft removal autogenous patch grafts are used to restore aortic and common femoral continuity so that limb circulation is assured through the native aorto-iliac-femoral arteries. Depending on the degree of occlusion of the native iliac arteries, in situ, semi-closed, oscillating-loop endarterectomy or autogenous arterial grafts (harvested from the occluded superficial femoral artery in the thigh) are effective in restoring limb perfusion through the native arterial segments. These procedures, although easy to describe, are among the most challenging reconstructive techniques known, and should only be considered if the surgeon has *considerable experience* with aorto-ilio-femoral endarterectomy in primary cases of atherosclerotic occlusive disease.

LIMITED (LOCALIZED) GRAFT LIMB INFECTION

When infection of a bifurcation prosthesis is confined to the distal portion of one limb, the body and contralateral graft limb can be preserved while unilateral extremity revascularization and graft limb removal are carried out.

The safest method for proving that the graft limb infection is truly localized is by direct operative inspection of the graft limb near its origin (aortic graft bifurcation) and confirmation of its *complete* incorporation. A retroperitoneal approach for this exposure is preferred and the graft can be divided and closed close to its origin and the distal end placed within the perigraft fibrous tunnel which is then closed, separating it from the contaminated graft distally in the groin. The retroperitoneal incision is then closed and sealed.

If a revascularization is required within the infected groin, then an autograft (artery or vein) is harvested through clean incisions and attached to the contralateral common femoral artery. It is then placed in a suprapubic tunnel and the incisions are closed and sealed. The infected groin is now opened and the graft anastomosis excised and the infected graft withdrawn from its retroperitoneal location. The autograft is retrieved within the suprapubic tunnel and anastomosed to the femoral artery, restoring circulation to that limb.

RESULTS

The principles of extremity revascularization and removal of the entire infected aortic graft have been used alone or together in managing 94 consecutive patients with this diagnosis referred to the UCSF during the last two decades. Forty patients have been treated in the past five-year period. Five patterns of operative management were identified in a recent review of this experience, as described in Table 24-1.

Table 24-1
Operative Management

None	Graft excision alone
Traditional	Graft excision and remote revascularization
Sequential	Remote revascularization and graft removal
Synchronous	Graft removal and autogenous in situ revascularization
Staged	Remote revascularization, later graft removal

Table 24-2

	No.	Mortality (%)	Amputation (%)	Infection (%)	Dehiscence (%)
None	15	20	47	—	13
Traditional	8	38	38	38	0
Sequential	37	30	11	19	14
Synchronous	17	29	29	—	6
Staged	17	18	18	6	12

The morbidity, amputation mortality, new prosthetic graft infection rates, and aortic stump dehiscence rate are shown in Table 24-2.

The past decade has seen the emergence of staged repair as the preferential strategy for aorto-femoral graft infection. A 7.5% mortality rate attests to the safety of this technique. All patients with any configuration of aorto-iliac or aorto-femoral graft infection can be successfully treated using the operative strategies that we have discussed. Remote prosthetic and in situ autogenous techniques allow limb revascularization in every patient. Graft removal with aortic reconstruction or interruption and secure closure are always feasible.

Late problems in our surviving patients are related to aortic stump dehiscence and infection of the remote prosthetic axillo-femoral graft. Stump dehiscence or blowout can be managed operatively by resection of the pararenal aortic cuff and submesenteric aortic closure without tension. Hepato-renal autograft bypass or spleno-renal bypass are available to re-perfuse the kidneys from new proximal arterial sources. Axillo-femoral failures from infection or occlusion can be managed by re-routing through a clean field or in-line conversion to an aorto-femoral bypass respectively.

The problem of aortic graft infection is representative of all problems facing the vascular surgeon who undertakes management of any infected vascular prosthesis. Revascularization of critical vascular beds by remote prosthetic grafts or in situ autogenous reconstruction are applicable in all circumstances. Removal of all the infected prosthetic material is essential but can be performed as a second stage in all patients unless life-threatening bleeding or limb- or organ-threatening ischemia dictates different priorities. Cure rates exceed 90% and operative mortality has fallen to below 10% in our recent experience. Late problems of stump dehiscence, prosthetic reinfection, and ischemia can be defined and appropriately and safely treated using innovative but proven reconstructive techniques.

ACKNOWLEDGMENT

Supported in part by the Pacific Vascular Research Foundation.

John Terblanche

25

The Management of Oesophageal Varices

INTRODUCTION

To review the management of oesophageal varices it is necessary to define how patients with varices present. They usually present to a surgeon because of acute variceal bleeding, either for emergency management at the time of the bleed or later once they have recovered for assessment for therapy to prevent recurrent variceal bleeds. Recent interest has been focused on preventing the first variceal bleed, with its attendant high mortality, by performing prophylactic procedures in patients in whom investigations reveal varices. Each will be considered separately, emphasising controversies and providing guidelines for management.

ACUTE VARICEAL BLEEDING

Initial Management

All patients with suspected acute variceal bleeding should be admitted to an intensive care unit in a hospital with an interest in liver disease. They require resuscitation with crytalloid fluids as well as with fresh frozen plasma, red blood cells, and platelets.

Most patients are treated initially with pharmacological agents to lower portal pressure.[1] Intravenous vasopressin administered as a continuous infusion at 0.4 units per minute remains the gold standard.[1] The addition of nitroglycerine given sublingually, by skin patch or by continuous intravenous infusion, potentiates the reduction in portal pressure while neutralising some of the side effects of vasopressin.[2,3] Combined vasopressin and nitroglycerine is the initial treatment of choice at present. The two other effective agents are expensive and require further evaluation before they can be accepted for routine use.[1] Glypressin, the synthetic analogue of vasopressin, has the advantage of apparently being as effective as a

VASCULAR SURGERY: ISSUES IN CURRENT PRACTICE
ISBN 0-8089-1839-7

continuous infusion of vasopressin when given as intermittent bolus doses of 2 mg, six hourly intravenously.[4] Early trials with somatostatin, which is not widely available, suggest it might also be superior to vasopressin.[5]

Emergency Endoscopy: Diagnostic and Therapeutic

Emergency endoscopy is essential in all patients with suspected variceal bleeding to confirm the diagnosis.[1] After excluding those patients who do not have varices, it should be possible to divide those with varices into three subgroups: those with varices, but who are bleeding from another lesion; patients actively bleeding from varices; and patients whose variceal bleeding has stopped. Although there may be difficulties in some cases in establishing a clear-cut diagnosis, only those patients who are bleeding, or who have bled, from varices require further management directed at their varices.

The author recommends that the diagnostic endoscopy be performed with one of the newer twin-channel fibreoptic endoscopes, so that immediate sclerotherapy can be undertaken whenever possible. This provides the best chance for early control of variceal bleeding and, by implication, must improve the patient's chance of surviving the acute variceal bleed. The technical details of the sclerotherapy procedure are presented later.

Balloon Tube Tamponade

A balloon tube for tamponade should only be inserted in patients with continued active variceal bleeding at the time of emergency diagnostic endoscopy, when it is not possible to control the acute bleed with sclerotherapy. If bleeding is stopped by sclerotherapy, or if bleeding stops spontaneously, balloon tube tamponade should not be used as it may be dangerous.[6] Tube tamponade can also cause significant local slough if used after sclerotherapy or continued for a prolonged period.

The author has only had experience with the Sengstaken–Blakemore modified four-lumen tube. The technical details of the insertion and care of the balloon tube have been presented elsewhere.[1] It should be inserted by the emergency endoscopist in those few patients who cannot be controlled by immediate sclerotherapy. It should also be used in recurrent acute variceal bleeding during the same hospital admission, particularly when two injection treatments have failed to control the acute bleed. Here the aim is to control the bleeding until a definitive surgical shunt or transection can be performed.[7]

Injection Sclerotherapy

Emergency sclerotherapy, whether used optimally at the time of emergency endoscopy[8,9] or subsequently,[10–13] remains the mainstay of therapy for controlling acute variceal bleeding. Early control of variceal bleeding is important to improve both early and long-term survival. There is increasing support for the concept that improving early survival after a variceal bleed is the best way to improve long-term survival.[14]

There are several technical variants of sclerotherapy but the best technique has still to be defined. Intending sclerotherapists are strongly advised to learn one technique well, preferably in a unit with extensive experience, and to apply it to their patients until the best technique is defined by controlled trials. Flexible endoscopes, without modification, should be used for free-hand injections, although there is still a place for the rigid endoscope in some cases of acute variceal bleeding which is difficult to control.[1,10] Sclerosant can be injected into the veins to cause thrombosis, thereby preventing recurrent bleeding, or next to the veins (paravariceal), producing local oedema which compresses the bleeding varix and later produces thickening of the overlying mucosa, or by a combined intra- and paravariceal technique.[1] The author favours a combined technique, using mostly intravariceal injections but combining this with paravariceal injections to control a local variceal bleeding point or bleeding from the needle puncture site. A wide variety of sclerosants have been advocated.[1] The substance used should be effective, but not excessively damaging to tissues if injected paravariceally. The author advocates 5% ethanolamine oleate, injecting up to 6 ml into each varix and injecting a further 0.5–1 ml paravariceally on either side of a bleeding point. Injections are localised to the lower oesophagus immediately above the oesophagogastric junction, and each variceal channel (usually three or four) is injected in turn, commencing with the varix which is bleeding, or which appears to have bled, so that immediate control is achieved. If the diagnostic endoscopy had not been completed prior to sclerotherapy, it is completed after sclerosing all the varices.

The main alternative solution for intravariceal injection is 5% sodium morrhuate. Sotredecal is too irritant and apparently associated with a higher complication rate. Other mixtures still have to be proven to be as effective as ethanolamine oleate or sodium morrhuate for intravariceal injection.

The most widely used solution for paravariceal injection is 0.5–1% polidocanol.[9] More concentrated solutions lead to complications, especially slough and stenosis.[13] The solution is usually injected in 0.5–1 ml boluses into each site between the varices, commencing at the oesophagogastric junction and repeating the procedure 30–50 times while progressing up the oesophagus in a helical fashion.[9]

Major groups have had success with intravariceal injections,[8,10,11] paravariceal injections,[9,13] or combined techniques[1,12] in managing acute variceal bleeding with control rates usually in excess of 90%. This is significantly better than the reported 40% control achieved with balloon tamponade prior to the widespread introduction of sclerotherapy.[15]

Emergency Shunts and Transection and Devascularisation Procedures

Although advocated as the initial therapy for acute variceal bleeding by some authors,[16,17] current view holds that these more extensive operations should be reserved for the rare failures of sclerotherapy.[1,7] The problem is to identify which patients are likely to fall into the 5–10% who will fail to respond to acute sclerotherapy. The Cape Town experience has been that patients who are not controlled after two acute injection treatments during a single hospital admission have a prohibitively high mortality of approaching 90%, if good-risk Child's A patients are excluded.[7] We therefore recommend that a recurrent bleed after a second acute injection should be treated with balloon tube tamponade, while the patient is resuscitated and subjected to an emergency shunt or transection operation.[1] Both emergency portacaval shunts[16,17] and emergency transection procedures[18-20] have their advocates. Until controlled trials define the best procedure for specific categories of patients, individual selection of what appears to be the best procedure for each patient is advised. The author favours either a standard portacaval shunt or an oesophageal transection using the staple gun. A devascularisation is added if the patient is fit enough for the more extensive procedure; otherwise the emergency treatment should be limited to staple gun transection.

Other Emergency Procedures

Percutaneous transhepatic obliteration of varices[21] has become less popular[22] and will probably disappear as a form of therapy because of a high rebleed rate, difficulty in repeating the procedure, and a high portal vein thrombosis rate.[22]

Other new procedures still have to be fully evaluated. These include laser coagulation and cautery. Their use cannot be justified other than in controlled trials undertaken by groups with experience in laser or cautery therapy for other upper gastrointestinal conditions with bleeding.

Advised Policy

Patients with suspected variceal bleeding should be admitted to an intensive care unit and actively resuscitated. A continuous intravenous infusion of 0.4 units per minute of vasopressin is commenced and combined with their sublingual or skin patch nitroglycerine administration. Emergency endoscopy must be available on a 24-hour call basis and be undertaken within 4–6 hours of the patient's admission. For patients with variceal bleeding, sclerotherapy should be performed at the same time. A Sengstaken balloon tube should only be inserted if active variceal bleeding cannot be controlled. In those few patients in whom Sengstaken tube control is required, urgent sclerotherapy should be performed 6–12 hours later, possibly with a rigid endoscope under general anaesthesia. However, the flexible endoscope is nearly as effective in this setting and should be used if expertise in rigid endoscopic sclerotherapy is not available. When the flexible scope is used for emergency sclerotherapy, a combined intravariceal with limited paravariceal injection technique using 5% ethanolamine oleate is recommended. Once variceal bleeding has been controlled, an early decision on subsequent therapy is required and a plan for future management must be formulated for each patient.

LONG-TERM MANAGEMENT

Should a patient who has bled from varices be subjected to specific treatment to prevent a recurrent bleed? A clear-cut answer cannot be given at present. The options are presented below. The fundamental question is what chance has the individual patient of having a life-threatening bleed in the future? This depends on many factors. The endoscopic criteria for high-risk patients defined by Paquet[23] and by Inokuchi's group[24,25] are detailed later in relation to prophylactic therapy. Long-term survival must depend on the severity and aetiology of the underlying liver disease. Different aetiologies of cirrhosis worldwide make studies from a variety of geographic areas difficult to compare. Child's grading or a modification[26,27] have been used but dissatisfaction has led to a search for other criteria for predicting survival.[28,29] Overall prognosis tends to be worse in communities where alcoholic cirrhosis predominates. It has been pointed out that in order to improve long-term survival it is necessary to improve survival for the early period after a variceal bleed.[14] The therapy required to achieve this has been presented above.

Conservative Therapy Only

Clearly conservative therapy directed at improving the underlying liver disease must be instituted in all patients. In alcoholic cirrhosis every effort must be made to persuade the patient to abstain from alcohol.

Is conservative therapy, awaiting the next variceal bleed, justified? The answer was yes when the various controlled trials were commenced. The results obtained in the four completed controlled trials comparing sclerotherapy with conservative management[30-33] have made it difficult to withhold therapy. Conservative therapy alone can only be justified in centres where a highly effective policy of emergency therapy is available, and such therapy would usually include emergency sclerotherapy. Even then, patients who present with repeated bleeds should be subjected to some form of treatment to prevent further bleeds, as each recurrent bleed carries its own risk of mortality.

Specific Medical Therapy

The era of specific medical therapy was heralded by Lebrec's papers on the use of propranolol to lower portal pressure and thereby presumably to lower the risk of recurrent variceal bleeds.[34,35] Others have questioned his results and pointed out that only Child's A grade risk patients were included and that patients bleeding from gastric erosions were also included.[36] The results of the controlled trial from London[37] did not support Lebrec's findings and thus the role of propranolol in long-term management is again in the melting pot.

Nevertheless, the concept of a simple form of drug therapy to prevent recurrent variceal bleeds is most appealing. Some form of pharmacological therapy is likely to be the treatment of the future. The ultimate drug will have to effectively diminish the risk of bleeding without serious side effects. Its mode of action need not necessarily be that of lowering portal pressure. There is increasing evidence suggesting other modes of action. An intriguing new area of research is into therapy which lowers oesophageal variceal pressure by constricting the lower oesophageal sphincter, a concept suggested some years ago by Miskowiak.[38]

Repeated Sclerotherapy

Innumerable uncontrolled series,[8,9,11,12,39] as well as four controlled randomised clinical trials,[30-33] have demonstrated that sclerotherapy is effective in eradicating oesophageal varices and preventing recurrent variceal bleeds, as long as follow-up is adequate. However, there is a question mark regarding its ability to improve survival. One controlled trial showed a highly significant improved survival,[32, 40] while two others required complex statistical analysis of the data to reach statistical significance,[31, 33] and the final trial did not show improved survival.[30] Criticisms have been levelled at all of these trials. Nevertheless, the ability of repeated sclerotherapy to improve survival, when compared with controls who have had the best emergency therapy for active bleeds, including sclerotherapy, has not been proven.[41]

Sclerotherapy has a number of advantages when compared with more major forms of therapy.[41] It is the simplest and most direct method of dealing with the problem of oesophageal varices. Morbidity and mortality are comparatively low. It does not affect liver function or increase the incidence of encephalopathy. It eradicates varices in most patients and prevents recurrent variceal bleeds with adequate follow-up. Also, when varices recur, as they invariably do, frequently only a single channel recurs and this recurrent varix is usually easy to re-eradicate.

Sclerotherapy also has problems. Portal hypertension persists and varices will, and do, recur. Life-long follow-up is required with repeated injections to prevent recurrent life-threatening bleeds. Unfortunately these repeated injections increase the chance of complications. Furthermore, during therapy, until the varices are eradicated, recurrent variceal bleeds continue.

The technical variants of sclerotherapy have been discussed. If emergency sclerotherapy has not been performed, the first injection should be undertaken as soon as possible to prevent a further life-threatening bleed. After emergency sclerotherapy, or after the first elective injection session, the patient should be re-endoscoped at one week. Any remaining varices should be injected unless overlying slough or ulceration prevents re-injection. In the latter situation any uncomplicated varices, not affected by the slough or ulceration, should be injected. Further endoscopy and injection should be undertaken at one to two weekly intervals until the varices are eradicated.[30, 32, 41, 42] After eradication the next endoscopy should be at three months and then at six or twelve monthly intervals. When recurrent varices occur, one or two weekly injections should be recommenced until eradication has been achieved once again.

Portosystemic Shunts

Shunts are the gold standard of therapy because a successful portosystemic shunt effectively prevents recurrent variceal bleeding.[43] Standard portacaval shunts are no longer widely practised because the results of controlled trials (predominantly in alcoholic cirrhotic patients) failed to show improved survival.[43] In addition the shunt is associated with a real and unpredictable risk of hepatic encephalopathy. The author believes that the major current role for standard portacaval shunting is in alcoholic cirrhotic patients who do not respond to repeated sclerotherapy.

The most widely advocated shunt today is the distal spleno-renal shunt of Warren and Zeppa. In theory this shunt selectively decompresses the oesophagogastric-splenic compartment while preserving mesenteric flow to the liver.[44] There are some problems with this shunt. It is more difficult to perform than a standard portacaval shunt, it is not applicable to all patients, especially those with severe ascites, and the maintenance of portal perfusion, as well as the ability to maintain separation between the two compartments, have been questioned.[45,46] A further drawback is that the excellent reported long-term results in nonalcoholic cirrhosis have not been confirmed in alcoholic cirrhotic patients.[47] This shunt requires further evaluation in controlled trials.

Mesocaval, central spleno-renal, and makeshift shunts all have their proponents. Most workers would, however, support the author's view that the choice at present lies between a standard portacaval shunt and the Warren–Zeppa shunt.

Devascularisation and Transection Operation

Staple gun oesophageal transection, with or without associated gastric and oesophageal devascularisation, is gaining widespread acceptance as an alternative form of therapy. Spence and Johnston of Belfast have achieved excellent medium- to long-term results using combined transection and devascularisation.[19] Transection alone is likely to be associated with early recurrent bleeds, as with the older under-running of varices and transection operations.[48] Remarkably good results are also being reported from Japan with extensive devascularisation and transection operations.[20,49] The author believes that the main role for these more extensive operations is in the management of patients who have failed to respond to repeated sclerotherapy. This, however, requires to be put to the test. A prospective randomised controlled clinical trial, comparing repeated sclerotherapy with transection and extensive devascularisation performed via the abdominal route, was commenced in Cape Town at the beginning of 1986 with the aim of assessing their roles in long-term management.

Other Procedures

None have yet gained widespread acceptance. Percutaneous transhepatic obliteration of varices has not proved successful in long-term management because of the difficulty in repeating the procedure and because of its complications.[22] No other new concept has been advocated recently.

Advised Policy

Currently most patients should be subjected to repeated sclerotherapy using one of the techniques and the timing schedule advised earlier. Individual patients should be considered for a Warren–Zeppa distal spleno-renal shunt or one of the transection and devascularisation operations. For the few patients in whom eradication of varices proves difficult with repeated sclerotherapy, or in whom sclerotherapy fails to prevent recurrent variceal bleeding, either a shunt or a devascularisation and transection operation is definitively indicated.

In alcoholic cirrhotic patients either a transection and devascularisation procedure or a standard portacaval shunt is to be preferred to a Warren–Zeppa shunt. For the future, simple pharmacological therapy has the greatest appeal. Drugs that lower portal pressure or which diminish oesophageal variceal pressure (such as by increasing the lower oesophageal sphincter tone) are being extensively evaluated. The results of these trials will require careful evaluation.

PROPHYLAXIS

Prophylactic therapy, including prophylactic sclerotherapy, is not justified outside of controlled clinical trials at present.[50] Prophylaxis in portal hypertension means treatment to prevent the first variceal bleed.

The concept of prophylactic therapy in cirrhotic patients is not new. Prophylactic portacaval shunts gained fairly widespread acceptance three decades ago in the height of the enthusiasm for portacaval shunts. They were abandoned when controlled clinical trials failed to show improved survival for shunted patients when compared with controls. In fact, survival was worse in the shunted patients in three of the four trials.[51–53]

A major problem in considering prophylaxis is the identification of patients with a high likelihood of a first bleed. In the prophylactic portacaval shunt controlled trials, only some 30% of the untreated patients actually bled from varices during the trial[51–53] and thus by inference 70% were treated unnecessarily. Recently, Paquet has identified endoscopic and haematological findings which place patients at high risk of a bleed. He defined high risk as patients with large varices, grade 3 or 4 by his classification, or with coagulation factors under 30%, or a combination of both.[23] In Japan Beppu and coworkers[25] and Inokuchi[24] used more complex endoscopic criteria to identify high-risk patients. However, the outcome of patients with portal hypertension varies widely in different geographical areas of the world due to differing aetiologies. This is highlighted by the variceal bleed rate in the two studies mentioned above. In Paquet's series untreated patients had a 66% bleed rate,[23] whereas only 19.2% of the Japanese control patients bled.[24]

The results of published prophylactic trials of sclerotherapy[23, 54] and major nondecompressive surgery[24] have been encouraging. Why then the author's pessimistic attitude? The low bleed rate in the Japanese surgical studies has already been emphasised.[24] A symposium in Munich in January 1986 addressed the problem, especially in relation to sclerotherapy.[50, 55] Paquet re-presented his trial in which 65 patients at high risk were randomised and in which he showed sclerotherapy to be superior, with a bleed rate of 6% versus 66% and a mortality of 6% versus 42% over a two-year period.[23] The published trial of Witzel, Wolbergs, and Merki included 109 patients followed for 25 months. They concluded that sclerotherapy was better based on a bleed rate of 9% versus 57% and a mortality of 21% versus 55%.[54] However, their patients were not selected as being at high risk for bleeding, and therefore the very high bleed rate in controls is surprising.[50] Criticisms were levelled at the published papers both at the Munich symposium[50] and in the correspondence columns of the Lancet.[56, 57] At the Munich symposium Burroughs of London reviewed the pitfalls in prophylactic treatment studies.[55] The natural history depends upon the type of patient included in the study, the geographic variation in pathology, and the degree of hepatic decompensation in individual patients. Burroughs summarised the risk factors for bleeding from varices as: the state of the varices, the state of the liver, and alcohol abuse. He presented guidelines for the design of prophylactic therapy studies. These were as follows: patient groups should be stratified for the above risk factors; follow-up, including endoscopy, must be the same in both groups because of the effect on compliance and the assessment of varices; and finally the treatment of acute bleeds must be optimal and the same in both groups.

At the Munich symposium seven other controlled trials were presented in preliminary form. Only one of these, under the direction of Fleig of Ulm, Germany, met Burroughs' criteria that the treatment of acute bleeds must be optimal and the same in both groups.[50, 55] The results of these trials were conflicting. The message from the Munich meeting has been summarised as indicating that prophylaxis, including prophylactic sclerotherapy, in patients with cirrhosis who have not yet bled from oesophageal varices is not justified outside of controlled clinical trials. Future controlled trials should only include patients at high risk of variceal bleeding and should be designed to stratify for risk factors, have similar follow-up, and the treatment of acute variceal bleeding should be the same in both groups, including the use of sclerotherapy when indicated. Based on the available data it is unlikely that prophylactic sclerotherapy will improve survival if the best available treatment is used for the first acute variceal bleed.[50]

ACKNOWLEDGEMENTS

The work presented and the author were supported by grants from the Staff Research Fund of the University of Cape Town, the South African Medical Research Council, the Ernest Oppenheimer Memorial Trust, and The Royal Society, London.

REFERENCES

1. Terblanche J, Bornman PC, Kahn D, Kirsch RE: The management of acute variceal bleeding, in Popper H, and Schaffner F, (eds): Progress in Liver Disease, Vol VIII. New York, Academic Press, 1986 (in press)
2. Groszman RJ, Kravetz, D, Bosch J, et al: Nitroglycerine improves the haemodynamic response to vasopressin in portal hypertension. Hepatology 2:757–762, 1982
3. Williams R: In discussion. Portal hypertension, in Kirsch RE, Kruskal JB, Csomos G, Terblanche J (eds): Liver Update, Vol 2. London, Bailliere Tindall, 1985, pp 157–196
4. Freeman JG, Cobden I, Lishman AH, Record CO: Controlled trial of terlipressin (glypressin) versus vasopressin in the early treatment of oesophageal varices. Lancet 2:66–68, 1982
5. Kravetz D, Bosch J, Teres J, et al: Comparison of intravenous somatostatin and vasopressin infusions in treatment of acute variceal haemorrhage. Hepatology 4:442–446, 1983
6. Chojkier M, Conn HO: Esophageal tamponade in the treatment of bleeding varices. A decadal progress report. Dig Dis Sci 25:267–272, 1980
7. Bornman PC, Terblanche J, Kahn D, et al: Limitations of multiple injection sclerotherapy sessions for acute variceal bleeding. S Afr Med J, 1986 (in press)
8. Lewis JW: Survival and rebleed after acute and chronic injection sclerotherapy, in Sivak MV (ed): Endoscopic Sclerotherapy of Esophageal Varices. New York, Praeger, 1984, pp 89–97
9. Paquet K-J: Endoscopic paravariceal injection sclerotherapy of the esophagus—Indications, technique, complications, results of a period of 14 years. Gastrointest. Endoscopy 29:310–315, 1983

10. Terblanche J, Yakoob HI, Bornman PC, et al: Acute bleeding varices. A five-year prospective evaluation of tamponade and sclerotherapy. Ann Surg 194:521–530, 1981

11. Spence RAJ, Anderson JR, Johnston GW: Twenty-five years of injection sclerotherapy for bleeding varices. Br J Surg 72:195–198, 1985

12. Soehendra N, de Heer K, Kempeneers I, Runge M: Sclerotherapy of esophageal varices: Acute arrest of gastrointestinal hemorrhage or long-term therapy? Endoscopy 15:136–140, 1983

13. Sorensen T, Burcharth F, Pedersen ML, Findahl F: Oesophageal stricture and dysphagia after endoscopic sclerotherapy for bleeding varices. Gut 25:373–377, 1984

14. Graham DY, Smith YL: The course of patients after variceal hemorrhage. Gastroenterology 80:900–909, 1981

15. Novis BH, Duys P, Barbezat GO, et al: Fibreoptic endoscopy and the use of the Sengstaken tube in acute gastrointestinal haemorrhage in patients with portal hypertension and varices. Gut 17:258–262, 1976

16. Orloff MJ, Bell RH, Hyde PV, Skivolocki WP: Long-term results of emergency portacaval shunt for bleeding esophageal varices in unselected patients with alcoholic cirrhosis. Ann Surg 192:325–340, 1980

17. Cello JP, Grendell JH, Crass RA, et al: Endoscopic sclerotherapy versus portacaval shunt in patients with severe cirrhosis and variceal hemorrhage. N Engl J Med 311:1589–1594, 1984

18. Orborne DR, Hobbs KEF: The acute treatment of haemorrhage from oesophageal varices: A comparison of oesophageal transection and staple gun anastomosis with mesocaval shunt. Br J Surg 68:734–737, 1981

19. Spence RAJ, Johnston GW: Results in 100 consecutive patients with stapled oesophageal transection for varices. Surg Gynecol Obstet 160:323–329, 1985

20. Sugiura M, Futagawa S: Results of six hundred thirty-six esophageal transections with paraesophagogastric devascularization in the treatment of esophageal varices. J Vasc Surg 1:254–260, 1984

21. Lunderquist A, Vang J: Transhepatic catheterization and obliteration of the coronary vein in patients with portal hypertension and esophageal varices. N Engl J Med 291:646–649, 1974

22. Bengmark S, Borjesson B, Hoevels J, et al: Obliteration of esophageal varices by PTP. A follow-up of 43 patients. Ann Surg 190:549–554, 1979

23. Paquet K-J: Prophylactic endoscopic sclerosing treatment of the esophageal wall in varices—A prospective controlled trial. Endoscopy 14:4–5, 1982

24. Inokuchi I: Prophylactic portal nondecompression surgery in patients with esophageal varices. Ann Surg 200:61–65, 1984

25. Beppu K, Inokuchi K, Koyanagi N, et al: Prediction of variceal hemorrhage by esophageal endoscopy. Gastrointest Endoscopy 27:213–218, 1981

26. Pugh RNH, Murray-Lyon IM, Dawson JL, et al: Transection of the oesophagus for bleeding oesophageal varices. Br J Surg 60:646–649, 1973

27. Terblanche J, Northover JMA, Bornman PC, et al: A prospective controlled trial of sclerotherapy in the long-term management of patients after esophageal variceal bleeding. Surg Gynecol Obstet 148:323–333, 1979

28. Clowes GHA, McDermott WV, Williams LF, et al: Amino acid clearance and prognosis in surgical patients with cirrhosis. Surgery 96:675–685, 1984

29. Garden OJ, Motyl H, Gilmour WH, et al: Prediction of outcome following acute variceal haemorrhage. Br J Surg 72:91–95, 1985

30. Terblanche J, Bornman PC, Kahn D, et al: Failure of repeated injection sclerotherapy to improve long-term survival after oesophageal variceal bleeding. A five year prospective controlled clinical trial. Lancet II:1328–1332, 1983

31. The Copenhagen Esophageal Varices and Sclerotherapy Project: Sclerotherapy after

first variceal hemorrhage in cirrhosis. A randomised multicenter trial. N Engl J Med 311:1594–1600, 1984

32. Westaby D, Macdougall BRD, Williams R: Improved survival following injection scler-otherapy for esophageal varices. Final analysis of a controlled trial. Hepatology 5:827–830, 1985

33. Korula J, Balart LA, Radvan G, et al: A prospective, randomized controlled trial of chronic esophageal variceal sclerotherapy. Hepatology 5:584–589, 1985

34. Lebrec D, Poynard T, Hillon P, et al: Propranolol for prevention of recurrent gastro-intestinal bleeding in patients with cirrhosis: a controlled study. N Engl J Med 305:1371–1374, 1981

35. Lebrec D, Poynard T, Bernuau et al: A randomised controlled study of propranolol for prevention of recurrent gastrointestinal bleeding in patients with cirrhosis: A final report. Hepatology 4:355, 1984

36. Conn HO: Propranolol in the treatment of portal hypertension: A caution. Hepatology 2:641–644, 1982

37. Burroughs AK, Jenkins WJ, Sherlock S, et al: Controlled trial of propranolol for the prevention of recurrent variceal hemorrhage in patients with cirrhosis. N Engl J Med 309: 1539–1542, 1983

38. Miskowiak K: How the lower oesophageal sphincter affects submucosal oesophageal varices. Lancet ii:1284, 1978

39. Rose JDR, Crane MD, Smith PM: Factors affecting successful endoscopic sclerotherapy for oesophageal varices. Gut 24:946–949, 1983

40. Macdougall BRD, Westaby D, Theodossi A, et al: Increased long-term survival in vari-ceal hemorrhage using injection sclerotherapy. Results of a controlled trial. Lancet 1:124–127, 1982

41. Terblanche J: The long-term management of patients after an oesophageal variceal bleed: The role of sclerotherapy. Br J Surg 72:88–90, 1985

42. Westaby D, Macdougall BRD, Melia W, et al: A prospective randomised study of two sclerotherapy techniques for esophageal varices. Hepatology 3:681–684, 1983

43. Conn HO: Therapeutic portacaval anastomosis: To shunt or not to shunt. Gastroenter-ology 67:1065–1073, 1974

44. Warren WD, Millikan WJ, Henderson JM, et al: Ten years portal hypertensive surgery at Emory. Results and new perspectives. Ann Surg 195:530–542, 1982

45. Fischer JE, Bower RH, Atamian S, Welling R: Comparison of distal and proximal sple-norenal shunts. A randomised prospective trial. Ann Surg 194:531–574, 1981

46. Maillard JN, Flemant YM, Hay JM, Chandler JG: Selectivity of the distal splenorenal shunt. Surgery 86: 663–671, 1979

47. Henderson JM, Millikan WJ, Wright-Bacon L, et al: Hemodynamic differences between alcoholic and non-alcoholic cirrhotics following distal splenorenal shunt—Effect on sur-vival? Ann Surg 198:325–334, 1983

48. Matory WE, Sedgwick CE, Rossi RL: Nonshunting procedures in management of bleeding esophageal varices. Surg Clin N Am 60:281–295, 1980

49. Inokuchi K: Present status of surgical treatment of esophageal varices in Japan: A nationwide survey of 3588 patients. World J Surg 9:171–180, 1985

50. Terblanche J: Sclerotherapy for prophylaxis of variceal bleeding. Lancet, 1986 (in press)

51. Jackson FC, Perrin EB, Smith AG, et al: A clinical investigation of the portacaval shunt. II. Survival analysis of the prophylactic operation. Am J Surg 115:22–42, 1968

52. Resnick RH, Chalmers TC, Ishihara AM, et al: A controlled study of the prophylactic portacaval shunt. A final report. Ann Int Med 70:675–688, 1969

53. Conn HO, Lindenmuth WW, May CJ, Rambsy GR: Prophylactic portacaval anasto-mosis. A tale of two studies. Medicine 51:27–40, 1972

54. Witzel L, Wolbergs E, Merki H: Prophylactic endoscopic sclerotherapy of oesophageal varices. A perspective controlled study. Lancet i:773–775, 1985
55. Abstracts. International symposium on prophylaxis of variceal bleeding, Munich, 24–25 January 1986
56. Burroughs AK, Hamilton G: Prophylactic endoscopic sclerotherapy of oesophageal varices. Lancet i:1105–1106, 1985
57. Hayes PC, Westaby D, Williams R: Prophylactic endoscopic sclerotherapy of oesophageal varices. Lancet i:1106, 1985

André Thevenet
and Bernard Albat

26

What is New in Brachiocephalic Disease?

Since successful extracranial arterial reconstruction was first performed three decades ago, the interest has been mainly concentrated on the diagnosis and surgical management of carotid bifurcation atherosclerosis. Changing concepts developed concerning pathogenetic mechanisms (thromboembolic, haemodynamic), with pathologic processes (stenosis, ulcerated plaque, intramural haemorrhage, luminal thrombi), indications (asymptomatic disease, TIA, progressing stroke, fixed neurologic deficit, associated coronary artery disease), and elements of surgical procedures (cerebral protection, endarterectomy, patch, bypass). Immediate and late results are well described. Therefore diagnosis and management of carotid disease are becoming less controversial.

Comprehensive and exhaustive contributions covering the field have recently been assembled in several books[1–5] which review the current state of knowledge.

In comparison, there is a limited experience in operations for occlusive diseases of the brachiocephalic vessels (the innominate, common carotid, subclavian, and vertebral arteries). However, during the last years, the techniques of arterial reconstructions of the great vessels of the aortic arch have been changed: the indications of direct transthoracic repair have been limited and extrathoracic bypass procedures have been very successful before the simplicity of arterial transposition was rediscovered. At the same time, vertebral artery surgery has been the beneficiary of the vogue of reimplantations while distal bypass favoured access to its third segment.

Long-term results of these operations provide the necessary information to recommend therapeutic options. Thus our review will be devoted to the surgery of the vertebral artery and the supraaortic trunks.

FREQUENCY

The frequency of brachiocephalic artery lesions reported by different authors is variable. Edwards and Mulherin[6] discovered subclavian or vertebral artery lesions in only 14% of 1700 cerebral angiograms.

VASCULAR SURGERY: ISSUES IN CURRENT PRACTICE
ISBN 0-8089-1839-7

Table 26-1
Extracranial Arterial Reconstruction Frequency
of Brachiocephalic Operations

	Wylie 1958–1978	Crawford 1958–1978	Thevenet 1962–1985
Carotid bifurcation	1769	602	1817
Vertebral	42	66	723
Supraaortic trunks	150	86	892
Total	1961	754	3432

During 20 years of experience with reconstructive surgery of the extracranial arteries, Wylie and Effeney[7] report 42 vertebral artery operations against 1769 carotid operations and 150 procedures on the supraaortic trunks. In the series reported by Crawford[8] between 1958 and 1978, 750 patients were operated upon, of whom 66 underwent vertebral operations, 602 carotid operations, and 86 supraaortic trunk operations. From 1962 to 1985 we performed 3432 cerebrovascular reconstructive procedures, 723 on the vertebral arteries, 1817 on the carotid bifurcation, and 892 on the supraaortic trunks. This demonstrates the attention we pay to the brachiocephalic arteries in the concept of total cerebral blood flow (Table 26-1).

Despite that, the experience is rather limited and operations on the brachiocephalic vessels are considered uncommon, approximately 10% at the University of California, San Francisco.[9]

In our recent experience (Table 26-2) from 1980 to 1985, the percentage of operations is 70% on carotid bifurcation, 10% on vertebral arteries, and 20% on great vessels of the aortic arch.

The frequency of involvement of branches of the aortic arch in our personal surgical experience from 1964 to 1984 is shown in Table 26-3.

Table 26-2
Extracranial Arterial Reconstruction

	1962–1985		1980–1985	
	Number	%	Number	%
Carotid bifurcation	1817	53	573	70
Vertebral	723	21	81	10
Supraaortic trunks	892	26	164	20
Total	3432		818	

Table 26-3
Supraaortic Trunks
Reconstruction 1964–1984

Innominate artery		87
Subclavian arteries	L	449
	R	223
Common carotid	L	60
	R	31
Total		850

Subclavian arteries are affected in 79% (53% for the left), common carotid in 10.7% (7% for the left), and innominate artery in 10.3%. Therefore, the left sub-clavian artery is involved by atherosclerosis five times more frequently than any other vessel, except the right subclavian artery (two times).

SURGERY OF THE VERTEBRAL ARTERY

Reconstructive surgery of the vertebral artery (VA) has not been as widely used as carotid surgery in the treatment of cerebrovascular disease.

In the case of symptoms of vertebrobasilar insufficiency, it is rarely a single lesion which is at fault, since there is usually a rich collateral circulation that com-pensates the brain supply.

Atheromatous obstructive disease of the vertebral arteries at their origin on subclavian arteries represents the most important cause of vertebrobasilar ischaemia. Usually there is a separate plaque at the narrowing but in advanced disease the entire subclavian artery is involved. More rarely, vertebral artery obstruction is caused by kinking, extraluminal compression due to fascial bands or bony cervical spurs, or by fibromuscular dysplasia and intramural dissection.

The role of the vertebral artery is often underestimated insofar as angiography offers a poor visualization of the arterial origin and the haemodynamic changes are difficult to evaluate because of the uncertain adequacy of the collateral supply, mainly of the posterior communicating arteries and the frequently associated carotid lesions.

The surgical procedure itself is debatable, since several techniques are available to restore cerebral blood flow.

Clinical Features

Different neurologic symptoms can be present either simultaneously or during subsequent ischaemic incidents. The most common clinical pattern is vertigo, visual disturbances, and headache, associated with balance instability. Positional changes of the head and neck can precipitate vertigo. However, transient ischaemic attacks are often unknown according to vague and confusing symptoms.

Investigating Procedures

Clinical examination, arterial blood pressure measurements in both arms, and auscultation over the great vessels are the first stage. Doppler measurements are not reliable because VA is anatomically deeply situated. Thus all patients have to undergo a complete angiographic evaluation of the brachiocephalic circulation in order to visualize the whole of the extra- and intracranial course of the cerebral vessels. Cervicothoracic and cranial seriographies are taken in different planes since highly stenotic lesions at the origin of the VA are not always appreciable on the frontal plane. The other interest of a complete arteriography is the visualization of associated carotid or innominate artery lesions.

Transcranial Doppler measurement (TDM) is performed every time that ver-tebrobasilar insufficiency is progressive or severe for elimination of cerebral lesion.

Indications

Neurologic status and artery lesions have to be discussed before surgical treatment.

Neurologic Status

1. The best indication is transient vertebrobasilar insufficiency. Surgical abstention consists of all extracranial reconstructive surgery: severe ischaemic attacks or progressive ischaemic attacks. In these cases TDM is very important to detect cerebral lesion after ischaemia.
2. Asymptomatic lesions of the vertebral arteries have to be corrected in patients operated on for another lesion of proximal vessels of the aortic arch or carotid and when there is a severe stenotic vertebral lesion which can develop a thrombosis.
3. The association of carotid and vertebral lesion is a real problem.
    (a) When vertebrobasilar symptoms are found we first correct the vertebral lesion, except of course when carotid stenosis is too important and haemodynamically critical.
    (b) When hemispheric symptoms are present the first lesion to be corrected is the carotid one. To improve the cerebral circulation in the case of inaccessible occlusion on a carotid and stenosis on the other, it should be better to first correct the vertebral artery lesion.

The benefit of surgery is limited by the diffuse nature of atherosclerotic disease, particularly when symptoms and carotid vertebral lesions are associated with bilateral lesions with nonsurgical intracranial lesions (syphon and basilar artery stenoses). Both vertebral and carotid artery obstructions are to be separately evaluated, considering that the involvement of one axis necessarily impairs the cerebral circulatory pool.

Arterial Lesions

Three different kinds of lesions are considered:

1. Atheromatous stenosis. Proximal lesions are the most frequent indications, but distal lesions or segmentary vertebral occlusion can now be corrected by means of distal VA bypass. In bilateral lesions, the dominant artery with the most severe stenosis has to be repaired first.
2. Kinkings. They involve the first few centimetres of the VA and are due to an elongation with sudden change of direction of the artery. The cause may be either an anatomic anomaly or an upward shifting of both the aortic arch and the subclavian artery due to pathologic changes of the cervical spine connected with old age. Sometimes, ostial atheromatous stenosis can be associated.
3. Extrinsic compressions. They are produced either on the first segment of the VA by nervous structures of the sympathetic cervical system (stellate ganglion) or within the transverse process by bony spurs.

Surgical Techniques

From a surgical point of view the VA can be reconstructed in its three extracranial segments.

Proximal Vertebral Segment[10-12]

On account of its deep location in the neck the origin of the VA can be approached through either a supraclavicular incision, or a left transpleural thoracotomy, or by splitting the sternum.

A transverse supraclavicular cervicotomy represents the routine approach of vertebral origin. Whenever supraaortic trunk lesions are associated, a thoracic approach is preferred.

A supraclavicular incision provides a good exposure of both the right and left VA. The clavicle is never resected. The two heads of the sterno-cleido-mastoid muscle are retracted. The omohyoid muscle is divided and the internal jugular vein and the vagus nerve are retracted medially. The phrenic nerve is exposed and the scalenus anticus muscle is only transected if necessary.

On the left side, the thoracic duct is identified, and either retracted or ligated and divided. The key to the VA approach is the division of the vertebral vein; this enables exposure of the subclavian artery, which is dissected and looped proximately and distally to the VA. The internal mammary artery and the thyrocervical trunk are rarely divided. The first 2–3 cm of the VA are then freed, starting from the origin.

According to the site and the nature of the lesions, there are different kinds of procedures, endarterectomy and vertebrocarotid transposition being the main methods:

1. *Endarterectomy.* Transclavian VA endarterectomy is the preferred technique for almost all atheromatous ostial lesions.

   Endarterectomy of the vertebral origin is performed through a longitudinal incision in the subclavian artery situated opposite the vertebral artery orifice. A cleavage plane is started along the upper edge of the incision or by developing a circular button around the vertebral orifice. Once started this plane is continued by coring out the atheromatous lesion, everting the VA in order to obtain an adequate end-point. The arteriotomy is closed with a simple running suture using a 7.0 absorbable monofilament or, rarely, when the subclavian artery wall is imperfect, by interposition of a Dacron patch. When the lesion is either limited to the vertebral orifice but involves the subclavian artery or it is ulcerated or calcified, a complete endarterectomy of the subclavian artery around the vertebral orifice is performed; interrupted "tack-down" sutures on the distal intima are inserted, if necessary.

   When subclavian artery occlusion is associated with vertebral stenosis, the subclavian artery is divided, obliterated up to the vertebral orifice, and reimplanted into the common carotid artery. In these cases carotid stump pressure measurements are always obtained and hypercapnia with hypoventilation is used for cerebral protection. No shunt is employed during vertebral or subclavian endarterectomy.

2. *Vertebrocarotid transposition.* This is the reimplantation of VA, which is divided near its origin, into the common carotid, as described by Edwards and Wylie. Reimplantation can be either direct into the external common carotid border or through a venous graft.

3. *Other procedures:*
   (a) Vertebrosubclavian angioplasty using patch (De Bakey) by performing vertical arteriotomy across vertebral and subclavian arteries.

(b)   Bypasses, not the prosthetic one initially suggested (Crawford[8]), but venous grafting connecting the subclavian artery to VA (Berguer[13]).

(c)   Vertebral artery reimplantation into the subclavian artery, used in some cases of VA kinkings with or without ostial stenosis associated after length excess resection.

(d)   Vertebrosubclavian side-to-side anastomosis in some kinds of loops.

(e)   Other corrective procedures can be mentioned: arteriolysis by nerve fibres section; scalenostomy associated with arteriopexis (power's procedure) when VA rises from the posterior subclavian border; arterioplasty using plication of the redundant VA and enlarging the ostium by a venous patch (Imparato[14]).

Middle Vertebral Segment (V2)

Usually it is not a surgical segment, except in the case of extrinsic compressions by the bony process, needing decompressive procedures to free the artery. The approach is then vertical, parallel to the anterior border of the sterno-cleido-mastoid muscle.

At the present time, long compression or stenosis between C6 and C2 are best managed with a bypass to the C1–C2 level.

Distal Vertebral Segment (V3)

Access to the distal extracranial VA segment at the C2–C1 spinal interspace is now a safe and well-described procedure (Berguer[13], Kieffer). Particular indications (arterio-venous fistulas, aneurisms, trauma, atheromatous proximal vertebral occlusions, diffuse disease) have emphasized its interest with the "occipital connection" which usually spares the distal segment of the VA.[13]

The incision is anterior to the sterno-cleido-mastoid muscle. The carotid bifurcation is first dissected. Then the distal VA is located in the upper end of the cutting. The transverse process of C1 is palpated behind the digastric muscle. The key to this approach is the anterior ramus of C2. When it is located, a guide is introduced between this nerve and the levator scapulac which is divided, opening the C1–C2 space. The muscle between the C1–C2 transverse processes is carefully excised. Behind the ramus appears the VA. The proximal part of the VA is occluded and the distal one is clamped and transposed anterior to the nerve. Ligation of occipital collateral branches may be used, if necessary.

Two kinds of reconstructive procedures may be employed:

1.   anastomosis from the VA to the common, external, or internal carotid using an autogenous venous graft;

2.   a direct anastomosis between the VA and the external or internal carotid.

Results

Results of vertebral artery surgery should be evaluated according to three different criteria: operative risk, arterial reconstruction, and neurologic results (Tables 26-4 and 26-5).

Table 26-4
Operations for Proximal Vertebral Artery Atherosclerosis

	Wylie 1979	Edwards 1983	Cooley 1984	Thevenet 1984	Imparato 1985
Endarterectomy	36	32		283	
Patch ± endarterectomy			15		
Reimplantation—carotid	3	283			4
Reimplantation—subclavian	3		21	14	
Resection-anastomosis	1				
Subclavian vertebral angioplasty					101
Graft			3		

Operative Risk

In all series the operative risk is very low. Mortality varies from 0 to 3%.

Postoperative neurologic deficit (1–4%) is always associated with multiple carotid and vertebral lesions. Local complications (Horner's syndrome, dysphonia, phrenic nerve paresis, lymph fistula) are noted but transient.

Arterial Reconstruction

The only method to evaluate the vertebral revascularization is the angiography. Reported series with such a control are rare. We reported on 96 patients with angiographic control.[11] The anatomic result was satisfactory in 81%, poor in 14% (residual irregularity or restenosis), and failure in 5%.

Neurologic Results

With a long follow-up, 80% of the patients in most of the published series showed favourable results (Table 26-5).

It is interesting to note in our last series of vertebral surgery comprising 29 patients (1984–1985) the percentage of the different procedures used, as shown in Table 26-6.

Table 26-5
Results of Surgery of Proximal Vertebral Artery

	Wylie	Edwards	Cooley	Thevenet	Imparato
Mortality (%)	2.3	0.2	0	0.6	3
Neurologic deficits (%)	4.7	0	2.5	1.2	0
Asymptomatic	76	68	82	68	
Improved	17	26		11	
Unchanged	7	6	18	9	
Follow-up (years)	8		12	9	

Table 26-6
Surgery of Vertebral Artery
1984–1985

	Number	%
Endarterectomy	12	41.4
Reimplantation—carotid	14	48.3
Distal reconstruction	3	10.3
Total	29	

SURGERY OF SUPRAAORTIC TRUNKS

Obstructive lesions of the brachiocephalic arteries are sometimes well tolerated because of other sources of collateral circulation. However, a number of patients have associated lesions with symptoms, either hemispheric or vertebrobasilar, others present symptoms of chronic cerebral hypoperfusion, and some are limited by different degrees of ischaemia in the upper extremities.

Extrathoracic repair for occlusion of the proximal brachiocephalic trunks had gained popularity because of a low mortality rate (5%) in contrast to the high mortality rate (20%) of the transthoracic repair as described in 1969 by Crawford and De Bakey. This is not true in our experience, reported in 1980,[15] with a 2% mortality rate for 189 intrathoracic repairs and a 0.9% mortality rate for 438 extrathoracic repairs. Moreover, Criado,[16] reviewing the English literature on extrathoracic procedures for aortic arch syndrome spanning the period 1962–1980 comprising 787 operations, reports a 1.9% mortality rate for carotid subclavian bypass. Furthermore, postoperative Doppler studies have shown in our experience that retrograde flow in extraanatomic bypasses is haemodynamically less effective for the cerebral circulation than the flow of direct revascularization. With recent knowledge of long-term results[17,18] it appears that direct operations are proving more durable than cervical bypass grafts.

Thus, there is a variety of surgical procedures to be considered when evaluating the best repair for an individual patient—not a single type.

To date no single method or combination of methods has replaced invasive contrast arteriography to identify lesions and vessel involvement to recommend arterial reconstructive surgery. Visualization of the entire arterial pattern, as much in the cervicothoracic pathway as in the intracranial one, is indispensable in determining operability of the patient. Occlusion of the proximal segment of either innominate artery or subclavian arteries can involve a reversal of vertebral artery flow with a siphoning effect on the cerebral circulation acting as a collateral supply to the arm, creating the so-called "subclavian steal syndrome".

The operative procedures of arterial reconstruction as well as surgical exposures depend essentially on the site, extent of the lesions, and character of single- or multiple-vessel disease. They can be large or of limited approach, intra- or extrathoracic, direct or extraanatomic repair.

Isolated Lesions

When general conditions permit, the direct approach to the lesion is preferable. The type of reconstruction is defined by the condition of the origin of the trunks of the aorta and the aortic involvement:

1. segmental not involving the origin (cul-de-sac visible on the angiogram): endarterectomy with or without patch;
2. limited to the origin with the normal aorta: endarterectomy plus patch across the origin onto the aorta or transposition after disobliteration;
3. extended to the aorta (aortic dome involvement): bypass from the aorta or cervical approach.

Innominate Artery[9, 19–21]

The vessel is approached through a median sternotomy. Endarterectomy is performed as the primary method of reconstruction every time there is no extension of atheroma into the aortic arch. When the plaque involves only the innominate orifice a special J clamp (Wylie) is placed onto a portion of aorta. The longitudinal arteriotomy is closed after endarterectomy by suturing a Dacron patch across the orifice. If the atheroma involves the aortic dome or if the left common carotid artery originates from the same orifice as the innominate a Dacron graft is sutured to the ascending aorta and distally to the bifurcation of the innominate artery in an end-to-end fashion. Following graft insertion, the proximal innominate artery is oversewn. Long-term results of these procedures are excellent.

In rare cases, in whom a transmediastinal approach is contraindicated, cervical extraanatomic bypasses can be carried out (carotid-carotid, subclavian-carotid, axillo-axillary, subclavian-subclavian). These techniques present the disadvantages of crossing the cervical region and leaving the source of emboli from the obstructive lesion in place.

The transsternal approach is associated with no greater mortality or morbidity than any of the extrathoracic procedures, regardless of the age of the patient.

Common Carotid Artery[9, 19]

Occlusion of the common carotid artery results either from a primary lesion at the origin of the left common carotid either from a retrograde thrombosis following progression of carotid bifurcation atheromatous disease. In the former situation patency of the internal and external carotid arteries is usually maintained. The left carotid artery is transected at the base of the neck and after thromboendarterectomy, transposed to the left subclavian artery by means of end-to-side anastomosis.

A carotid-carotid bypass is indicated only if the left subclavian artery is not suitable.

In the case of retrograde thrombosis, the carotid bifurcation is first explored and after bifurcation endarterectomy, a retrograde thromboendarterectomy of the common carotid is carried out.

Subclavian Artery[9, 19, 22]

Occlusive disease of the proximal left subclavian artery is the most common involvement of the brachiocephalic vessels. In a number of cases, subclavian artery occlusions are asymptomatic unless there is concomitant carotid disease. However, symptoms can be observed including arm claudication, microemboli to the fingers, vertebrobasilar insufficiency (direct reduction of flow in a dominant vertebral artery or steal syndrome).

There are three principal reconstructive techniques available for single subclavian artery lesion:

1. Endarterectomy shares many advantages in limited lesions, sparing the innominate artery bifurcation on the right and the first centimetre of origin on the left. A simple supraclavicular approach permits adequate exposure on both sides despite a deeper situation on the left. Retrograde endarterectomy of the left subclavian artery is reserved for lesions involving the vertebral ostium and extending to the proximal segment, leaving the aortic origin free.

    We do not use the transthoracic endarterectomy through a left thoracotomy any more. This technique provides excellent long-term results but better options are available for single lesion.

2. Transposition operation by end-to-side anastomosis of the transected subclavian artery proximal to the origin of the vertebral artery to the ipsilateral common carotid artery can be considered as close as possible to the "ideal procedure" (safe, effective, without prosthetic or autogenous material, excellent long-term relief).

    Subclavian-carotid transposition makes possible the enlargement of the vertebral orifice by vertebrosubclavian endarterectomy or carotid anastomosis of a subclavian arteriotomy extended to the first centimetre of the vertebral artery.

    It is the procedure of choice in isolated proximal lesions of the subclavian arteries.

3. Extrathoracic bypasses.[16, 19] Extraanatomic revascularization procedures for brachiocephalic artery lesions are numerous. The carotid-subclavian bypass has gained a wide clinical experience and proved the absence of carotid steal. Another development concerns the carotid-axillary bypass with avoidance of subclavian exposure complications.

    Other bypasses, like the axillo-axillary and subclavian-subclavian bypasses, are simple but involve some disadvantages, including length and cross-over position as well as interference with the performance of a median sternotomy for a later coronary artery bypass or aorto distal artery bypass for progression of aortic arch disease.

    These latter procedures must be considered as compromise and restricted to situations where local or general conditions of the patient preclude performance of the unilateral operations.

    In view of the patency rates achieved by extrathoracic bypass, use of a vein graft is undesirable (18–45% of thrombosis).[16, 22] The graft material of choice is prosthetic Dacron tube of 8 mm.

Multiple Lesions[18, 23, 24]

The multiple-branch involvement as a pattern of brachiocephalic arterial disease poses difficult judgement decisions and presents the most difficult operative challenge in reconstructive surgery of extracranial vessels. However, it is an imperative indication for revascularization.

An extrathoracic repair is precluded since these procedures require the availability of one patent arch vessel. In some situations axillary or subclavian bypass can be carried out with the addition of a carotid bypass, but the procedure is more complicated and more vulnerable than direct repair.

Two types of operative procedures were employed in our experience, all performed through a median sternotomy:

1. Endarterectomy of aortic dome and origin of supraaortic trunks under circulatory arrest with profound hypothermia[23] is ideally suited in good-risk patients with limited lesions at the origin of the aortic branches, extending into the upper part of the aorta in a single atheromatous block.
2. Multiple bypass grafts originating from the ascending aorta with segmental endarterectomies and transposition of the left common carotid artery, as necessary,[24] represents the best method in more diffuse atherosclerotic involvement.

These procedures provide lasting functional improvement and long-term arterial patency.

Takayasu–Onishi arteritis[25]

Supraaortic Takayasu arteritis is a rare but not exceptional disease and is to be considered as being responsible for almost 10% of the obstructive lesions of the supraaortic trunks. The preferential involvement concerns the subclavian artery extended to axillary and brachial arteries in isolated lesions. Multiple involvement includes the common carotid arteries sparing carotid bifurcations as well as vertebral arteries at their origin.

In single lesions, carotido-subclavian or carotido-brachial bypasses are used. In multiple diseases, transsternal revascularization with aorto-distal bypass originating from the ascending aorta, associated if necessary with segmental endarterectomies (vertebro-subclavian, carotid bifurcation) or carotid-axillary or brachial bypasses, represents the best procedures.

Results

Reconstructive surgery of the supraaortic trunks, transthoracic or extrathoracic is very gratifying. Relief of symptoms is obtained in 94–83% of the patients[15, 17, 18, 24] with long-term follow-up. Operative mortality is low (1.1% in 850 personal reconstructions). In proximal obstruction of the subclavian artery, endarterectomy and transposition produce better long-term patency and results than extrathoracic bypass.[22]

The results of a comparative study concerning 294 cervical reconstructions between 1973 and 1980 with three types of operations (190 endarterectomies, 61

Table 26-7

Isolated Subclavian Artery Reconstruction 1973–1980
Results (follow-up 4–12 years; mean 8 years)

	Endarterectomies $N = 190$	Carotid Transpositions $N = 61$	Bypass $N = 43$
Hospital mortality	1 (0.52%)	0	0
Late mortality	20 (10.5%)	2 (3.2%)	5 (11.6%)
Early thrombosis	8 (4.2%)	0	2 (4.6%)
Late thrombosis	4 (2.1%)	0	5 (11.6%)
Asymptomatic	162 (85.2%)	56 (91%)	26 (60.5%)

transpositions, and 43 extrathoracic bypasses) which were followed up between 4 and 12 years, mean 8 years, are shown in Table 26-7.

During the last few years, 1981–1985, due to these results, the percentage of different procedures have changed: transposition 66%, endarterectomy 23.4%, and bypass 10.6% (Table 26-8).

In multiple-vessel occlusive disease, the surgical management used in our experience is listed in Table 26-9. Results of these reconstructions, with a follow-up from 2–18 years, mean 8 years, are summarized in Table 26-10.

Table 26-8

Isolated Subclavian Artery Reconstruction

	1973–1980		1981–1985	
	Number	%	Number	%
Endarterectomy	190	64.6	22	23.4
Transposition (carotid anastomosis)	61	20.8	62	66
Extrathoracic bypass	43	14.6	10	10.6
Total	294		94	

Table 26-9

Multiple Arch Vessel Occlusive Disease; Surgical Management

	Atheroma	Aortitis
Circulatory arrest (profound hypothermia)		
Endarterectomy—aortic dome	12	
Aortoplasty + LCC transposition	1	1
Multiple bypasses	17	10
+ Endarterectomy	(7)	(5)
+ LCC transposition	(6)	
Sequential endarterectomy	11	
+ LCC transposition	(4)	
	41	11

Table 26-10
Multiple Arch Vessel Reconstruction Results 1964–1982

| | Atheroma | | | | |
	Endarterectomy Circulatory Arrest	Multiple Bypass	Sequential Endarterectomy	Aortitis	Total
No patients	13	17	11	11	52
Hospital mortality	1			1	2
Patency	12	17	11	10	50
Asymptomatic	11	17	11	9	48
Late mortality	3	3	4	1	11
Follow-up (years)	2–16	2–14	2–18	2–12	8 (mean)

In summary, surgical means at the level of supraaortic trunks are various. There is no exclusive or systematic method. Eclectic choice of the best option remains individual, related to the lesional and clinical situations of the patient. Intrathoracic repair remains the method of choice for treatment of innominate artery and proximal multiple-vessel lesions.

Single involvement of other branches of the aortic arch is relieved by the cervical approach.

REFERENCES

1. Warlow Ch, Morris PJ (eds): Transient Ischemic Attacks. Marcel Dekker, 1982
2. Greenhalgh RM (ed): Extra-anatomic and Secondary Arterial Reconstruction. Pitman Publishing, 1982
3. Bergan JJ, Yao JST (eds): Cerebrovascular Insufficiency. Grune and Stratton, 1983
4. Berguer R, Bauer RB (eds): Vertebrobasilar Arterial Occlusive Disease. Raven Press, 1984
5. Courbier R (ed): Basis for a Classification of Cerebral Arterial Diseases. Excerpta Medica, 1985
6. Edwards WH, Mulherin JL: The surgical reconstruction of the proximal subclavian and vertebral artery. J Vasc Surg 2:634–639, 1985
7. Wylie EJ, Effeney DJ: Surgery of the aortic arch branches and vertebral arteries. Surg Clin N Am 54:669–680, 1979
8. Crawford ES: Complications of arch and vertebral operations, in Complications of Vascular Surgery, Grune and Stratton, 1980, pp 245–257
9. Ehrenfeld WK, Rapp JH: Direct revascularization for occlusion of the trunks of the aortic arch. J Vasc Surg 2:228–230, 1985
10. Roon AJ, Ehrenfeld WK, Cooke PB, Wylie EJ: Vertebral artery reconstruction. Ann J Surg 138:29–36, 1979
11. Thevenet A, Ruotolo C: Surgical repair of vertebral artery stenosis. J Cardiovasc Surg 25:101–110, 1984
12. Reul GJ, Cooley DA, Olson SK, et al: Long term results of direct vertebral artery operations. Surg 96:854–862, 1984
13. Berguer R: Distal vertebral artery bypass: Technique, the "occipital connection" and potential uses. J Vasc Surg 2:621–626, 1985

14. Imparato AM: Vertebral arterial reconstruction: A nineteen-year experience. J Vasc Surg 2:626–634, 1985
15. Thevenet A: Chirurgie des lésions obstructives des troncs supra-aortiques. Med et Hyg 38:4154–4160, 1980
16. Criado FJ: Extra-thoracic management of aortic arch syndrome. Br J Surg 69(Suppl):545–551, 1982
17. Vogt DP, Hertzer NR, O'Hara PJ, Beven EG: Brachiocephalic arterial reconstruction. Ann Surg:196–541, 1982
18. Crawford ES, Stowe CL, Powers RW: Occlusion of the innominate, common carotid and subclavian arteries: Long term results of surgical treatment. Surg 94:781–791, 1983
19. Moore WS: Extra-anatomic bypass for revascularization of occlusive lesions involving the branches of the aortic arch. J Vasc Surg 2:230–232, 1985
20. Brewster DC, Moncure AC, Darling RC, Ambrosino JJ, Abbott WM: Innominate artery lesions: Problems encountered and lessons learned. J Vasc Surg 2:99–110, 1985
21. De Sobrega RC, Lopez Collado M, Matas Docampo M, et al: Surgery of the innominate artery. J Cardiovasc Surg 27:31–37, 1986
22. Gerety RL, Andrus CH, May AG, Rob ChG, Green R, DeWeese JA: Surgical treatment of occlusive subclavian artery disease. Circulation 64(Suppl):228–230, 1981
23. Thevenet A: Surgical management of atheroma of the aortic dome and origin of supra-aortic trunks. World J Surg 3:187–195, 1979
24. Thevenet A: Chirurgie des lésions multiples des troncs supra-aortiques à leur origine. Chirurgie 106:491–501, 1980
25. Thevenet A: Upper limb arteritis in Takayasu's disease. Int Angio 4:335–340, 1985

Ralph G. DePalma

27

Surgery for Vasculogenic Impotence

Within the past decade increasing attention has been directed toward operations to correct impotence due to vascular causes. This interest stemmed from two observations: first, procedures to correct aorto-iliac occlusive and aneurysmal disease in and of themselves often provoked postoperative impotence[1,2] and, second, the discovery of a subset of patients with isolated occlusion of the pudendal arteries as a cause of impotence.[3,4] As a result of efforts to improve the quality of life, techniques of aorto-iliac reconstruction evolved to minimize postoperative sexual dysfunction.[5-8] These same reconstructive methods also offered the prospect of restored sexual function in some men. The maintenance of an intact autonomic nervous system and internal iliac artery flow are the two important principles involved in obviating sexual dysfunction and restoring normal function after aorto-iliac surgery.

There has also been progress in delineating the problem of pudendal arterial occlusion in recent years. An important relationship between risk factors for atherosclerosis and impotence has been suggested.[9,10] Pudendal and penile arteriopathies can be demonstrated anatomically by selective internal iliac angiography,[11,12] and cavernosography provides information about venous drainage.[13] Physiologically, the use of artificially induced pharmacologic erection now provides information about the hemodynamics of erection.[14,15] The ability to demonstrate the physiologic effects of vascular lesions and display their anatomy stimulated development of microvascular operations upon the pudendal artery and its branches as well as upon the penile venous drainage.[16]

CASE SELECTION AND CAUSES OF VASCULOGENIC IMPOTENCE

Detailed knowledge of the vessels involved is integral to rational treatment of vasculogenic impotence. Table 27-1 provisionally classifies the causes of vasculogenic impotence based on current knowledge. Arterial vasculogenic impotence has

Table 27-1

Vasculogenic Impotence: Provisional Classification, 1986

Arterial
Large vessel: aorta and branches to division of internal iliac
Small vessel: proper pudendal artery and branches
Combined: aortic aneurysm or ulcerated plaque with distal embolization
Cavernosal
Fibrosis idiopathic or postpriapic
Peyronie's disease with mechanical deficit and/or venous leakage
Other refractory states of unknown etiology
Venous
Congenital: cavernosum-spongiosum leakage
Acquired: venous insufficiency

been known since the time of Leriche[17] who listed erectile failure as the first symptom in men with the syndrome named after him. Occlusions of the proper pudendal artery and its distal branches have been recently demonstrated by selective angiography techniques; we have become aware that aortic aneurysms or ulcerated plaques can cause distal embolization into the pudendal artery. While screening patients for the chief complaint of vasculogenic impotence we have uncovered occult aortic aneurysms not previously diagnosed. Thus, the symptom of impotence can be a harbinger of lethal undetected aortic disease and also, in some men, is associated with coronary disease.[18]

In spite of adequate inflow, factors at the cavernosal level might also inhibit normal erection, e.g., diabetic neuropathy or Peyronie's disease. Normal penile erection involves neurally regulated arterial flow increase into the corpus cavernosum and the corpus spongiosum with concomitant obstruction of venous outflow from the corpus cavernosum. It is now believed that this process depends mainly upon relaxation of smooth muscle within the erectile tissue of the corpora cavernosa.[19, 20] Penile blood flow during erection has been studied by several investigators[21–23] and exhibits unique characteristics. At rest, flow is estimated at 6–10 ml/min, whereas to obtain an erection flows from the proximal arterial system of 120 ml/min are required. During maintenance of erection flows of about 30 ml/min occur.

Table 27-2 summarizes the characteristics of penile hemodynamics once erection has been obtained. These data obtain from Lue's elegant studies[24] of nerve-stimulated erection in subhuman primates. With full erection there is closure of the cavernosal venous drainage and pressurization of the corpus cavernosum within the tunica albuginea. There is no flow in the internal iliac arteries during diastole; however, during systole there is flow presumably supplying the glans and spongiosum. At full erection systolic pressures at or even slightly above systemic, blood is

Table 27-2

Penile Blood Flow during Erection

Closure of cavernosal vein drainage
No flow in diastole
Some flow in systole (mainly spongiosal tissue)
Anticoagulant activity in stagnant cavernosal blood

stagnant in the corpora. There appears to be an anticoagulant activity within this blood which prevents thrombosis, an observation which is easily confirmed by aspiration of the corpus during full erection.

Factors at the cavernous level such as fibrosis of the normally reactive smooth muscle or neural deficits can inhibit the normal erectile process. Peyronie's disease is believed to be a vasculitis with a mechanical defect in the lining of the corpus cavernosum. We have observed, using cavernosography, that this condition creates a syndrome of rapid venous leakage about the inflamed plaques. There also exist other refractory states of the corpus cavernosum of unknown etiology.

As a result of investigation of patients with primary impotence,[25] leakage from the normally impervious corpus cavernosum into the spongiosum was discovered and corrected. Another subset of patients, mainly middle-aged men, exists in whom there is venous leakage mainly in the area of the dorsal vein and also at the crura of the corpora cavernosa.[26] The diagnosis of this condition requires cavernosography using dilute radioopaque contrast medium. Operations to correct venous leakage have been met with success provided arterial inflow and cavernosal physiology are adequate.[13, 26] In selecting procedures to treat vasculogenic impotence each of these factors must be considered and investigated. A further complicating facet of this field is that there may be combinations of neurovascular factors which contribute to erectile failure.

Surgery of impotence can be divided into general subsets, each with particular clinical characteristics. Patients with aorto-iliac disease present mainly with complaints of peripheral ischemia related to their lower extremities. They require correction of proximal aorto-iliac lesions using techniques which spare autonomic nervous fibers insofar as possible and restore flow into the internal iliac arteries. A few of these patients complain only of impotence and exhibit stenosis of one or both internal iliac arteries. These lesions can be corrected by endarterectomy or a bypass graft via an extraperitoneal approach. Among this group of patients there exist also individuals who exhibit stenotic disease involving the division of the internal iliac artery into its anterior and posterior branches. When the internal pudendal artery arises high from the anterior division of the internal iliac, endarterectomy is also possible. A small subset of men exists in whom renal artery stenosis is the main problem. Treatment with antihypertensive agents has rendered such patients physiologically impotent. The ideal patient for correction of renal artery stenosis will have had the condition for three years or less and be in the age range of 30–50 years. Relief of the renal artery stenosis will allow moderation of the antihypertensive drugs and usually normal postoperative erectile function.

Impotence occurring postoperatively or due to atheroembolism is best treated by a penile prosthesis. This alternative offers the best prospect for immediate postoperative coital function currently available. There are a variety to choose from and rigid, semirigid, and inflatable prosthesis have been recently discussed.[27, 28] In spite of the advantage of immediate coital sufficiency, there are disadvantages. Once a prosthesis has been inserted the cavernosal tissues will have been destroyed and the patient will always require a prosthesis for normal intromission. Both inflatable and rigid prostheses exhibit a finite postoperative failure rate. Many men will not accept a prosthesis; these individuals with proper screening become candidates for microvascular surgery of the distal pudendal artery. Finally, men exhibiting venous leaks, when properly selected, by confirming good inflow and normal neurophysiology, are gratifying subjects for operation. Cavernosography to demonstrate the venous leak under artificial erection or tumescence is required preoperatively.[13] With these qualifications about proper case selection, operations which prevent sexual dysfunction or restore sexual function will be discussed.

LARGE VESSEL RECONSTRUCTIONS FOR IMPOTENCE

Table 27-3 summarizes procedures which are applicable to patients with impotence. As mentioned previously, patients requiring aorto-iliac or aorto-femoral bypass are symptomatic due to peripheral ischemia or have aneurysms. The procedures are modified to avoid postoperative sexual disability or to restore function. These operative principles involve dissections to preserve both vascular and neural elements of the erectile process. The operation must restore or maintain the iliac flow, avoid atheroembolism into the internal iliac bed during flushing, and remove atheromatous material which might later embolize into the pudendal arteries. As a result of empirically based observations on the distribution of atherosclerosis, which often involves the external iliac artery, aorto-femoral bypass rather than aorto-iliac bypass emerged as a preferred procedure in most cases of occlusive disease. A common accompaniment of aorto-femoral procedures is postoperative impotence based on failure to provide retrograde perfusion via a seriously diseased external iliac artery. In aneurysm surgery aorto-iliac anastomoses just proximal to the bifurcation of the common iliac artery are associated with a lesser incidence of impotence.[1] Unfortunately, disease of the external iliacs may not permit proximal anastomosis and would compromise lower extremity circulation. Thus, aorto-femoral operations are tailored to provide internal iliac artery perfusion by adding an extra limb to the graft or combining the operation with side-to-side anastomoses and internal iliac endarterectomy. There exist other cases in which a proximal iliac anastomosis can be selected if the pattern of atherosclerosis permits.

In young patients endarterectomy is a favored procedure when there is discrete segmental involvement proximal to the common iliac bifurcation and when soft atheromatous lesions with minimal calcifications exist. Successful proximal thromboendarterectomy maintains axial flow both to the internal and external iliac and the system offers an important advantage in properly selected cases. Cases suitable for endarterectomy are reported to be more common in the European experience.[4]

We have described favorable results on sexual function using femoro-femoral reconstructions at times combined with transluminal angioplasty of the donor vessel.[29] This operation may offer slightly less long-term patency than aorto-femoral bypass, but is a useful option in patients in whom postoperative sexual function is an important consideration. Axillo-femoral bypass has not been a particularly

Table 27-3
Large Vessel Reconstructions for Impotence

Aorto-iliac or aorto-femoral bypass
Internal iliac endarterectomy or bypass
Femoro-femoral reconstruction
Transluminal angioplasty
Profundoplasty in conjunction with other inflow procedures

favored approach of this author's because of the necessity for frequent reoperations. Flannigan and coworkers,[30] however, showed that this reconstruction combined with profundoplasty restored sexual function via collaterals which arise from the profunda, even when both internal iliac arteries were occluded. The importance of restoring adequate profunda inflow by extending the aorto-femoral graft hood onto this vessel is consistent with our previous experience.[7,8]

In young men one patent internal iliac artery usually suffices for normal sexual function. The importance of intact iliac artery circulation has been underscored by the recognition that a second renal transplant usually causes impotence when a second internal iliac artery is divided for end-to-end anastomosis to the donor kidney.[31] In our clinic we have employed end-to-side anastomoses to the iliac artery to avoid this complication. Methods to correct post second renal transplant impotence by internal iliac to distal pudendal artery bypass have also been described.[32]

Patients discovered to have an abdominal aortic aneurysm require operation by virtue of the presence of this lesion itself. In these cases we do not recommend selective arteriography to visualize the distal reaches of the internal iliac and the pudendal artery. Selective pudendal arteriography may cause atheroembolism as the catheters are manipulated through the extensively diseased distal abdominal aorta. Conventional aortography with the catheter positioned just above the lesion and oblique pelvic views suffice. The anatomy of the distal pelvic vessels should be studied preoperatively to make the best possible estimate of the method of distal anastomosis. The author recommends aortography prior to aneurysm repair in almost all cases and most particularly in those where postoperative sexual function is a concern.

An inlay technique for abdominal aortic aneurysm repair is utilized. The initial dissection is carried out to minimize interference with the neural fibers and preserve the nerves passing within the inferior mesenteric artery. Therefore there is little dissection on the left and the orifice of the inferior mesenteric artery is sutured from within the aneurysm. The inlay type of aneurysm reconstruction expedites surgery and minimizes blood loss and postoperative sexual dysfunction. In the course of operating recently on four men with aneurysms in whom impotence was the presenting complaint, the author has noted restoration of sexual function in only one patient postoperatively. In the three remaining patients there was no improvement in spite of particular efforts to preserve neural fibers and internal iliac flow. If postoperative sexual function is a concern in any patient about to undergo aorto-iliac surgery a prosthesis ought to be discussed with the patient preoperatively as one cannot predict return of erectile function. Erectile failure in preoperatively impotent aneurysm patients can be due to internal iliac occlusion, distal occlusion of the pudendal, possibly atheroembolism, or neuropathy. We now investigate these patients using pre- and postoperative vascular laboratory measurements, artificial erection, and pudendal somatosensory evoked potentials.[33]

SMALL VESSEL ARTERIAL RECONSTRUCTION FOR IMPOTENCE

Table 27-4 lists various small vessel reconstructions used to treat arterial impotence due to arteriopathy or traumatic disruptions of the internal pudendal artery or its branches. At the outset it should be recognized that the unique hemodynamics

Table 27-4

Small Vessel Reconstruction
for Impotence

Arterialization of corpus cavernasum
Arterialization of deep dorsal vein
Bypass into pudendal artery
Bypass into dorsal artery
Bypass into deep cavernosal artery

---

of penile erection require an anastomosis which at rest delivers a low flow (6–8 ml), is capable of then increasing to a relatively high flow of 120 ml/min or more to obtain erection, and then maintaining an intermediate flow of 30 ml/min during sustained erection. Further, the neural and venous components of the erectile process must also be relatively intact. These physiologic requirements and the unique anatomy of the penile arteries themselves require special considerations when such operations are contemplated.

There exist as yet no long-term data on the patency of these bypasses, nor in the author's experience is long-term patency of epigastric to dorsal artery anastomoses inevitably related to potency. The surgical experiences described, as with any developing surgical procedure, are still anecdotal. In their early evolutions, direct corporal revascularization vein grafts from the femoral artery and the inferior epigastric artery were used as unilateral or bilateral implants. The vein bypasses were too large and resulted in priapism. In the author's personal experience with direct bilateral inferior epigastric artery to corpora cavernosa anastomoses the results were remarkably successful for three to four months, and then closure was documented by recurrence of the impotence, loss of pulse wave recordings, and arteriography.[6] The author then applied anastomosis of the inferior epigastric artery to vein patches on the corpora cavernosa. There was initial success in two patients and serious priapism occurred in another patient which required ligation of the arterial graft. This complication, also described by Puech-Leao, Puech-Leao, and Albers,[34] probably occurs because blood is delivered directly into the cavernous space at too high a flow and overriding normal neural control.

End-to-end or side-to-side anastomoses of one inferior epigastric artery to one dorsal artery may be rational; these are capable of providing retrograde perfusion of the deep cavernosal artery. These operations are not difficult to perform under magnification, but no follow-up longer than $2\frac{1}{2}$ years is available. Puech-Leao, Puech-Leao, and Albers[34] record early successful results of these procedures. Goldstein, Martara, and Krane reported in 1984[35] improved erectile function in 11 of 14 young patients with traumatic occlusive disease and poor results in older patients with atherosclerotic disease. The latter is consistent with the author's experience in two cases in whom patency could be ascertained with Doppler probes, but with no improvement in erectile function. Direct arterial anastomoses to the cavernosal artery have been described, but the size of this vessel, i.e., less than 0.2 mm, probably precludes long-term successful microvascular anastomoses. Shaw and Zorgniotti[36] mentioned an instance in which this was recently done. Crespo and coworkers[37] have described multiple microvascular anastomoses to both dorsal and cavernosal arteries using vein grafts. No life table or long-term patency data are available about the results of these procedures.

VIRAG'S OPERATION

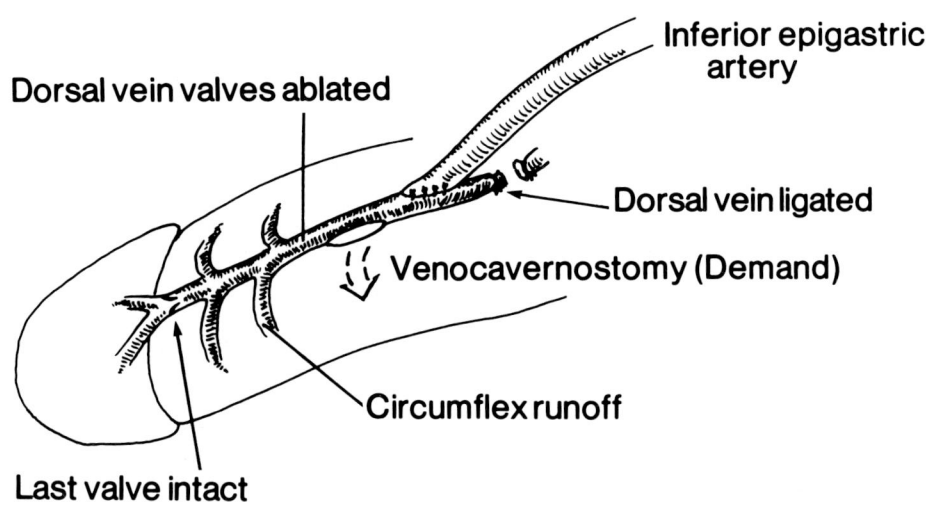

Fig. 27-1. Schematic drawing of R. Virag's fifth variant of inferior epigastric artery to dorsal vein anastomosis for penile revascularization.

Among the more promising recent operations is arterial bypass into the dorsal vein of the penis, as illustrated in Fig. 27-1. This operation, the fifth of a number of arterial-venous variations described by Virag and coworkers,[16] consists of the following elements: ligation of the proximal dorsal vein with destruction of the two distal valves and a venocavernosostomy which possibly provides demand flow during erection. One complication of this operation is edema of the glans penis and for that reason the distal valve is left intact. The arterio-venous anastomosis allows a constant high flow delivery by the inferior epigastric artery but provision is made for runoff via the circumflex veins. The venocavernosostomy provides an inflow capability which may be demand regulated. It is also possible that the operation effectively exerts a favorable effect on the venous dynamics during erection. This operation is being evaluated prospectively by its originator and a group of American surgeons interested in this problem.

VENOUS INTERRUPTION

As initially described by Ebbejoh and Wagner,[25] congenital leaks from the normally impervious corpus cavernosum into the glans penis resulted in primary impotence. This condition was corrected by cavernosal repair. Recently patients with acquired venous leakage from the corpus cavernosum have been characterized using artificial erection and dynamic cavernosography. This diagnostic procedure is performed after intracavernous injection of papaverine or passive roller pump induced erection. A #20 scalp vein needle is then inserted behind the corona and 20% Renografin (Squibb) diluted with intravenous saline is injected under fluoroscopic control. Multiple films are exposed to detect sites of leakage from the corpus cavernosum. A positive study is illustrated in Fig. 27-2. Wespes and Schulman[13] using a

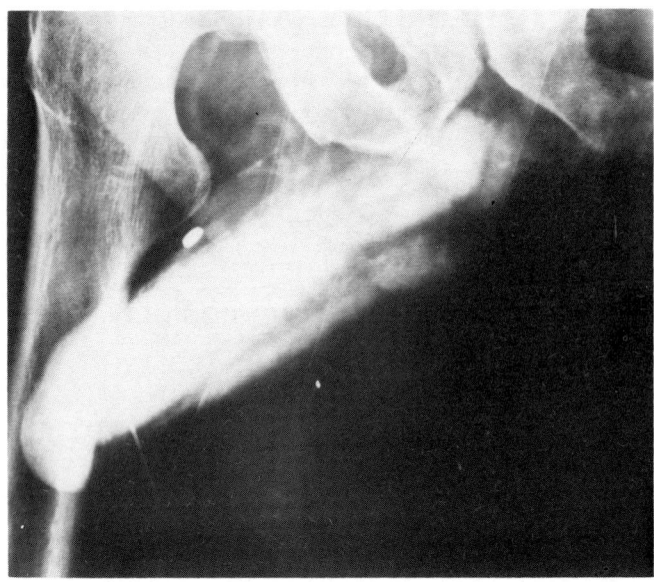

Fig. 27-2. Venous leakage demonstrated from deep dorsal vein after intracavernous injection of papaverine and infusion of 20% Renografin (Squibb). Preoperative arterial studies negative and artificial erection studies characteristic of venous insufficiency.

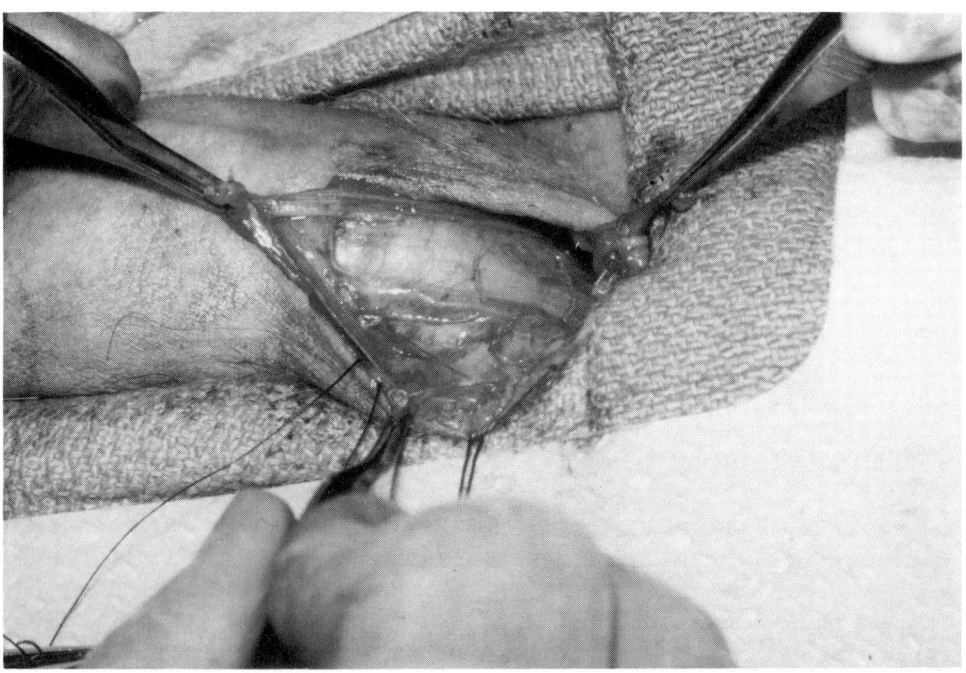

Fig. 27-3. Operative photograph from same patient as Fig. 27-2. Resection of deep dorsal vein and ligation of all communicators. Patient reports continued normal function one year postoperatively.

roller pump with cavernous pressure monitoring detected similar venous leaks; after ligation of the dorsal vein to correct leaks they reported satisfactory results in 16 of 20 patients short term. The patient illustrated in Fig. 27-3 was also benefited by this procedure. These procedures involve resection of the dorsal vein and ligation of all superficial and deep communicating veins about the base of the penis. Venous leaks have been described at the ventral surface of the penis deep in the perineum near the proximal crura. Effective surgical exposures have not yet been developed to permit direct interruption of incompetent veins in this area.

The diagnosis and treatment of impotence has yielded much new information about normal erectile anatomy and physiology. The microvascular interventions in this area are still developmental. Given the option of prosthetic implantation, there is virtually no case of erectile failure that cannot be successfully treated, but ideal therapy involves an accurate diagnosis of the cause or causes of erectile failure in each individual. It should be noted that combined arterial, venous, and neural abnormalities coexist; this complicates case selection. Surgical methods to restore sexual function which involve standard operations on the large vessels are straight-forward and require some additional attention to detail during operations for lower extremity ischemia or aneurysms. Treatment of the other causes of vasculogenic impotence, i.e., isolated pudendal arteriopathy, cavernosal disorders, and venous insufficiency, require specialized examinations to clarify abnormal physiology. As these diagnositc methods improve, a more precise application of medical and surgical therapy for vasculogenic impotence will ensue.

REFERENCES

1. May AG, DeWeese JA, Rolo CG: Changes in sexual function following operation on the abdominal aorta. Surgery 65:41–47, 1969
2. Sabri S, Cotton LT: Sexual function following aorto-iliac reconstruction. Lancet ii:1218–1219, 1971
3. Zorgniotti AW, Rossi G (eds): Vasculogenic Impotence. Springfield, Thomas, 1980, 343 pp
4. Michal V: Arterial disease as a cause of impotence. Clin Endocrinol Metab 11:725–748, 1982
5. Weinstein MH, Machleder HI: Sexual function after aorto-iliac surgery. Ann Surg 181:787–790, 1974
6. DePalma RG, Kedia K, Persky L: Vascular operations for preservation of sexual function, in Bergan JJ, Yao JST (eds): The Surgery of the Aorta and Its Body Branches. New York, Grune and Stratton, 1979, pp 277–296
7. DePalma RG: Aorto-iliac dissection principles, in Zorgniotti A, Rossi G (eds): Vasculogenic Impotence. Springfield, Thomas, 1980, pp 299–308
8. DePalma RG: Prevention of sexual dysfunction in aorto-iliac surgery, in Jamieson C (ed): Current Operative Surgery. Eastbourne, E Sussex, Bailliere Tindall, 1985, pp 80–96
9. Virag R, Bouilly P, Frydman D: Is impotence an arterial disorder? Lancet 181–184, January 26, 1985
10. Virag R, Bouilly P, Frydman D: About arterial risk factors and impotence. Lancet 1109–1110, May 11, 1985
11. Ginestie JF, Romieu A: Radiologic Exploration of Impotence. The Hague, Martinus Nijhoff, 1978

12. Juhan CM, Hughet JF, Clerissi JA, Courjaret P: Classification of internal pudendal artery lesions in one-hundred cases, in Zorgniotti AW, Rossi G (eds): Vasculogenic Impotence. Springfield, Thomas, 1980, pp 153–168

13. Wespes E, Schulman CC: Venous leakage: Surgical treatment of a curable case of impotence. J Urol 133:796–798, 1985

14. Virag R, Spencer PP, Frydman D: Artificial erection in diagnosis and treatment of impotence. Urology 24:157–161, 1984

15. Virag R, Frydman D, Legman M, et al: Intracavernous injection of papaverine as a diagnostic and therapeutic method in erectile failure. Angiology 35:79–87, 1984

16. Virag R, Frydman D, Legman H, et al: Possibilities chirurgicales dans l'impuissance vasculaire. Gaz Med de France 90:2031–2038, 1983

17. Leriche R: Des obliterations arterielles hautes (obliteration de la terminasion de l'aorte) comme causes des insufficances circulatoires des membres inferieurs. Bull Mem Soc Chir 49:1404, 1923

18. DePalma RG, Edwards C: Noninvasive evaluation of erectile dysfunction and intracorporal papaverine injection, in Virag R, Virag H (eds): Proceedings of First World Conference on Impotence. Paris, Editions du Ceri (in press).

19. Goldstein AMB, Meehan JP, Zakhary R, et al: New observations on microarchitecture of corpora cavernosa in man and possible relationship to mechanism of erection. Urology 20:259–266, 1982

20. Brindley GS: Neurophysiology of erection. Abstr Proc First World Meeting Impotence, Paris, 1984, p 17

21. Michal V, Simana J, Rehak J, et al: Haemodynamics of erection in man. Physiologia Bohemoslavaca 32:497–499, 1983

22. Wagner G, Urenholdt F: Blood flow measurement by the clearance method in human corpus cavernosum in the flaccid and erect states, in Zorgniotti AW, Rossi G (eds): Vasculogenic Impotence. Springfield, Thomas, 1980, pp 41–46

23. Shirai M, Ishii N: Haemodynamics of erection in man. Arch Androl 6:27–32, 1981

24. Lue TF, Takamura T, Schmidt RA, et al: Hemodynamics of erection in the monkey. J Urol 130:1237–1241, 1983

25. Ebbehoj J, Wagner G: Insufficient penile erection due to abnormal drainage of cavernous bodies. Urology 13:507–510, 1979

26. Virag R: Syndrome d'erection instable par insufficiance veineuse. J Mal Vasc 6:121–124, 1981

27. Finney RP: Rigid and semirigid penile prostheses, in Bennett AH (ed): Management of Male Impotence. Baltimore, Williams and Wilkins, 1982, pp 198–209

28. Bennett AH: The inflatable and malleable prostheses, in Bennet AH (ed): Management of Male Impotence. Baltimore, Williams and Wilkins, 1982, pp 210–218

29. Merchant RF Jr, DePalma RG: The effects of femoro-femoral grafts on postoperative sexual function: Correlation with penile pulse volume recordings. Surgery 90:962–970, 1981

30. Flannigan DP, Schuler JJ, Keifer T, et al: Elimination of iatrogenic impotence and improvement of sexual function following aorto-iliac revascularization. Arch Surg 117:544–550, 1982

31. Gittes RF, Waters WB: Sexual impotence: The overlooked complication of a second renal transplant. J Urol 121:719–210, 1979

32. Billet A, Dagher FJ, Queral LA: Surgical correction of vasculogenic impotence in a patient after bilateral renal transplantation. Surgery 91:108–112, 1982

33. Haldeman S, Bradley WE, Bhatia NN, et al: Pudendal evoked responses. Arch Neurol 39:280–283, 1982

34. Puech-Leao LE, Puech-Leao, Albers MTV: Impotencia sexual vasculogenica: Diagnostico e tratamento. Sao Paulo, Brazil, Sarvier, 1981.

35. Goldstein I, Martara R, Krane RJ: Microsurgery for atherosclerotic and non atherosclerotic occlusive disease. Oral communication: Proceedings of the First World Meeting on Impotence, Paris, June 1984

36. Shaw WW, Zorgniotti AW: Surgical techniques in penile revascularization. Urology 23:76–78, 1984

37. Crespo E, Soltanik E, Bove D, Farrell G: Treatment of vasculogenic sexual impotence by revascularizing cavernous and/or dorsal arteries using microvascular techniques. Urology 20:271–275, 1982

PART V

Venous and Pulmonary Embolism Problems

J. T. Hobbs

28

Can We Prevent Recurrence of Varicose Veins?

Primary varicose veins are due either to incompetence of valves in the perforating veins or to weakness of the vein wall and surrounding supporting tissues. The most common site of incompetence is the termination of the long or short saphenous veins.

In secondary varices the damaged deep veins following venous thrombosis produce their most serious effects through incompetence of the distal perforating veins which in turn leads to skin changes in the lower leg. Another cause of secondary varices is arterio-venous fistulae, either congenital or traumatic, where the undamped arterial pressure reaches the venous system.

In an ideal world, recurrence of significant primary varices can be prevented by correct surgery but the less troublesome, though more disfiguring, dilated superficial veins cannot be eliminated because the skin and subcutaneous tissues cannot be changed. Obviously, recurrence of secondary varices due to the postthrombotic syndrome or congenital arterio-venous fistulae (Klippel–Trenaunay syndrome) cannot be prevented because the underlying cause persists. Varices secondary to traumatic arterio-venous fistulae will not recur when the fistula is closed.

In practice, even those significant primary varices which should be cured will have a high recurrence rate because of inadequate surgery, which has resulted from poor supervision and teaching. Varicose vein patients are seen in both the general and vascular surgical clinics where the more serious leg and life-threatening conditions rightly demand most attention, leaving patients with vein problems to be seen by the junior trainee surgeons. These inexperienced doctors are not supervised and so when they become seniors they are not able to teach the next generation!

When the primary problem is not recognised or treated correctly the further venous disease is a continuation or persistence of the original problem rather than a recurrence. True recurrence cannot be prevented because the condition did not exist

VASCULAR SURGERY: ISSUES IN CURRENT PRACTICE
ISBN 0-8089-1839-7

at the time of treatment and only after pregnancy or some other cause will new varices appear in a new territory or in the previously unaffected contralateral leg. If the problem is dilated superficial veins or venules, they can be eliminated by sclerotherapy, but recurrence in new areas cannot be prevented.

This review is therefore concerned with failure of primary treatment rather than the continuation of an incurable and unpreventable disease process.

ASSESSMENT

Venous problems require accurate treatment with careful assessment, detailed planning, and precise execution if good results are to be consistently obtained. Much of surgery is based on the history and clinical findings supplemented by the results of investigations, particularly radiology, and the incision is fairly standard with the procedure being varied according to the findings. However, vein surgery requires more detailed planning.

In venous disease the leg must be carefully assessed after the patient has stood for a sufficient period of time. The knee must be slightly flexed to relax the popliteal fascia so that the termination of the short saphenous vein can be palpated. A careful mapping of the superficial veins combined with sliding palpation should enable most points of control, presumably including all incompetent perforator sites, to be located. Sometimes examination with Doppler ultrasound will assist the clinical inspection. If damage to the deep veins is suspected, venography is necessary to demonstrate the patency of the deep veins and their valvular function. The degree of impairment can be quantified by venous pressure studies. Frequently the failure of treatment arises from inadequate initial examination and it is not uncommon for surgeons to operate on a leg which they have never seen before. It is essential that the surgeon examines the leg with the patient standing prior to operation and the surgeon should be the person who marks the leg because there may be little to see when the leg is horizontal or slightly elevated.

INJECTION–COMPRESSION

Sclerotherapy is often discredited because either it is used in the wrong situation or the technique is inadequate. The aim of sclerotherapy is to obliterate the lumen of abnormally dilated superficial veins by replacement with fibrous tissue. If a large thrombus is allowed to form in the vein it is painful, often resulting in discolouration, and it is likely that recanalisation will occur and probably with additional valve damage. This is more likely when injections are made with the patient standing to facilitate placement of the needle in the vein lumen which is then distended. To overcome the problem of dilution in the larger blood volume the amount of sclerosant is increased, resulting in a more extensive inflammatory process and sometimes the toxic effects of overdose. If the leg is not bandaged effectively the thrombotic process may extend and if compression is removed early the inflammatory process of superficial thrombophlebitis may be excessive.

For these reasons effective sclerotherapy requires the injections of a small volume of sclerosant into a collapsed vein (leg horizontal) at the marked parts of

Table 28-1
Ten-year Results of Surgery and
Sclerotherapy of Varicose Veins with
Proximal Incompetence

	Operation (%)		Injection (%)	
	Success	Failure	Success	Failure
1 year	96	4	91	9
5 years	79	21	30	70
10 years	71	29	6	94

From Hobbs JT: Surgery or sclerotherapy for varicose veins:
10 year results of a random trial, in Tesi M, Dormandy J
(eds): Superficial and Deep Venous Diseases of the Lower
Limbs. Milan, Edizione Minerva Medica, 1984, pp 243–248.

control (intended to include the sites of all incompetent perforating veins) followed by compression of the vein until the occlusion is permanent; bandaging is required for two to six weeks depending upon the size of the vein and local reaction. Whenever compression can be maintained for a sufficient period of time good results can be obtained.

The successful treatment of varicose veins requires either adequate surgical treatment or sclerotherapy and sometimes both. It is surprising that there is still so much difference of opinion as to which method of treatment should be used. Controlled trials have shown that a good initial result will be achieved by sclerotherapy when proximal incompetence is present, but there is a marked falloff with time which was not seen when treatment was by surgery (Table 28-1).[1]

These results have been confirmed in trials in Copenhagen[2] and Sweden.[3] The late results of the random trial showed that dilated superficial veins and incompetent lower leg perforating veins are best treated by sclerotherapy because adequate compression can be maintained.

SURGERY

When there is proximal incompetence surgery is the only effective method of treatment which will give long-lasting success.

Sapheno-femoral Junction

The most common cause of significant primary varicose veins is incompetence at the sapheno-femoral junction. Theoretically it should not be difficult to achieve a flush sapheno-femoral ligation because the level at which the long saphenous vein joins the femoral vein is very constant although there is much variation in the position and number of its tributaries. Despite this there is an unacceptably high recurrence rate and, surprisingly, recurrence is not uncommon after surgery by experienced general or vascular surgeons. The groin skin fold is not a reliable landmark because in obese people the sapheno-femoral junction is well above this level whereas in thin people there is a danger of making the incision too high. The sapheno-femoral junction is best located by using the pubic tubercle as a marker; the fossa ovalis is felt as a depression about 2.5 cm below and 3.5 cm lateral to this bony point and is medial to the pulsation of the femoral artery. It is recognised that all tributaries must be divided to achieve a flush ligation on the femoral vein and it must also be remembered that some of the tributaries join the femoral vein separately from the long saphenous vein.

In discussing the surgical management of recurrent varicose veins one expert[4] believed that to avoid the risk of damage surgeons should be taught to avoid exposing the femoral veins but to ligate and transfix the saphenous vein within 1 cm of the femoral vein and ligate all of the tributaries which join the long saphenous vein in this area. He preferred to leave any tributaries joining at, or near, the junction, believing that damage to the femoral vein was more serious. He also stated that a repeat operation was much simpler after a previous low incision. Transfixion of the vein is not necessary and can be complicated by tearing if the vein is fragile. Patients with recurrence of the long saphenous vein are often found to have low incisions and clearly the previous surgery must have left many tributaries. Both the lateral and medial sides of the femoral vein are easily seen through relatively small incisions, even in fat legs. It is essential that the incision is correctly placed and retractors are effectively used. Sometimes the long saphenous vein is duplicated and sometimes the lateral tributaries join the femoral vein collectively but separate from the saphenous vein. In a review of vein surgery the recurrence rate after sapheno-femoral ligation was found to be as high as 50%, which the investigator[5] rightly claimed as unacceptable for a nonessential operation. Obviously ligation at the sapheno-femoral junction must be flush and include all tributaries if recurrence is to be prevented.

In another study[6] 1000 Mexican soldiers were reviewed 9–18 years after long saphenous vein surgery and the recurrence rate differed with experience, being 14% for experienced surgeons (operating time 2 hours), 13% for trainee surgeons under supervision (operating time 3.2 hours), and 17% for unsupervised junior surgeons (operating time 1.2 hours).

Flush ligation at the sapheno-femoral junction is apparently simple but this is not always so, even by expert hands. The most common error seen after competent vascular surgeons have dealt with the sapheno-femoral junction is a persistence of the antero-lateral tributary (Fig. 28-1). This large vein is easily flattened against the side of the femoral vein when the long saphenous vein is drawn up to ligate it. The lateral vein must be sought and found. The postero-medial tributary often joins the long saphenous vein a little way below the sapheno-femoral junction and can usually be found by retracting the lower edge of the incision. It often continues down to join the short saphenous vein and is best divided and ligated to avoid the possibility of haematoma formation after the long saphenous vein is stripped, because this vein is above the level of bandaging.

Even when all of the tributaries are divided with a flush ligation there can be recurrence because of the normal drainage, but with a slightly atypical anatomical arrangement.

Most often the superficial inferior epigastric, superficial circumflex iliac and antero-lateral veins join separately (Fig. 28-2A). However, apart from sometimes being duplicated, it is not uncommon for the circumflex iliac vein and antero-lateral vein to form a single common lateral tributary (Fig. 28-2B). Sometimes both the

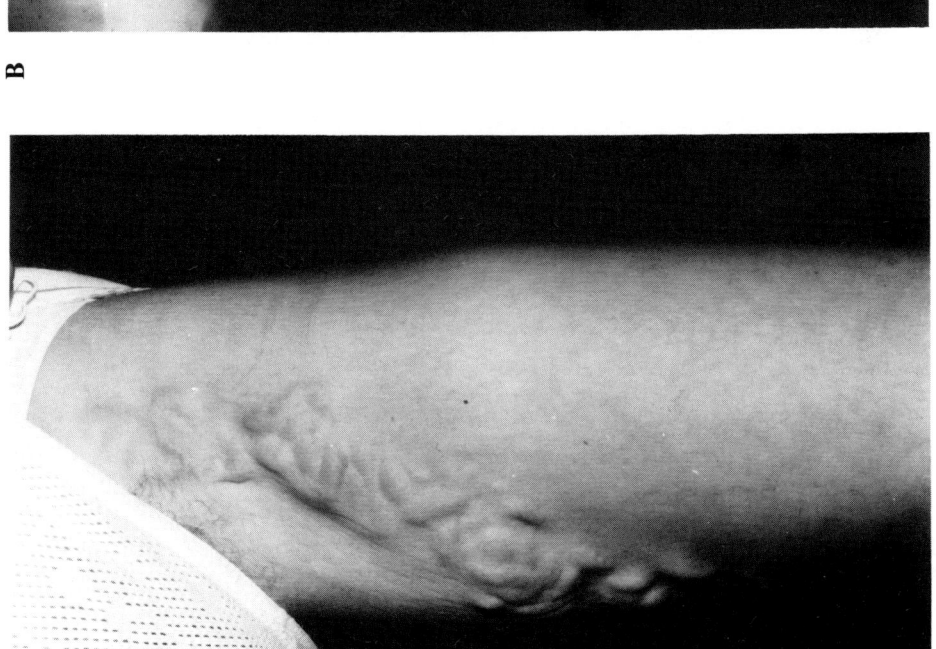

B

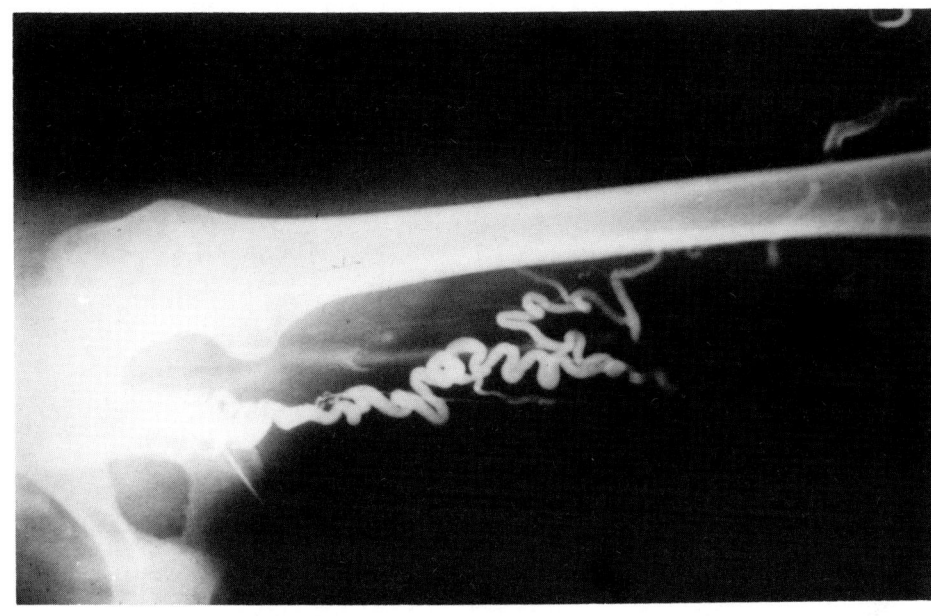

A

Fig. 28-1. (A) Recurrent varicose veins due to persistence of the lateral tributary at the groin. (B) Venogram showing persistent antero-lateral tributary.

359

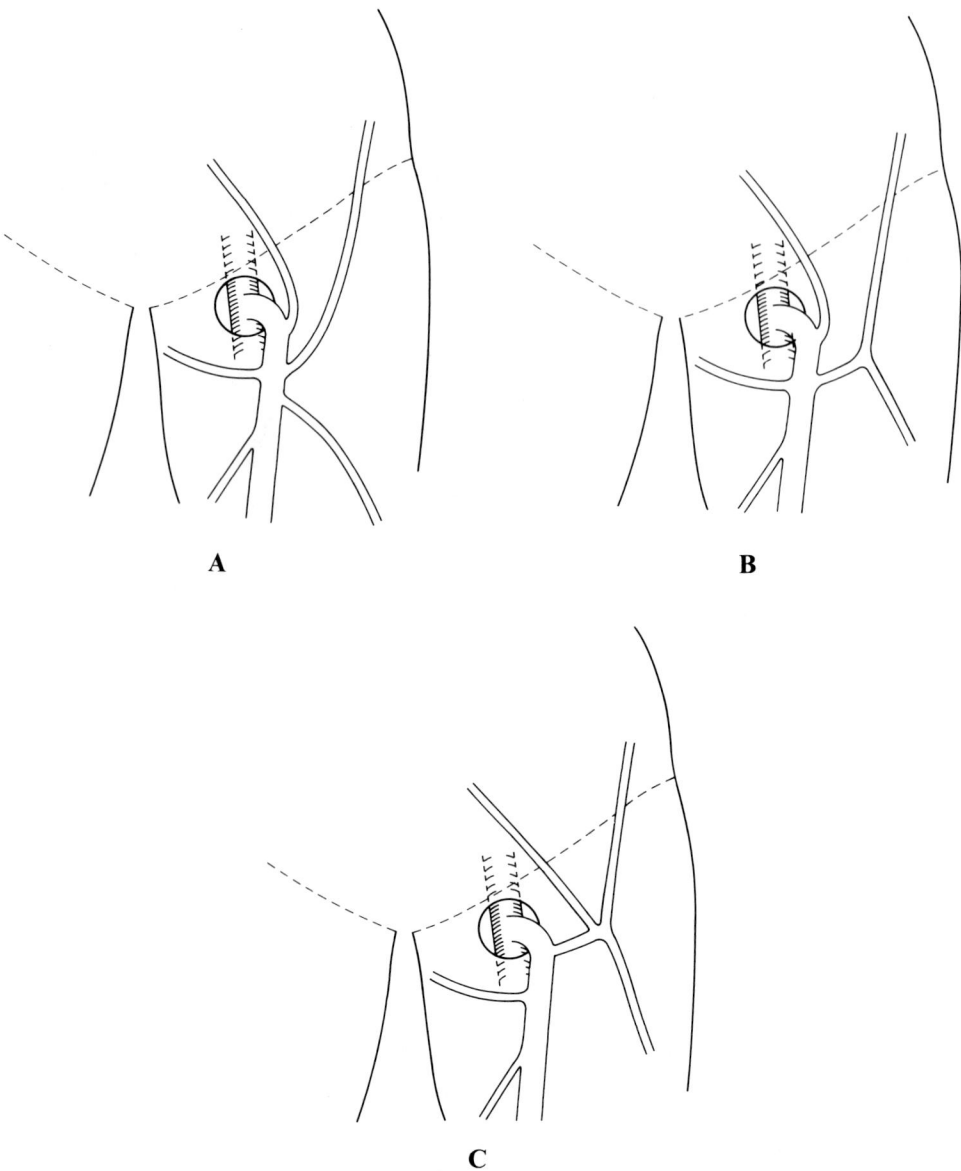

Fig. 28-2. The tributaries of the termination of the long saphenous vein: (A) normal, (B) double lateral, (C) triple lateral.

inferior epigastric and circumflex iliac veins join the antero-lateral vein to form a single large lateral tributary (Fig. 28-2C).

In this situation if only the lateral vein is ligated (Fig. 28-3A), the normal venous drainage from the skin and subcutaneous tissue of the lower abdominal wall, flank, and buttock will pass down to the groin and then cause dilatation of the antero-lateral vein. It is therefore essential to find and ligate all three tributaries separately as in Fig. 28-3B.

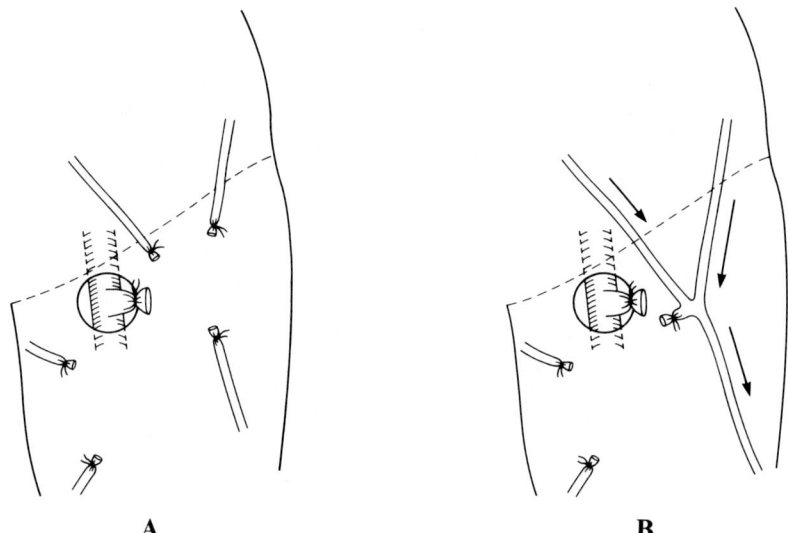

Fig. 28-3. Ligation of the lateral tributaries of the termination of the long saphenous vein:
(A) correct, (B) incorrect.

Long Saphenous Vein

There is now much academic support for not stripping the long saphenous vein because it is unnecessary, since the defect, i.e., the sapheno-femoral incompetence, has been eliminated and the long saphenous vein provides a useful donor for arterial surgery where it is associated with better patency rates than all other graft materials. This case is grossly overstated because the vast majority of vein patients are women who never require arterial surgery and male patients only present for vein surgery when the problem is gross and such pathological veins are unsuitable for arterial replacement. Only abnormal veins should be removed and the long saphenous vein is stripped down to just below the knee where the posterior arch vein, anterior tibial tributary, and perforating vein just below the knee (Boyd's) are included. The long saphenous vein in the lower leg is protected in a fascial tunnel and does not connect with any direct perforating veins. It can therefore be left, avoiding incisions at the ankle and the risk of damaging lymphatic vessels or the saphenous nerve. This part of the long saphenous vein can be used for coronary artery surgery. Furthermore, the perforating veins in the lower leg join the posterior arch vein, not the long saphenous vein. Stripping in a downward direction avoids damage to the lymphatics and nerves and longer lengths of tributaries are removed.

Some academic surgeons recommend flush sapheno-femoral ligations followed by sclerotherapy for all other veins. This is cumbersome, combining the most disabling part of both techniques. All other incisions can be less than 1 cm and only the bandages on the thigh are associated with discomfort and problems. Leaving the long saphenous vein in situ increases the chance of recurrence because there is a large vein for any persistent tributaries at the groin to rejoin and produce an early gross recurrence (Fig. 28-4).

If there are significant incompetent perforating veins in the thigh (Dodd's), leaving the long saphenous vein in the thigh is associated with early gross recur-

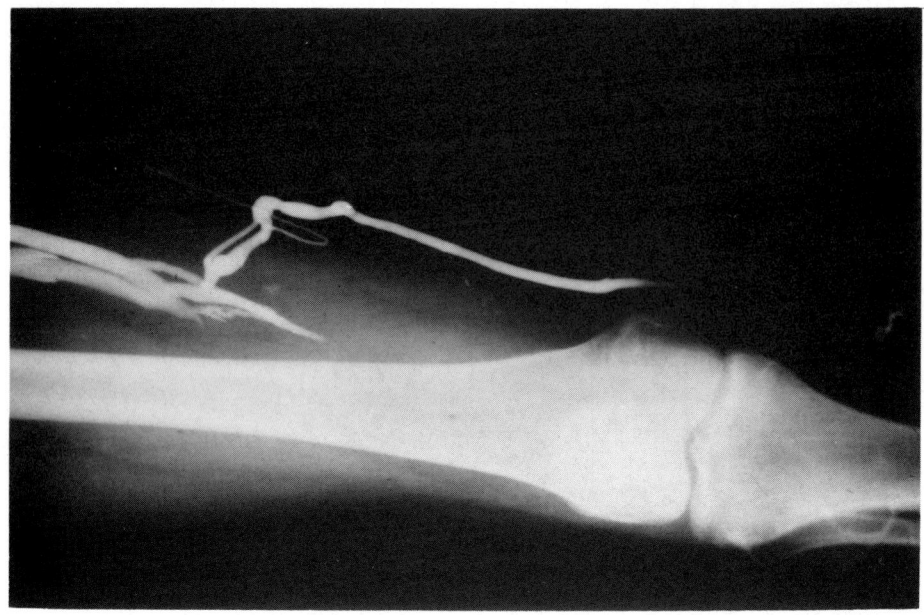

Fig. 28-5. Recurrence of long saphenous vein from incompetent mid-thigh perforating vein.

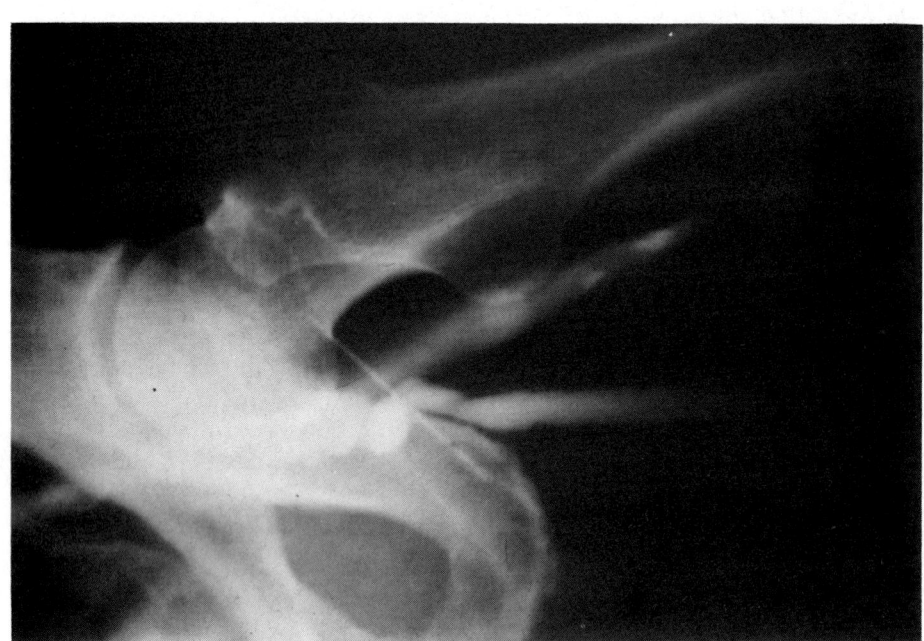

Fig. 28-4. Venogram showing persistent LSV after previous sapheno-femoral ligation.

rence (Fig. 28-5). In a random trial Jacobsen[2] compared full surgery, groin tie plus injection, and only injection in three matched groups, each comprising 160 patients with incompetence of the long saphenous vein. When reviewed at three years the success rate was 89.9% for full surgery, 65.2% for groin tie plus sclerotherapy, and 36.6% for sclerotherapy alone.

Perivulval Veins

It is not uncommon for varices to appear on and around the vulva during pregnancy and these may be associated with dilated veins over the buttock and down the back of the thigh. Sometimes these veins arise from sapheno-femoral incompetence via the superficial external pudendal vein, in which case standard surgery is effective. However, often there is an association with a retroverted uterus and large veins can be demonstrated in the broad ligament by direct venography (Fig. 28-6), retrograde selective venography, or peruterine venography.

Often there are veins on the posterior thigh but frequently the long saphenous vein territory is involved and proximally, instead of crossing the adductor tendon to join the sapheno-femoral junction, the veins terminate in the perivulval region (Fig. 28-7), communicating with the internal iliac vein via the internal pudendal or obturator veins and sometimes the inferior gluteal veins.

In most instances these veins are at the posterior part of the vulva but sometimes the anterior part of the labia is involved and venography will then demonstrate varices in the round ligament (Fig. 28-8), which communicate with the ovarian vein and are comparable with varicocele in the male, except that in women they are more common on the right side and often bilateral.

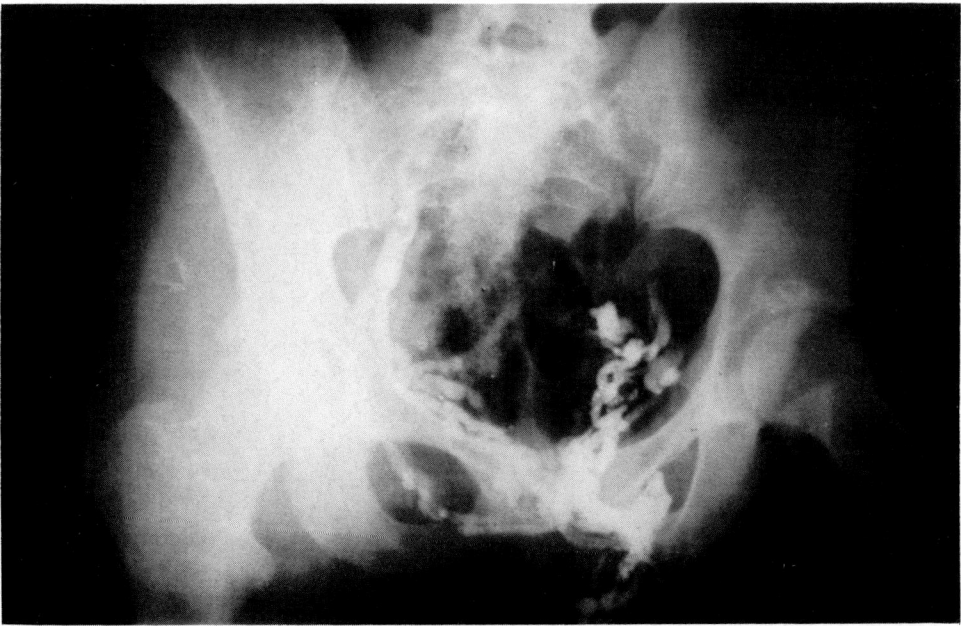

Fig. 28-6.   Venogram after injection of contrast into a left perivulval vein showing varices in the broad ligaments.

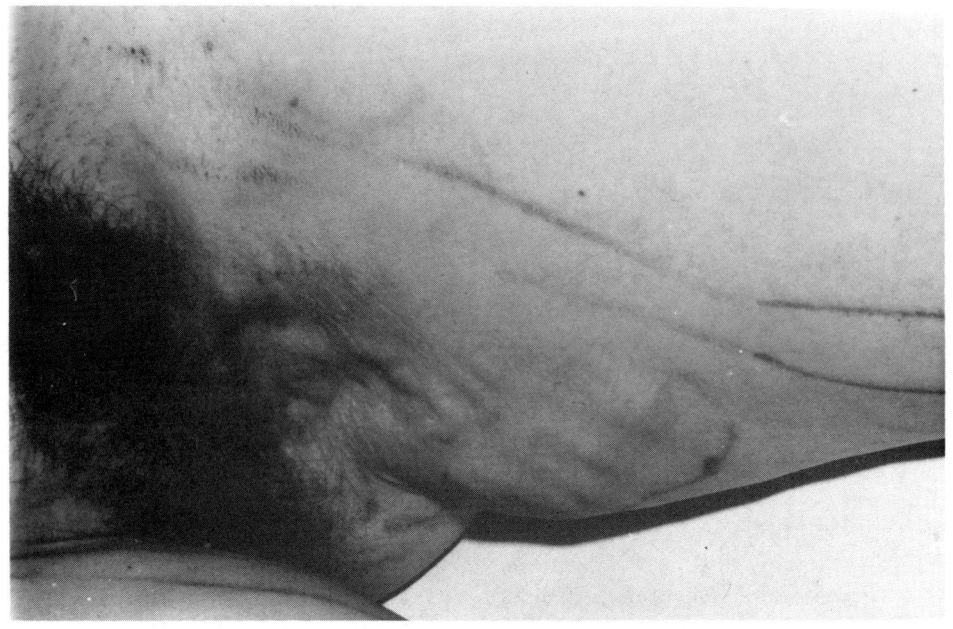

A

B

Fig. 28-7. (A) Long saphenous vein terminating proximally by communicating with varices in perivulval region (patient horizontal). (B) Venogram of veins seen in A.

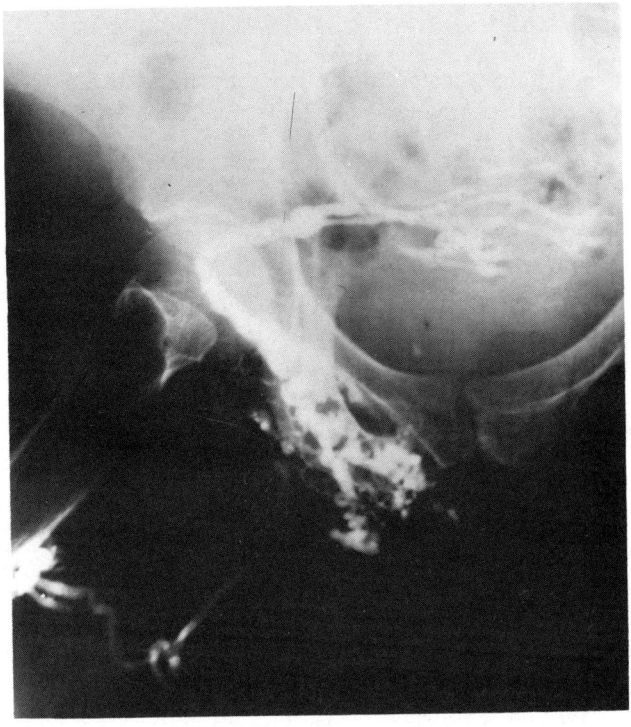

A

B

Fig. 28-8. (A) Venogram after injection of contrast into right-sided anterior vulval varices showing filling of round ligament veins and ovarian vein. (B) Cross section of round ligament (1.5 cm diameter) showing dilated veins.

To prevent recurrence these veins must be identified and dealt with while treating the leg veins. Further pregnancies are associated with an early recurrence of vulval varices.

Lateral Thigh Veins

It is often taught that large veins on the lateral aspect of the thigh are associated with the Klippel–Trenaunay syndrome, and although veins are frequently found in this situation such congenital vascular malformations are rare. It is possible to overlook a pale pink skin flush in some hairy male legs where there is no obvious soft tissue or bony enlargement and veins therefore recur because the underlying arterio-venous malformations cannot be eliminated.

However, the vast majority of veins on the lateral aspect of the thigh are associated with incompetence of the sapheno-femoral junction affecting only the antero-lateral vein, but the long saphenous vein and other tributaries have competent valves (Fig. 28-9).

If there is a large vein extending up to the sapheno-femoral junction the diagnosis is obvious. However, often in fat female thighs the only veins present are on the lateral aspect of the thigh extending down to the lateral calf and then to the anterior or posterior surface of the lower leg. The proximal antero-lateral tributary is not seen or the vein communicates with the long saphenous vein in the mid-thigh and the incompetent proximal segment of this vein is overlooked (Fig. 28-9B). The proximal communications of these veins can only be clearly demonstrated by venography which is best done as a one-shot on-table X-ray, injecting contrast media directly into the varicose vein (varicogram). Sometimes the lateral vein arises from the sapheno-femoral junction via the postero-medial tributary of the long saphenous vein.

Occasionally patients are seen who have persistent veins on the lateral aspect of the thigh despite numerous scars from several operations (Fig. 28-10A). Venography in such cases has demonstrated that these veins communicate with the profunda femoris vein via a large incompetent perforating vein which passes through the fascia lata (Fig. 28-10B).

The fascial defect is often above the clinical determined highest part of the vein. Guided by the X-ray a small vertical incision can be made to expose the fascial defect (Fig. 28-10). On ligating and dividing this perforating vein its proximal part retracts and the fascial defect is easily closed. The remaining vein can then be removed via several small incisions. Any smaller tributaries can later be eliminated by sclerotherapy. Once the fascial defect has been obliterated a good long-term result can be expected in such cases.

Short Saphenous Vein

Occasionally veins on the medial or lateral aspect of the lower thigh communicate with the sapheno-popliteal area, even though the short saphenous vein is normal. Varicosities on the medial or lateral aspect of the lower leg may also be associated with the sapheno-popliteal area.

The short saphenous vein is often overlooked because examination of the leg is inadequate. The proximal half of the short saphenous vein is beneath the strong

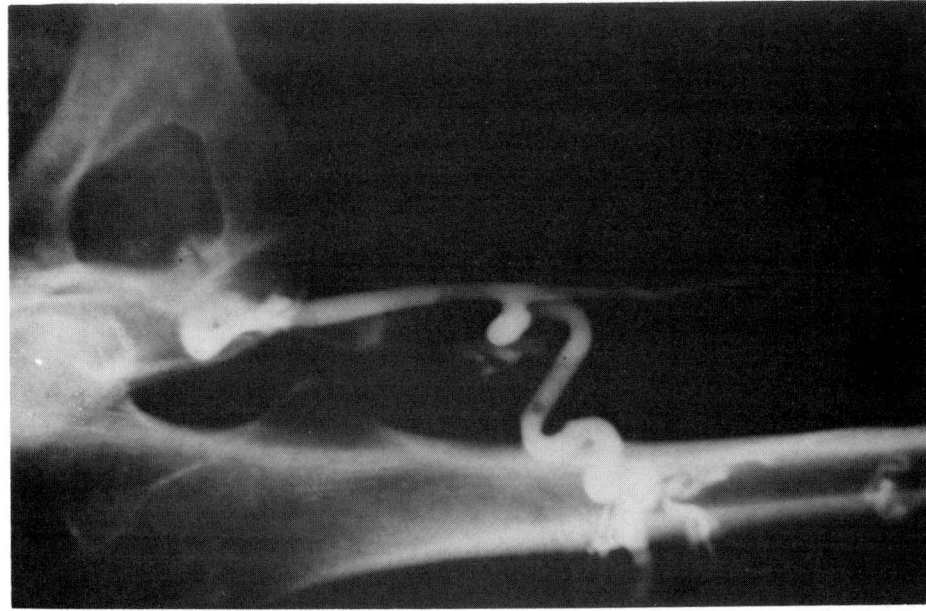

B

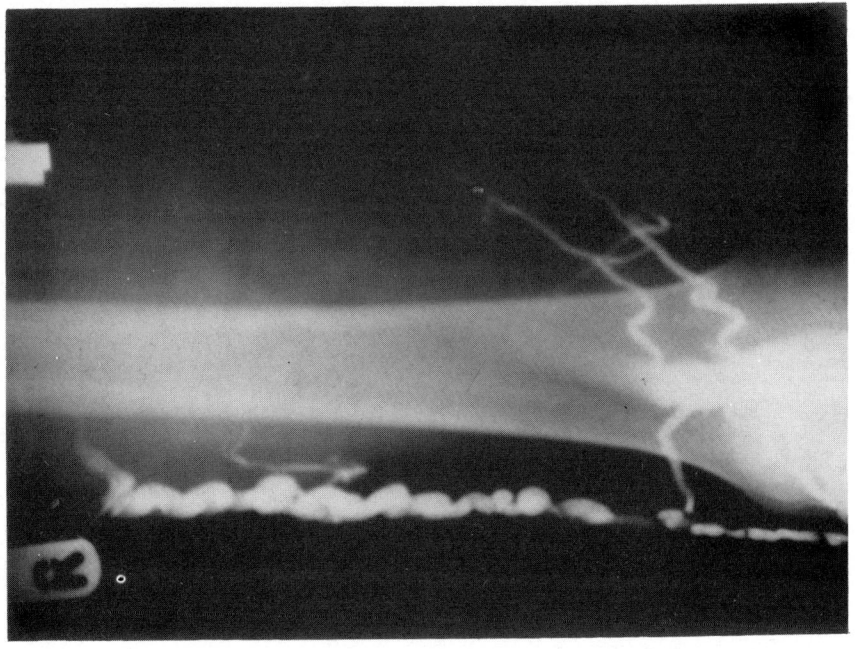

A

Fig. 28-9. (A) Venogram showing varicose lateral tributary on thigh with distal re-entry to tributaries of long saphenous vein in lower thigh an communications to the popliteal vein. (B) Venogram showing lateral veins communicating with long saphenous vein in mid-thigh.

367

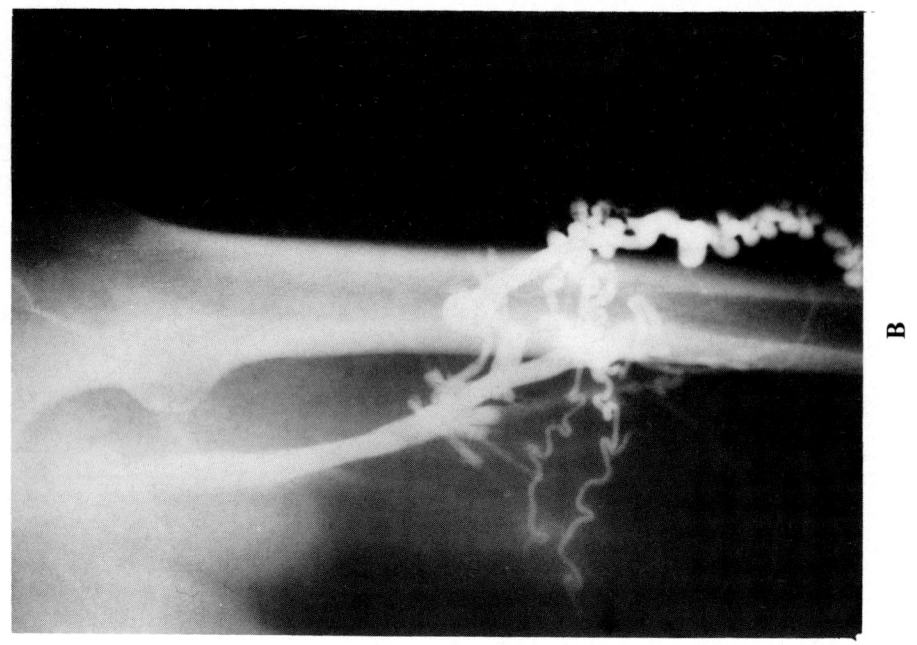

B

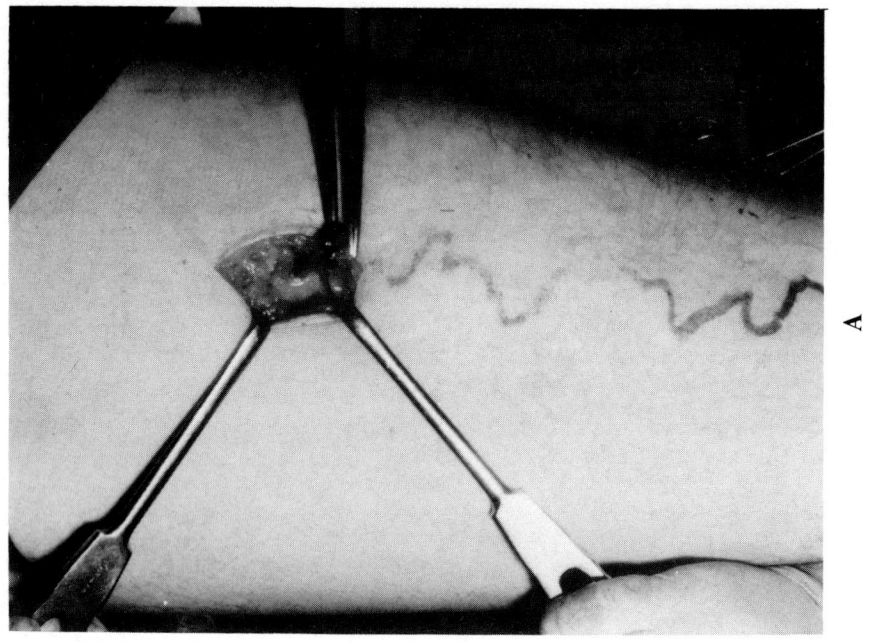

A

368

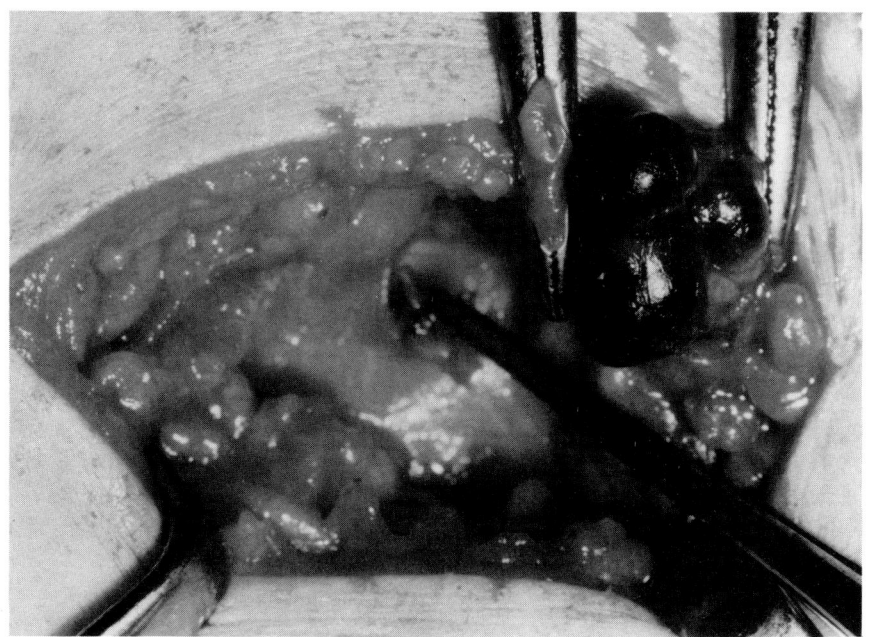

C

Fig. 28-10. (A) Lateral surface of thigh showing recurrent varices with scars of two previous operations. Incision exposing vein passing through fascia lata. (B) Venogram showing lateral vein joining profunda femoral vein. (C) Close-up of incision showing vein divided with clamp on proximal stump in fascial defect of fascia lata.

369

deep fascia and even a grossly dilated short saphenous vein cannot sometimes be felt until the knee is slightly flexed to relax the popliteal fossa. Often recurrent veins in the long saphenous vein territory are associated with an incompetent short saphenous vein which has been missed. The diagnosis of short saphenous vein incompetence may be assisted by examination with Doppler ultrasound, but this may produce errors because of variations in the anatomy.[7] Many surgeons do not appreciate the wide variations in the level and patterns of termination of the short saphenous vein. It is generally taught that it is sufficient to divide and tie this vein beneath the deep fascia. However, this is associated with a significant recurrence rate and it was because of the frequency of seeing many such cases who had previously been treated by competent vascular surgeons that peroperative venography was introduced[8] and is now widely practised. This simple technique enables accurate surgery through small incisions often well above the popliteal skin crease. It is claimed that the popliteal fossa must be explored until the sapheno-popliteal junction is found,[9] but often the short saphenous vein does not communicate with the popliteal vein.

Embryologically the short saphenous vein was the postaxial vein of the hind limb and drained into the internal iliac vein. In 1926, Kosinski[10] suggested that the subsequent transformation into a short saphenous vein terminating at the popliteal vein was an adaptation to the elongation and relative rigidity of the hind limb. Hence, although the majority of short saphenous veins terminate at the popliteal vein, it is not unusual to find the short saphenous vein ending in the mid-thigh by communicating with the deep femoral vein, the superficial femoral vein, or the long saphenous vein. Sometimes the short saphenous vein continues up to join the long saphenous vein in the groin and occasionally it joins the internal iliac vein via the internal pudendal, gluteal, or sciatic veins. The various terminations of the short saphenous vein have been reported by several workers who all found a similar distribution. Peroperative venography has been used in more than 1500 operations since 1970 and 860 were to demonstrate the short saphenous vein. Some of these variations in relation to surgery were recently reported.[11] Various extensive incisions have been described to enable adequate exploration of the popliteal fossa. However, peroperative venography enables accurate surgery through small incisions placed precisely from the X-ray findings.

A true sapheno-popliteal junction is present in 60% with the level of this junction between 2 and 7 cm above the knee joint (half of these are between 3 and 5 cm) (Fig. 28-11A). In another 30% there is no communication to the popliteal vein, but the short saphenous vein continues into the thigh and terminates high by joining the long saphenous vein, usually via the postero-medial tributary at the groin (Fig. 28-11B), sometimes via the posterior vein to the deep femoral vein or to tributaries of the internal iliac vein. The remaining 10% terminate in the calf either by joining the long saphenous vein or by joining the gastrocnemius vein via a mid-calf perforator. Venography is therefore essential to accurately determine the pattern and level of the sapheno-popliteal junction and is especially useful when treating recurrent vein problems (Fig. 28-12).

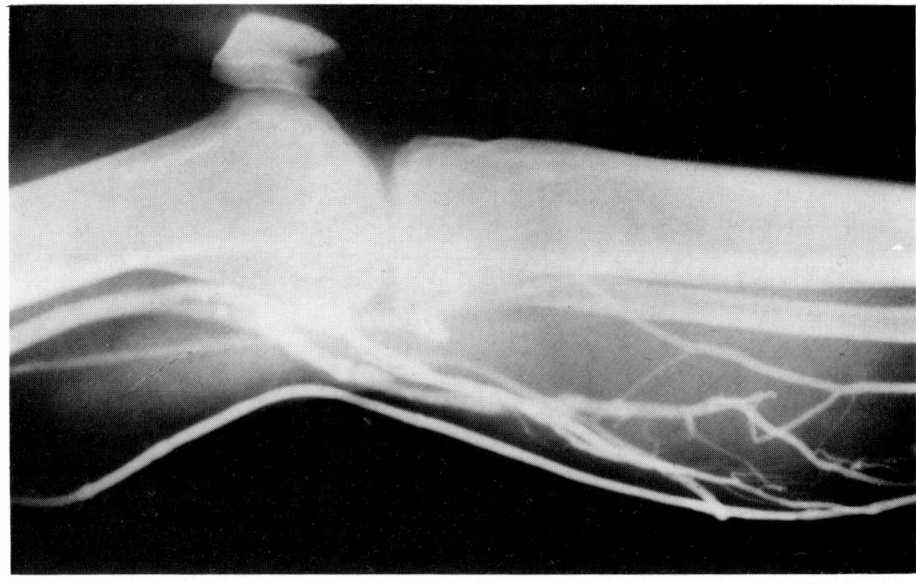

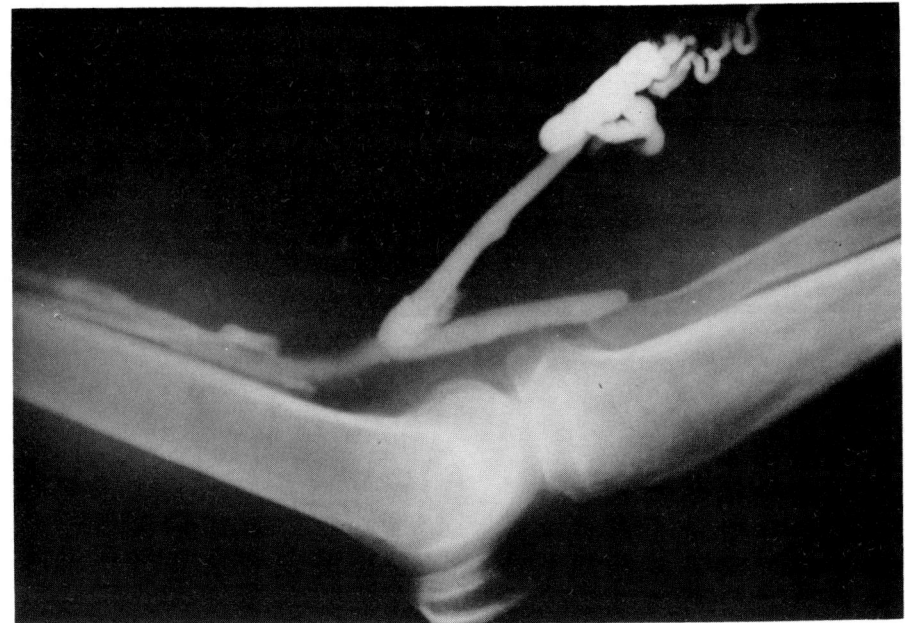

Fig. 28-11. (A) Peroperative venogram showing typical sapheno-popliteal junction and varicosities of short saphenous vein. (B) Venogram showing short saphenous continuing up to postero-medial tributary of LSV with no communication to popliteal vein; the gastrocnemius veins are filled via the mid-calf perforating vein.

371

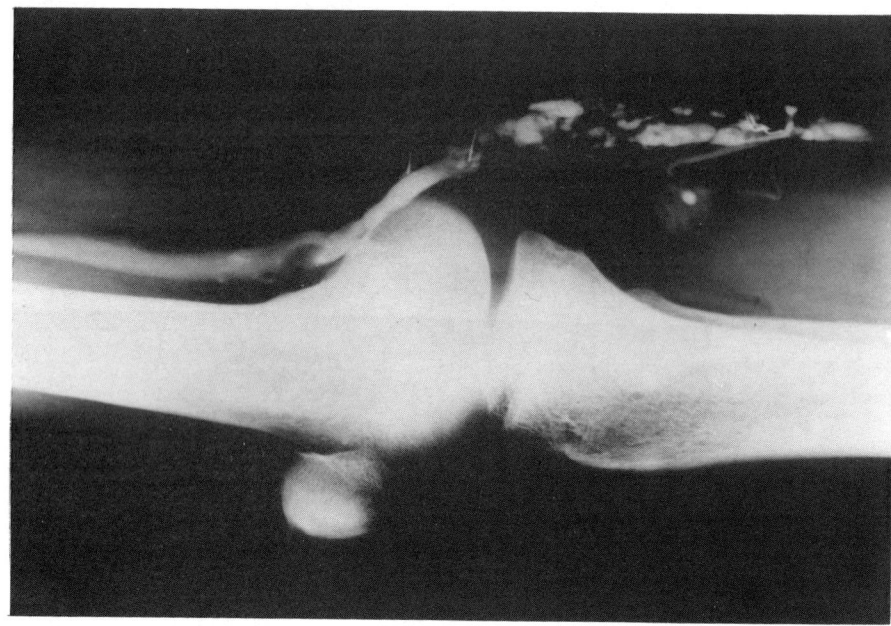

B

A

Fig. 28-12. Peroperative venogram showing sapheno-popliteal junction above previous ligation with recurrent varices: (A) rejoining persistent SSV, (B) in territory of SSV.

CONCLUSION

Many so-called recurrent varicose veins are really persistent veins because the previous surgery was inadequate and failed to eliminate the problem. Dilated superficial veins and venules cannot be permanently cured because there is an inherent weakness of the skin and supporting tissue of the superficial veins. Secondary veins associated with the postthrombotic syndrome or congenital arterio-venous fistula are best controlled by sclerotherapy because the underlying problem cannot be removed.

The majority of significant vein problems are associated with incompetence of the perforating veins, the most important of which are the termination of the saphenous veins. These should be cured if properly treated; this requires careful examination, precise planning, and accurate execution. Because experience takes so long to acquire and patients should not suffer during this training phase, better teaching of the assessment and management of venous disease is essential if recurrence is to be minimised.

REFERENCES

1. Hobbs JT: Surgery of sclerotherapy for varicose veins: 10 year results of a random trial, in Tesi M, Dormandy J (eds): Superficial and Deep Venous Diseases of the Lower Limbs. Milan, Edizione Minerva Medica, 1984, pp 243–248
2. Jacobsen BH: The value of different forms of treatment for varicose veins. Br J Surg 66:182–184, 1979
3. Neglen P, Einarsson E, Jonsson B, Eklof B: Socio-economic benefits of ambulatory surgery or compression sclerotherapy (CST) of varicose veins. Ab Book of 1st UK Meeting Union Internationale de Phlebologie, London, 1985, pp 18–11
4. Lord JW Jr: The surgical management of recurrent varicose veins, in Bergan JJ, Yao ST (eds): Venous Problems. Chicago, Year Book Publishers, 1978, Ch 6, pp 85–88
5. Harper DR: Presented at Colloquium on Surgery of the Venous System, Royal College of Surgeons of Edinburgh, 8 January 1985
6. Villavicencio JL: Presented at International Vascular Symposium, London, 17 September 1981
7. Hobbs JT: Errors in the differential diagnosis of incompetence of the popliteal vein by Doppler ultrasound. J Cardiovasc Surg 27:169–174, 1986
8. Hobbs JT: Peroperative venography to ensure accurate sapheno-popliteal ligation. Br Med J 1:1578–1579, 1980
9. Rivlin S: Primary varicose veins. Surg Rev 2:331–333, 1981
10. Kosinski C: Observations on the superficial venous system of the lower extremities. J Anat 60:131–142, 1926
11. Hobbs JT: A new approach to short saphenous vein varicosities, in Bergan JJ, Yao ST (eds): Surgery of Veins. Orlando, Grune and Stratton, 1985, pp 301–321

Russell D. Hull
and Gary E. Raskob

29

Prevention of Venous Thromboembolism

INTRODUCTION

Pulmonary embolism has long been recognized as one of the most important complications of both medical and surgical patients, and it remains the commonest preventable cause of death in hospital, being responsible for 100,000 or more deaths each year in the United States.[1] Many of these embolic deaths occur in terminally ill patients, but a significant proportion occur in patients who would otherwise have survived to lead a normal life, e.g., in patients undergoing elective major surgery. In the absence of prophylaxis, the frequency of postoperative fatal pulmonary embolism ranges from 0.1–0.8% in patients undergoing elective general surgery[2,3] to 0.3–1.7% in patients undergoing elective hip surgery[4] to 4–7% in patients undergoing emergency hip surgery.[5,6]

The majority of patients who die from pulmonary embolism do so suddenly with little or no warning, and, in many cases, a diagnosis of pulmonary embolism is not established until after the patient's death.[1] Therefore, the prevention of deaths due to pulmonary embolism lies with the vigorous use of prophylactic measures rather than therapy. Although anticoagulant therapy is highly effective for preventing death and morbidity from venous thromboembolism, two-thirds of patients who die from pulmonary embolism succumb within 30 minutes after the acute event[7] before anticoagulant treatment can be initiated or take effect. It should be emphasized that effective prophylaxis against venous thromboembolism is now available for most high-risk patients and the use of primary prophylaxis is a much more effective approach for preventing death and morbidity from pulmonary embolism than is treatment of the established event. It has been estimated that the routine use of effective prophylactic measures in patients undergoing elective general surgery, for example, could prevent 4000–8000 postoperative deaths each year in the United States.[8]

Many hospitals lack an organized strategy for preventing venous thromboembolism.[9,10] There are several reasons for this apparent oversight. First, because death from pulmonary embolism is a relatively rare event in an individual surgeon's experience, a busy surgeon may have to operate on a large number of patients before being reminded of the lethality of pulmonary embolism. Second, there are doubts about the safety of antithrombotic drugs and the effectiveness of all forms of prophylaxis. Finally, at the institutional level, there has been a reluctance to add interventions whose cost-effectiveness has not been adequately evaluated.[9,10]

The purpose of this article is to provide an overview of the currently available approaches for preventing venous thromboembolism (venous thrombosis and/or pulmonary embolism).

RISK FACTORS FOR VENOUS THROMBOEMBOLISM

A number of clinical risk factors for venous thromboembolism have been identified and include advanced age, previous venous thromboembolism, prolonged immobility or paralysis, malignant disease, obesity, varicose veins, oral contraceptive use, and congestive heart failure.[11,12] In addition, certain surgical procedures such as orthopaedic surgery to the lower limbs, or extensive pelvic or abdominal surgery for advanced malignant disease, are associated with a particularly high risk of postoperative venous thromboembolism.

Table 29-1
Classification of the Risk of Postoperative Venous Thromboembolism

Risk Category	Risk of Venous Thromboembolism (%)		
	Calf Vein Thrombosis	Proximal Vein Thrombosis	Fatal Pulmonary Embolism
High risk 1. General surgery in patients >40 years with recent history of DVT or PE 2. Extensive pelvic or abdominal surgery for malignant disease 3. Major orthopaedic surgery of lower limbs	40–80	10–20	1–5
Moderate risk* 1. General surgery in patients >40 years lasting 30 min or more	10–40	2–10	0.1–0.7
Low risk 1. Uncomplicated surgery in patients <40 years with no additional risk factors 2. Minor surgery (i.e., less than 30 min) in patients >40 years with no additional risk factors	<10	<1	<0.01

* Risk is increased by advancing age, malignancy, prolonged immobility, cardiac failure, and varicose veins.

In general, patients can be classified as either low, moderate, or high risk for developing venous thromboembolism;[12] this classification is summarized in Table 29-1.

Low-risk patients are those under the age of 40 without additional risk factors who have an uncomplicated elective abdominal or thoracic surgical procedure or those over the age 40 without additional risk factors who have minor elective abdominal or thoracic surgery (i.e., surgery under general anaesthesia for less than 30 minutes). In the absence of prophylaxis, these patients have less than a 10% risk of developing calf vein thrombosis, less than a 1% risk of developing proximal venous thrombosis (thrombosis involving the popliteal or more proximal deep veins of the leg), and less than a 0.01% risk of fatal pulmonary embolism.[12]

Moderate-risk surgical patients are defined as those patients over the age of 40 who have elective general abdominal or thoracic surgery performed under general anaesthesia which lasts for at least 30 minutes. The risk of venous thromboembolism in these patients is increased by advancing age, the presence of malignancy, prolonged bedrest, extensive surgical dissection, large bowel surgery, varicose veins, and obesity.[11] In the absence of prophylaxis, patients in the moderate-risk category have a 10–40% risk of developing calf vein thrombosis, a 2–10% risk of proximal vein thrombosis, and a 0.1–0.7% risk of fatal pulmonary embolism.[12] High-risk surgical patients are those who have a history of recent venous thromboembolism who require surgery, and those who undergo extensive pelvic or abdominal surgery for advanced malignant disease, or major orthopaedic surgery of the lower limbs. In the absence of prophylaxis, these patients have a 40–80% risk of developing calf vein thrombosis, a 10–20% risk of proximal vein thrombosis, and a 1–5% risk of fatal pulmonary embolism.[12]

APPROACHES TO THE PROPHYLAXIS OF VENOUS THROMBOEMBOLISM

Two approaches can be taken to prevent fatal pulmonary embolism. These approaches are *primary prophylaxis* using either drugs or physical methods which are effective for preventing deep vein thrombosis and pulmonary embolism, and *secondary prevention* by the early detection and treatment of subclinical venous thrombosis (before pulmonary embolism occurs) by screening patients postoperatively with objective diagnostic tests (e.g., ^{125}I-fibrinogen leg scanning) that are sensitive for venous thrombosis. Primary prophylaxis is likely to be more effective, less expensive, and is the prophylaxis of choice in most clinical circumstances.[9,10,12] The ideal primary prophylactic approach should be effective, free of clinically important side effects, and well accepted by patients, nurses, and medical staff. It should also be easily administered, inexpensive, and require minimal monitoring. Secondary prevention by screening should never replace primary prophylaxis, and is reserved for those patients in whom effective primary prophylaxis is either contra-indicated or unavailable. Postoperative screening may also be used to supplement primary prophylaxis in very high-risk patients, e.g., those who have suffered a recent episode of venous thrombosis and who require surgery.

A number of primary prophylactic approaches have been evaluated by randomized clinical trials and are effective for preventing venous thrombosis and pulmonary embolism. The most thoroughly tested approaches are low-dose sub-cutaneous heparin,[13,34] intermittent pneumatic compression of the legs,[35–48] oral anticoagulants,[5,49–56] and intravenous dextran.[19,33,57–64] Other promising approaches include adjusted doses of subcutaneous heparin,[65] graduated compression stockings,[66,67] and combined modalities such as the combination of the veno-constrictor dihydroergotamine (DHE) and low doses of heparin,[68,69] and the combination of intravenous dextran plus intermittent pneumatic compression.[70] Antiplatelet agents, such as aspirin, have a very limited role for preventing venous thromboembolism.[12,70–85] Although none of the above approaches meet all of the criteria for an ideal prophylactic approach, most of these criteria are met by low-dose heparin or intermittent pneumatic compression.

The effectiveness and safety of the alternative prophylactic approaches varies for the different risk categories and also according to different surgical groups (e.g., general surgical patients versus patients undergoing hip surgery). Selection of the most appropriate preventative approach for different clinical settings is an important aspect of prophylaxis (see "Choice of Prophylaxis for the Alternative-risk Categories and Different Surgical Groups").

Pathophysiologic Basis for the Alternative Prophylactic Measures

Venous thrombi usually develop at sites of slow or disturbed flow and begin as small deposits of platelets, fibrin, and red cells in venous valve cusp pockets or in the intramuscular sinuses of the leg veins.[86] As the thrombus grows, it occludes the lumen of the vein producing stasis, and then extends both proximally and distally as a coagulation thrombus composed of red cells with interspersed fibrin. The mechanisms which are recognized to be important in the pathogenesis of venous thrombo-embolism are venous stasis, activation of blood coagulation, and vascular endothelial damage.[86] The primary prophylactic methods which have been evaluated clinically have been directed at one or more of these pathogenic factors and include anticoagulants which counteract the activation of blood coagulation; drugs which suppress platelet function and the interaction of platelets with the damaged vessel wall; and mechanical devices which prevent venous stasis in the leg veins increasing venous flow in the lower extremities. On theoretical grounds, combined prophylactic approaches which interact against two or more of the above pathogenic factors for venous thromboembolism are attractive. For example, the combination of low-dose heparin with the venoconstrictor dihydroergotamine (DHE) prevents the activation of blood coagulation and also counteracts venous stasis in the leg veins.

Low-dose Heparin

Low-dose heparin prevents thrombosis by inhibiting the blood coagulation cascade. It markedly accelerates the rate of inhibition by antithrombin III of the coagulation factors XII_a, XI_a, IX_a, X_a, and thrombin. Because the activation process is amplifed by each successive step in the coagulation cascade, much lower doses of heparin are required to inhibit the initiation of blood coagulation than are required for the treatment of established venous thromboembolism.[12]

Low-dose subcutaneous heparin is usually given in a dose of 5000 units two hours preoperatively, and then either 12 hourly or 8 hourly postoperatively. This form of prophylaxis is not only effective for preventing calf vein thrombosis but is also effective for preventing proximal vein thrombosis and major pulmonary embolism.[12–25, 29] It is one of the measures of choice for preventing thromboembolism in moderate- and high-risk general surgical patients.[9, 10, 12–25, 29, 33] Although low-dose heparin prophylaxis is effective, its acceptance has been delayed and its use somewhat limited by the fear that it induces bleeding. This fear is not supported by the evidence to date, and, in particular, the use of 5000 units of heparin every 12 hours has not been associated with a clinically or statistically significant increased risk of bleeding in general surgical patients.[12, 13] However, because of the potential for bleeding, it should not be used in patients undergoing cerebral, eye, or spinal surgery. In patients undergoing hip surgery or prostatic surgery, low-dose heparin is of limited effectiveness and is not the prophylaxis of choice in these two patient groups.[12, 26–28, 30, 41]

Low-dose heparin has the advantage that it does not require anticoagulant monitoring and is administered by a relatively simple and convenient method.

Intermittent Pneumatic Leg Compression

Intermittent pneumatic leg compression prevents venous thrombosis by enhancing blood flow in the deep veins of the legs, thus preventing venous stasis. It also increases blood fibrinolytic activity and this effect may contribute to its anti-thrombotic properties.[12] Intermittent pneumatic leg compression is an attractive form of prophylaxis which is effective for preventing venous thrombosis in moderate-risk general surgical patients and in patients undergoing neurosurgery, major knee surgery, prostatic surgery, and pelvic surgery.[34–48] It is the prophylaxis of choice in a number of patient groups in which low-dose heparin is either contra-indicated or ineffective.[12, 39–43] In patients undergoing hip surgery, intermittent pneumatic compression of the calf has been shown to prevent calf vein thrombosis, but it is relatively ineffective in preventing thigh vein thrombosis.[12] Recently, a combined calf and thigh intermittent compression device has been produced which may be more effective in preventing thigh vein thrombosis in patients undergoing hip surgery.[46]

Intermittent pneumatic leg compression is virtually free of clinically important side effects and offers a valuable alternative to patients who have a high risk of bleeding. It may produce discomfort in the occasional patient, and in patients with overt evidence of leg ischaemia caused by peripheral vascular disease, intermittent pneumatic compression should not be used. A variety of well-accepted, comfortable, and effective intermittent pneumatic devices are currently available, which may be applied preoperatively, at the time of operation, or in the early postoperative period. Intermittent pneumatic compression should be continued for the entire period while the patient is confined to bed and until the patient is fully ambulant.

Oral Anticoagulants

Oral anticoagulants prevent thrombosis by inhibiting the synthesis of functionally active vitamin-K-dependent coagulation factors II, VII, IX, and X. Multiple studies have established the effectiveness of oral anticoagulants for preventing venous thrombosis and pulmonary embolism.[5, 49–56] When administered in doses which prolong the prothrombin time to 1.5–2 times control (using rabbit brain thromboplastin), oral anticoagulants are highly effective both for preventing post-operative venous thromboembolism (in all risk categories)[5, 49–56] and for preventing recurrent venous thromboembolism in patients with established proximal vein thrombosis.[87] Prophylaxis with oral anticoagulants can be commenced pre-operatively, at the time of operation, or in the early postoperative period. The use of oral anticoagulants commenced at the time of surgery or early postoperatively may not prevent the formation of small venous thrombi which form soon after surgery because the anticoagulant effect is not achieved until the third or fourth postoperative day. However, prophylaxis with oral anticoagulants commenced at the time of surgery or in the early postoperative period is effective for inhibiting the extension of these thrombi and has the potential to prevent clinically significant venous thromboembolism.

Oral anticoagulant prophylaxis, when administered preoperatively or at the time of surgery in doses that prolong the prothrombin time to 1.5–2 times control (using rabbit brain thromboplastin, corresponding to an international normalized ratio of 4–7), may be associated with a higher frequency of clinically important bleeding complications than the other prophylactic modalities in current use, and the perceived risk of bleeding complications has limited the acceptance of oral anti-coagulant prophylaxis. A recent study[56] in patients undergoing major orthopaedic surgery of the lower limbs has provided important new information about the relationship between the intensity of the anticoagulant effect and the effectiveness and safety of oral anticoagulant prophylaxis. In a randomized clinical trial of 100 patients, Francis and coworkers compared the efficacy and safety of warfarin sodium with dextran 40 for preventing venous thrombosis in patients undergoing elective total hip or knee replacement (a high-risk group).[56] A low dose of warfarin was started 10–14 days preoperatively and the dose of warfarin was adjusted to maintain the prothrombin time (using rabbit brain thromboplastin) between 1.5 and 3 seconds longer than the control at the time of surgery. Immediately after surgery, the dose was increased to prolong the prothrombin time to 1.5 times control. Thus, warfarin was administered in a two-step regimen with the intent to avoid bleeding complications while retaining effectiveness for preventing venus thrombosis. The overall frequency of venous thrombosis and the frequency of proximal vein throm-bosis were both statistically and clinically significantly lower in patients receiving the two-step warfarin prophylactic regimen. Postoperative bleeding was similar and infrequent (4%) in both treatment groups. These findings indicate that by decreasing the intensity of the anticoagulant effect of warfarin, the risk of bleeding can be substantially reduced while retaining effectiveness for preventing venous thrombo-embolism. The results of Francis and coworkers are supported by the findings of Taberner and coworkers in general surgical patients[55] and by the results of a recent randomized trial of less intense warfarin for the long-term treatment of established proximal vein thrombosis.[87]

At present, oral anticoagulant prophylaxis is not accepted as a routine form of prophylaxis because of the increased risk of major clinical bleeding, although it is regarded by some authorities as the prophylactic measure of choice in patients undergoing hip surgery. Oral anticoagulant prophylaxis is relatively inconvenient because it requires careful anticoagulant monitoring with frequent prothrombin times.

Dextran

Dextran is a glucose polymer which was introduced as a volume expander and was subsequently evaluated as an antithrombotic agent. Two sizes of dextran polymer have been used clinically: dextran 70 with a mean molecular weight of 70,000 and dextran 40 with a mean molecular weight of 40,000. The antithrombotic properties of dextran have been attributed to a number of actions including decreased blood viscosity, reduced platelet interaction with the damaged vessel wall, and an increased susceptibility for fibrin clots formed in the presence of dextran to undergo fibrinolysis.

Dextran 40, administered intravenously in a volume of 500 millilitres over four to six hours commencing at the time of operation and then daily for two to five days postoperatively, is an effective form of prophylaxis in moderate-risk general surgical patients and in patients undergoing hip surgery.[12, 19, 33, 57–64] Dextran is well tolerated by most patients, but its use may be complicated by volume overload in patients who have impaired cardiac function, particularly in the elderly patient with unrecognized cardiac impairment. Hypersensitivity reactions to dextran occur as an uncommon side effect. By comparison with low-dose subcutaneous heparin, the administration of dextran is relatively inconvenient, requiring the maintenance of an intravenous line.

Adjusted-dose Subcutaneous Heparin

Moderate adjusted doses of subcutaneous heparin is a promising approach to prophylaxis in high-risk patients in whom low-dose heparin is of limited effectiveness or is ineffective (e.g., hip surgery). Leyvarz and coworkers[65] have reported a randomized trial in patients undergoing elective hip surgery using a prophylactic approach which overcame the thrombotic tendency by increasing the dose of subcutaneous heparin to a level that restores towards normal the shortened activated partial thromboplastin time which occurs in response to operation, without producing therapeutic anticoagulation. These investigators demonstrated that the shortening of the activated partial thromboplastin time that occurs during the first postoperative week can be restored to normal, and venous thrombosis prevented, by using adjusted doses of subcutaneous heparin. Seventy-nine patients undergoing elective hip arthroplasty were randomly allocated to receive either fixed low-dose (3500 IU) heparin subcutaneously every eight hours or to the alternate approach utilizing an initial dose of 3500 IU which was then adjusted to maintain the activated partial thromboplastin time between 31.5 and 36 seconds. Subcutaneous heparin prophylaxis was commenced in both groups two days preoperatively and was continued for at least seven to nine days postoperatively. From the day of surgery to the eighth day postoperatively, patients receiving the adjusted heparin regimen required progressively more heparin to maintain the activated partial thromboplastin time in the prescribed range. Venography revealed deep vein thrombosis in only 5 of 38 patients (14%) in the adjusted heparin group compared with 16 of 41 patients (39%) in the fixed low-dose heparin group ($p < 0.01$).[65] The frequency of proximal vein thrombosis (thrombosis involving the popliteal, femoral, or iliac veins) was strikingly reduced in the adjusted heparin group (5%) compared with the fixed low-dose heparin group (32%) ($p < 0.003$). The increased protection provided by adjusted-dose subcutaneous heparin was not associated with an increased frequency of bleeding complications. The number of units of blood transfused, the frequency of postoperative wound hematomas, and the drop in hemoglobin levels were identical in the two groups. Based on the findings of Leyvarz and workers, it appears that adjusted-dose heparin prophylaxis is an effective and safe method for preventing venous thrombosis in patients undergoing elective total hip replacement. Further randomized clinical trials are required to confirm these results and determine the place of adjusted-dose subcutaneous heparin prophylaxis in other high-risk patient groups.

Graduated Compression Stockings

Graduated compression stockings reduce venous stasis in the limb by applying a graded degree of compression to the ankle and the calf, with greater pressure being applied more distally in the limb. Recent studies have demonstrated graduated compression stockings to be effective for preventing postoperative venous thrombosis in low-risk general surgical patients.[66, 67] Graduated compression stockings are inexpensive and provide a convenient form of prophylaxis which is free of clinically important side effects. However, the effectiveness of graduated compression stockings for preventing venous thromboembolism in moderate- and high-risk patients is currently uncertain.[12]

Aspirin

The antithrombotic effect of aspirin has been attributed to its modulation of platelet function by inhibiting the synthesis of prostaglandins and related compounds (i.e., thromboxane A_2) in platelets.[12] It was originally hoped that the antiplatelet action of aspirin would provide effective prophylaxis against postoperative venous thromboembolism. Aspirin prophylaxis, although inexpensive and highly convenient, has limited application, if any, because of its relative ineffectiveness. The randomized clinical trials performed to date have produced conflicting results.[12, 70–85] At best, aspirin may be effective for preventing venous thrombosis in men undergoing elective hip surgery, but conflicting findings have also been reported in this patient group.[12, 77–85]

Based on the reported differential effect of aspirin on platelet thromboxane production and on prostacyclin generation by the vessel wall, the hypothesis has been advanced that low doses of aspirin would be more effective in antithrombotic prophylaxis than medium or high doses. Harris and coworkers[70] have recently reported a randomized trial comparing the effectiveness of 0.3 g of aspirin daily with 1.2 g of aspirin daily for preventing venous thrombosis infollowing elective hip surgery. The overall frequencies of venous thrombosis is the low-dose and high-dose aspirin groups were 61 and 60% respectively.[70] These findings indicate that the lower dose of aspirin has no prophylactic advantage.

Combined Prophylactic Modalities

The use of combined prophylactic approaches (e.g., low-dose heparin plus dihydroergotamine (DHE) or low-dose heparin plus intermittent pneumatic compression) is based on the concept that venous thromboembolism can be more effectively prevented by counteracting two or more of the pathogenic factors promoting the development of postoperative venous thrombosis.[12,86] There is currently only limited data on the effectiveness of combined prophylactic modalities. Recent data suggest that the combined use of low-dose heparin plus DHE is more effective in reducing the frequency of venous thrombosis than an equivalent dose of low-dose heparin alone.[68,69] Promising results have also been obtained with the use of intermittent pneumatic compression combined with intravenous dextran in patients undergoing elective hip replacement. Harris and workers[70] evaluated the effectiveness and safety of external pneumatic compression of the calf and thigh combined with a three-day course of low molecular weight dextran. The combined modality of leg compression and dextran resulted in a striking reduction in the frequency of postoperative venous thrombosis (a frequency of 21%) which was both statistically and clinically significant compared with the relatively high frequencies of postoperative venous thrombosis in the regular-dose aspirin (1.2 g a day) and low-dose aspirin (0.3 g) groups (60 and 61% respectively). The combination of external pneumatic compression using a device with four chambers compressing the calf and two compressing the thigh (with sequential filling in a distal to proximal direction), with intravenous dextran, was effective in preventing both calf and proximal venous thrombi. Dextran appeared to be associated with excessive bleeding when administered in doses of more than 500 ml during the operation; when administered in lesser doses, excessive bleeding was not observed.

CHOICE OF PROPHYLAXIS FOR THE ALTERNATIVE-RISK CATEGORIES AND DIFFERENT SURGICAL GROUPS

The applicability of the different forms of prophylaxis varies among the different risk categories and according to the particular surgical procedure.[12] The definition of low-, moderate-, and high-risk surgical patients, and the risk of venous thromboembolism in each of these categories, is summarized in Table 29-1. Within the moderate- and high-risk categories, the choice of prophylaxis is influenced by the type of surgical procedure and by the risk of bleeding. The recommended prophylactic approaches for the alternative patient risk categories and surgical group are summarized in Table 29-2.

Elective General Abdominal and Thoracic Surgery

The definition of low, moderate, or high risk in patients undergoing elective general abdominal or thoracic surgery is outlined in Table 29-1. In low-risk patients, early ambulation should be encouraged, and it would be reasonable to use graduated compression stockings as the only form of prophylaxis, provided the patient does not develop complications which require confinement to bed.

Moderate-risk general surgical patients should be given prophylaxis either with low-dose heparin or with intermittent pneumatic compression. Dextran is an effective alternative but is slightly more expensive and is less convenient because it must be administered by intravenous infusion.

Table 29-2

Recommended Prophylactic Approaches for the Alternative
Patient Risk Categories and Different Surgical Groups

Risk Category	Recommended Approach(es)
Low risk	Graduated compression stockings
Moderate risk	
General abdominal or thoracic surgery*	Low-dose heparin
	Intermittent pneumatic compression
	Dextran
Neurosurgery	Intermittent pneumatic compression
Genitourinary surgery	Intermittent pneumatic compression
High risk	
General abdominal or thoracic surgery	Oral anticoagulants
	Low-dose heparin (q8h) ± intermittent pneumatic compression
	Low-dose heparin + DHE
	Adjusted-dose heparin
Elective hip surgery	Oral anticoagulants
	Adjusted-dose heparin
	Dextran ± intermittent pneumatic compression
Fractured hip	Oral anticoagulants
	Dextran
Major knee surgery	Intermittent pneumatic compression

* In patients with a high risk of bleeding (e.g., spinal anasthaesia), intermittent pneumatic
compression is the prophylaxis of choice.

The relative effectiveness of the different forms of prophylaxis has not been
specifically compared in high-risk general surgical patients. On the basis of current
evidence, one of the following regimens is recommended:

1. Oral anticoagulants commenced a number of days preoperatively and adjusted
   to maintain the prothrombin time (using rabbit brain prothromboplastin) at
   1.5–3 seconds longer than control at the time of surgery. Immediately preoperatively, the dose should be increased to prolong the prothrombin time 1.5–2
   times control. This approach could be combined with intermittent pneumatic
   compression which is commenced at the time of surgery.
2. Low-dose heparin using the eight-hourly regimen. If the promising results of the
   combination of low-dose heparin and dihydroergotamine are confirmed, then
   this combination could be used in these patients.
3. External pneumatic compression combined with low-dose heparin.
4. Adjusted-dose heparin, commenced two days preoperatively and adjusted to
   maintain the activated partial thromboplastin time between 31.5 and 36
   seconds.
5. A combination of any of the above four methods of primary prophylaxis with
   ^{125}I-fibrinogen leg scanning to detect patients who break through prophylaxis.

Hip Surgery

Patients undergoing elective total hip replacement and patients who sustain a
fractured hip are at particularly high risk of postoperative venous thromboembolism. Unprotected, over 50% of these patients develop venous thrombosis, 20%

develop proximal vein thrombosis, and between 1 and 5% suffer fatal pulmonary embolism.[4, 18, 26-28, 30, 64, 65, 70]

At present, based on the data reported in the literature, four approaches to primary prophylaxis have been shown to be effective in patients undergoing elective hip surgery. These four approaches are: .

1. oral anticoagulants;
2. intravenous dextran;
3. adjusted-dose subcutaneous heparin;
4. intravenous dextran plus intermittent pneumatic compression.

Further clinical trials will no doubt modify the above recommendations, but given the potentially serious nature of venous thromboembolic disease and the demonstrated effectiveness of these approaches, it is clearly imprudent to withhold prophylaxis while awaiting further information.

Intermittent pneumatic compression alone, using a calf and thigh device, may be effective but requires more extensive evaluation. To date, the results with both low-dose heparin and aspirin prophylaxis have been inconsistent, and neither of these two approaches should be used.[12, 26-28, 30, 77-85] Screening with combined impedance plethysmography and ^{125}I-fibrinogen leg scanning plus routine venography at a fixed interval postoperatively will provide early detection of venous thrombosis,[88] but this approach is expensive and logistically demanding.

Oral anticoagulants are most effective when treatment is commenced preoperatively or at the time of surgery, but in the past this approach has been associated with an increased risk of bleeding which is considered unacceptable by most orthopaedic surgeons. Recent data[64] indicate that the risk of bleeding with warfarin can be reduced to less than 5%, without loss of effectiveness, by monitoring warfarin to achieve a less intense anticoagulant effect preoperatively, and then increasing the dose postoperatively to prolong the prothrombin time to 1.5 times control (using rabbit brain thromboplastin). This approach reduced the frequency of venous thrombosis from 51 to 21%; importantly, the frequency of proximal vein thrombosis was reduced to 2%.[64] Alternatively, oral anticoagulants may be commenced 48 hours postoperatively in a dose which is aimed to prolong the prothrombin time to approximately 1.25-1.5 times control (using rabbit brain thromboplastin) on the fourth to fifth postoperative day, but the effectiveness of this approach for preventing venous thromboembolism has not been demonstrated in a controlled randomized study.

Dextran, commenced preoperatively and then on alternative days until the patient is fully ambulant, is also effective;[54-56] promising results have been obtained when intermittent pneumatic compression is combined with intravenous dextran.[70] The risk of bleeding associated with dextran can be minimized by using no more than 500 ml preoperatively. The use of adjusted-dose subcutaneous heparin in patients undergoing elective hip surgery is also particularly attractive as this approach is effective (reducing the frequency of proximal vein thrombosis to 5%) and is not associated with an increased risk of serious bleeding complications.[65]

In patients undergoing surgery for fractured hip, either warfarin or dextran provide effective protection against venous thromboembolic complications. At present, neither are widely used in this patient group due to the fear of bleeding complications. The risk of bleeding associated with warfarin sodium can be substantially reduced by using a less intense warfarin regimen.[64, 87] Patients who sustain a fractured hip are frequently elderly and are at particular risk for volume overload with dextran prophylaxis; in these patients, the less intense warfarin regimen is preferred.

Major Knee Surgery

Patients undergoing major knee surgery (e.g., total knee replacement, tibial osteotomy, etc.) are at high risk for postoperative venous thromboembolism (Table 29-1). In the absence of prophylaxis, 60–70% of patients undergoing total knee replacement or elective tibial osteotomy develop calf vein thrombosis and 20% develop proximal vein thrombosis. External pneumatic compression is highly effective in these patients and is the prophylactic measure of choice.[42] An external compression device is available which can be worn either under plaster casts or back slabs, and can be applied in the operating theatre over a bandage and beneath a plaster cast. In most patients, external pneumatic compression should be continued for seven to ten days postoperatively, at which time many patients are no longer immobilized while others have walking plaster casts. In this latter group, prophylaxis should be continued with oral anticoagulants or adjusted subcutaneous heparin until the plaster cast is removed because, in the absence of prophylaxis, these patients remain at risk for developing late venous thromboembolic complications.

Neurosurgery

In the absence of prophylaxis, the frequency of venous thromboembolism in patients having neurosurgical procedures varies between 20 and 25%. Anticoagulants are potentially dangerous in this patient group because even minimal intracranial bleeding could have serious consequences. External pneumatic compression is effective in these patients and is the prophylactic method of choice.[39,40,43]

Genitourinary Surgery

Patients having a transurethral resection of the prostate have a 7–10% risk of developing ^{125}I-fibrinogen leg scan-detected calf vein thrombosis, while those having retropubic prostatectomy or an equivalent operation have a 25–50% chance (moderate risk) of developing fibrinogen leg scan-detected calf vein thrombosis. Low-dose heparin is of limited effectiveness in patients undergoing open prostatectomy. Intermittent pneumatic compression is effective in these patients and is the method of choice.[12,41]

High-risk Medical Patients

Myocardial Infarction

Between 20 and 40% of patients who sustain acute myocardial infarction develop calf venous thrombosis. Low-dose heparin is effective in reducing the frequency of leg scan-detected venous thrombosis in these patients[29,89] but there is no evidence that this approach is effective in preventing systemic embolism. Patients with acute transmural myocardial infarction are at high risk of developing mural thrombosis and systemic embolism, and should be treated with a combination of full doses of heparin and oral anticoagulants commencing at the time of admission to hospital. Heparin therapy can then be stopped after three to five days and oral anticoagulants continued for three to four weeks. Alternative approaches which are likely to be as effective include:

1. oral anticoagulants administered on admission and then daily with the aim of increasing the prothrombin time to 1.5 times control value (rabbit brain thromboplastin) after four or five days or
2. subcutaneous heparin in doses of 12,500 units every 12 hours while the patient remains in hospital.

In both patients, anticoagulant prophylaxis should be continued for three to four weeks. The moderate-dose subcutaneous heparin regimen is particularly useful if facilities for laboratory monitoring are not available. Patients with subendocardial myocardial infarction have a lower risk of systemic embolism and, in these patients, it would be reasonable to direct prophylaxis against venous thromboembolism by using low-dose heparin while they remain in hospital.

Stroke

Approximately 60% of all patients who sustain paralytic stroke develop leg scan-detected venous thrombosis.[90,91] Although not definitely established, it is likely that either external pneumatic compression or low-dose heparin would be effective in preventing serious venous thromboembolism in this patient group. External pneumatic compression has the theoretical advantage of not exposing the patient to the risk of intracerebral hemorrhage.

THE COST-EFFECTIVENESS OF PROPHYLAXIS

An extensive and comprehensive body of literature deals with the efficacy and safety of the various prophylactic measures; however, relatively little attention has been addressed to the economic implications of prophylaxis. In many hospitals, the lack of an organized strategy for the prevention of venous thromboembolism has been due, in part, to a reluctance to add new interventions whose cost-effectiveness has not been adequately evaluated. Cost-effectiveness analysis provides a formal method for ranking the alternative prophylactic modalities in terms of both their cost and effectiveness.

The cost incurred by applying an approach for preventing venous thrombo-embolism can be categorized as follows:

1. the cost of the prophylactic agent or measure;
2. the cost of side effects induced by the prophylactic measure;
3. the diagnostic cost of confirming the presence of venous thromboembolism in patients who develop clinically suspected venous thrombosis or pulmonary embolism;
4. the cost of treating deep vein thrombosis and nonfatal pulmonary embolism;

5. the cost of side effects of treatment in patients who develop venous thrombosis or pulmonary embolism;

6. the cost of excess hospital days in patients requiring treatment of deep vein thrombosis or pulmonary embolism.

In the context of prophylaxis of venous thromboembolism, the desired health effect is measured in terms of the number of deaths due to pulmonary embolism averted. The "best" prophylactic strategy would prevent the maximum number of deaths from pulmonary embolism at a minimum cost.

Two published reports have addressed the issue of cost-effectiveness of the alternative approaches for preventing venous thromboembolism in general surgical patients.[9,10] The cost-effectiveness of primary prophylaxis with either low-dose subcutaneous heparin, intravenous dextran, or intermittent pneumatic compression, and of secondary prevention by screening with ^{125}I-fibrinogen leg scanning are shown in Table 29-3. The cost-effectiveness of these alternative prophylactic measures are compared with the "no-program" approach (i.e., the approach of not using prophylaxis, other than early ambulation and treating those patients who develop venous thromboembolism).

The results of cost-effectiveness analysis in general surgical patients outlined in Table 29-3 warrant three conclusions. First, the use of "no prophylaxis" is ineffective, resulting in unnecessary loss of life, and is costly due to the diagnostic and treatment costs incurred by the substantial proportion of patients who develop venous thromboembolism. Second, primary prophylaxis with low-dose subcutaneous heparin is highly cost-effective for preventing fatal pulmonary embolism in general surgical patients; dextran prophylaxis is also effective, but considerably more expensive. Intermittent pneumatic leg compression is relatively inexpensive, but to date its effectiveness for preventing fatal pulmonary embolism has not been evaluated in a randomized clinical trial and must be inferred, based on the knowledge that it is effective for preventing deep vein thrombosis. For this reason, in general surgical patients, intermittent pneumatic compression should be confined to those patients at high risk of bleeding in whom low-dose heparin is contraindicated (e.g., patients undergoing spinal anaesthesia). Third, primary prophylaxis with active measures is considerably more cost-effective than secondary prevention by screening

Table 29-3

Total Cost of the Alternative Prophylactic Strategies
per Thousand General Surgical Patients

	Cost*	
Strategy	$Cdn(1985)	$US(1985)
Traditional ("no prophylaxis") approach	97,126	112,875
[125]I-fibrinogen leg scanning	425,873	720,293
Intravenous dextran	163,620	220,729
Intermittent pneumatic compression	64,067	118,862
Low-dose subcutaneous heparin	48,269	121,274

* Costs are expressed in Canadian dollars as reported by Hull and coworkers (CMAJ 127:990–995, 1982)[10] and in US dollars as reported by Salzman and Davies (Ann Surg 191:207–218, 1980)[9] which have been adjusted to reflect 1985 costs.

with ^{125}I-fibrinogen leg scanning, because this latter approach necessitates full-dose anticoagulant treatment of a large number of patients with subclinical venous thrombosis.

The cost-effectiveness analysis outlined above does not take into account the economic loss to society of those patients dying from massive pulmonary embolism, and when these costs are taken into account, the burden to society is even greater.

As further data from randomized clinical trials become available, it will also be possible to evaluate the cost-effectiveness of the alternative prophylactic approaches in the various risk categories and other surgical groups. In the final analysis, however, the decision to use prophylaxis should not be based on economic grounds, but on avoiding the tragic and unnecessary loss of life due to massive pulmonary embolism.

REFERENCES

1. Dalen JE, Alpert JS: Natural history of pulmonary embolism. Prog Cardiovasc Dis 17:259, 1975
2. Skinner DB, Salzman EW: Anticoagulant prophylaxis in surgical patients. Surg Gynecol Obstet 125:741, 1967
3. Shepard RM, White HA, Shirkey AL: Anticoagulant prophylaxis of thromboembolism in post-surgical patients. Am J Surg 112:698, 1966
4. Coventry MB, Nolan DR, Beckenbaugh RD: "Delayed" prophylactic anticoagulation: A study of results and complications in 2,012 total hip arthroplasties. J Bone Joint Surg 55A:1467, 1973
5. Eskeland G, Solheim K, Skjorten F: Anticoagulant prophylaxis, thromboembolism and mortality in elderly patients with hip fractures: A controlled clinical trial. Acta Chir Scand 131:16, 1966
6. Kakkar W, Stamatakis JD, Bentley PG, Lawrence D, deHass HA, Ward VP: Prophylaxis for post-operative deep-vein thrombosis. JAMA 241:39, 1979
7. Donaldson GA, Williams C, Scanell J, Shaw RS: A reappraisal of the application of the Trendelenburg operation to massive fatal embolism. N Engl J Med 268:171, 1963
8. Fratantoni J, Wessler, S: Prophylactic therapy of deep-vein thrombosis and pulmonary embolism. DHEW Publication No (NIH) 76–866, Washington DC, United States Government Printing Office, 1975
9. Salzman EW, Davies GC: Prophylaxis of venous thromboembolism: Analysis of cost-effectiveness. Ann Surg 268:171, 1980
10. Hull R, Hirsh J, Sackett DL, Stoddart G: Cost-effectiveness of primary and secondary prevention of fatal pulmonary embolism in high-risk surgical patients. CMAJ 127:990–995, 1982
11. Carter C, Gent M: The epidemiology of venous thrombosis, in Coleman RW, Hirsh J, Marder V, Salzman EW (eds): Hemostasis and Thrombosis: Basic Principles and Clinical Practice. JB Lippincott Co, 1982, pp 805–819
12. Salzman EW, Hirsh J: Prevention of venous thromboembolism, in Coleman RW, Hirsh J, Marder V, Salzman EW (eds): Hemostasis and Thrombosis: Basic Principles and Clinical Practice. JB Lippincott Co, 1982, pp 986–999
13. International Multicentre Trial: Prevention of fatal post-operative pulmonary embolism by low doses of heparin. Lancet 2:45, 1975
14. Gordon-Smith IC, Le Quesne LP, Grundy DJ, Newcombe JF: Controlled trial of two regimens of subcutaneous heparin in prevention of post-operative deep-vein thrombosis. Lancet 1:1133, 1972

15. Kakkar W, Spindler J, Flute PT, Corrigan T, Fossard DP, Crellin RQ: Efficacy of low-doses of heparin in prevention of deep-vein thrombosis after major surgery: A double-blind randomized trial. Lancet 2:101, 1972

16. Nicolaides AN, Dupont PA, Desais S, Douglas JN, Fourides G, Lewis JD, Dodsworth H, Luch KJ, Jamieson CW: Small doses of subcutaneous sodium heparin in preventing deep venous thrombosis after major surgery. Lancet 2:890, 1972

17. Ballard RM, Bradley-Watson PJ, Johnston FD, Kenney A, McCarthy TG, Campbell S, Weston J: Low doses of subcutaneous heparin in the prevention of deep-vein thrombosis after gynecological surgery. J Obstet Gynecol Br Commonw 80:469, 1973

18. Lahnborg G, Friman L, Bergstrom K, Lagergren H: Effect of low-dose heparin on incidence of post-operative pulmonary embolism detected by photoscanning. Lancet 1:329, 1974

19. Scottish study: A multi-unit controlled trial: Heparin versus dextran in the prevention of deep-vein thrombosis. Lancet 2:118, 1974

20. Albernethy EE, Hartsuck JM: Post-operative pulmonary embolism: A prospective study utilizing low-dose heparin. Am J Surg 128:739, 1974

21. Covey TH, Sherman L, Baue E: Low-dose heparin in post-operative patients. Arch Surg 110:1021, 1975

22. Rosenberg IL, Evans M, Pollock AV: Prophylaxis of post-operative leg vein thrombosis by low-dose subcutaneous heparin or pre-operative calf muscle stimulation: A controlled clinical trial. Br Med J 1:649, 1975

23. Gallus AS, Hirsh J, O'Brien SE, McBridge JA, Tuttle RJ, Gent M: Prevention of venous thrombosis with small subcutaneous doses of heparin. JAMA 235:980, 1975

24. Gruber UF, Duckert F, Fridrich R, Torhorst J, Rem J: Prevention of post-operative thromboembolism by dextran 40, low doses of heparin or xantinol nicotinate. Lancet 1:207, 1977

25. Groot Schuur Hospital Thromboembolus Study Group: Failure of low-dose heparin to prevent significant thromboembolic complications in high-risk surgical patients: Interim report of post-operative trial. Br Med J 1:1447, 1979

26. Morris GK, Henry APJ, Prestion BJ: Prevention of deep-vein thrombosis by low-dose heparin in patients undergoing total hip replacement. Lancet 2:797, 1974

27. Hampson WGJ, Harris FC, Lucas HK, Roberts PH, McCall IW, Jackson PC, Powell NL, Staddon GE: Failure of low-dose heparin to prevent deep-vein thrombosis after hip replacement arthroplasty. Lancet 2:795, 1974

28. Venous Thrombosis Clinical Study Group: Small doses of subcutaneous sodium heparin in the prevention of deep-vein thrombosis after elective hip operations. Br J Surg 62:348, 1975

29. Gallus AS, Hirsh J, Tuttle RJ, Trebilcock R, O'Brien SE, Carroll JJ, Minden JH, Hudecki SM: Small subcutaneous doses of heparin in prevention of venous thrombosis. N Engl J Med 288:545, 973

30. Manucci PM, Citterio LA, Panajotopoulos N: Low-dose heparin and deep-vein thrombosis after total hip replacement. Thromb Haemost 36:157, 1976

31. Negus D, Friedgood A, Cox SJ, Peel ALG, Wells BW: Ultra-low-dose intravenous heparin in prevention of post-operative deep-vein thrombosis. Lancet 1:891, 1980

32. Moskovitz, PA, et al: Low-dose heparin for prevention of venous thromboembolism in total hip arthroplasty and surgical repair of hip fractures. J Bone Joint Surg 60A:1065–1070, 1978

33. Gruber UF, Seldeen T, Brokop T, et al: Incidence of fatal post-operative pulmonary embolism after prophylaxis with dextran-70 and low-dose heparin. Br Med J 1:69, 1980

34. Clarke-Pearson DL, et al: Venous thromboembolism prophylaxis in gynecologic oncology: A prospective, controlled trial of low-dose heparin. Am J Obstet Gynecol 145:606, 1983

35. Sabri S, et al: Prevention of early postoperative deep-vein thrombosis and intermittent compression of the leg during surgery. Br Med J 4:394–396, 1971

36. Hills NH, Pflug JJ, Jeyasingh K, Boardman L, Calman JS: Prevention of deep-vein thrombosis by intermittent pneumatic compression of calf. Br Med J 1:131, 1972

37. Roberts VC, Cotton LT: Prevention of postoperative deep-vein thrombosis in patients with malignant disease. Br Med J 1:358, 1974

38. Clarke WB, MacGregor AB, Prescott RJ, Ruckley CV: Pneumatic compression of the calf and post-operative deep-vein thrombosis. Lancet 2:5, 1974

39. Turpie ACG, Gallus A, Beattie WS, Hirsh J: Prevention of venous thrombosis in patients with intracranial disease by intermittent pneumatic compression of the calf. Neurology 27:435, 1977

40. Skillman JJ, Collins RE, Coe NP, Goldstein BS, Shapiro RM, Zervas NT, Bettmann MA, Salzman EW: Prevention of deep-vein thrombosis in neurosurgical patients: A controlled, randomized trial of external pneumatic compression boots. Surgery 83:354, 1978

41. Coe NP, Collins REC, Klein LA, Bettmann MA, Skillman JJ, Shapiro RM, Salzman EW: Prevention of deep-vein thrombosis in urological patients: A controlled, randomized trial of low-dose heparin and external pneumatic compression boots. Surgery 83:220, 1978

42. Hull RD, Delmore TJ, Hirsh J, Gent M, Armstrong P, Lofthous R, MacMillan A, Blackstone I, Reed-Davis R, Detwiller RC: Effectiveness of intermittent pulsatile elastic stockings for the prevention of calf and thigh vein thrombosis in patients undergoing elective knee surgery. Thromb Res 16:37, 1979

43. Turpie ACG, et al: Prevention of venous thrombosis by intermittent sequential calf compression in patients with intracranial disease. Thrombo Res 15:611–616, 1979

44. Borow M, Goldson H: Post-operative venous thrombosis. Am J Surg 141:245–251, 1981

45. Butson ARC: Intermittent pneumatic calf compression for prevention of deep venous thrombosis in general abdominal surgery. Am J Surg 142:525–527, 1981

46. Hartman JT, et al: Cyclic sequential compression of the lower limb in prevention of deep venous thrombosis. J Bone Joint Surg 64A:1059–1062, 1982

47. Caprinin JA, et al: Thrombosis prophylaxis using external compression. Surg 156:599–604, 1983

48. Clarke-Pearson DL, et al: Prevention of venous thromboembolism by external pneumatic calf compression in patients with gynecologic malignancy. Obstet Gynecol 63:92–98, 1984

49. Sevitt S, Gallagher NG: Prevention of venous thrombosis and pulmonary embolism in injured patients: Trial of anticoagulant prophylaxis in middle-aged and elderly patients with fractured neck of femur. Lancet 2:981, 1959

50. Borgstram S, Greitz T, Vander Linden W, Molin J, Rudics I: Anticoagulant prophylaxis of venous thrombosis in patients with fractured neck of the femur: A controlled clinical trial using venous phlebography. Acta Chir Scand 129:500, 1965

51. Hamilton HW, Crawford JS, Gardiner JH, Wiley AM: Venous thrombosis in patients with fracture of the upper end of the femur. J Bone Joint Surg (Br) 52:268, 1970

52. Pinto DJ: Controlled trial of an anticoagulant (warfarin sodium) in the prevention of venous thrombosis following hip surgery. Br J Surg 57:349, 1970

53. Hume M, Kuriakose T, Xavier ZL, Turner RH: ^{125}I-fibrinogen and the prevention of venous thrombosis. Arch Surg 107:803, 1973

54. Morris GK, Mitchell JR: Warfarin sodium in the prevention of deep venous thrombosis and pulmonary embolism in patients with fractured neck of femur. Lancet 2:869, 1976

55. Taberner DA, Poller L, Burslem RW, Jones JB: Oral anticoagulants controlled by the British comparative thromboplastin versus low-dose heparin in prophylaxis of deep-vein thrombosis. Br Med J 1:272–274, 1978

56. Francis CW, Marder VJ, Evarts M, Yaukoolbodi S: Two-step warfarin therapy: Prevention of postoperative venous thrombosis without excessive bleeding. JAMA 249:374–378, 1983

57. Bonnar J, Walsh J: Prevention of thrombosis after pelvic surgery by British dextran 70. Lancet 1:614, 1972

58. Bonnar J, Walsh JJ, Haddon M: Thromboembolism following radical surgery for carcinoma prevention by dextran 70 infusion during and immediately after operation. Proc 4th Congr Int Soc Thromb Haemost (Vienna) 278A:1973

59. Carter AE, Eban R: The prevention of post-operative deep venous thrombosis with dextran 70. Br J Surg 60:681, 1973

60. Becker J, Schampi B: The incidence of post-operative venous thrombosis of the legs: A comparative study on the prophylactic effect of dextran 70 and electrical calf muscle stimulation. Acta Chir Scand 139:357, 1973

61. Kline A, Hughes LE, Campbell H: Dextran 70 in prophylaxis of thromboembolic disease after surgery: A clinically oriented randomized double-blind trial. Br Med J 2:109, 1975

62. Ahlberg A, Nylander G, Robertson B, Cronberg S, Nilsson IM: Dextran in prophylaxis of thrombosis in fractures of the hip. Acta Chir Scand (Suppl) 387:83, 1968

63. Johnsson SR, Bygdeman S, Eliasson R: Effect of dextran of post-operative thrombosis. Acta Chir Scand (Suppl) 387:80, 1968

64. Evarts CM, Feil EJ: Prevention of thromboembolic disease after elective surgery of the hip. J Bone Joint Surg (Am) 53:1271, 1971

65. Leyvarz PF, Richard J, Bachmann F, et al: Adjusted versus fixed dose subcutaneous heparin in the prevention of deep-vein thrombosis after total hip replacement. N Engl J Med 309:954–958, 1983

66. Scurr JH, Ibrahim SZ, Faber RG, LeQuesne LP: The efficacy of graduated compression stockings in the prevention of deep-vein thrombosis. Br J Surg 64:371, 1977

67. Scholz PM, Jones RH, Sabiston DC: Prophylaxis of thromboembolism. Adv Surg 13:115–143, 1979

68. Kakkar W, Stamatakis JD, Bentley PG, et al: Prophylaxis for post-operative deep-vein thrombosis: Synergistic effect of heparin and dihydroergotamine. JAMA 241:39–42, 1979

69. Multicenter Trial Committee: Dihydroergotamine-heparin prophylaxis of post-operative deep-vein thrombosis. JAMA 251:2960–2966, 1984

70. Harris WH, Athanasoulis CA, Waltman AC, Salzman EW: Prophylaxis of deep-vein thrombosis after total hip replacement: Dextran and external pneumatic compression compared with 1.2 or 0.3 gram of aspirin daily. J Bone Joint Surg 67A:57–62, 1985

71. O'Brien JR, Tulevski V, Etherington M: Two in-vivo studies comparing high and low aspirin dosage. Lancet 1:399, 1971

72. Medical Research Council: Report of the Steering Committee: Effect of aspirin on post-operative venous thrombosis. Lancet 2:441, 1972

73. Clagett GP, Salzman EW: Prevention of venous thromboembolism, in Sonnenblick EH, Lesch M (eds): Progress in Cardiovascular Diseases, vol XVIII. New York, Grune and Stratton, 1975, p 345

74. Renney JTG, O'Sullivan EF, Burke PF: Prevention of post-operative deep-vein thrombosis with dipyridamole and aspirin. Br Med J 1:992, 1976

75. Loew D, Brucke P, Simma W, Vinazzer H, Dienstl E, Boehme E: Acetylsalicylic acid, low-dose heparin and a combination of both substances in the prevention of post-operative thromboembolism: A double-blind study. Thromb Res 1:81, 1977

76. Plante J, Boneu B, Vaysse C, Barret A, Gouzi M, Bierne R: Dipyridamole aspirin versus low doses of heparin in the prophylaxis of deep venous thrombosis in abdominal surgery. Thromb Res 14:399, 1979

77. Wood EH, Prentice CRM, McGrouther DA, Sinclair J, McNicol GP: Trial of aspirin and RA233 in prevention of post-operative deep-vein thrombosis. Thromb Diathes Haemorrh 30:18, 1973

78. Harris WH, Salzman EW, Athanasoulis C, Waltman AC, Baum S, DeSanctis RW: Comparison of warfarin, low-molecular-weight dextran, aspirin, and subcutaneous heparin prevention of venous thromboembolism following total hip replacement. J Bone Joint Surg (Am) 56:1552, 1974

79. Soreff J, Johnsson H, Diener L, Goransson L: Acetylsalicylic acid in a trial to diminish thromboembolic complications after elective hip surgery. Acta Orthop Scand 46:246, 1975

80. Dechavanne M, Ville D, Viala JJ, Kher A, Faivre J, Pousset MB, Dejour H: Controlled trial of platelet antiaggregating agents and subcutaneous heparin in prevention of post-operative deep-vein thrombosis in high-risk patients. Haemostasis 4:94, 1975

81. Jennings JJ, Harris WH, Sarmiento A: A clinical evaluation of aspirin prophylaxis of thromboembolic disease after total hip arthroplasty. J Bone Joint Surg 58A:926, 1976

82. Morris GK, Mitchell JRA: Preventing venous thromboembolism in elderly patients with hip fractures. Studies of low-dose heparin, dipyridamole, aspirin, and flurbiprofen. Br Med J 1:535, 1977

83. Harris WH, Salzmann EW, Athansoulis CA, Waltman AW, DeSanctis RW: Aspirin prophylaxis of venous thromboembolism after total hip replacement. N Engl J Med 297:1246, 1977

84. Stamatakis JD, Kakkar W, Lawrence D, Bentley PG, Nairn D, Ward V: Failure of aspirin to prevent post-operative deep-vein thrombosis in patients undergoing total hip replacement. Br Med J 1:1031, 1978

85. Hume M, Donaldson WR, Suprenant J: Sex, aspirin and venous thrombosis. Orthop Clin Am 3:761, 1978

86. Thomas DP: Pathogenesis of venous thrombosis, in Coleman RW, Hirsh J, Marder V, Salzman EW (eds): Hemostasis and Thrombosis: Basic Principles and Clinical Practice. JB Lippincott Co, 1982, pp 820–830

87. Hull R, et al: Different intensities of oral anticoagulant therapy in the treatment of proximal vein thrombosis. N Engl J Med 307:1676–1681, 1982

88. Hull, R, Hirsh J, Sackett DL, et al: The value of adding impedance plethysmography to ^{125}I-fibrinogen leg scanning for the detection of deep-vein thrombosis in high-risk surgical patients: A comparative study between patients undergoing general surgery and hip surgery. Thrombosis Res 15:227–234, 1979

89. Warlow C, Terry G, Kenmure ACF, Beattie AG, Ogston D, Douglas AS: A double-blind trial of low doses of subcutaneous heparin in the prevention of deep vein thrombosis after myocardial infarction. Lancet 2:436, 1973

90. Warlow C, Ogston D, Douglas AS: Deep-vein thrombosis of the leg after strokes. Part 1. Incidence and predisposing factors. Br Med J i:1178–1183, 1976

91. McCarthy St, Turner JJ, Robertson D, Hawkey CJ, Macey DJ: Low-dose heparin as a prophylaxis against deep-vein thrombosis after acute stroke. Lancet II:800–801, 1977

Joerg Dieter Gruss

30

Does Surgery Have a Place in Acute Venous Thrombosis?

INTRODUCTION

In the German Federal Republic, with a population of about 60 million, there are about 5 million people suffering from chronic venous insufficiency. In the large majority of them (80% of cases) this is part of a postthrombotic syndrome—i.e., it results from previous phlebothrombosis (Widmer: Basle study[1] and Fischer: Tübingen study[2]). Despite the general acceptance and systematic use of antithrombotic prophylaxis, every year 25,000 patients in the Federal Republic still die of pulmonary embolism. Both these facts underline the relevance and importance of acute venous thrombosis and its impact on social medicine and the economy. The occurrence of fatal pulmonary embolism and the development of postthrombotic syndromes can only be reduced or prevented by aggressive treatment of acute phlebothrombosis.[3-6] The problems of acute phlebothrombosis were the subject of an international German-speaking interdisciplinary discussion between experts in the field, which took place in Munich on 29 November 1985 on the occasion of the first annual meeting of the German Society for Vascular Surgery; much of the material of the present paper derives from the results of this discussion. The participants were: for vascular surgery, U. Brunner (Switzerland), H. Denck (Austria), J. D. Gruss (GFR); for conservative angiology, H. Böhme and A. Kriessmann (both from GDR).[7] The value of any treatment method (specifically, of thrombectomy, fibrinolysis, and heparin therapy) must be assessed in the light of the results obtained with each treatment and the risks involved in it.

DIAGNOSIS

The success of any form of aggressive treatment for acute venous thrombosis depends on the time elapsed before treatment is instituted. In any patient in whom there is the slightest suspicion of acute thrombosis, therefore, the aim must be to

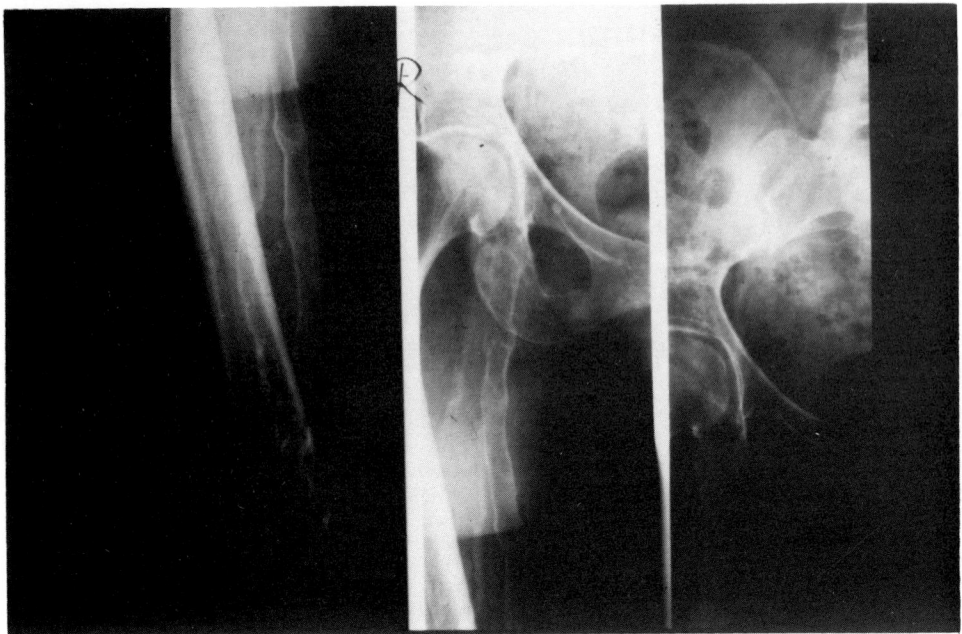

Fig. 30-1. Ascending phlebography of an acute fresh thrombosis. The preservation of the valves seems to be the most reliable sign of a recent thrombosis.

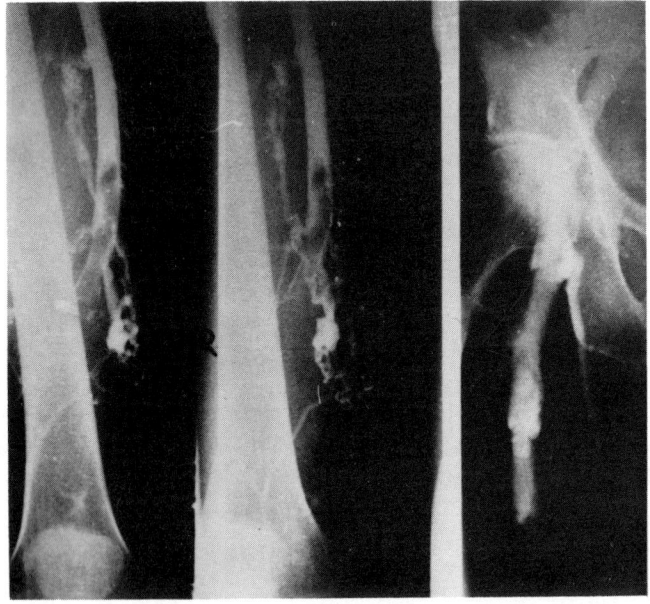

Fig. 30-2. Ascending phlebography of a six month old femoral thrombosis. The so-called floating thrombus does not allow the diagnosis of a fresh thrombosis.

carry out immediate ascending phlebography in order to confirm or exclude this possibility. All other (noninvasive) methods, such as Doppler ultrasound or venous occlusion plethysmography, carry too high an error rate to be used for therapeutic decisions in the acute situation.[8-11] Ultrasound studies can yield false–negative results in the presence of paired popliteal or femoral veins. Ascending phlebography (Fig. 30-1), furthermore, can produce decisive information on the site of thrombotic occlusion, and thus essentially decides the type of treatment to be used. Our experience over the last few years has shown that phlebograms only allow very tentative conclusions to be drawn about the age of a thrombus. The "dome" phenomenon and "contour signs" of a so-called floating thrombus (Fig. 30-2) can frequently be demonstrable for six weeks and may even be seen after six months.[12] A certain amount of information is provided by the extent of the collateral circulation. However, the most reliable data on the age of a thrombosis are provided by a careful history. The choice of therapy is therefore decided on the basis of the history and the ascending phlebogram. Only phlegmasia cerulea dolens is treated surgically by many operators without a phlebogram. It must be stressed that clinical examination, so frequently mentioned in this context, is generally unhelpful in the diagnosis of acute phlebothrombosis—particularly in bedridden patients, e.g., after orthopaedic, posttraumatic, or gynaecological surgery; on the slightest suspicion of thrombosis it is always essential to clarify the situation with a phlebogram.

THERAPY

Comparative studies have shown that fibrinolysis and surgical thrombectomy produce practically identical results. The risks and complications of the two procedures are also of the same order.[7] Treatment with heparin alone as a therapeutic manoeuvre is no longer an acceptable alternative to aggressive treatment. The choice between thrombolytic therapy and surgery depends on regional factors and also on whether the patient is admitted to a department of conservative angiology or to a vascular surgical unit. During the past few years the following therapeutic schedule has become established in our department. Isolated crural vein thrombosis with occlusion of up to three veins is treated on an outpatient basis with self-injected heparin (2×7500 units b.d.) and elastic compression. It is essential to carry out check phlebograms at three days and one week in order to ensure that the thrombosis has not extended into the popliteal vein. Venous thrombosis in the leg, with occlusion of more than three crural veins, is treated by fibrinolysis.[7]

If the phlebographically demonstrated thrombus already extends into the popliteal vein, or if the popliteal vein is itself occluded, then in our view there is an indication for thrombectomy—as with all other extensive occlusions of the femoropopliteal or iliac venous segments.[12] An exception to this rule is recurrent thrombosis in the presence of a preexisting postthrombotic syndrome; such cases are treated with fibrinolysis. Floating thrombi in mobile vein segments (i.e., at the level of the knee and hip joints) are associated in our view with a particularly high risk of embolism. We therefore consider that thrombectomy is indicated in all cases of fresh phlebothrombosis (not over 10 days old) at or above the level of the popliteal vein; also in phlegmasia cerulea dolens (perhaps even without ascending phlebography); following unsuccessful fibrinolysis even after the 10-day limit; and in thrombosis progressively extending from the crural veins into the mobile segment of the popliteal vein. In contrast to fibrinolysis, there is no hard-and-fast age limit to this approach. Advanced tumour cachexia is regarded as a contraindication to surgery.

OPERATIVE TECHNIQUE

Thrombectomy is performed in the anti-Trendelenburg position, with the head end of the operating table elevated and with continuous positive-pressure (PEEP) ventilation (Fig. 30-3). Depending on the site of occlusion, the vein may be mobilized via a high inguinal incision in the groin, or via a longitudinal tibial incision below the knee joint. Denuding of the vein is performed as sparingly as possible in order not to damage the adventitial sheath. The vein is clamped with moistened soft elastic tapes or Hydragrip clamps. The vein and phlebotomy margins are handled as little as possible with so-called atraumatic instruments. Disobliteration of the venous channel is carried out with a Fogarty balloon catheter. Only in exceptional cases is it useful to use a ring-stripper to help scrape off tightly adherent thrombi from the vein wall. For extensive occlusions of several days' standing it is useful to expose the vein below the knee joint and in the groin. A major advance in this context has been the new Fogarty catheter with a tip that can be unscrewed; this makes it possible always to pass the balloon catheter only in the direction of the valves. A further major advance has been the routine use of the Cellsaver in all venous thrombectomies; this can practically obviate the use of donor blood.[8-13]

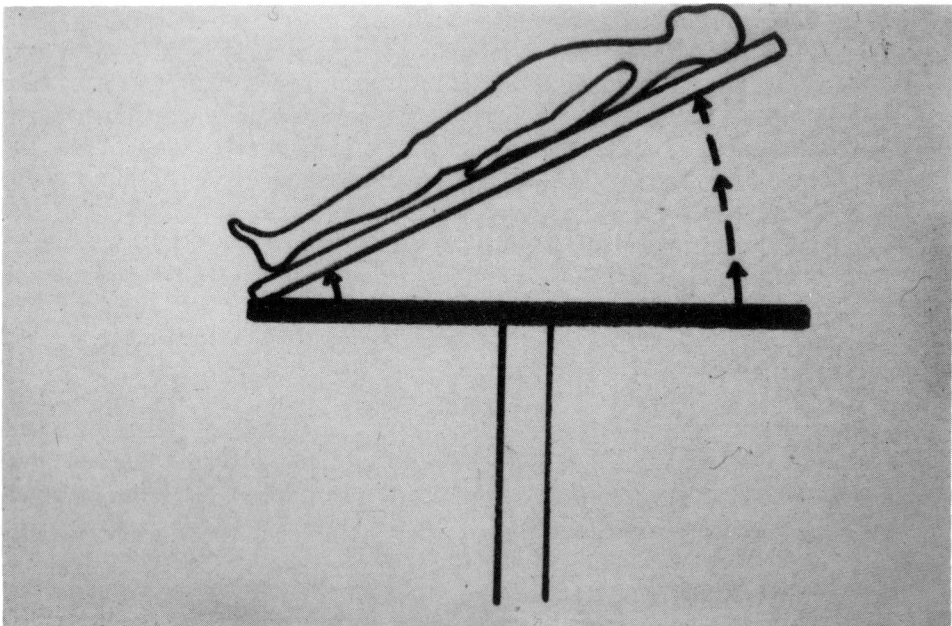

Fig. 30-3. Patient's position during thrombectomy. Original drawing from Gruss JD, Laubach K: Modifikation der Operationstechnik bei tiefer Becken- und Oberschenkelvenenthrombose. Thoraxchirurgie 19:508, 1971.

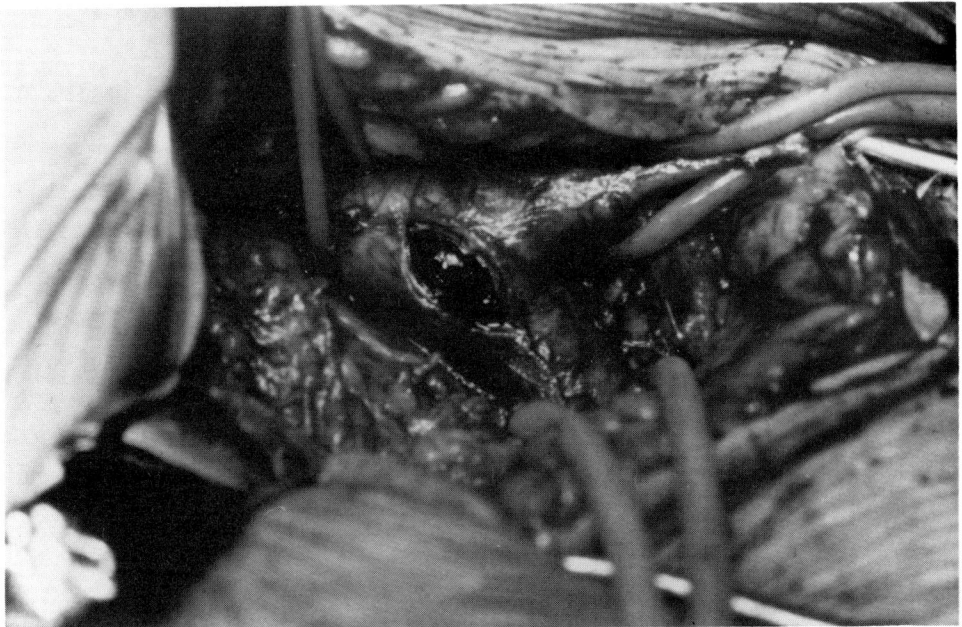

Fig. 30-4. For the thrombectomy the common femoral vein is opened by a longitudinal phlebotomy. Bleeding control is done by moistened rubber tapes.

This approach has enabled fresh phlebothrombosis with preservation of the valves to be treated by a very limited surgical procedure. Phlebotomy of the popliteal vein is always carried out transversely (Fig. 30-4). The femoral vein can be opened longitudinally or transversely, as preferred, depending on whether it is necessary to perform thrombectomy of the profunda femoris or long saphenous veins as well. Disobliteration of the crural veins is performed by manual massage of the calf and application and unwinding of an Esmarch bandage. It has also occasionally proved useful to open a posterior tibial vein behind the medial malleolus and to pass a Fogarty catheter of the type described from there up into the popliteal vein. A point of decisive importance, even with thromboses that are not very recent, is to disobliterate the areas of confluence, both in the crural and inguinal veins. For thromboses of long standing, or where disobliteration of the venous channels has been incomplete, a temporary arterio-venous fistula is fashioned. Originally we created inguinal AV fistulae for old pelvic vein thromboses by implanting the long saphenous vein into the common femoral artery (Fig. 30-5).[14,15] Later we spared the long saphenous vein itself and used a high saphenous tributary for the AV fistula (Fig. 30-6). We had initially postulated that there would be a "water vacuum pump"-like effect on deeper vein segments, i.e., on the superficial femoral vein, but no such effect could be demonstrated—indeed, check phlebography and arterio-venography showed that an AV fistula in the groin actually reduced return flow from the deeper venous segments (Fig. 30-7). We therefore adopted a suggestion of Brunner and created an AV fistulae at the level of the adducter canal, using a small twig of an artery for the fistula.[16] However, difficulties with the closure of such AV fistulae have now led us to site fistulae, if possible, at the lowest point of the thrombosis, i.e., behind the medial malleolus, between a posterior tibial vein and the

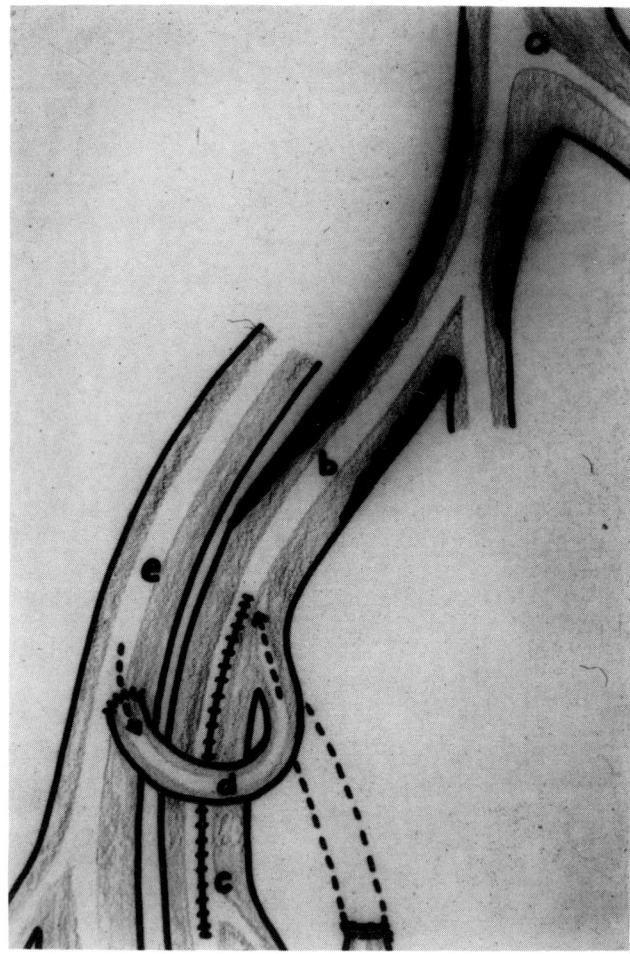

Fig. 30-5. The technique of the first AV fistula. Original drawing from Gruss JD, Laubach K: Modifikation der Operationstechnik bei tiefer Becken- und Oberschenkelvenenthrombose. Thoraxchirurgie 19:508, 1971.

posterior tibial artery (Fig. 30-8). The fistula is fashioned by dividing a posterior tibial vein transversely and implanting it transversely end-to-side in the posterior tibial artery.[15, 17]

The results of thrombectomy are documented by intraoperative phlebograms or by check phlebograms on the first postoperative day. Anticoagulation with heparin is started on the operating table. Heparin dosage is increased progressively from 15,000 to 40,000 units over the next few days. If wound healing proceeds uneventfully, the patient is changed to a dicoumarol preparation, with an overlap period, starting on day 6. An elastic compression bandage is applied on the operating table, except in patients with an AV fistula at the malleolar level. About one week postoperatively, after resolution of oedema and with the leg still in the postoperative elevated position, a class III compression stocking is made to measure. Once again, this does not apply to patients with peripheral AV fistulae.

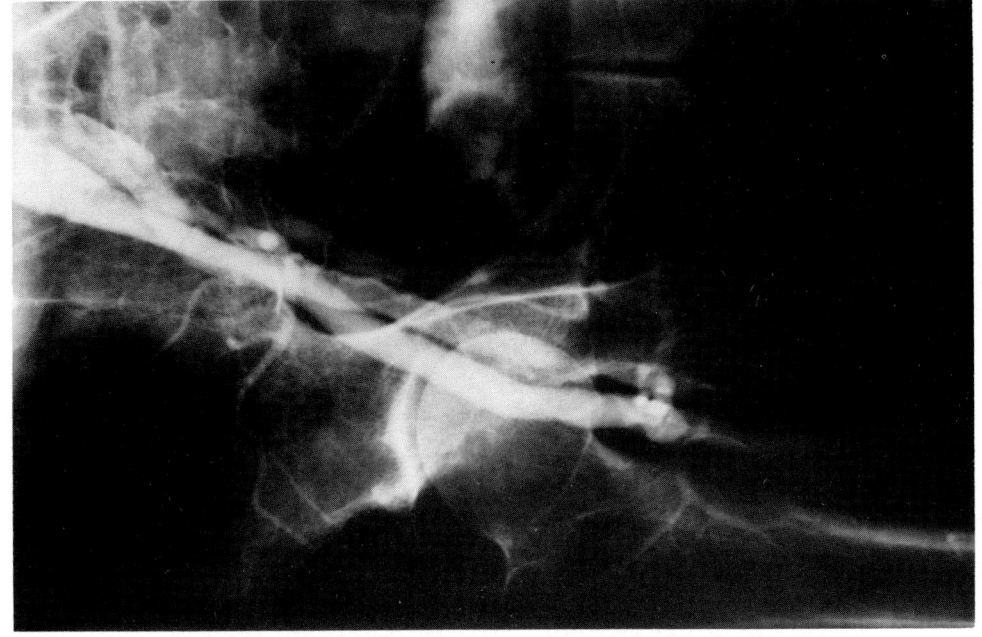

Fig. 30-7. Arteriovenogram showing a functioning AV fistula at the groin level with a perfect recanalization of the iliac vein.

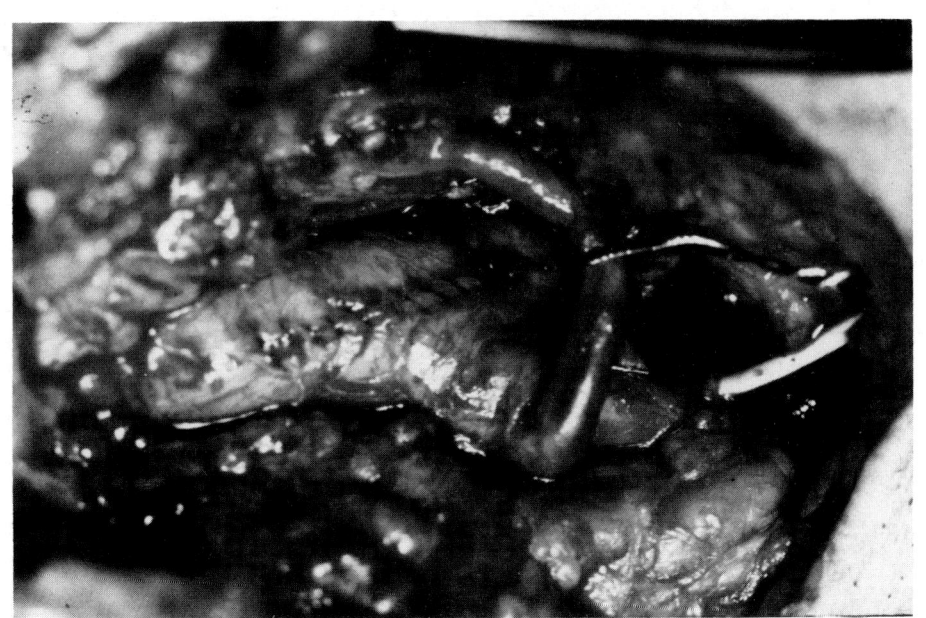

Fig. 30-6. Our current AV fistula technique using a tributary of the greater saphenous vein. The fistula is marked with a wire loop.

401

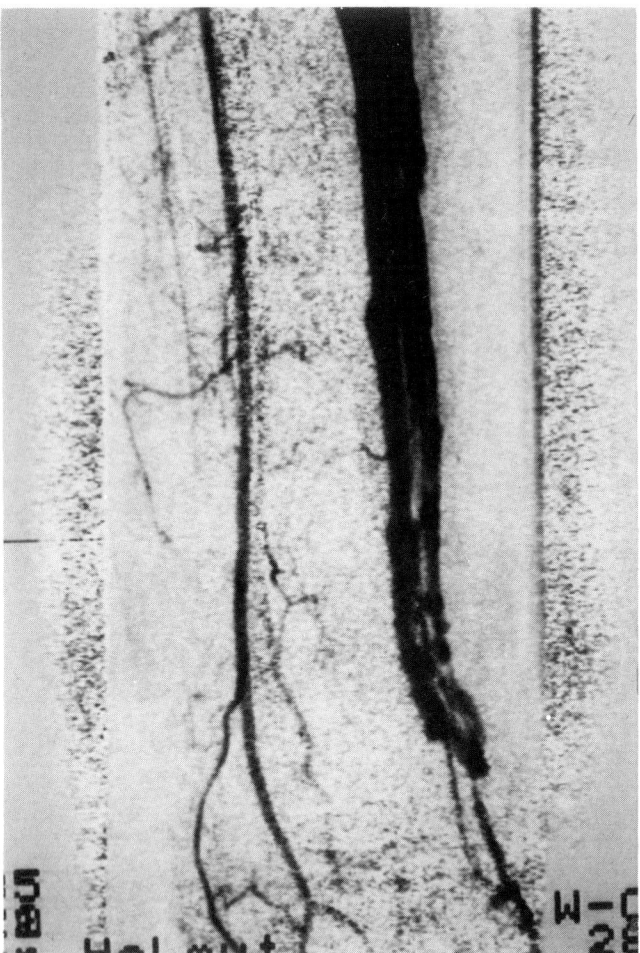

Fig. 30-8. Arteriovenogram showing function of an AV fistula between the posterior tibial artery and a posterior tibial vein. Good recanalization of the whole vein segment.

In phlegmasia cerulea dolens the arterial as well as the venous system is involved, both by reflex spasm and by compression within fascial compartments. These pathophysiological events prohibit the creation of temporary AV fistulae. It has, however, proved useful, particularly in severe cases with early venous gangrene, to carry out extensive fasciotomy in the leg. Four of our own cases showed rapid progression of venous gangrene of the foot, despite successful venous thrombectomy with fasciotomy. In three cases, continuous high-dose intraarterial prostaglandin E_1 infusion via a fine plastic catheter resulted in preservation of a functional extremity.[18] A striking feature in these patients was the fact that only a few hours after the beginning of the PGE_1 infusion, the feet become warm, the skin became pink, and the necrotic process was halted. In the fourth patient, treatment was started too late and a through-knee amputation could not be avoided.

Temporary AV fistulae lead to improved recanalization and collateral vascularization. We know of evidence demonstrating complete recanalization of the posterior vein group produced by peripheral AV fistulae behind the medial malleolus, in inoperable cases. The small number of patients involved makes it impossible as yet to give a final verdict on peripheral AV fistulae as a sole therapeutic manoeuvre long-standing phlebothrombosis.

POSTOPERATIVE COURSE AND RESULTS

Anticoagulation and compression are continued in principle for at least six months. Other centres recommend at least a year.[7,16] Temporary AV fistulae are closed two to three months after initial surgery.[12] In the groin, the locating and interruption of the fistula are facilitated if it is marked with a wire loop brought into the subcutaneous tissue.[13] For AV fistulae behind the medial malleolus it is sufficient to apply a tight elastic compression bandage or to provide a class III compression stocking.

The compression effect is generally sufficient to close distal AV fistulae. Only in three cases was surgical exposure and ligation necessary. The duration of anticoagulation and compression treatment depends on the results of treatment. For postoperative monitoring, venous occlusion plethysmography is much more helpful than check phlebography.[4] The vascular morphology—i.e., the quality of recanalization and collateral formation—does not run parallel with functional parameters, which

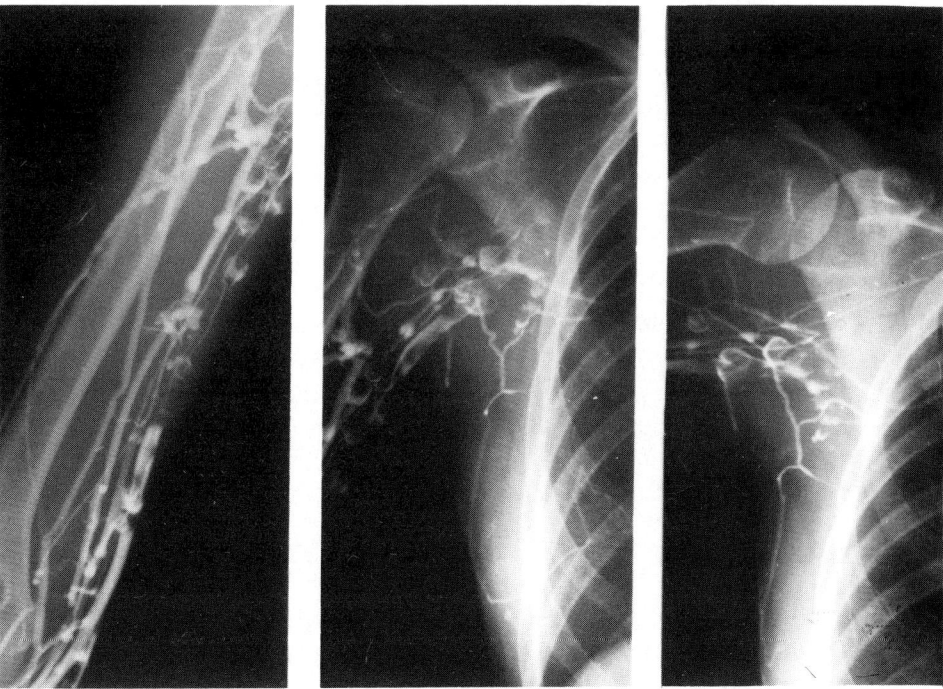

Fig. 30-9. Ascending phlebography showing an acute axillary and subclavian vein thrombosis (19 year old girl).

can be objectively measured by phlebodynamometry and venous occlusion plethysmography.[19] The qualitative value of the information from both these techniques is identical. In our hands, light reflection rheography has proved unsuitable for monitoring such patients. In venous occlusion plethysmography, the venous capacity and maximal outflow are less informative than the volume curve on stress by standing on tiptoe or knee-bending. The curve of volume reduction on stress largely corresponds to the venous pressure curve under exercise. The amplitude of the volume wave with each muscular contraction reflects the extent of valve destruction, as does the refilling time. In the presence of an unfavourable plethysmogram, anticoagulation and compression are continued. Functional studies are repeated at six-month intervals. In our experience, after anticoagulation has been continued for two years there is no further benefit to be expected from it, and it is then discontinued. In long-standing phlebothrombosis, where the operation can only be designated as an attempted thrombectomy with inadequate recanalization and insufficient collateral vascularization, compression must be maintained lifelong. Five years postoperatively, 82% of our thrombectomy patients show a normal venous occlusion plethysmogram and do not need compression stockings; 18% have a more or less marked postthrombotic syndrome, requiring long-term use of class III compression stockings. No patient has leg ulcers.

Crural venous thrombosis in combination with thrombosis of the popliteal vein carries a very high risk of later leg ulceration.[3,4] We would therefore like to consider our cases of crural vein and popliteal vein thrombosis separately; the number of these patients is too small for percentage figures to be given. Out of 44 patients who had surgery for crural and popliteal thrombosis, 34 need no compression treatment and do not have a postthrombotic syndrome, eight have a moderate-grade postthrombotic syndrome with a tendency to oedema formation and skin pigmentation, requiring class III compression stockings, and two have a significant postthrombotic syndrome with permanent oedema, skin fibrosis, and secondary varicose veins. No patient has developed a leg ulcer.

Caval plication has no place in the treatment of acute thrombosis of the veins of the pelvic and lower limbs.[20–22]

UPPER LIMB THROMBOSIS

The vast majority of arm vein thrombosis, unlike those of the pelvic and lower limb veins, have a single clinically discernible cause. In the case of the lower limbs one must think of May's venous spur, iatrogenic or traumatic lesions, or antithrombin III deficiency; acute subclavian or axillary vein occlusion, on the other hand, always obliges one to think of a thoracic outlet syndrome. The aim of treatment is therefore twofold: (1) to restore the venous circulation; (2) to remove the cause of thrombosis.[23–25]

Our procedure is as follows. After phlebographic confirmation of acute thrombosis, thrombectomy is carried out starting from the bicipital sulcus. Restoration of the venous circulation by fibrinolysis is an alternative option. A decisive factor is postoperative check phlebography with the arm in abduction and elevation, which

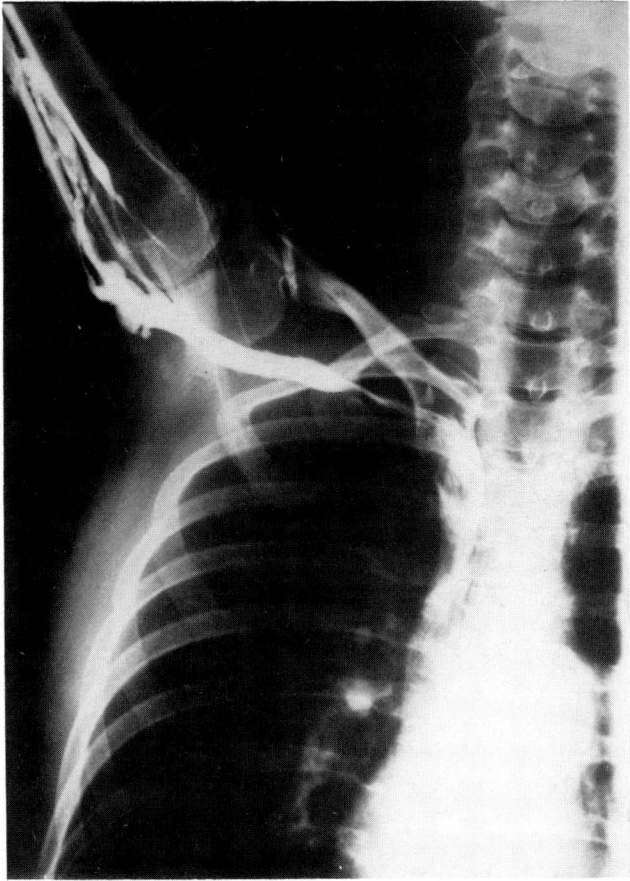

Fig. 30-10.   After thrombectomy the compression of the vein by the first rib is documented
by another phlebography in the elevation and abduction position (same patient).

demonstrates a compression effect on the subclavian vein by the first rib or an
anomalous band in some 75% of our patients. In such cases it is essential to carry
out transaxillary resection of the first rib, if necessary with excision of a cervical rib
and all anomalous bands, within the first 24 hours. It is not uncommon for renewed
thrombosis to occur between the first and second operation. In these cases repeat
thrombectomy must be carried out via a transaxillary approach. Subsequent management is as described for acute lower limb and pelvic vein thrombosis. Complications occur much more rarely after acute arm vein thrombosis. Thus only 1%
of all fatal pulmonary emboli originate in the arms. Phlegmasia cerulea dolens of
the upper extremity is exceptionally rare. A postthrombotic syndrome in the arm
only rarely causes lasting functional impairment, invalidity, and dependence on
treatment. It is therefore only necessary in exceptional cases to create a temporary
AV fistula after carrying out thrombectomy or fibrinolysis followed by resection of
the first rib, or to perform reconstructive procedures on the long-term occluded
subclavian vein.

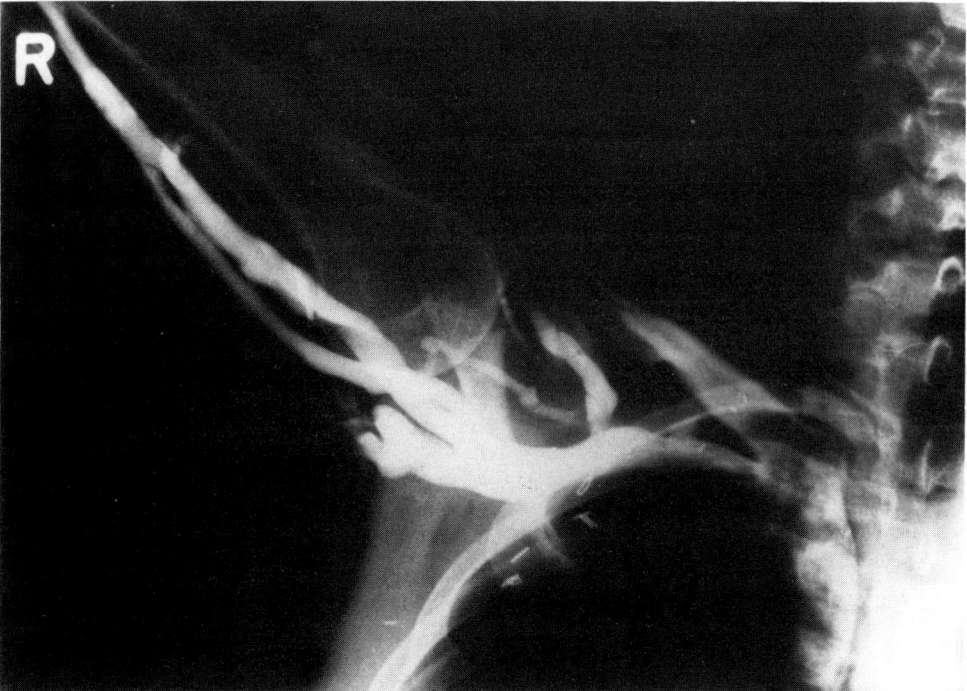

Fig. 30-11. Postoperative phlebogram after thrombectomy and second thrombectomy with patch angioplasty at the level of the compression and resection of the first rib.

REFERENCES

1. Widmer LK, Stähelin HB, Nissen C, DaSilva A: Venen-, Arterien-Krankheiten, koronare Herzkrankheit bei Berufstätigen. Prospektiv-epidemiologische Untersuchung Basler Studie I–III 1959–1978. Bern, Verlag Hans Huber, 1981
2. Fischer H, Biland L, DaSilva A, Herwig E, Mehringer G, Mucker A, Widmer MTH, Scheibler P, Widmer LK: Venenleiden. Eine repräsentative Untersuchung in der Bevölkerung der Bundesrepublik Deutschland (Tübinger Studie). München–Wien–Baltimore, Urban u Schwarzenberg, 1981
3. Zimmermann B: Thromboselokalisation und klinisches Bild des postthrombotischen Syndroms. Phlebol u Proktol 14:38, 1985
4. Salzmann P: Gibt es eine Korrelation zwischen dem postthrombotischen Syndrom und dem Ausmaß der Veränderungen des tiefen Venensystems? Phlebol u Proktol 14:34, 1985
5. Netzer CO, v Rudowski A, Hinz A, Sturm B: Zur Prognose des spät- und postthrombotischen Zustandes. Phlebol u Proktol 14:28, 1985
6. Gruss JD: Operative Maßnahmen am tiefen Venensystem bei der chronisch venösen Insuffizienz, in Gruss JD, Bartels D, Valencia (eds): Gefässchirurgie Interdisziplinär 1984. TM-Verlag, 1985, p 139
7. Denck H, Böhme H, Brunner U, Gruss JD, Kriessmann A: Interdisziplinäres Gespräch 29.11.1985: Bein- und Beckenvenenthrombosen. Angio (in press)
8. Gruss JD: Der heutige Stand der rekonstruktiven Venen-chirurgie. Schwerpunktmed 6:21, 1983
9. Neimann HL: Venography in acute and chronic venous disease, in Bergan JJ, Yao JST (eds): Surgery of the Veins. Orlando–San Diego–New York–London–Toronto–Montreal–Sydney–Tokyo, Grune and Stratton, 1985, p 73

10. Hull RD, Hirsh J: Diagnostic techniques in venous thrombosis, in Bergan JJ, Yao JST (eds): Surgery of the Veins. Orlando–San Diego–New York–London–Toronto–Montreal–Sydney–Tokyo, Grune and Stratton, 1985, p 47

11. Barnes RW: Noninvasive tests for chronic venous insufficiency, in Bergan JJ, Yao JST (eds): Surgery of the Veins. Orlando–San Diego–New York–London–Toronto–Montreal–Sydney–Tokyo, Grune and Stratton, 1985, p 99

12. Bartels D, Gruss JD: Operative treatment of acute thrombosis of the popliteal vein. First United Kingdom Meeting of the Union Internationale de Phlebologie, London, 16–20 September 1985.

13. Simmenroth HW, Scholl W, Bartels D, Vargas-Montano H, Gruss JD: Einsparung von Fremdblut durch autologe intraoperative Retransfusion am Beispiel des aortofemoralen Bifurkationsbypass. Angio 6:83, 1984

14. Gruss JD, Laubach K: Modifikation der Operationstechnik bei tiefer Becken- und Oberschenkelvenenthrombose. Thoraxchirurgie 19:508, 1971

15. Gruss JD, Bartels D, Tsafandakis E, Ohta T, Schlechtweg B: The av-fistula operation technique, in May R, Weber J (eds): Pelvic and Abdominal Veins. Progress in Diagnostics and Therapy. International Congress Series 550, Amsterdam–Oxford–Princeton, Excerpta Medica, 1981, p 215

16. Brunner U: Chirurgie der akuten Femoroiliakalvenenthrombose, in May R (ed): Chirurgie der Bein-und Beckenvenen. Stuttgart, Georg Thieme Verlag, 1974, p 115

17. Eklof B, Einarsson E, Plate G: Role of thrombectomy and temporary arteriovenous fistula in acute iliofemoral venous thrombosis, in Bergan JJ, Yao JST (eds): Surgery of the Veins. Orlando–San Diego–New York–London–Toronto–Montreal–Sydney–Tokyo, Grune and Stratton, 1985, p 131

18. Gruss JD: Treatment of the severely ischaemic limb by intra-arterial prostaglandin, in Jamieson CW (ed): Vascular Surgery. London–Philadelphia–Toronto–Mexico City–Rio de Janeiro–Sydney–Tokyo–Hong Kong, Baillière Tindall, 1985, p 54

19. Gruss JD, Bartels D, Vargas-Montano H: Über den Einsatz von PGE_1 bei der Phlegmasia cerulea dolens. Hamburg, Tagung Vereinigung nordwestdeutscher Chirurgen, 5–7 December 1985

20. Nicolaides AN, Zukowski, A, Lewis R, Kyprianou P, Malouf GM: Venous pressure measurements on venous problems, in Bergan JJ, Yao JST (eds): Surgery of the Veins. Orlando–San Diego–New York–London–Toronto–Montreal–Sydney–Tokyo, Grune and Stratton, 1985, p 111

21. Greenfield LJ: Results of catheter embolectomy and greenfield filter insertion, in Bergan JJ, Yao JST (eds): Surgery of the Veins. Orlando–San Diego–New York–London–Toronto–Montreal–Sydney–Tokyo, Grune and Stratton, 1985, p 479

22. Roehm JOF, Gianturco C, Barth MH: Percutaneous interruption of the inferior vena cava: The bird's nest filter, in Bergan JJ, Yao JST (eds): Surgery of the Veins. Orlando–San Diego–New York–London–Toronto–Montreal–Sydney–Tokyo, Grune and Stratton, 1985, p 487

23. Flinn WR, Yao JST, Bergan JJ: Direct vena cava interruption, in Bergan JJ, Yao JST (eds): Surgery of the Veins. Orlando–San Diego–New York–London–Toronto–Montreal–Sydney–Tokyo, Grune and Stratton, 1985, p 497

24. Roos DB: Thoracic outlet syndromes, in Machleder HI (ed): Vascular Disorders of the Upper Extremity. Mount Kisco, New York, Futura Publishing Company, 1983, p 91

25. Gruss JD, Bartels D, Karadedos C, Tsafandakis E, Straubel H, Ohta T: Unser Behandlungskonzept beim akuten Verschluß der Vena subclavia. Phlebol u Proktol 10:25, 1981

26. DeWeese JA: Management of subclavian venous obstruction, in Bergan JJ, Yao JST (eds): Surgery of the Veins. Orlando–San Diego–New York–London–Toronto–Montreal–Sydney–Tokyo, Grune and Stratton, 1985, p 365

C. V. Ruckley

31

Can We Help the Postphlebitic Limb?

A broad definition of the postphlebitic syndrome will be adopted. In clinical practice it is difficult to do otherwise. When a patient presents with the symptoms and signs of chronic venous insufficiency it may not be possible to ascertain what role, if any, venous thrombosis has played in the pathogenesis. The features are generally nonspecific: a heavy, aching limb with varicose veins and skin changes including eczema, pigmentation, atrophie blanche, and ulceration in the gaiter area. Exceptionally the symptoms include venous claudication, swelling, and cyanosis indicating major outflow obstruction which can be related to a definite episode of ilio-femoral thrombosis. However, recanalisation or collateral development eventually minimise the obstructive component. Valvular incompetence is by far the predominant haemodynamic disorder and it makes little practical difference to management whether the defect is congenital or acquired.

PREVENTION

One of the justifications for an active approach to the treatment of acute deep venous thrombosis (DVT) has been the expectation that the surgical removal or rapid dissolution of thrombus would minimise valve damage and preserve function. Supporting evidence is limited since few centres have sufficient numbers of patients or completeness of follow-up.

Venous thrombectomy has fallen from favour in all but a few centres. The relatively good long-term results reported by some authors[1-6] have been balanced by other series in which there are high complication rates in the acute phase[7] and high reocclusion rates,[7-9] which have led the authors to limit the indications for surgery to limb-threatening thromboses, i.e., phlegmasia caerulea dolens and impending venous gangrene. It has to be borne in mind that these latter conditions are usually associated with advanced malignancy.

VASCULAR SURGERY: ISSUES IN CURRENT PRACTICE
ISBN 0-8089-1839-7

A seed of doubt as to whether thrombectomy should be abandoned remains from the observations by several authors that when the operation does succeed, specifically in those patients whose veins have been shown to remain phlebographically patent on late follow-up, the postphlebitic syndrome is likely to be avoided or ameliorated.[2, 3, 4, 6, 10]

Thrombolytic therapy has also waned in popularity in recent years on account of its high complication rates and limited success in relation to cost. The principal obstacle in DVT, unlike arterial thrombosis, is that there is often a delay of several days between the onset of the thrombosis and the development of symptoms. Consequently the thrombus, or a substantial proportion of it, is not susceptible to lysis. Even when complete early lysis is obtained the evidence for long-term benefit from thrombolytic therapy is not plentiful. Common and coworkers assessed the clinical and phlebographic outcome at a mean of seven months in 15 streptokinase(SK)-treated patients compared with 12 treated with heparin.[11] They observed that the superior phlebographic clearance obtained with SK corresponded with clinical outcome. Johansson, Ericson, and Zetterquist also related the success of lysis to clinical outcome in a review of 19 patients followed for between 6 and 50 months.[12] Eight patients whose follow-up phlebograms were normal were free of postphlebitic symptoms and they also had normal outflow capacity and valvular function, as demonstrated by venous occlusion plethysmography. Johansson and coworkers carried out foot volumetry and phlebography in 19 patients 8–14 years after treatment with heparin or SK (not randomised).[13] They found fewer postthrombotic symptoms in patients who had had successful lysis.

Unfortunately these optimistic early results have not been borne out by more recent studies. Norgren and Widmer carried out foot volumetry on 21 patients 2–9 years after treatment with SK.[14] They found normal venous function in two out of four who had had successful lysis of femoral thrombi but in all 17 patients who had had both femoral and calf thrombi the expelled volumes were abnormally low, regardless of whether or not lysis had been achieved. Albrechtsson and coworkers reported that at an average of 29 months after SK treatment for phlebographically proven DVT only two out of 35 patients were without symptoms or signs of venous insufficiency and had normal findings on plethysmography and foot volumetry.[15]

One may conclude that while thrombectomy or thrombolytic therapy can remove or ameliorate postthrombotic symptoms in the acute stage, and possibly reduce the danger of major embolism, they make little difference in the majority of patients to the development of chronic venous insufficiency.

Should the new generation of thrombolytic agents such as acylated plasminogen-streptokinase[16, 17] and tissue plasminogen activator[18] prove more effective than streptokinase alone in achieving early lysis then the question of late sequelae will have to be examined afresh.

Heparin is the mainstay of treatment in the acute stage. It is usually followed by a course of oral anticoagulants. Whether prolonging the course of anticoagulants protects against the development of postthrombotic syndrome is not known. Since the process of organisation and canalisation take place over many weeks or months[19] there are theoretical grounds for continuing anticoagulants for six months or more. Hull and coworkers compared warfarin sodium with low-dose heparin in the long-term treatment of venous thrombosis. They found that when thrombi extended into the popliteal vein or above, recurrences were frequent when low-dose heparin was given but no recurrences occurred on warfarin therapy.[20] Holgrem and coworkers compared one month versus six months of warfarin treatment in patients with symptomatic DVT. During a one-year follow-up there were 17 symptomatic recurrences with no differences between the treatment groups.[21]

MANAGEMENT

Assessment

In the early stages after a DVT swelling, heaviness and aching on standing may be the only symptoms. Secondary varicose veins usually take months or years to develop while the changes of lipodermatosclerosis may not develop until 10 or even 20 years have elapsed.[22] From time to time, however, one sees patients who develop the full postphlebitic syndrome, including ulceration, within a few months of the acute thrombotic episode.

Since in the majority of patients graduated elastic compression is all that is required to ameliorate symptoms and to prevent progression, radiological or laboratory investigations are usually not necessary. In more severely affected legs, especially in younger patients, they are valuable.

The choice of phlebographic technique and the quality of the examination are all important. Nonirritant contrast medium should be used.[23] Ascending phlebography may delineate outflow obstruction satisfactorily but will usually require to be supplemented by contralateral perfemoral phlebography if the pelvic veins and cava are to be properly visualised. The demonstration of valve incompetence in the deep system requires descending phlebography. Secondary varicose veins, especially those of the recurrent variety, may require varicography to detect the deep connections of thigh varices, while calf perforators are best delineated by the ascending technique.

The assessment of reflux at the sapheno-femoral junction, the sapheno-popliteal junction, and at perforator sites can be made easily and quickly in the clinic with a portable directional Doppler. The patency and competence of the deep veins can be assessed by the same means.[24]

To assess the nature and severity of the haemodynamic derangement direct pressure measurements have largely been replaced by noninvasive methods. These include foot volumetry, photoplethysmography, and strain-gauge plethysmography. Their principal place is in the assessment of the severity of outflow obstruction or of reflux and they are particularly valuable, being readily repeatable, for monitoring the progression of disease and the response to treatment.

In the late stages of chronic venous insufficiency investigations take on a somewhat different role. Population studies of patients with chronic leg ulcers indicate that only about two-thirds give a history of venous disease.[25] Of these approximately half are purely of venous aetiology while the remainder are of mixed aetiology. This is predominantly an elderly population with a peak prevalence in the 70–75 age group. Since elastic compression is the standard treatment for venous ulcers the most important aetiological factor to recognise is arterial insufficiency either in the form of atherosclerosis or of arteritis. Measurement of the Doppler resting pressure index is the most useful noninvasive test where the pulses are impalpable. Evidence of arteritis should be sought by appropriate serology.

TREATMENT

The Whole Patient

The haemodynamic disorder in chronic venous insufficiency is compounded by a variety of factors of which obesity and locomotor disorders, notably arthropathy, are the most important. Chronic venous ulcer is seldom seen in a lean and fit individual. It follows that potentially there is a great deal that can be achieved by conservative measures such as weight control and physiotherapy. In practice this approach proves to be fruitless in a disappointingly high proportion of patients, partly because of age and partly because there is often an element of psychological inadequacy or self-neglect which has given rise to the peripheral complications in the first place.

In some patients the postthrombotic syndrome is the result not of a single thrombosis but of recurrent episodes. Malignant disease should always be considered. The first essential, in order to avoid the unnecessary administration of anticoagulants, is to distinguish between an exacerbation of symptoms and a true recurrence of acute thrombosis. Phlebography in these circumstances may be difficult to interpret. Leclerc and coworkers have advocated a system of initial screening with impedance plethysmography and ^{125}I-fibrinogen scanning.[26] If recurrent thromboses are confirmed a haematological screen should be carried out for a hypercoagulable state. This topic has been comprehensively reviewed by Schafer.[27] In the author's experience the cause of recurrent thromboses remains obscure in the majority of patients.

The Limb

Care of the limb afflicted with chronic venous insufficiency comprises physiotherapy, control of oedema, skin care, and correction of superficial venous hypertension.

In the elderly patient the abnormalities of gait, so common in patients with ulcer, may be beyond correction, but improvements may be made in the function of the calf muscle pump by increased joint mobility and by muscle-building exercise. Oedema should be controlled in the first instance by posture and exercise. Pneumatic compression or bandaging of the elevated limb under skilled supervision can be successful. Attempts to reduce oedema solely by tight bandaging are dangerous. Diuretics are not appropriate for the long-term control of venous or lymphatic oedema.

Once controlled, oedema may be contained in a graduated elastic compression stocking whose main function is to counteract the venous hypertension. It has been demonstrated that to give maximal benefit compression should be greatest at the ankle and diminishing as it ascends the leg.[27] It has also been shown that graduated stockings with ankle pressures between 30 and 50 mmHg increased the expelled volume and extended the refilling times in postphlebitic patients.[29] However, there is little guidance to be found on the appropriate pressures for different grades of severity and different types of patients. Indeed, it has not even been proven that elastic support is superior to nonelastic support. In practice one prescribes the grade of stocking which the patient can don and wear with comfort. In the great majority of patients these simple measures provide relief of symptoms and protection from complications.

PHARMACOLOGICAL AGENTS

There are two approaches to medical treatment which appear to have a sound experimental basis. The first is fibrinolytic enhancement designed to reverse the process of pericapillary fibrin cuff formation which has been observed in the lipo-sclerotic tissues of the ulcer-bearing area in chronic venous insufficiency.[30] Treatment of lipodermatosclerosis with stanozolol has been shown to be effective,[31] but a similar effect in the ulcerated limb has yet to be proven.

The increased capillary permeability which occurs in chronic venous hypertension and which is responsible for the chronic inflammatory changes in the skin and subcutaneous tissues can, in experimental models, be inhibited by hydroxy-ethylrutosides.[32, 33] A reduction in oedema has been reported in patients with chronic venous insufficiency treated with hydroxyethylrutosides.[34]

SURGERY

Provided that the deep veins have been shown by phlebogram to be patent, the skin and subcutaneous tissues may be protected from the effects of venous hypertension by interception of the communications between deep and superficial systems. This at least is the theoretical basis of ligation of the perforators in the calf.[35, 36] Whether, in the absence of graduated compression, this operation prevents ulcer recurrence remains a matter for debate. It may depend on whether there is simply perforator incompetence as distinct from perforator incompetence combined with deep reflux. Early reports of good results[37–42] have been followed by others reporting high recurrence rates and advocating noninterference with perforators.[43–47] There is a need for prospective studies in which postoperative ulcer recurrence is related to competence of the deep system. Of crucial importance is the careful separation of chronic ulcers into different pathological groups, not only in terms of the patterns of venous insufficiency but also of associated diseases.[48] Negus and Friegood, in reporting that 83% of 91 ulcers remained healed after vein surgery when followed up for a mean of more than three years, have underlined the particular healing problems presented by ulcers in the presence of rheumatoid disease.[49]

VENOUS RECONSTRUCTION

Patency and valvular competence are the two functional requirements of the deep system. As noted earlier obstruction in the deep veins is relatively rare among patients with chronic venous insufficiency. Whether it can be relieved by surgical reconstruction depends on the level of the block, the pressure differential, and whether the inflow and outflow channels are patent. Where the popliteal and tibial veins are chronically occluded reconstruction is not possible and surgery on superficial varicosities is likely to aggravate the disability.

Since it is valvular incompetence in the deep veins which is the most important lesion in chronic venous insufficiency, valve repair or replacement offers the greatest theoretical attraction in the treatment of this disease. This is dealt with in the following chapter.

It is clear, however, that the great majority of patients with chronic venous insufficiency, whether it is "postphlebitic" or not, are neither suitable for venous reconstruction nor do they need it. They can be helped by simple commonsense measures supplemented, in judiciously selected patients, by properly executed surgery to the superficial veins and the perforators.

REFERENCES

1. Harris EJ, Brown WH: Patency after thrombectomy for iliofemoral thrombosis. Ann Surg 167:91–97, 1968
2. DeWeese JA, Adams JT, Rogoff SM: Restoration and maintenance of venous patency in venous thrombosis: Anticoagulation, thrombectomy and partial venous interruption. Pacific Med Surg 75:77–82, 1967
3. Mavor GE, Galloway JMD: Iliofemoral venous thrombosis. Br J Surg 56:45–52, 1969
4. Provan JL, Rumble EJ: Re-evaluation of thrombectomy in the management of iliofemoral venous thrombosis. Canad J Surg 22:378–381, 1979
5. Goto H, Wada T, Matsumoto A, Matsumura H, Soma T: Iliofemoral venous thrombectomy. J Cardiovasc Surg 21:341–346, 1980
6. Andriopoulos A, Wirsing P, Botticher R: Results of iliofemoral venous thrombectomy after acute thrombosis. J Cardiovasc Surg 23:123–124, 1982
7. Johansson E, Nordlander S, Zetterquist S: Venous thrombectomy in the lower extremity—clinical, phlebographic and plethysmographic evaluation of early and late results. Acta Chir Scand 139:511–516, 1973
8. Lansing AM, Davis WM: Five year follow up study of ilio-femoral venous thrombectomy. Ann Surg 168:620–626, 1974
9. Raithel D, Sohnlein B: Limited indication for venous thrombectomy. J Cardiovasc Surg 22:511, 1981
10. Eklof B, Einarsson E, Plate G: Role of thrombectomy and temporary arteriovenous fistula in acute iliofemoral venous thrombosis, in Bergan JJ, Yao JST (eds): Surgery of the Veins. Grune and Stratton, 1985, pp 131–144
11. Common HH, Seaman AJ, Rosch J, Porter JM, Dotter CT: Deep vein thrombosis treated with streptokinase or heparin. Angiology 27(11):645–654, 1976
12. Johansson E, Ericson L, Zetterquist S: Streptokinase treatment of deep venous thrombosis of the lower extremity. Acta Med Scand 199:89–94, 1976
13. Johansson L, Nylander G, Hedner U, Nilsson IM: Comparison of streptokinase with heparin: Late results in the treatment of deep venous thrombosis. Acta Med Scand 206:93–98, 1979
14. Norgren L, Widmer, LK: Venous function evaluated by foot volumetry in patients with a previous deep venous thrombosis treated with streptokinase. VASA 7(4):412–414, 1978
15. Albrechtsson U, Anderson J, Einarsson E, Eklof B, Norgren L: Streptokinase treatment of deep venous thrombosis and the postthrombotic syndrome. Arch Surg 116:33–37, 1981

16. Smith RAG, Dupe RJ, English PD, Green J: Fibrinolysis with acylenzymes: A new approach to thrombolytic therapy. Nature 290:505–508, 1981

17. Prowse CV, Hornsey V, Ruckley CV, Boulton FE: A comparison of acylated streptokinase plasminogen complex and streptokinase in human volunteers. Thromb Haemostas 47:132–135, 1982

18. Collen D: Human tissue type plasminogen activator: From the laboratory to the bed side. Circulation 72:18–20, 1982

19. Pathology of venous thrombosis. Chapter in Hume M, Sevitt S, Thomas DP (eds): Venous Thrombosis and Pulmonary Embolism, vol 2. Harvard, 1970, pp 25–53

20. Hull R, Delmore T, Genton E, et al: Warfarin sodium versus low dose heparin in the long term treatment of deep venous thrombosis. New Engl J Med 301:855–858, 1979

21. Holgrem K, Andersson G, Fagrell B, et al: One month versus six month therapy with oral anticoagulants after deep vein thrombosis. Acta Med Scand 218:279–284, 1985

22. Bauer G: A roentgenological and clinical study of the sequels of thrombosis. Acta Chir Scand (Suppl) 86:74, 1942

23. Albrechtsson U, Olsson CG: Thrombosis after phlebography: A comparison of two contrast media. Cardiovasc Radiol 2:9–14, 1979

24. Barnes RW: Non invasive diagnostic techniques in peripheral vascular disease. Am Heart J 97:241–258, 1979

25. Callam M, Ruckley CV, Harper DR, Dale JJ: Chronic ulceration of the leg: Extent of the problem and provision of care. Br Med J 1985:1855–1856, 1985

26. Leclerc JR, Jay RM, Hull RD, Hirsh J: Recurrent leg symptoms following deep vein thrombosis. A diagnostic challenge. Arch Int Med 145:1867–1869, 1985

27. Schafer AI: The hypercoagulable states. Ann Int Med 102:814–828, 1985

28. Fernandes é Fernandes J, Horner J, Needham T, Nicolaides AN: Value of graduated compression stockings in venous disorders of the legs. Br Med J 1980:820–821, 1980

29. Jones NAG, Webb PJ, Rees RI, Kakkar VV: A physiological study of elastic compression stockings in venous disorders of the legs. Br J Surg 1980:569–572, 1980

30. Burnand KG, Clemensen G, Whimster I, et al: The effect of sustained venous hypertension in the skin capillaries of the canine hind limb. Br J Surg 69:41–44, 1982

31. Burnand KG, Clemensen G, Morland M: Venous lipodermatosclerosis treated by fibrinolytic enhancement and elastic compression. Brit Med J 280:7–11, 1980

32. Svensjo E, Arfors K-E, Arturson G, Bergqvist D, Rutili G: Effects of O-(beta-hydroxy-ethyl)-rutoside on macromolecular permeability in the hamster cheek pouch microvasculature, in Kappert (ed): New Trends in Venous Disease. Berne Hans Huber, 1977, pp 296–301

33. Hilton JG: Dose related inhibition by intravenous hydroxyethylrutosides of plasma volume loss after thermal injury, in Hydroxyethylrutosides in Vascular Disease. Academic Press, 1981, pp 15–18

34. Bergqvist D, Hallböök T: A double blind trial of O-(beta-hydroxyethyl)-rutosides in patients with chronic venous insufficiency, in Hydroxyethylrutosides in Vascular Disease. Academic Press, 1981, pp 31–32

35. Linton R: The communicating veins of the lower leg and the operative technique for their ligation. Ann Surg 107:582–587, 1938.

36. Cockett FB and Elgan Jones DE: The ankle blow out syndrome: A new approach to the varicose ulcer problem. Lancet 1:17–23, 1953

37. Cranley JJ, Krause RS, Strasser ES: Chronic venous insufficiency of the lower extremity. Surgery 49:48–58, 1961

38. Hansson LO: Venous ulcers of the lower limb. Acta Chir Scand 128:269–277, 1964

39. Bertelsen S, Gamelgaard A: Surgical treatment of postthrombotic leg ulcers. J Cardiovasc Surg 6:452, 1965

40. Silver D, Gleyston JJ, Rhodes GR, et al: Surgical treatment of the refractory postphlebitic ulcers. Arch Surg 103:554–557, 1971

41. Field P, Van Boxall P: The role of the Linton flap procedure in the management of stasis dermatitis and ulceration in the lower limb. Surgery 70:920–926, 1971
42. Arnoldi IC, Haeger K: Ulcus cruris venosum-crux medicorum Lakartidnningen 64:2149–2157, 1967
43. Racek E: A critical appraisal of the role of ankle perforators for the genesis of venous ulcers in the lower leg. J Cardiovasc Surg 12: 45–51, 1971
44. Burnand KG, Lea Thomas M, O'Donnel E, et al: Relation between post-phlebitic changes in the deep veins and results of surgical treatment of venous ulcers. Lancet 1:936–938, 1976
45. Lumley JSP: Surgical treatment of varicose veins, in Marston A (ed): Contemporary Operative Surgery. London, Northwood Books, 1979
46. Strandness DE, Theile DL: Selected Topics in Venous Disorders. New York, Futura, 1981
47. Browse NL, Burnand KG: The cause of venous ulceration. Lancet 2:243–245, 1982
48. Ruckley CV, Dale JJ, Callam MJ, et al: Causes of chronic leg ulcer. Lancet 2:615–616, 1982
49. Negus D, Friegood A: The effective management of venous ulceration. Br J Surg 70:623–627, 1983

Simon G. Darke

32

Reconstructive Surgery for Chronic Venous Insufficiency of the Lower Limb

INTRODUCTION

Reconstructive surgery for chronic venous insufficiency of the lower limb is undertaken to overcome obstruction or to restore valvular competence. Obstruction is usually the sequela of previous thrombosis, but may occasionally be due to malignant infiltration or compression. It is now recognised that deep valvular incompetence (DVI) is more commonly due to an inherent or "primary" weakness, although it may also be the result of previous thrombotic episodes. Technical innovations over the last 10 years have led to renewed interest in the possibilities of repairing this defect.

The indications for and limitations of venous reconstruction for outflow obstruction and similar aspects of venous surgery have recently been comprehensively and authoritatively documented.[1,2] It is not intended, therefore, to focus on this aspect but instead to discuss the unresolved questions that surround surgery for DVI.

A consecutive series of patients with chronic venous disorders of the lower limb are reported, in which the prevalence and, in particular, likely clinical significance of DVI is assessed. This is established by correlating the clinical state with investigative findings, assessing the benefits of conventional saphenous and perforator surgery in the presence of coexistent DVI, and by quantifiable tests of venous function. The pathogenesis and diagnosis will be discussed, along with the technical options, and reported results of valve surgery to date. Comments will derive both from review of the existing literature and from the author's experience. By these means it is hoped to rationalise the selection of patients for these procedures and develop a general strategy for management of chronic venous insufficiency of the lower limb.

VASCULAR SURGERY: ISSUES IN CURRENT PRACTICE
ISBN 0-8089-1839-7

CLINICAL MATERIAL

Patients with chronic venous disorders can, for convenience, be divided into those with primary varicose veins and those with complex problems. The latter group comprises both the skin changes of venous insufficiency culminating in ulceration, and the syndrome of pain and swelling of the leg. These may occur separately, or coexist.

Over a 30-month period a consecutive series of patients with chronic venous disorders has been studied. These patients were referred to one surgeon with an interest in arterial and venous disorders. A total of 594 patients have been assessed. Table 32-1 shows the categories into which these patients have been divided. Those who, on clinical grounds, were thought to have primary and uncomplicated varicose veins are not considered further.

Table 32-1
Thirty-Month Study—Consecutive Series

Total number of patients	594
Patients with primary varicose veins	466
No saphenous incompetence 46	
Saphenous incompetence 420	
Patients with complex disorders	128 (145 limbs)
48 limbs ulcer	(26 women, mean age 56)
52 limbs ulcer pain and swelling	(22 women, mean age 54)
45 limbs pain and swelling alone	(22 women, mean age 40)

All those with "ulcer" had current ulceration or lesions that had only healed within the previous three months. Those designated as having the "pain and swelling" syndrome had both measurable calf oedema (and, in some, in the thigh as well) and described pain, often provoked by exercise, and in excess of the ache which may be associated with primary and uncomplicated varicose veins. Thus, three groups of patients were identified on clinical grounds and are studied and compared:

1. There were 42 patients with 48 limbs with ulcer alone. In 14 limbs there was a past history of deep vein thrombosis and in 16 limbs a family history of similar disorders.
2. There were 46 patients with 52 limbs with ulcer and pain and swelling as well. In 20 limbs there was a family history of similar disorders and in 15 a past history of deep venous thrombosis.
3. There were 39 patients with 45 limbs with isolated pain and swelling syndrome. They tended to be a little younger than the other groups. In 17 limbs there was a family history of a similar disorder. There was a past history of deep venous thrombosis in 11 legs.

All these patients have been studied by clinical assessment, Doppler ultrasound, to demonstrate saphenous and popliteal vein incompetence,[3–5] and by ascending and descending venography,[6] to identify ankle perforator incompetence, postphlebitic damage to calf, thigh, and pelvic veins, and superficial and deep femoral reflux.

RESULTS

By these means a variety of abnormalities may be recognised. These are summarised in Table 32-2.

Table 32-2

Abnormalities	Modes of Recognition
Long saphenous incompetence	Clinical Doppler
Short saphenous incompetence	Doppler
Ankle perforator incompetence	Ascending venography Doppler
Postphlebitic damage to Calf veins Thigh veins Pelvic veins	Ascending venography
Popliteal vein incompetence	Doppler Duplex
Superficial and deep femoral vein incompetence	Descending venography Duplex scan

Incidence of Femoral Incompetence

In this study, venographic evidence of femoral reflux of grade II[7,8] has arbitrarily been regarded as clinically significant.

Table 32-3 shows the incidence of grade II or greater reflux in the superficial femoral vein alone, the superficial and deep femoral vein, and in the deep femoral vein alone, in the three groups of patients studied. A total of 65 limbs out of the 145 exhibited incompetence. In 54 this was confined to the superficial femoral vein. In eight this was in both superficial and deep femoral veins. Finally, there were three patients in which the only identified abnormality was incompetence of the deep femoral vein itself. These patients complained of pain and swelling in the thigh. Examination revealed oedema, warmth, and dilated varicosities confined to the thigh. The author has been unable to find a description of this recorded in the literature.

Table 32-3
Femoral Incompetence

	Ulcer	Ulcer, Pain and Swelling	Pain and Swelling
Total number of limbs	48	52	45
SFV alone	16	22	16
SFV + DFV	0	5	3
DFV alone	0	0	3

SFV = superficial femoral vein
DFV = deep femoral vein

Correlation between Venographic Evidence of Femoral Incompetence and Doppler Evidence of Popliteal Reflux

Of the 65 patients with femoral incompetence of grade II or greater severity, 49 had associated reflux in the popliteal vein on Doppler. There were a further 19 patients with Doppler evidence of reflux, but with competent valves above, as shown on venography. Details of patients with superficial, deep, and popliteal incompetence in the three groups of patients is shown in Table 32-4.

Table 32-4
Correlation between "Venographic Incompetence" of the Superficial Femoral Vein (SFV), Deep Femoral Vein (DFV) and "Ultrasound Incompetence" of the Popliteal Vein (PV)

	Ulcer Alone		Ulcer, Pain, and Swelling		Pain and Swelling		Total	
	Number	%	Number	%	Number	%	Number	%
	48	100	52	100	45	100	145	100
SFV + PV	9	17	20	39	10	23	39	27
PV alone	6	11	6	11	7	16	19	13
SFV alone	7	15	2	4	6	11	15	10
SFV + PV + DFV	0	0	5	10	3	7	8	5
DFV + PV	0	0	0	0	2	4	2	1
DFV alone	0	0	0	0	1	2	1	0.5
SFV + DFV	0	0	0	0	0	0	0	0

This degree of correlation between these two means of investigation is of relevance. It implies that what is demonstrated on X-rays is of haemodynamic significance. Furthermore, the Doppler popliteal reflux test is simple, noninvasive, quick, and easy to perform. It can be used to screen patients. (There were no patients within the group designated as having primary and uncomplicated varicose veins in whom popliteal incompetence was demonstrated.)

That femoral and popliteal reflux may be demonstrated independently has been reported by others. Taheri, Lazar, and Elias[9,10] have described a group of patients who have a competent femoral and upper superficial femoral valves but incompetent popliteal valves below this level. This was demonstrated by serial injections of dye following retrograde catheterisation through the transbrachial route. Nicolaides[11] has made similar observations with duplex studies.

Pathogenesis: Relationship of DVI to Previous Thrombosis

Venographic evidence of previous deep vein thrombosis, although not quantifiable, can be separated anatomically into changes in the calf, thigh, and iliac systems. Of the 145 limbs studied this was present in 31. It was confined to the calf in 10, present in calf and thigh in 9, calf, thigh, and iliac system in 3, thigh alone in 5, iliac system alone in 3, and thigh and iliac systems in 1. There was no difference in the

Table 32-5

Incidence and Distribution on Venographic Evidence of
Previous DVT

	All Limbs	Ulcer Alone	Ulcer, Pain, and Swelling	Pain and Swelling Alone
Total limbs studied	145	48	52	45
Calf alone	10	4	3	3
Calf and thigh	9	3	3	3
Calf, thigh, and iliac	3	2	0	1
Thigh alone	5	2	3	0
Iliac alone	3	0	2	1
Thigh and iliac	1	0	1	0

incidence and distribution between the three groups of patients; details of this are given in Table 32-5. Included among these cases with a damaged deep venous system are two due to trauma.

There were 15 patients in this group with grade II or greater femoral reflux on venography. In common with previous authors,[12–15] therefore, in 50 of the 65 patients in this series of DVI there was no evidence demonstrable on X-rays of previous deep venous thrombosis. These data support the view that there is a "primary" or inherent weakness in the valve or vein wall which accounts for the abnormality. It is, of course, possible that in a proportion of limbs, previous thrombosis had damaged the cusps and this was not apparent on the X-ray. However, findings at operation and histological studies of excised segments have, in the author's experience, failed to suggest any unsuspected previous thrombosis in the few cases where it was appropriate to make these assessments. This view is supported by Raju.[15]

The possibility that primary DVI might in itself predispose to thrombotic incidents has also been suggested.[15] The author has anecdotal evidence to support this view, in the form of three patients reported here:

1. A 25-year-old man presented with pain, swelling, and ulceration in the left leg which followed a compound fracture of the tibia and fibula, complicated by an ilio-femoral thrombosis two years earlier. Venography confirmed postphlebitic damage to calf, thigh, and iliac vessels with associated deep reflux. An incidental finding in his opposite normal limb was popliteal reflux on routine testing with the Doppler. Venography confirmed superficial femoral reflux. There was no evidence of previous thrombosis in this limb.

2. A previously fit 36-year-old man awoke with a painful swollen left leg and was referred as a possible spontaneous deep vein thrombosis. This was confirmed on ascending venography. There were no demonstrable predisposing factors. In the opposite asymptomatic limb there was popliteal reflux on routine Doppler testing, with grade III superficial femoral reflux on descending venography, without evidence of previous thrombosis.

3. A 52-year-old man with known chronic venous insufficiency with pain and swelling syndrome had two years previously undergone venography which had shown grade III reflux in the superficial femoral vein associated with popliteal

reflux on Doppler. There were no other abnormalities and no sign of previous deep vein thrombosis. No surgical treatment was undertaken. He presented as an emergency with an acute exacerbation of pain and swelling in the leg and ascending venography demonstrated thrombosis, apparently "spontaneous", in the calf and thigh.

CLINICAL RELEVANCE OF DEEP INCOMPETENCE

The demonstration of DVI is not in itself evidence that it is necessarily of relevance. The likely clinical significance can be best determined by assessing this finding in the context of other coexistent abnormalities which might also be contributory. Various combinations were found and in most instances there was more than one disorder. These are analysed in the patients with ulcer, with or without pain and swelling, and those with the pain and swelling syndrome alone.

LIMBS WITH VENOUS ULCERATION, WITH OR WITHOUT PAIN AND SWELLING SYNDROME

There were a total of 100 limbs studied in this group. The combinations of abnormalities are shown in Table 32-6. There were six limbs with perforator incompetence alone. In 29 limbs there was a combination of saphenous (only two short saphenous) and perforator incompetence. There were 23 patients with postphlebitic damage and 11 with associated superficial femoral incompetence in addition to a variety of saphenous and popliteal incompetence. The remainder exhibited a combination of DVI, perforator incompetence, and, in some, saphenous incompetence.

In all these patients, therefore, there are demonstrable abnormalities independent of deep incompetence, which are regarded as causative factors in the develop-

Table 32-6
Incidence, Venographic and
Doppler Incompetence:
Ulcerated Limbs with or
without Pain and Swelling

Total number of limbs studied	100
Perf. alone	6
Perf. saph.	29
Perf. saph. SFV + PV	16
Perf. saph. SFV	7
Perf. saph. PV	8
Perf. SFV + PV	11
Phlebitic ± other (11 with SFV)	23

Perf. = perforator
Saph. = sapheno-femoral (two short
saphenous)
SFV = superficial femoral vein
PV = popliteal vein (Doppler)

ment of venous ulcer. On this evidence alone, the precise pathogenic significance of DVI remains uncertain. Further information is sought from determining the effects of surgery.

Strategy for Management of Venous Ulcer: Relative Significance of Saphenous and Perforator Incompetence, DVI, and Postphlebitic Damage

In the author's view saphenous ligation remains the main therapeutic tool, appropriate to at least 30% of cases, and probably more. Its value in venous ulceration has been presented in more detail elsewhere.[16] In 29% of the limbs with ulcer, saphenous and perforator incompetence were the only abnormalities. It must therefore be recognised that ulceration may occur in the presence of competent deep veins, and without evidence of previous thrombosis. Preoperative vein pressure measurements in this group of patients indicate that groin ligation and limited stripping can be expected to reestablish relatively normal venous haemodynamics. It is concluded that associated perforator incompetence is of secondary importance. This group of patients are the easiest to treat and offer the best chance of a successful outcome. Those with isolated perforator incompetence and normal deep veins (6%) can be expected to respond to appropriate ligation.[17]

Twenty-three per cent with ulcer combine saphenous and perforator incompetence with DVI without evidence of previous thrombosis. This group is currently being studied further. Preliminary results of pressure measurements, photoplethysmography, and clinical assessment before and after saphenous and perforator ligation suggest that in a proportion, improvement from these procedures can be expected. However, in common with other workers,[14] there are limbs within this group that are not or have not been apparently improved by this approach, and in these it can be reasonably assumed that DVI is relevant.

This view is supported by the observation that there are patients within this group who have recurrent or persistent ulceration in spite of saphenous ligation performed several years previously.

Of the 100 limbs studied with ulcer, 18 had recurred after previous excision of the long saphenous system some years earlier. Two further cases were in association with subfascial ligation, making 20 in all. Seven of these patients had evidence of previous deep vein thrombosis. There were therefore 13 patients with primary DVI who fall within the category on which discussion centres. In four, ulceration persisted in spite of apparently adequate saphenous ligation. In nine there was recurrent sapheno-femoral incompetence. These data are summarised in Table 32-7. The morphology of saphenous recurrence was typical, showing bizarre tortuous veins reconnecting with distal superficial varicosities.

What is the significance of persistent ulceration after saphenous ligation? In the four without recurrent saphenous incompetence, DVI or possibly perforator incompetence would seem to be critical factors. Of those with recurrence of saphenous incompetence it may be the development of further saphenous reflux per se that has led to further ulceration. Alternatively, saphenous surgery may have been of limited effect in these limbs, with both recurrent ulcer and saphenous incompetence attributable to deep reflux. This issue requires further study.

Table 32-7
Recurrent Ulceration after Previous Saphenous
Ligation: Incidence in 100 Consecutive Limbs

Abnormalities Detected	Number of Limbs	Previous Saphenous Ligation	Recurrent Saphenous Incompetence
Primary saphenous and/or perforator incompetence	35	0	0
Primary DVI ± saphenous perforator incompetence	42	13	9
Postphlebitic ± other	23	6	1

Nonetheless, these data indicate that there is a recognisable group of patients with ulcer in whom DVI is likely to be relevant. These patients might therefore benefit from some form of valve surgery. The position in some patients with combined perforator and deep incompetence (11% of the total) is probably similar.

There were 23 limbs with postphlebitic changes, in 11 of which DVI was apparent. It is difficult to assess the significance of this finding in this group because of the widespread damage and often obstructive elements that exist among these patients. This is discussed further, below.

LIMBS WITH ISOLATED PAIN AND SWELLING SYNDROME

There were 45 limbs studied. The combinations are listed in Table 32-8. For the purposes of this analysis, the presence of ankle perforating incompetence has been ignored as it is thought that this is unlikely to be of relevance in this syndrome. There were 14 patients in whom the only abnormality was DVI and thus it seems this abnormality was a causative factor.

Table 32-8
Venographic Abnormalities—Limbs with Pain
and Swelling Syndrome (Perforator
Incompetence Excluded)

	Number	%
Total number of limbs	45	100
Isolated femoral incompetence	14	31
Isolated saphenous incompetence	10*	22
Postphlebitic changes ± other	8	18
Multiple incompetence	7	15
Isolated popliteal incompetence	3	6.5
Saphenous and popliteal incompetence	3	6.5

* Three with short saphenous vein incompetence.

Of the remainder there were nine limbs in which symptoms could only be ascribed to saphenous incompetence (short saphenous in one). There were eight patients in whom there was postphlebitic damage. In two this was an isolated finding; in two it was associated with both long saphenous and femoral incompetence; in one there was recurrence of saphenous incompetence; in two there was coexistent popliteal incompetence; in one isolated femoral incompetence; and in one femoral and popliteal incompetence. There were six patients with incompetence in the popliteal vein and in three limbs this was associated with saphenous incompetence. In the other three this was an isolated finding. There were a further seven patients with a wide variety of abnormalities.

Tests of Venous Function in Patients with Isolated Deep Venous Incompetence

Photoplethysmography and ambulant dorsal foot vein pressure studies were undertaken on selected patients. In these, investigations had revealed neither saphenous incompetence nor venographic evidence of previous deep vein thrombosis which might influence results. All these patients had grade III or greater reflux in the superficial femoral vein of inherent origin. Some had associated perforator incompetence.

These tests were undertaken in conjunction with and without the application of a tourniquet placed above the ankle and inflated to 120 mmHg to eradicate the effects of ankle perforator incompetence. Where this manoeuvre resulted in an improved performance, this reading was utilised. The results are compared with a group of normal limbs matched for age and sex. Table 32-9 shows the outcome of this investigation. Significant dysfunction in limbs with DVI is apparent.[18] Similar results are reported by Nicolaides,[11] Queral and coworkers,[19] and Eriksson and Almgren.[14]

Table 32-9
Studies of Venous Function: Patients with Isolated Primary
Deep Venous Incompetence

	Number of Limbs	PPG Recovery Time ($\pm$SD) (sec)	Pressure Fall on Exercise (%)
Primary DVI	8	26 (4)	2 (3)
Control	6	7 (2)	38 (6)

EVALUATION OF VALVULAR RECONSTRUCTION

Evidence demonstrating the effects of valve surgery should validate and correlate three aspects, both in the immediate postoperative period and in the long term:

1. to demonstrate technical success;
2. to demonstrate an improvement in quantifiable tests of venous haemodynamics, between pre- and postoperative studies;
3. to evaluate improvement in symptoms and signs.

Patients complain of skin changes, culminating in ulceration and/or the symptoms of pain and swelling. Although the principal aim of any therapeutic manoeuvre is relief of these, they are difficult to assess objectively and document. Ferris and Kistner[20] have suggested a comprehensive scheme by which this might be achieved. Venous ulcers tend to heal and break down again spontaneously. The period of leg elevation and relative immobilisation that is attendant on operative procedures will have brought about improvement irrespective of the effect of valve surgery. Furthermore, other measures to sustain healing may have been introduced, such as enthusiastic nursing care and the use of support stockings. Thus, not only short-term but long-term follow-up are mandatory. The symptoms of pain and swelling and "venous claudication" are subjective and difficult to quantify.

Indications for surgery need to be clearly defined, with documentation of associated venous abnormalities. Synchronous employment of other surgical techniques such as ligation of incompetent saphenous and perforating veins confuse the issue.

Comparisons of these results, between those with inherent weakness and postphlebitic disease, and for the relief of pain and swelling as opposed to skin ulceration, are desirable because differences might exist.

SURGICAL OPTIONS

Brachial Valve Transplant

This procedure was first advocated by Taheri.[21] It consists of the excision of a segment of brachial vein containing one or two valves and the insertion of this into the superficial femoral or popliteal vein. The approach for the latter is similar to that employed for femoro-popliteal bypass. It is a straightforward procedure to perform.

The veins of the arm function at a lower pressure than the legs and the transplanted valves are thus subjected to greater forces. This theoretical disadvantage is exacerbated by the fact that the majority of these patients have inherent weakness of their vein or valve wall—a weakness which may be manifest generally and thus apply equally to the transposed valve. This technique might therefore be better applied to those patients with reflux attributable to postphlebitic disease, in whom it is often the only option anyway, although increased susceptibility to further thrombosis may be a risk.

Free transplant runs the theoretical risk of ischaemic damage due to disruption of the blood supply with consequent damage to the valve cusps (see Fig. 32-1).

Eriksson and Almgren[14] have reported the results of nine valve transplants with a minimum follow-up of six months and in some cases longer. All these patients had grade IV reflux and early postoperative Doppler analysis, and descending venography confirmed function of the valves. Symptomatic relief at six months was present in five out of the nine patients. In these there was improvement in their venous function studies. At later follow-up a number of these have become incompetent, however.

Taheri[22,23] has reported his experience of valve interposition. The indications for surgery are not clear although the majority would seem to have been for the

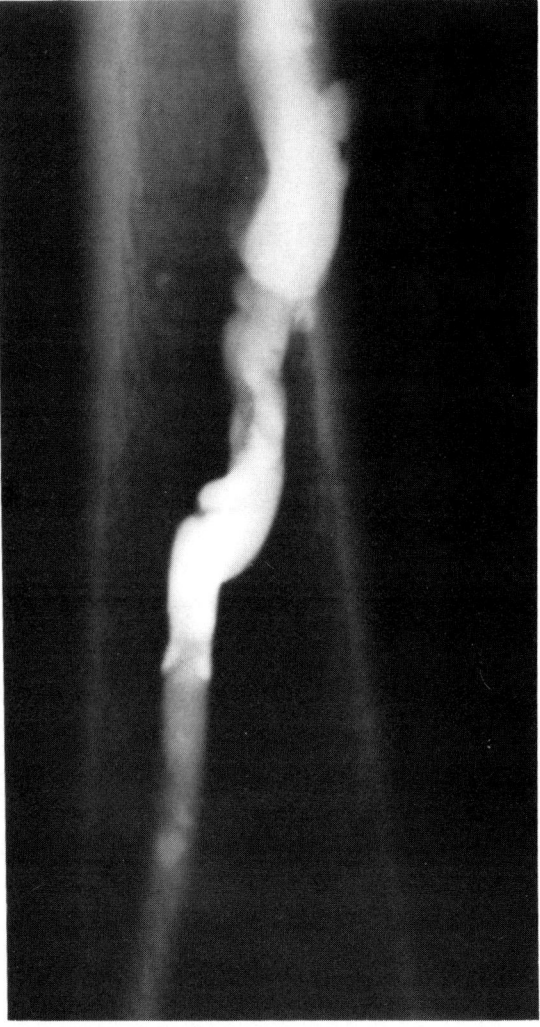

Fig. 32-1. Segment of superficial femoral vein one year after implantation of brachial valve for incompetence following previous deep vein thrombosis. Recurrent incompetence can be seen (although this initially proved to be competent in the early postoperative period) and what appears to be contraction and fibrosis of the transplanted valve cusps.

pain and swelling syndrome. Only 18 of the 52 patients had previous ulceration. The immediate postoperative descending venograms confirmed competence and patence in the great majority—28 out of the 31 limbs studied. Postoperative venous pressure studies were inclusive and difficult to interpret. Unfortunately in this large group of patients, long-term follow-up has only been performed by correspondence. The majority are said to have reported "improvement or complete relief". Those with leg ulcers healed in 17 out of 18 patients. The duration of follow-up of these patients is not stated.

Vein Transposition

The incompetent vein, usually the superficial femoral, is divided and reinserted, end-to-side, to incorporate a competent valve in an adjacent vein. This may be the deep femoral, but the long saphenous has also been used. There are a number of technical variations which can be employed to accomplish this.[13,24] While transposition to the long saphenous vein is a relatively easy procedure there may be doubts as to whether the greater part of the limb's venous return can be accommodated by this channel. Theoretically this might lead either to thrombosis or dilatation of the saphenous and subsequent incompetence of the valve incorporated in the system. Thus transposition to the deep femoral vein, which is usually competent (see Table 32-2), on the face of it would appear more promising.

The concept of transposition to any alternative vein carries the same disadvantage as vein transplant. The newly incorporated valve may be susceptible, in due course, to inherent weakness that existed within the valves of the superficial femoral system (see Fig. 32-2).

Ferris and Kistner[20] report the results of 14 transposition procedures. Two of these were from deep femoral vein to long saphenous vein and one from long saphenous vein to deep femoral. The technical objective for these is not clear. The majority were for the relief of ulceration. Some patients had synchronous interruption of saphenous and perforating veins and it is uncertain as to what extent this component influenced the clinical results, and the evaluation of pre- and postoperative haemodynamic data. Early postoperative venography was performed on most patients and, in these, competence of the inserted valve was confirmed. There was late follow-up available in seven, four of which showed no deterioration in function.

Queral[24] reports haemodynamic measurements, ultrasound, and ascending and descending venography, on a selected group of patients undergoing valvular transposition in whom it was the only procedure undertaken. Four were for ulcer and eight for pain and swelling. Two of the limbs were to the deep femoral vein, the remainder were to the long saphenous vein. In nine of the 12 limbs, deep incompetence was due to postphlebitic damage, as demonstrated on ascending venography. Postoperatively, descending venography showed competence in all but one, apart from two which had thrombosed. There was significant improvement in postoperative PPG assessments, but venous pressure studies failed to show any improvement. The author's interpretation of these findings was that in the postphlebitic limb the extent of venous dysfunction is such that the inclusion of a single competent valve at groin level was insufficient—a point also made by Malette.[25]

These same limbs were then followed up and reported by Johnson and coworkers[26] 18 months after surgery. No patient attained normal venous pressures at any time after surgery and improvement of venous refilling time was transient, nine of the 12 limbs having reverted to preoperative abnormal levels. Unfortunately, descending venography at late follow-up was only available in two limbs. These were patent and still competent.

Valve Repair

The concept that the cusps of the incompetent valve might be sutured and rendered functional was reported by Kistner.[7] The technique has been described and illustrated in detail.[13] This procedure is only applicable to those valves with

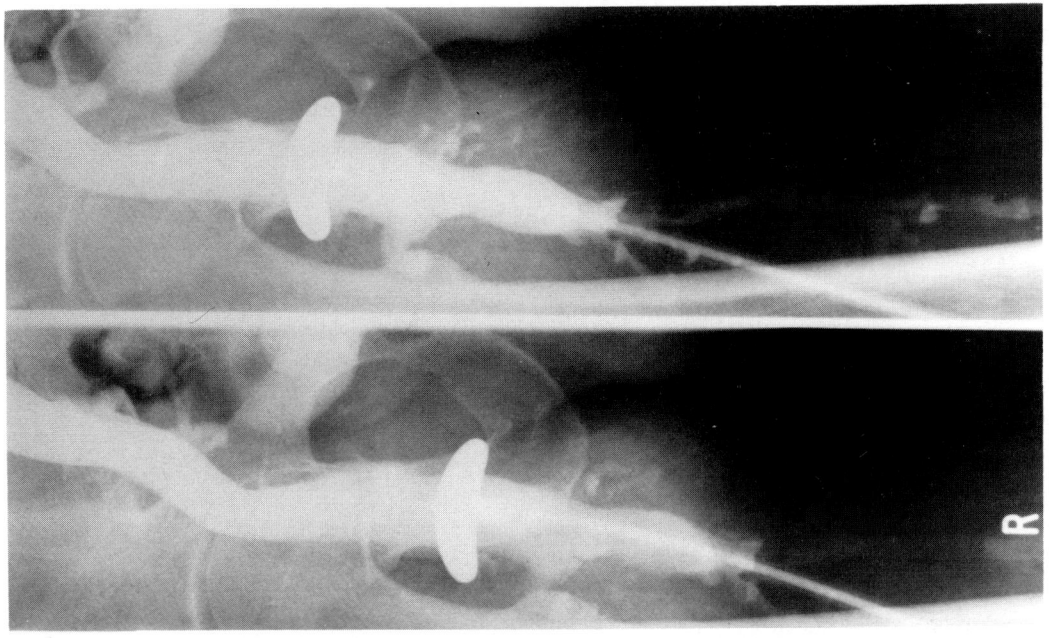

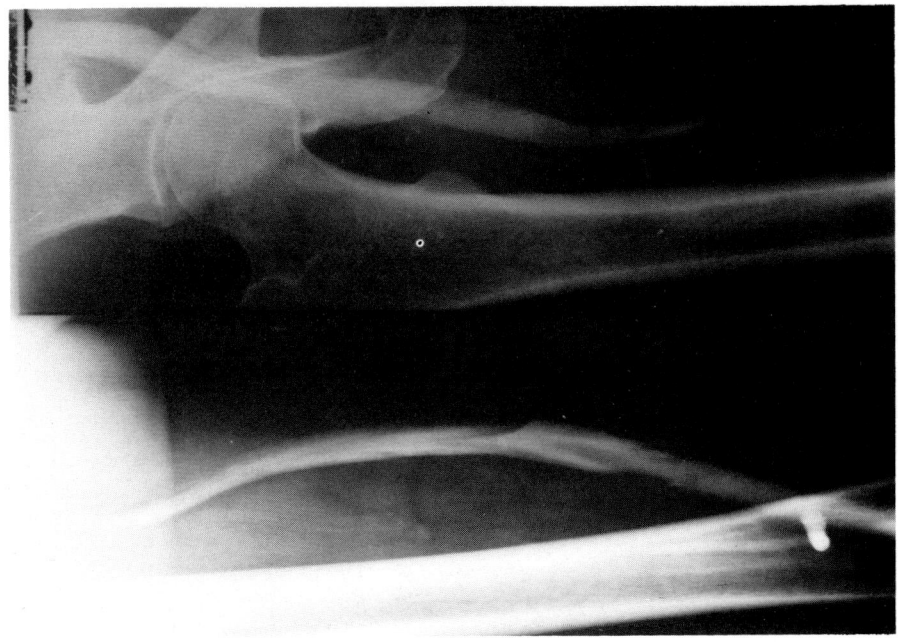

Fig. 32.2. (A) Patent superficial femoral to deep femoral transposition three months postoperatively. (B) Descending venogram at the same time on the same patients showing competence of the femoral system.

429

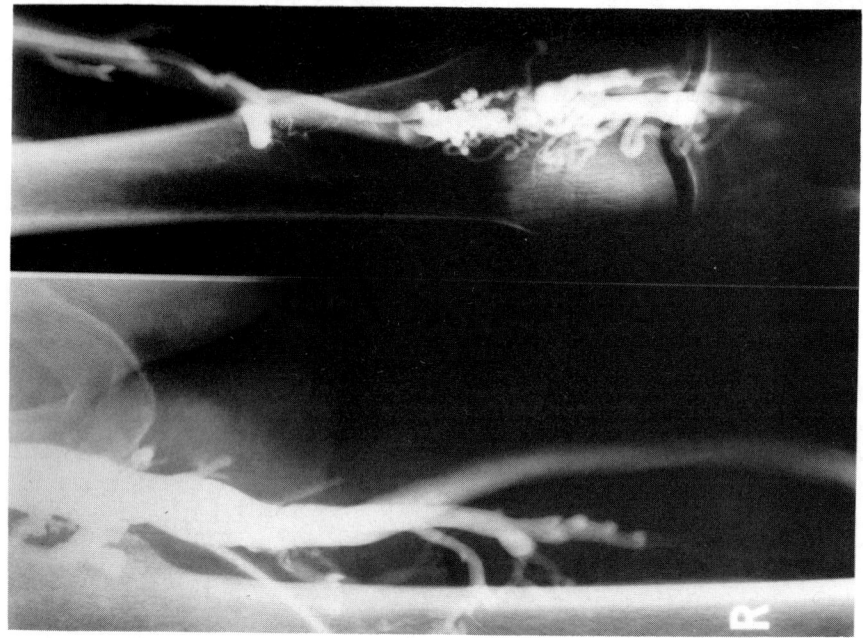

Fig. 32-2. (C) Descending venogram three years later after recurrence of symptoms and ulceration showing that the deep femoral valve has now become incompetent with descent dye into the popliteal vein and early recurrent short saphenous incompetence.

(C)

430

primary weakness which is the greater proportion. Those damaged by previous thrombosis are not suitable. The author has no personal experience of this technique. Inherent weakness is not, per se, altered and the possibility of recurrent laxity and reflux must exist.

Eriksson and Almgren[14] have reported the results of 18 direct valve repairs with a follow-up of not less than six months. Early Doppler analysis confirmed competence in the postoperative period. Associated perforator and saphenous incompetence had been eliminated prior to valve surgery. In general there was good late symptomatic relief of symptoms in 73% of cases and, in particular, they were able to show significant improvement and recovery time in venous pressure movements. However, this was confined to those limbs in which there was competence of the deep femoral vein. These authors conclude that this indicates the importance of the deep femoral vein in venous haemodynamics. Alternatively, it may be a reflection of widespread incompetence throughout the limb and it indicates the degree of valvular dysfunction. At 11 months follow-up, five late failures were observed, with a recurrence of symptoms and return to the preoperative level of venous pressure measurements.

Ferris and Kistner[20] have described their experience of 32 valve repairs principally for ulceration. An undetermined factor is the number in whom synchronous interruption of saphenous and perforating veins was undertaken, although it is conceded that a significant proportion underwent perforator interruption. This makes evaluation of the observed improvement both of symptomatic relief and of pre- and postoperative haemodynamic data difficult to evaluate. Early postoperative venography confirmed that the great majority of repair valves were competent and in 17 patients descending venograms were performed 2–13 years after surgery. In 15 of these the repair appeared to have remained stable, although there was deterioration of valve function in two.

These authors emphasise the need for synchronous interruption of perforators. However, the question must be posed as to whether the perforator ligation alone would have been sufficient to have achieved ulcer healing, particularly as they state that in a proportion of cases in which the incompetent deep system alone was repaired, the results were not so good. They conclude that valve repair produced a durable result.

Jones, Elliott, and Kerstein[27] reported the results in five patients of triangular venous valvular plasty. The technique is to excise a wedge of vein and to reef this, thus narrowing the vein at the point of the valve. No details of follow-up are given.

All authors report a surprisingly and acceptably low incidence of postoperative thrombosis with these three procedures.

Ligation of the Superficial Femoral or Popliteal Vein

This procedure was suggested by Bauer[28] and would seem to have merit if the valves within the deep femoral system, through which the venous return would be substantially rerouted, were competent. The long-term results of this procedure have been documented and found to be disappointing.[29] This may be due to the outflow obstruction produced by this procedure or to the progression of valve incompetence within the profunda system, or both.

SUMMARY

1. A consecutive series of patients with chronic venous insufficiency of the lower limb are presented. Patients were found to fall into three broad and roughly equal groups: those with apparently primary saphenous and perforator incompetence and normal deep veins; those with widespread primary incompetence of both deep and saphenous and perforating veins; those with changes due to previous thrombotic episodes.

2. Out of the 145 studied, 65 were found to have reflux in the femoral system on descending venogram.

3. In common with other authors, over 75% of these patients' with femoral incompetence was found to be unassociated with previous deep vein thrombosis and would appear to have an inherent weakness of the vein or valve wall, so-called "primary" deep venous incompetence (DVI). The possibility that primary DVI in itself predisposes in turn to thrombosis is discussed.

4. A degree of correlation between venographic reflux and incompetence in the popliteal vein on Doppler ultrasound was demonstrated. It is recognised, however, that incompetence may be identified in either segment independently of the other. In 19 limbs there was isolated popliteal reflux.

5. In a proportion of patients venous insufficiency occurred in the presence of an apparently normal deep venous system. The therapeutic value of saphenous ligation in these limbs is emphasised.

6. All patients with venous ulcer associated with DVI had at least one other demonstrable abnormality in venous function which could have accounted for skin changes. However, in some patients with pain and swelling syndrome the only recognisable abnormality of likely significance was primary DVI.

7. Among those with ulceration and primary DVI a group of patients can be identified who are apparently not benefited either in retrospect or prospectively by conventional ligation of coexistent incompetence of saphenous and perforator veins.

8. Patients with isolated primary DVI have been demonstrated to have disordered venous function studies.

9. It can be concluded from the above that in a proportion of patients, primary DVI is of pathogenic significance. Those patients with DVI due to previous deep vein thrombosis are more difficult to assess because of the often widespread nature of postphlebitic damage and the obstructive element that may coexist.

10. Transposition, interposition, and valve repair surgery have been reviewed. It has a surprisingly low incidence of perioperative thrombosis. All three techniques have been shown to have a high initial technical success rate.

11. There is some evidence that symptoms are relieved and that haemodynamic functions can be restored to normal by these forms of surgery.

12. Follow-up reveals some late valve failures. Of the three procedures, valve repair is possibly the most durable.

13. The long-term symptomatic relief is better in those with primary DVI, especially if reflux is confined to the superficial femoral vein. Those with associated deep femoral vein incompetence, or reflux due to previous deep vein thrombosis and valve damage, fair less well, perhaps due to the widespread nature of the venous problems.

14. There is enough evidence to pursue this form of surgery in selected patients. Further progress will only be made if there is systematic case selection and critical and objective short- and long-term assessment.

REFERENCES

1. Halliday P, Harriss J, May J: In Bergan JJ, Yao JST (eds): Surgery of the Veins. Grune and Stratton, 1985, pp 241–254
2. Gruss JD: In Bergan JJ, Yao JST (eds): Surgery of the Veins. Grune and Stratton, 1985, pp 255–266
3. Chan A, Chisholm I, Royle JP: The use of directional Doppler ultrasound in the assessment of sapheno-femoral incompetence. Aust NZ J Surg 53:399–402, 1983
4. McIrvine AJ, Corbett CRR, Aston ND, Sherriff EA, Wiseman PA, Jaemieson CW: The demonstration of sapheno-femoral incompetence; Doppler ultrasound compared with standard clinical tests. Br J Surg 71:506–508, 1984
5. Nicolaides AN, Miles C, Zimmerman H: The non-invasive assessment of venous insufficiency, in Greenhalgh RM (ed): Hormones and Vascular Disease. Bath, Pitman Press, 1981, pp 219–237
6. Darke SG, Andress MR: In Greenhalgh RM (ed): Diagnostic Techniques and Assessment Procedures in Vascular Surgery. Grune and Stratton, 1985
7. Kistner RL: Surgical repair of the incompetent femoral vein valve. Arch Surg 110:1336–1342, 1975
8. Herman RJ, Neiman HL, Yao JST, Egan TJ, Bergan JJ, Melave SR: Descending venography: A method of evaluating lower extremity venous valvular function. Radiology 137(i):63–69, 1980
9. Taheri SA, Lazar L, Elias SM: Surgical treatment of post-phlebitic syndrome. Br J Surg 69 (Suppl):59–62, 1982
10. Taheri SA, Lazar L, Elias SM: Status of vein valve transplant after 12 months. Arch Surg 117:1313–1317, 1982
11. Nicolaides AN: 1986 (personal comments)
12. Kistner RL: Primary venous valve incompetence of the leg. Am J Surg 140:218–224, 1982
13. Kistner RL, Ferris: Technique of surgical reconstruction of femoral vein valves, in Bergan JJ, Yao JST (eds): Operative Techniques in Vascular Surgery. Grune and Stratton, 1980, pp 291–300
14. Eriksson I, Almgren B: The influence of the profunda femoris vein on venous haemodynamics of the limb. 1986 (in press)
15. Raju S: Venous insufficiency of the lower limb and stasis ulceration. Ann Surg 197:688–697, 1983
16. Sethia KK, Darke SG: Long saphenous incompetence as a cause of venous ulceration. Br J Surg 71:754–755, 1984
17. Negus D, Friedgood A: The effective management of venous ulceration. Br J Surg 70:623–627, 1983
18. Lansdown M, Darke SG: 1986 (in press)
19. Queral LA, Whitehouse WM, Flinn WR, Neiman NL, Yao JST, Bergan JJ: Surgical correction of chronic deep venous insufficiency by valvular transposition. Surgery 87:688–695, 1980
20. Ferris, Kistner RL: 1982
21. Taheri SA: 1975
22. Taheri SA, Heffner R, Meenaghan MA, et al: In Bergan JJ, Yao JST (eds): Surgery of the Veins. Grune and Stratton, 1984

23. Taheri SA, Prendergast DR, Lazar E, Pollack LH, Meenaghan MA, Shores RM, Budd T, Taheri P: Vein valve transplantation. Am J Surg 150:201–202, 1985

24. Queral LA: Correction of deep venous insufficiency by valvular transposition, in Bergan JJ, Yao JST (eds): Operative Techniques in Vascular Surgery. Grune and Stratton, 1980, pp 301–305

25. Malette WG: In discussion. Waddell WG, Pruhomne P, Ewing JB, et al: Venous valve transplantation in post-phlebitic and post-thrombotic veins. Arch Surg 95: 833, 1967

26. Johnson ND, Queral LA, Flinn WR, Tao JST, Bergan JJ: Late objective assessment of venous valve surgery. Arch Surg 116:1461–1466, 1981

27. Jones JW, Elliott F, Kerstein MD: Triangular venous valvuloplasty. Arch Surg 117:1250–1251, 1982

28. Bauer G: The aetiology of leg ulcers and their treatment by resection of the popliteal vein. J Internat Chirugie 8:937–961, 1948

29. Lindhagen A, Hallbrook T: Venous function in the leg 20 years after ligation and partial resection of the popliteal vein. Acta Chir Scand 148:131–134, 1982

30. Lodin A, Lindvall N: Congenital absence of valves in the deep veins of the leg. A factor in venous insufficiency. Arch Derm Venereol 41 (Suppl 45):1–90, 1961

V. V. Kakkar

33

Can Death from Pulmonary Embolism be Prevented?

Deep vein thrombosis of the lower extremities is a common, age-related phenomenon manifested by focal intravascular coagulation in which the mechanism is obscure, the clinical recognition elusive, the recurrence rate high, and mortality unpredictable. Apart from the immediate risk to life, one must also consider the late sequelae of extensive deep vein thrombosis—swelling of the legs, varicose veins, ulceration, and other trophic changes which represent an equally distressing situation. It is often asked whether postoperative pulmonary embolism is preventable and, furthermore, whether it is worth preventing, since the mortality due to this complication is extremely low and all prophylactic measures require supervision, extra work, organisation, and vigilance. The data presented in this chapter support the argument that not only should this complication be prevented but also that several prophylactic measures are now available which make prevention a practical proposition. Therefore, the most rational approach would seem to be that of developing an effective method of prophylaxis if the mortality due to pulmonary embolism and the misery due to the postphlebitic syndrome are to be significantly reduced. If such a method is to be adopted on a wide scale, it must fulfil the following criteria: it must be simple, safe and effective; it must be applicable to all types of patient at risk of developing deep vein thrombosis; and it must cover the period of risk, which in surgical patients has been shown to extend from the time of operation through the first 7 to 10 postoperative days.

The efficacy of several prophylactic measures in preventing death due to postoperative pulmonary embolism has been recently assessed in numerous clinical trials. These include oral anticoagulants, low-dose heparin, and dextran (usually dextran-90). However, low-dose heparin has been most extensively investigated and at present is the most commonly used prophylactic therapy against postoperative pulmonary embolism. Therefore, the data of studies using this form of prophylaxis are analysed to answer the critical question—can death from pulmonary embolism be prevented?

VASCULAR SURGERY: ISSUES IN CURRENT PRACTICE
ISBN 0-8089-1839-7

Table 33-1
Effectiveness of Low-dose Heparin in the Prevention of Postoperative Deep Vein Thrombosis

Reference	Patient Population	Number of Patients	Frequency of Thrombosis (%)		
			Controls	LDH	Significance
Abernethy and Hartsuck[23]	General surgery	125	5	6	NS
Ansay et al[24]	General surgery	50	63	26	$p < 0.05$
Ballard et al[25]	Gynaecology	110	29	4	$p < 0.01$
Bergqvist and Hallbook[26]	General surgery	97	27	13	$p < 0.05$
Cerrato, Ariano, and Fiacchino[27]	Neurosurgery	100	34	6	$p < 0.005$
Clarke-Pearson et al[28]	Gynaecologic malignancy	185	12	15	NS
Coe et al[29]	Urology	52	25	21	NS
Covey, Sherman, and Baue[30]	General surgery	105	10	8	NS
Gallus et al[31]	General surgery	209	15	1	$p < 0.001$
Gallus et al[31]	General surgery	782	16	4	$p < 0.05$
Gordon-Smith et al[32]	General surgery	150	42	14[a] 8[b]	$p < 0.003$ $p < 0.001$
Groote Schuur Hospital[33]	Abdominal surgery	199	27	12	$p < 0.007$
Gruber et al[34]	General surgery	194	36	13	$p < 0.005$
Hedlund and Blomback[35]	Urology	59	46	21	NS
International Multicentre Trial[36]	General surgery	1292	25	8	$p < 0.005$
Jackaman, Perry, and Siddons[37]	Thorax surgery	183	51	28	$p < 0.005$
Joffe[38]	General surgery	120	51	9	$p < 0.0005$
Kakkar et al	General surgery	78	42	8	$p < 0.001$

Study	Type of surgery				
Kettunen et al[39]	General surgery	200	41	8	$p < 0.001$
Kraytman et al[40]	General surgery	50	63	26	$p < 0.05$
Kutnowski et al[41]	Urology	47	36	9	$p < 0.05$
Lahnborg et al[42]	Abdominal surgery	112	20	5	$p < 0.05$
Lawrence et al[43]	Abdominal surgery	242	17	7	$p < 0.05$
Multiunit Controlled Trial[44]	General surgery	160	43	15	$p < 0.05$
	Gynaecology	55	14	0	$p < 0.05$
	Thorax surgery	38	44	15	$p < 0.05$
Nicolaides et al[45]	General surgery	251	24	1	$p < 0.0001$
Plante et al[46]	General surgery	108	21	7	$p < 0.05$
Rem et al[47]	General surgery urology	178	36	13	$p < 0.001$
Rosenberg et al[48]	General surgery	154	44	7	$p < 0.001$
Sebeseri, Kummer, and Zingg[49]	Urology	65	58	12	$p < 0.01$
Strand, Bank-Mikklesen, and Lindewald[50]	General surgery	100	20	6	$p < 0.05$
Taberner et al[51]	Gynaecology	57	23	6	$p < 0.05$
Torngren and Forsberg[52]	Abdominal surgery	124	33	16	$p < 0.05$
Williams[53]	Abdominal surgery	44	33	0	$p < 0.02$
Wu, Tsapogas, and Jordan[54]	Abdominal surgery	88	14	0	$p < 0.01$

* The ^{125}I-fibrinogen test was used to detect DVT.

† In total, three doeses of low-dose heparin.

‡ Low-dose heparin for five days.

Table 33-2

Effect of Low-dose Heparin on the Proximal Extension of Thrombi in the Popliteal, Femoral, and Iliac Veins in Patients Undergoing Abdominal Surgery

Reference	Control Group			Heparin Group		
	Number of Patients	DVT	Number with Extension	Number of Patients	DVT	Number with Extension
Corrigan, Kakkar, and Fossard[55]	434	121	29	320	23	1
Nicolaides et al[45]	122	29	9	128	11	0
Gallus et al[56]	408	66	12	412	13	3
Kakkar, Corrigan, and Fossard[2]	667	164	49	625	48	5
Total	1631	380	99	1485	95	9
Percentage	—	23.3	6	—	5.79	0.6

PREVENTION OF DEEP VEIN THROMBOSIS

Early classic autopsy studies established the connection between emboli in the lungs and thrombi in the lower limbs. Therefore, it can be argued that prevention of such thrombi should also lead to reduction in the incidence of fatal pulmonary embolism. In the early 1970s, many studies demonstrated the efficacy of low-dose subcutaneous heparin in preventing postoperative deep vein thrombosis (DVT) after nonorthopaedic surgery (Table 33-1). These included 34 randomised clinical trials involving 6163 patients, and DVT was diagnosed by means of leg scanning with the ^{125}I-fibrinogen uptake test (FUT). In 29 trials, there was a significant reduction in the incidence of DVT in patients receiving low-dose heparin prophylaxis.

Few physicians would deny that venous thrombosis, although very common, is generally a benign disease. With the use of the ^{125}I-fibrinogen test and phlebography, it has been shown that in surgical patients the majority of thrombi form in the calf veins. A surprisingly high proportion of these thrombi undergo spontaneous lysis. In about 20% of patients these thrombi extend more proximally from the calf into the popliteal, femoral, and iliac veins. In this group with thrombosis extending proximally, pulmonary embolism occurs in almost 50%. Only a very small proportion prove fatal.[1] The effect of low-dose heparin prophylaxis on the extension of venous thrombosis was evaluated in four of the larger studies of patients undergoing elective abdominal surgery, which together included more than 3000 patients (Table 33-2). Of 1631 control patients, thrombi were detected in 380, while extension of thrombus occurred in 99, or 6%. In contrast, of 1485 patients receiving heparin, thrombi were detected in 95 and extension occurred in only nine, or 0.6%. The difference in the frequency of extending thrombi between the two groups was statistically significant, not only in the aggregate of these four studies but in each of the individual trials as well.

PREVENTION OF FATAL PULMONARY EMBOLISM

Because fatal pulmonary embolism (PE) is uncommon, a large-scale multicentre trial is needed to assess potential differences in mortality between treated patients and controls. The most comprehensive trial of low-dose heparin prophylaxis against fatal PE is from King's College Hospital, London, and is known as the International Multicentre Trial. The results of this study, published in 1975,[2] provide a foundation for current recommendations concerning postoperative prophylaxis. The study was carried out in 28 centres in a randomised controlled design. Eligible patients were over the age of 40 years and were scheduled to undergo elective major surgery. Those undergoing emergency surgery and those receiving anticoagulant therapy were excluded.

Patients in the treatment group received 5000 units of subcutaneous calcium heparin two hours preoperatively and every eight hours thereafter for seven days. If a patient was still confined to bed at the end of this period, the therapeutic regimen was continued until the patient became ambulatory. Control patients did not receive any specific prophylaxis. Randomisation provided treatment and control groups that were well matched for baseline characteristics.

Each centre's pathologist was asked to record causes of death. Uniform criteria were established for determining that PE was the cause of death, i.e., if necropsy revealed massive fresh emboli in the pulmonary trunk, in the main pulmonary artery, or in at least two lobar arteries, and if no other possible cause of death was found.

Analysis of the results in the first 2000 patients indicated a substantially greater benefit from heparin than had been envisaged at the planning stage. The incidence of fatal pulmonary embolism in the control group was approximately 1%, rather than 0.5% as was originally thought. The intake to the trial was therefore closed when 4471 patients had been admitted. Three hundred and ten patients were excluded from the analysis for several reasons, leaving 4121 patients in whom the protocol had been correctly followed—2076 in the control group and 2045 in the heparin group. The two groups were well matched for age, sex, weight, blood group, and other factors that could predispose to the development of venous thrombo-embolism. One hundred and eighty patients (4.4%) died during the postoperative period, 100 in the control group and 50 in the heparin group. Of the patients who died, 72% from the control group and 66% from the heparin group had necropsy examination. At necropsy, 16 patients in the control group and two in the heparin group were found to have died as a result of acute massive pulmonary embolism ($p < 0.005$). In addition, emboli found at necropsy in six patients in the control group and three in the heparin group were considered either contributory to death or an incidental finding, since death in these patients was attributed to other causes (Table 33-3). The findings were again significant ($p < 0.005$) when all cases of pulmonary embolism were considered together. One of the 350 patients excluded from the trial also died from pulmonary embolism. This patient had received heparin. Even if this patient is included in the analysis, the results are still highly significant ($p < 0.005$). In addition, 24 patients in the control group and eight in the heparin group were treated for clinically suspected pulmonary embolism; this difference again is statistically significant ($p < 0.005$). DVT was detected at necropsy in 24 patients in the control group and six in the heparin group ($p < 0.005$). Thirty-two

Table 33-3

Causes of Death in Patients with Nonfatal Pulmonary Emboli

	Control	Heparin
Number of deaths	100	80
Number of necropsies	72	53
Causes of death		
Pulmonary embolus	16	2
Pneumonia	13	11
Myocardial infarction	13	7
Peritonitis	9	7
Pulmonary oedema	3	5
Carcinomatosis	5	5
Septicaemia	4	3
Hepatic failure	1	2
Renal failure	0	2
Haemorrhage	5	4
Others	3	5

patients in the group and 11 in the heparin group developed DVT that was confirmed by venography ($p < 0.005$). In addition, 24 patients in the control group and eight in the heparin group were treated for clinically suspected pulmonary embolism. The difference in the number of patients requiring treatment for DVT or pulmonary embolism or both in the two groups was again significant ($p < 0.005$).

No therapeutic trial has ever escaped some form of adverse criticism; this is true of all the trials involving an evaluation of antithrombotic agents. Of the criticisms levelled against this study, only three are considered to be pertinent to an evaluation of the accuracy of the conclusions:

1. Was the autopsy rate high enough to avoid imbalances between autopsied and nonautopsied cases?
2. To what extent did errors in pathological interpretation influence the results?
3. To what extent could bias have influenced the results?

Responses to these questions have been adequately summarised by Sherry.[3] The autopsy rate of 70% is high enough to exclude imbalance as a likely source of error. As for the second point, some error in pathological interpretation is possible, but considering the competence of the pathologists, the error must be relatively small compared with the striking differences between the groups. Finally, as to the influence of bias, this is of no influence when death is used as the end-point.

A subsequent report from one of the participating centres of the International Multicentre Trial was by Gruber and coworkers.[4] As already indicated, the major end-point of the trial was fatal pulmonary embolism diagnosed at autopsy. Pulmonary embolism was considered to have caused the patient's death if the necropsy revealed massive fresh emboli in the pulmonary trunk, in the main pulmonary artery, or in at least two lobar arteries, and no other cause of death was found. Subsequently, it was claimed by Gruber and coworkers that multiple peripheral emboli may also cause death and hence should be considered fatal. Using this revised criterion for fatal pulmonary embolism, they reported that in six of 94 patients who received heparin the cause of death was acute pulmonary embolism. These data were inconsistent with their previous reports[5] and with the study design that was returned to the multicentre trial centre. They proposed that another multicentre trial be undertaken to resolve this issue. Therefore, a Second International Multicentre Trial was organised by these authors using the same protocol as in the first trial. A total of 4352 patients were admitted to this prospective randomised multicentre trial, which was designed to compare the prophylactic efficacy of dextran-70 and low-dose heparin against fatal pulmonary embolism after elective operations for general, orthopaedic, urological, and gynaecological diseases. The results of this study were reported in January 1980.[6] Of 3984 patients correctly admitted to the study, 1993 were allocated to receive dextran and 1991 to receive low-dose heparin. Of 75 patients who died within 30 days after operation, 38 had been given dextran and 37 low-dose heparin. Necropsy was performed in 33 and 32 of these cases respectively. The pulmonary arteries were dissected down to small segmental vessels. Cases of pulmonary embolism were divided into three groups: (1) those in which no other cause of death was found, (2) those in which pulmonary embolism was considered to be a contributory cause of death, and (3) those in which pulmonary embolism was regarded as incidental. Emboli found at autopsy were considered to be the sole cause of death in only three of 1991 patients who received

Table 33-4
Effect of Heparin, Dihydroergotamine (DHE), and the Fixed
Combination in the Prophylaxis of Postoperative Deep Vein
Thrombosis Diagnosed by the ^{125}I-Fibrinogen Uptake Test

Reference	Number of Patients	DVT	Number of Patients	DVT	Statistical Significance (p Value)
	Control		DHE		
Fey et al[57]	75	43 (57%)	73	24 (32%)	0.001
Muhe et al[58]	75	33 (44%)	75	18 (24%)	0.01
Buttermann et al[59]	49	17 (34.7%)	57	5 (8.8%)	0.001
	Heparin		DHE		
Kakkar et al[12]	50	2 (4%)	50	10 (20%)	0.05
	Heparin		Heparin + DHE		
Kakkar et al*[12]	50	26 (52%)	50	10 (20%)	0.05
Koppenhagen et al[60]	162	32 (19.8%)	150	13 (8.7%)	0.0
Kunz et al[61]	88	13 (14.8%)	90	6 (6.7%)	0.05
Westerman et al*[14]	63	29 (46%)	61	12 (25%)	0.05
Sagar et al*[62]	25	8 (32%)	25	4 (16%)	0.01

* Includes patients who had total hip replacement and diagnosis of DVT established by phlebography
with ^{125}I-fibrinogen test.

heparin. Another three patients in the heparin group had pulmonary embolism as a
contributory cause of death. Thus, the total incidence of pulmonary embolism
demonstrated at autopsy was six of 1991 patients. These figures are the same as
reported by us in 1975.

Furthermore, a statistical overview (undertaken by the Clinical Trial Service
Unit, Radcliffe Infirmary, Oxford, UK) of the randomised controlled trials of low-
dose heparin prophylaxis where PE mortality was not the main end-point supports
the results of the multicentre trial. Correspondence with the investigators yielded
cause-specific mortality by allocated treatment for all randomised patients. An overview of these results indicated 29 control PE allocated deaths and only six treatment
PE allocated deaths ($p < 0.001$). In addition, nonfatal PE was moderately reduced,
as was death from causes other than PE (Table 33-4). In most of these trials, it
might have been fairly obvious which patients were receiving active treatment,
which could have biased the assessment of nonfatal PE and, to a lesser extent, of
whether deaths were due to PE, though total mortality was also significantly
reduced ($p < 0.03$).

COMBINATION OF DIHYDROERGOTAMINE AND HEPARIN

Changes in blood coagulation and stasis in the deep veins of the lower limbs
are both considered to be important factors in the pathogenesis of deep vein thrombosis. It is therefore logical to propose that prophylaxis might be better achieved by
methods that minimise or eliminate both of these factors rather than counteracting
either factor alone.

Dihydroergotamine (DHE) is a potent vasoconstrictor in humans.[7] Its site of action seems to be the capacitance vessels of the limbs. Dihydroergotamine administered subcutaneously has been shown to increase the velocity of venous flow in the major veins of the lower limbs by constricting the capacitance vessels while exerting a negligible influence on resistance vessels and capillary filtration.[8] A single injection of 0.5 mg of DHE has been shown to increase the mean calf muscle blood flow significantly, an effect that persists for up to 5 hours.[9] It has also been shown that DHE enhances the synthesis of prostaglandins, and this may affect platelet function. Furthermore, several workers have also shown that administration of drugs that affect vascular motility increases the plasminogen activator from the vein wall.[10,11] Therefore, it is possible that DHE, by producing vasoconstriction through its action on adrenoreceptors of the vein wall, may enhance release of plasminogen activator and thus increase fibrinolytic activity.

Heparin–Dihydergot, a fixed combination of either 5000 or 2500 IU of heparin sodium with 0.5 mg of dihydroergotamine mesylate, is available in single-dose vials as the sterile, lyophilised mixture. This preparation has been developed to overcome the physicochemical incompatibility of the available parental formulations of both sodium and calcium heparin with that of dihydroergotamine mesylate.

Fourteen clinical trials of heparin–dihydroergotamine in a variety of patient populations have been reported. Objective methods were used for diagnosis, such as the fibrinogen uptake test, and for venography (Table 33-4). All of these trials were randomised, with one exception. In general, the addition of dihydroergotamine reduced by a further 50% the already lowered incidence of deep vein thrombosis detected when heparin alone was used. Four further clinical trials in which deep vein thrombosis was detected by the ^{125}I-fibrinogen test and venography performed in orthopaedic patients confirm the superiority of the antithrombotic effect of the combination compared with heparin alone.[9,12–14] Patients admitted to these four trials who received heparin alone had approximately a 45% incidence of DVT compared with 20% among those receiving the combination. There was no recognised difference in the amount of operative or postoperative blood loss in the two treatment groups, although heparin concentration in the plasma was significantly higher in the patients who received the combined treatment.[12]

LOW MOLECULAR WEIGHT HEPARIN

Commercially available heparin represents a heterogeneous mass, the result of randomness in the biosynthetic process. Therefore, heparin is considered to be a family of straight-chain anionic polysaccharides, more specifically, glycosaminoglycan (GAG) sulphate esters of highly variable molecular weight, averaging 9000 to 15,000 but ranging from 3000 to 40,000. Heparin has the ability to form a complex with antithrombin III, but only a specific portion of the heparin in clinically used preparations binds strongly to antithrombin III. With affinity chromatography on purified, matrix-bound antithrombin, heparin can be divided into one fraction (about one-third of the total amount) with high affinity to antithrombin III and high anticoagulant activity and one virtually inactive fraction with low affinity for antithrombin III.[15,16]

According to these hypotheses, low molecular weight heparin should possess antithrombotic properties, possibly without causing excessive bleeding.

The efficacy and safety of a low molecular weight (LMW) heparin fraction in preventing postoperative venous thromboembolism was assessed in a double-blind, randomly allocated trial, and in an "open" study.[17] Of 395 patients included in the double-blind trial, 199 received unfractionated (UF) calcium heparin and 196 the LMW heparin fraction. The data were analysed on an "intention to treat" basis. The two groups were well matched for risk factors which could predispose to the development of venous thrombosis. Fifteen (7.5%) of 199 patients receiving UF heparin and five (2.5%) of 196 patients in the LMW heparin group developed DVT ($p < 0.05$). There was no significant difference between the two groups in terms of excessive incisional or total blood loss during surgery, postoperative drainage, or wound haematoma formation. Of 910 patients included in the "open" study who received a single injection of LMW heparin every day, 30 (3.2%) died during the postoperative period; in none of the autopsied patients were pulmonary emboli detected. Thirty-one (3.4%) patients developed isotopic DVT; 27 (2.9%) were receiving prophylaxis at the time the DVT was diagnosed. Thirty-six (3.9%) patients developed wound haemotoma; 25 (12.4%) of those were in the 201 undergoing surgery for gynaecological conditions and 11 (1.5%) in the 709 patients having general abdominal surgery. This difference is statistically significant ($p < 0.001$). The results of a double-blind trial indicate that a single daily injection of 1850 APTT units (7500 antifactor Xa units) of an LMW heparin is more effective than 10,000 APTT units of commercially available UF heparin in preventing postoperative DVT. The findings of the "open" study suggest that this regimen also provides an effective prophylaxis against postoperative major pulmonary embolism.

COMPLICATIONS OF LOW-DOSE HEPARIN PROPHYLAXIS

The risk of haemorrhage is the main limitation on the routine use of anticoagulants for the prevention of thromboembolic disease in surgical patients. One definite criterion for evaluating this risk is the frequency of wound haematoma formation.

Two studies in which large numbers of patients were investigated reported a significant difference between the number of patients receiving heparin and the number of their control counterparts who developed wound haematomas.[12,18] However, a recent double-blind study failed to confirm such a difference. The reason for this discrepancy arises from the fact that in the International Multicentre Trial[2] and the study reported by Gallus and coworkers[19] heparin was administered every eight hours, whereas Kiil and coworkers gave it every 12 hours. Similar results have been reported by other workers. It seems that there is a small but definite risk of bleeding when an eight-hour regimen is used, but not when a 12-hour regimen is followed.

A much higher incidence of bleeding complications has been observed in some of the studies reported in the United States.[20] This difference could be due to several factors. Plasma heparin levels after subcutaneous administration depend not only on the molecular weight but also on the type of heparin salt used and the standard that is used by manufacturers for the calibration of heparin. Unfortunately, two standards are used: American heparin is calibrated according to the USP unit, which in the past has been 15% more potent than the international unit (IU) established by the World Health Organisation. Most European studies have been carried out using heparin calibrated in international units. The difference between the two standards is relatively small, but together with other factors likely to affect heparin absorption, it may give rise to sufficiently higher levels to produce serious bleeding. Currently, the difference between the two units is less. The USP unit is now only 6–7% more potent than the international unit.

Another important factor that might have contributed to the higher incidence of bleeding complications reported from the United States relates to the concentration of heparin solution used. The use of multidose vials is inconvenient and wasteful, and at times may lead to bleeding from the accidental administration of large amounts of heparin. Ampules made specifically for prophylactic use are now available. They contain 5000 units of either the calcium or sodium salt of heparin in 0.2 ml aqueous solution. The widespread use of such specially prepared ampules has certainly reduced the frequency of bleeding complications.

Ecchymosis at the injection site has also been observed more frequently when the sodium salt of heparin has been used. Such differences could be due to the fact that the sodium and calcium salts of heparin behave differently when administered subcutaneously. A comparative trial showed that the calcium salt caused significantly less ecchymosis at the site of injection than the sodium salt.[21] Of 266 subcutaneous injections (133 each of sodium heparin and calcium heparin), sodium heparin caused local bruising greater than 0.5 cm in diameter in 7%, less than 0.5 cm in 47%, and none at all in 46%, whereas calcium heparin produced local bruising over 0.5 cm in diameter in 3%, under 0.5 cm in 22%, and no bruising in 75% ($p < 0.001$). Pain was rarely reported. When present, it was not significantly different in patients receiving the two heparin preparations and was not related to the formation or size of haematomas.

ADOPTION OF LOW-DOSE HEPARIN PROPHYLAXIS

The value of low-dose heparin in the prophylaxis of postoperative deep vein thrombosis can no longer be seriously disputed. For prophylactic therapy to be widely adopted, it must be easily administered, readily available, of low cost, and, above all, of minimal risk. The basic question is the benefit–risk ratio. There is now good reason to believe that the potential benefits of prophylactic low-dose heparin far outweigh the risk of haemorrhage. An 88% reduction in the incidence of fatal pulmonary embolism, for example, can be achieved at the cost of a 2.5% increase in the incidence of postoperative bleeding, largely in the form of wound haemotoma formation. A question is whether this form of prophylaxis is being adopted on a large scale to protect high-risk individuals—not just those with surgically approachable lesions, but also those with medical conditions such as myocardial infarction, congestive heart failure, arrhythmias, stroke, pulmonary insufficiency, and illnesses requiring periods of prolonged immobilisation. Two recent surveys tend to suggest that this form of prophylaxis is now being used more widely. All 236 clinics in Sweden dealing with general, urological, orthopaedic, and gynaecological surgery were sent a questionnaire concerning their policy about prophylaxis against throm-boembolism.[22] In all, 94% replied, and 76% claimed to use some kind of prophy-laxis. Decisive factors for the adoption of routine prophylaxis and prophylactic methods in current use varied among the four specialities. In the survey, 90% of the general surgery clinics, 87% of the urological surgery clinics, 100% of the ortho-paedic surgery clinics, and 97% of the gynaecological surgery clinics replied. Several pharmacological agents were used as prophylaxis against postoperative venous thromboembolism. These included oral anticoagulants, low-dose heparin, acetylsali-cylic acid, and the combination of dihydroergotamine and heparin. Low-dose heparin was used in 78% of the general surgery patients, 54% of the urological surgery patients, only 39% of the orthopaedic surgery patients, and 69% of the gynaecological surgery patients.

In a second survey,[23] 752 orthopaedic and 663 general surgeons were sent a questionnaire asking how they attempted to prevent venous thromboembolism. The survey concerned prophylaxis offered routinely to elderly patients with hip fractures, to patients undergoing elective hip replacement arthroplasty, and to patients under-going major abdominal and thoracic operations. Approximately 70% of those ques-tioned replied. The general surgeons returned 521 questionnaires, for an effective response rate of 78%. The orthopaedic surgeons returned 605 questionnaires, and 47 surgeons did not complete that part of the questionnaire which dealt with patients who had hip fractures, either because their practice did not include such patients or because they were involved in clinical trials of prophylactic agents. Simi-larly, 59 surgeons did not complete the section concerning patients undergoing elec-tive hip replacement arthroplasty. Thus, the effective response rate was 74% for hip fractures and 73% for hip replacements. The survey showed that more general sur-geons provide routine prophylaxis than do their orthopaedic colleagues. The differ-ence was attributable mainly to the popularity of low-dose heparin among general surgeons. That low-dose heparin prophylaxis is effective in general surgical patients has been detailed widely, and the consensus seems to be in its favour. The safety and simplicity of the method were persuasive factors and accounted for the fact that a quarter of all the general surgeons who replied use low-dose heparin routinely as the sole method of prophylaxis.

The routine use of oral anticoagulants has been recommended for nearly 20 years for the prevention of venous thromboembolic complications. In the Nether-lands, for instance, more than 60% of surgeons routinely use this form of prophy-laxis. Yet in the United Kingdom, none of the 515 surgeons undertaking general abdominal surgery indicated that they use oral anticoagulants, compared with 128 (24.8%) who reported that they use low-dose heparin routinely as the sole method of prophylaxis. This trend surely must be considered as a major breakthrough when one considers that the objective evidence of the effectiveness of this form of prophy-laxis has been accumulated only during the past few years. The survey undertaken by Morris[22] suggests that published evidence concerning the prevention of venous thromboembolism has only had a limited influence on surgical practice in the United Kingdom, and the question has arisen as to whether the published evidence that supports the prophylaxis is convincing. To those who find it so, the inaction of the surgeons who do not employ prophylaxis may be regarded as negligence. However, those who are familiar with the literature and do not provide prophylaxis may choose not to do so for two reasons. First, there is a great discrepancy between the ubiquity of venous thromboembolism and the relative infrequency with which it causes death. Second, an individual surgeon, no matter how extensive a personal practice, will never recognise the success of prophylactic action, yet will invariably be reminded of failures. In view of such circumstances, what should be the role of a practising clinician? The published evidence and the clinical experience with low-dose heparin prophylaxis should now be used to influence the methods used by surgeons for preventing fatal pulmonary embolism occurring after operations.

REFERENCES

1. Kakkar VV, Howe CT, Flanc C: Natural history of postoperative deep vein thrombosis. Lancet 2:230, 1969
2. Kakkar VV, Corrigan TP, Fossard DP: Prevention of fatal postoperative pulmonary embolism by low doses of heparin. Lancet 2:45, 1975
3. Sherry S: Prophylactic therapy on deep vein thrombosis and pulmonary embolism. DHEW Publication No (NIH) 76-866, 1975, p 229
4. Gruber UF, Fridrich R, Ducker F, et al: Prevention of postoperative thromboembolism by dextran 40, low doses of heparin, or xantinol nicotinate. Lancet 1:207, 1977
5. Rem J, Duckert F, Fridrich R, et al: Low dose heparin in prevention of postoperative venous thrombosis. Schweiz Med Wochenschr 105:827, 1975
6. Gruber UF, Saldeen T, Brokop T, et al: Incidence of fatal postoperative pulmonary embolism after prophylaxis with dextran 70 and low dose heparin: An International Multicentre Study. Br Med J 280:69, 1980
7. Aellig WH: Untersuchung über die venenkonstringierende Wirkung von Ergotverbindungen in Menschen. Triangle 14:39, 1975
8. Mellander S, Nordenfelt I: Comparative effects of dihydroergotamine and noradrenaline on resistance, exchange and capacitance fractions in the peripheral circulation. Clin Sci 39:183, 1970
9. Stamatakis JD, Kakkar VV, Lawrence D, et al: Synergistic effect of heparin and dihydroergotamine in the prophylaxis of postoperative deep vein thrombosis, in Past HW, Maurer G (eds): Postoperative Thromboembolie-prophylaxe. Stuttgart, Schattauer Verlag, 1977, p 109
10. Aberg M, Nilsson IM: Fibrinolytic response to venous occlusion and vasopressin in health and thrombotic disease, in Davidson JF, et al (eds): Progress in Chemical Fibrinolysis and Thrombolysis. New York, Raven Press, 1975, pp 301–309
11. Mannucci PM, Aberg M, Nilsson IM, et al: Mechanism of plasminogen activator and factor VIII increase after vasoactive drugs. Br J Haem 30:81, 1974
12. Kakkar VV, Stamatakis JD, Bentley PG, et al: Prophylaxis for postoperative deep vein thrombosis. Synergistic effect of heparin and dihydroergotamine. JAMA 241:39, 1979
13. Sagar S, Nairn D, Stamatakis JD, et al: Efficacy of low-dose heparin in prevention of extensive deep vein thrombosis in patients undergoing total hip replacement. Lancet 1:1153, 1976
14. Westerman K, Trentz O, Prestschner P, et al: Use of heparin–Dihydergot in total hip replacement surgery, in Past HW, Maurer FK (eds): 6th Rotherburger Colloquium. Stuttgart, Schattauer Verlag, 1977, p 146
15. Anderson LO, Barrowcliffe TW, Holmer E, et al: Anticoagulant properties of heparin fractionated by affinity chromatography and by gel filtration. Thrombosis Res 9:575, 1976

16. Hook M, Bjork I, Hopwood J, et al: Anticoagulant activity of heparin. Separation of high-activity species by affinity chromatography on immobilized antithrombin. Fed Eur Biochem Sco LeH 66:70, 1976

17. Kakkar VV, Murray WJG: Efficacy and safety of law molecular weight heparin (CY 216) in preventing postoperative venaus thromboembolism: a cooperative study. Br J Surg 72:786–791, 1985

18. Godal HC: Report to the International Committee on Haemostasis and Thrombosis, from the working party on clinical aspects of heparin. Philadelphia, 2 July 1977

19. Gallus AS, Hirsh J, O'Brien SE, et al: Prevention of venous thrombosis with small subcutaneous doses of heparin. JAMA 235:1980, 1975

20. Pachter ML, Riles TS: Low dose heparin. Bleeding and wound complications in the surgical patient. Ann Surg 186:669, 1977

21. Whitehead MI, McCarthy TG: A comparative trial of subcutaneous sodium and calcium heparin as assessed by local haematoma formation and pain, in Kakkar VV, Thomas DP (eds): Heparin: Chemistry and Clinical Use. London, Academic Press, 1976, pp 361–366

22. Morris GK: Prevention of venous thromboembolism. Lancet 1: 572, 1980

23. Abernethy EA, Hartsuck JM: Postoperative pulmonary embolism. A prospective study utilizing low dose heparin. Am J Surg 128:739, 1974

24. Ansay J, Fastrez R, Kutnowski M, et al: Prevention des thromboses veineuses profondes postoperatoires par l'heparine sous-cutanee a faibles doses. Ann Chir 31:263, 1977

25. Ballard RM, Bradley-Watson PJ, Johnstone FD, et al: Low doses of subcutaneous heparin in the prevention of deep vein thrombosis after gynaecological surgery. J Obstet Gynaecol Br Commonw 80:469, 1973

26. Bergqvist D, Hallbook T: Prophylaxis of postoperative venous thrombosis in a controlled trial comparing dextran 70 and low-dose heparin. World J Surg 4:239, 1980

27. Carrato D, Ariano C, Fiacchino F: Deep vein thrombosis and low-dose heparin prophylaxis in neurosurgical patients. J Neurosurg 49:378, 1978

28. Clarke-Pearson DL, Coleman RE, Synan IS, et al: Venous thromboembolism prophylaxis in gynaecologic oncology: A prospective, controlled trial of low-dose heparin. Am J Obstet Gynecol 145:606, 1983

29. Coe NP, Collins REC, Klein LA, et al: Prevention of deep vein thrombosis in urological patients: A controlled, randomized trial of low-dose heparin and external pneumatic compression boots. Surgery 83: 230, 1978

30. Covey TH, Sherman L, Baue AE: Low-dose heparin in postoperative patients. A prospective coded study. Arch Surg 110:1021, 1975

31. Gallus AS, Hirsch J, O'Brien SE, et al: Prevention of venous thrombosis with small, subcutaneous doses of heparin. JAMA 235:1980, 1976

32. Gordon-Smith IC, Grundy DJ, Le Quesne LP, et al: Controlled trial of two regimens of subcutaneous heparin in prevention of postoperative deep vein thrombosis. Lancet 1:1133, 1972

33. Groote Schuur Hospital Thromboembolus Study Group: Failure of low-dose heparin to prevent significant thromboembolic complications in high-risk surgical patients. Interim report of a prospective trial. Br Med J 1:1447, 1979

34. Gruber UF, Duckert F, Fridrich R, et al: Prevention of postoperative thromboembolism by dextran 40, low doses of heparin, or xantinol nicotinate. Lancet 1:207, 1977

35. Hedlund PO, Blomback M: The effect of prophylaxis with low dose heparin on blood coagulation parameters. A double blind study in connection with transvesical prostatectomy. Thromb Haemost 41:337, 1979

36. International Multicentre Trial: Prevention of fatal postoperative pulmonary embolism by low doses of heparin. Lancet 2:45, 1975

37. Jackaman FR, Perry BJ, Siddons H: Deep vein thrombosis after thoracotomy. Thorax 33:761, 1978

38. Joffe S: Drug prevention of post-operative deep vein thrombosis. A comparative study of calcium heparinate and sodium pentosan polysulphate. Arch Surg 111:37, 1976

39. Kettunen K, Poikolainen E, Karjalainen P, et al: Prophylaxis of deep vein thrombosis with small doses of subcutaneous heparin (in Finnish). Duodecim 90:834, 1974

40. Kraytman M, Kutnowski M, Ansay J, et al: Prophylaxie par l'heparine sous-cutanee a faibles doses des thromboses veineuses postoperatoires. Acta Chir Belg 5:519, 1976

41. Kutnowski M, Valendris M, Steinberger R, et al: Prevention of postoperative deep vein thrombosis by low-dose heparin in urological surgery. A double-blind, randomized study. Urol Res 5:123, 1977

42. Lahnborg G, Bergstrom K, Friman L, et al: Effect of low-dose heparin on incidence of postoperative pulmonary embolism detected by photoscanning. Lancet 1:329, 1974

43. Lawrence JD, Xabregas A, Gray L, et al: Seasonal variation in the incidence of deep vein thrombosis. Br J Surg 64: 777, 1977

44. Multiunit Controlled Trial: Heparin versus dextran in the prevention of deep vein thrombosis. Lancet 2:118, 1974

45. Nicolaides AN, Dupont AN, Desai S, et al: Small doses of subcutaneous sodium heparin in preventing deep venous thrombosis after major surgery. Lancet 2:890, 1972

46. Plante J, Boneu B, Vaysse C, et al: Dipyridamole–aspirin versus low doses of heparin in the prophylaxis of deep vein thrombosis in abdominal surgery. Thromb Res 13:399, 1979

47. Rem J, Duckert F, Fridrich R, et al: Subkutane klein heparindosen zur thrombose-prophylaxe in der allgemeinen chirurgie und urologie. Schweiz Med Wschr 105:827, 1975

48. Rosenberg IL, Evans M, Pollock AV: Prophylaxis of postoperative leg vein thrombosis by low dose subcutaneous heparin or preoperative calf muscle stimulation: A controlled clinical trial. Br Med J 1:649, 1975

49. Sebeseri O, Kummer H, Zingg E: Controlled prevention of postoperative thrombosis in urological diseases with depot heparin. Eur Urol 1:229, 1975

50. Strand, L, Bank-Mikklesen OK, Lindewald H: Small heparin doses as prophylaxis against deep vein thrombosis in major surgery. Acta Chir Scand 141:624, 1975

51. Taberner DA, Poller L, Burslem RW, et al: Oral anticoagulants controlled by the British comparative thromboplastin versus low-dose heparin in prophylaxis of deep vein thrombosis. Br Med J 1:272, 1978

52. Torngren S, Forsberg K: Concentrated or diluted heparin prophylaxis of postoperative deep venous thrombosis. Acta Chir Scand 144:283, 1978

53. Williams HT: Prevention of postoperative deep vein thrombosis with perioperative sub-cutaneous heparin. Lancet 2:950, 1971

54. Wu TK, Tsapogas MJ, Jordan FR: Prophylaxis of deep venous thrombosis by hydroxy-chloroquine sulfate and heparin. Surg Gynecol Obstet 145:714, 1977

55. Corrigan TP, Kakkar VV, Fossard DP: Low dose subcutaneous heparin—optimal dose regimen. Br J Surg 61:320, 1974

56. Gallus AS, Hirsh J, Tuttle RJ, et al: Small subcutaneous doses of heparin in prevention of venous thrombosis. New Engl J Med 288:545, 1973

57. Fey KH, Herzfeld U, Saggau W, et al: Postoperative Thromboseprophylaxe durch Tonisierung des kaudalen Venensystems. Ein neues medikamentoses Behandlungsprinzip. Med Klin 70:1553, 1975

58. Muhe, Burghardt KH, Kolb W, et al: Eine neue Methode zur Prophylaxe post-operative Veninthrombosen. Klinikartz 4:88, 1975

59. Butterman G, Thiesinger W, Oeschler H, et al: Untersuchungen über die postoperative Thromboembolieprophylaxe nach einem neuen medikamentösen Behandlungsprinzip. Dtsch Med Wochenschr 100:2069, 1975

60. Koppenhagen K, Wiechmann A, Frey E, et al: Klinisch-experimentelle Ergebnisse mit Heparin-Dihydroergotamin. Dtsch Med Wochenschr 102:1374, 1977

61. Kunz S, Drahne A, Briel RC: Prophylaxe der postoperative Thromboembolie. Erfahrungen mit Heparin-Dihydergot in der Gynakologie, in Past HW, Mauer G (eds): Postoperative Thromboembolie-prophylaxe. Stuttgart, Schattauer Verlag, 1977, p 275
62. Sagar S, Massey J, Sanderson JM: Low-dose heparin prophylaxis against fatal pulmonary embolism. Br Med J 4:257, 1975

Alfred V. Persson
and Christine A. Persson

34

Medical Therapy for Deep Venous Thrombosis

INTRODUCTION

Deep venous thrombosis (DVT) is a critical problem encountered by most physicians at one time or another. Many factors contribute to thrombosis, including immobilization, chemical or mechanical injury, varicose veins, blood dyscrasias, dehydration, compression, oral contraceptives, and other estrogen compounds. Thrombosis can occur in patients of all ages and in conjunction with a variety of illnesses. Although prophylaxis is the best treatment, DVT is still a major medical problem and demands aggressive management.

This chapter will address the medical treatment of deep venous thrombosis. Prophylaxis, diagnosis, and surgical treatment are discussed in other chapters.

PLANNING THERAPY

Before the options for treatment are considered, a firm diagnosis must be established using an objective method. Clinical impression is correct in only 50% of cases[1] but is useful because the diagnosis is more likely in the right setting. For example, a postoperative obese, sedentary patient is a prime candidate for deep venous thrombosis, while a thin, active patient rarely develops DVT. Patients at high risk to DVT should be aggressively evaluated if any signs or symptoms of DVT develop.

The diagnosis of deep venous thrombosis can be established by the use of non-invasive methods such as impedance plethysmography (IPG), phleborheography (PRG), or Doppler ultrasound examination. More recently, B-mode ultrasound has been utilized to make this diagnosis. If these methods are inconclusive or not available, venography must be performed to confirm the diagnosis of deep venous thrombosis before treatment is begun. *It is inappropriate to treat a patient by any method without a firm diagnosis.*

HYPERCOAGULABLE STATES

Patients with inherited clotting factor deficiencies warrant special mention. This group includes patients with a positive family history of recurrent "spontaneous" deep venous thrombosis or pulmonary embolus, onset of DVT or PE at a young age, multiple episodes, and venous thrombosis in unusual locations.[2] Currently available tests may reveal deficiencies in antithrombin III, protein C, and protein S. Complete evaluation is necessary to plan long-term anticoagulation therapy for these patients. Maintenance of long-term anticoagulation therapy (warfarin) is mandatory or thrombotic episodes will recur. It is also important to evaluate other family members for these deficiencies. Whether to treat an asymptomatic family member is controversial. However, our practice is to treat such individuals. It is very important to recognize these patients to prevent recurrence and to prevent unusual complications.

While on coumadin patients with protein C deficiencies can develop skin necrosis. It appears that the "coumadin-foot" is isolated to these patients.[3] Generally, coumadin should be continued because the risk of recurrent thrombosis and pulmonary embolus is significantly greater than the incidence of skin necrosis.[4] Of course, if the complication develops, the medication must be discontinued. Because the above tests are invalid if the patient is undergoing any form of anticoagulation therapy, the tests must be performed before the onset of therapy. When planning therapy for a patient with DVT it is important to elicit a complete history and have a high index of suspicion.

Pulmonary Emboli

It is estimated that 200,000 people die each year in the United States of pulmonary embolus.[5] Many of these patients have preexisting fatal conditions, and the pulmonary embolus simply precipitates the final event. Other patients are in good general health and develop deep venous thrombosis associated with a self-limiting benign problem. It is in these patients that a fatal pulmonary embolus is particularly tragic.

Postphlebitic Syndrome

The postphlebitic syndrome, the second most common complication of DVT, is caused by retrograde venous flow, decreased venous return, venous hypertension, and a decrease in the lymphatic return—all caused by destruction of the venous valves occurring with the initial phlebitis or secondary to dilatation of the collateral venous circulation beyond the capacity of the valves, with the exception of decreased venous return. This is caused by occlusion of the lymphatic channels secondary to the inflammatory process.[6]

The postphlebitic syndrome usually appears several years after the initial insult to the veins—long after both the patient and primary physician are satisfied with the initial result.

When planning therapy, the acute problem, as well as the long-term sequalae, should be considered. Although the immediate problems of increased venous pressure, lymphatic blockage, and pain must be addressed, one must not forget the long-term sequalae of this common problem.

ACUTE THERAPY

Acute therapy is aimed at relieving pain, halting the thrombotic process, and improving the lymphatic drainage. Pain is not caused by the inflammatory reaction but by distension of the veins. When the intraluminal clot is removed surgically or medically and the veins return to normal size, the pain resolves. Nonsteroidal inflammatory agents do little to relieve the pain.

Nonsteroidal anti-inflammatory drugs are not beneficial in decreasing the anti-inflammatory response seen in acute deep venous thrombosis. Antibiotics are like-wise not useful in this setting unless the patient has septic phlebitis. Deep venous thrombosis is primarily a thrombotic process and not an infective problem.

ADMINISTRATION OF ANTICOAGULANTS

The most commonly employed agent in the treatment of acute deep venous thrombosis is heparin. Its function is to arrest the thrombotic process. Most phys-icians administer heparin by continuous intravenous infusion because it is the safest method of administration.[7] Patients are monitored by frequent determinations of the partial thromboplastin time (PTT) or thrombin clot time. Sufficient heparin is administered to keep the PTT level at 2–2.5 times control. If the patient is otherwise medically sound and there is no undue risk of bleeding, we administer a bolus of heparin at the start of therapy, usually 5000–10,000 units depending on the weight of the patient. However, if there is concern about bleeding (i.e., recent trauma or recent surgery with large areas of dissection), we generally do not administer the bolus dose. The bolus of heparin brings the patient into therapeutic range almost immediately. The administration of the maintenance dosage of heparin only will bring the patient into therapeutic range slowly and avoid overdosing, and thus decrease the incidence of bleeding. The average 75 kg patient requires between 800 and 1000 units of heparin per hour.

Heparin can also be administered by intermittent intravenous bolus or inter-mittent subcutaneous injections. Although all three methods of administration are equally effective, the continuous intravenous dosage has been found to be safest as it avoids the peaks and troughs in blood levels associated with intermittent adminis-tration.[7]

MAINTENANCE THERAPY

The usual course of treatment is heparin administered for 7–10 days, followed by coumadin for 3–6 months. We generally start coumadin on the second day of therapy when the patients' sensitivity to anticoagulants has been established. The standard dose is 10 mg of coumadin each day for three to four days until the pro-thrombin time is 1.5–2 times the control. The average maintenance dose is 5–7.5 mg. Heparin is administered for 48 hours after the prothrombin time has reached thera-peutic levels. There are very few reports in the literature to indicate the length of coumadin treatment following an acute episode of deep venous thrombosis. The best evidence, however, indicates a minimum of three months.[8] Most physicians, including the authors, continue coumadin for six months, unless the patient develops complications. The prothrombin time is monitored by weekly or bimonthly measurements, seeking a level of 1.5 times the control. This dose of coumadin has proven equally effective in maintaining the patient at a level 2.5–3 times the control.[7] There have been few problems with bleeding, other than those associated with direct trauma.

FIBRINOLYTIC THERAPY

Three fibrinolytic drugs are available for use in the treatment of deep venous thrombosis: streptokinase, urokinase, and tissue plasminogen activator (t-PA). Streptokinase and urokinase have been commercially available in the United States for nearly 10 years and for over 20 years in Europe, providing widespread clinical experience with their use. We feel that fibrinolytic therapy, as opposed to heparin therapy, is the treatment of choice because it has the potential to achieve the goals of preserving the valves, therefore restoring the patient to normal physiology.

The contraindications to fibrinolytic therapy are recent childbirth, cerebrovascular accident within six months, blood dyscrasias, GI bleed within three weeks, vascular reconstructive surgery with placement of an artificial graft within three months, and liver disease. Fibrinolytic agents are generally quite safe; we have used these agents in over 200 patients with only two incidences of serious bleeding.

Streptokinase is used in preference to urokinase because urokinase is six times more expensive. All studies comparing the two agents demonstrate equally efficacious results. Urokinase is also used in patients who have developed allergies to streptokinase, particularly patients who had previous therapy with streptokinase within the last year. The antibodies to streptokinase that these patients develop do not cause an anaphylactic-type reaction, but do render the drug ineffective.

Tissue-type plasminogen activator (t-PA) is an experimental drug. Although the reports on its use on coronary thrombosis have been exciting,[9,10] there is very little work reported on its use in the treatment of deep venous thrombosis. The difficulty in procuring t-PA and the associated expense may limit its use. However, the human t-PA gene has recently been cloned and production of large quantities of t-PA should be forthcoming. This is one of the more exciting uses of recombinant DNA technology. At this early stage it is not possible to answer questions concerning formation of antibodies, long-term results, or future costs of the agent. Like all new therapies, these questions will be answered with time and the performance of properly controlled studies.

MECHANISM OF ACTION OF FIBRINOLYTIC AGENTS

Before describing the various dosage schedules, it is appropriate to discuss the mechanism of actions of fibrinolytic agents. An understanding of the pharmacokinetics provides the rationale for various treatment regimens and dosage schedules.

Streptokinase, urokinase, and t-PA function by activating the body's own fibrinolytic system. Plasmin is a naturally occurring enzyme that depolymerizes

$$Plasminogen + streptokinase = activator$$

$$Plasminogen + activator = plasmin$$

$$Fibrin + plasmin = split\ products$$

Fig. 34-1. Mechanism of action of streptokinase.

fibrin and other protein clotting factors. Streptokinase is an indirect activator; it first binds with plasminogen to form an activator. This activator binds with more plasminogen to form plasmin. Plasmin is the active agent that lyses the fibrin in the clot and forms fibrin split-products (Fig. 34-1). Urokinase is a direct activator, converting plasminogen to plasmin without the intermediate step. Smaller dosages of urokinase are used to obtain a lytic effect. In the treatment of deep venous thrombosis, both urokinase and streptokinase are administered intravenously. Both agents cause a systemic fibrinolytic state at therapeutic dosages by activating free plasminogen and plasminogen within the clot.

Tissue-type plasminogen activator (t-PA) is a direct activator of plasminogen. It has a greater affinity for plasminogen bound to fibrin in the clot than for free plasminogen in the serum. It therefore causes an essentially localized fibrinolysis at therapeutic levels. In human studies, t-PA has been used primarily in the treatment of coronary thrombosis.[11-14] There has been a minimal systemic fibrinolytic state created, as determined by measurement of thrombin clot time, fibrinogen, and alpha antiplasmin levels. Reports have been published on animal studies for the treatment of venous thrombosis which indicate successful lysis of the clots.[15] However, only isolated reports exist of t-PA used in the treatment of deep venous thrombosis and pulmonary embolism in humans;[16] its safety and efficacy in treatment of deep venous thrombosis has yet to be proven. When the marketing of t-PA for clinical use is permitted, some of the problems associated with streptokinase and urokinase caused by the systemic fibrinolytic state may be avoided.

All fibrinolytic agents depolymerize the protein-based clotting factors (II, VII, IX, X) and are therefore active anticoagulants as well as thrombolytic agents. It is therefore redundant and unnecessary to administer heparin in conjunction with a fibrinolytic agent.

DOSAGE SCHEDULES OF FIBRINOLYTIC AGENTS

Three dosage schedules exist for the clinical administration of streptokinase and urokinase. The method that has recently received the most attention is the administration of low doses of the drugs directly into the thrombosed vessel via a catheter. Frequent fluoroscopic examinations are used to determine the efficacy and duration of the infusion. This method is used primarily for interarterial thrombosis and is rarely used to treat deep venous thrombosis. This method is reported to be superior to other methods of administration. The literature provides mixed reports on the effectiveness of this dosage schedule,[17-19] but it is quite clear that there is

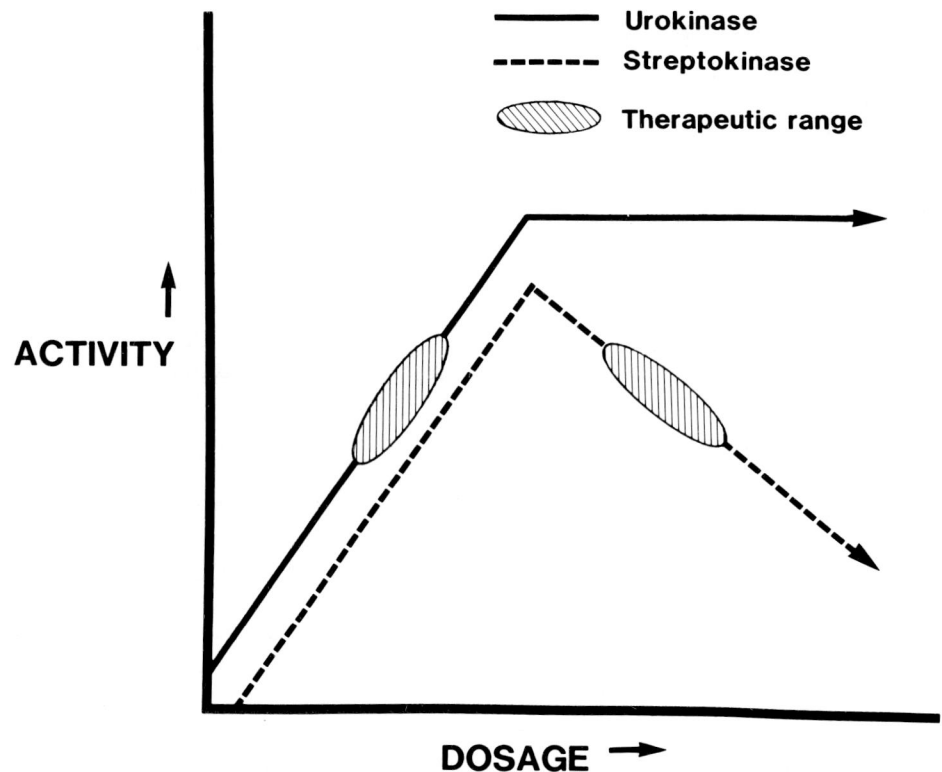

Fig. 34-2. Relationship between fibrinolytic activity and the dosages of urokinase and streptokinase. Elipses indicate the therapeutic ranges for continuous-dose therapy as recommended in package inserts.

also a marked increase in bleeding, generally 20–30% (mostly around the administration catheter). This was the same experience noted in the early Streptokinase–
Urokinase Pulmonary Embolism Trial reporting on the efficacy of fibrinolytic
therapy in patients with pulmonary embolus.[20,21] Although the results were very
promising, the incidence of bleeding around the administration catheters was high.
It was not until the agents were administered into a peripheral vein that these drugs
provided better results and gained popularity. For patients with DVT these drugs
are usually administered intravenously, preferably through a vein in the non-
dominant forearm.

The standard and most commonly used method of administration is by continuous intravenous infusion.[22] The dosage is 250,000 units of streptokinase during the
first hour followed by 100,000 units per hour. The loading dose is given to overcome
antistreptokinase antibodies and to push the activity curve over the peak onto the
right-hand side of the curve (Fig. 34-2). This is a very effective dosage regimen and
carries a relatively low incidence of bleeding complications.[23] Its major drawbacks
are increased expense (because of the large amounts of drug used) and an "exhaustion phenomenon" which commonly develops after three to four days of use. The
exhaustion phenomenon occurs because all circulating plasminogen has been activated and the body depends exclusively on the production of new plasminogen in

the blood for further activity. The 100,000 units of streptokinase per hour often equals the amount of plasminogen produced. The patient, therefore, has an abundance of circulating activator and a relatively low amount of plasmin because of the preferential affinity of streptokinase to form activator and then to form plasmin.

Urokinase, a direct activator, is administered with a loading dose of 2000 units per pound of patient weight over the first 30 minutes, followed by 2000 units per pound per hour for the course of the therapy.[22]

The lytic state (achieved by either agent) is generally maintained for at least four to five days when treating patients with DVT. The PTT and fibrinogen level should be measured once a day to verify that a lytic state is being maintained. The exact level is not important, only verification that the exhaustion phenomenon has not occurred. After a full course of fibrinolytic therapy, the patient must be maintained on anticoagulants or the vessel will re-clot. Three months minimum, or better six months, of coumadin is necessary (as in the treatment of patients managed with heparin). Two to three days of heparin therapy are usually required before the patient's prothrombin time is at an adequate therapeutic level, at which time coumadin therapy begins.

The third method of administration is called burst therapy. We developed this dosage schedule approximately four years ago and have used it to treat our last 50 patients.[24–26] The dosage schedule is 250,000 units of streptokinase over the first hour, followed by 100,000 units per hour for five hours. The infusion is then discontinued for 12 hours to allow the liver to replenish the circulating plasminogen. Therapy is then continued with 250,000 units of streptokinase mixed with 50 ml of normal saline infused over one hour twice a day, usually at 9 AM and 6 PM. This intermittent burst therapy is equally effective when compared to the standard dosage schedules[24–26] and has the advantage that it has eliminated the exhaustion phenomenon. Burst therapy is especially useful in patients with large volumes of clot associated with deep venous thrombosis; therapy can be continued as long as necessary. Burst therapy is also less expensive than the other dosage schedules, as less drug is used. In addition, we have had fewer febrile reactions associated with fibrinolytic therapy.

We have administered urokinase in a similar burst manner; beginning with 2000 units of drug per pound over the first 30 minutes, followed by 2000 units per pound per hour for four hours. The infusion is then discontinued for 12 hours and 2000 units per pound is administered over one hour twice a day.

Patients are followed by serial noninvasive tests and therapy is continued for 24 hours after a normal test, or seven days if no improvement has been demonstrated. Therapy is not halted before seven days because we have treated several patients who appeared to be resistant to therapy until the sixth or seventh day when they started to show improvement.

Approximately three years ago we made another change in our method of administration of fibrinolytic therapy; we no longer proceed from streptokinase to heparin to coumadin. Patients are given 10 mg of coumadin 12 hours before the last burst of fibrinolytic agent. This is generally in the evening when the patient has received maximum benefit from the lytic state. Administering coumadin stops the production in the liver of the vitamin K dependent coagulation factors (II, VII, IX, X). When the final burst of fibrinolytic agent is given the next morning, these protein-based coagulating factors are depolymerized and the patient will generally

Table 34-1
Vitamin K Dependent
Protein; Clotting Factors in
Biologic Half-Life Hours*

Factor	Hours
Prothrombin (II)	67–106
Factor VII	4–6
Factor IX	24
Factor X	?24–60

Adapted from Wintrobe MM, Lee GR, Boggs DR, et al: Clinical Hematology, 8 ed. Philadelphia, Lea and Febiger, 1981, p 407.
* Biologic half-life as distinguished from overall in vivo half-life or half disappearance time. Question mark indicates insufficient data or significant disagreement between published figures.

have a prothrombin time of 1.5–2 times control by the following evening (or 24 hours after the administration of a single 10 mg dose of coumadin). The reason for the usual three to four day delay in the prothrombin time coming into therapeutic range is not because coumadin is slow to act but because of the half-life of the circulating coagulation factors that were present when the first dose was given (Table 34-1).[27] By administering coumadin in this manner most patients who are admitted and treated require only one week of hospitalization, rather than the standard two or three weeks for heparin therapy. This has considerably decreased the cost of treating acute deep venous thrombosis.

TREATMENT OF EDEMA

Equally important in the treatment of deep venous thrombosis is the control of edema. This is not affected by any anticoagulant. The lymphatics are blocked primarily because of the inflammatory reaction to the clot in the vein. By removing the clot with fibrinolysis one hopes to decrease this reaction and to increase the flow of lymph in the lymph channels. The swelling is also secondary to the increased venous pressure itself. Our patients are kept at bedrest, with heels higher than hips, from the very onset of therapy. The legs are wrapped with elastic bandages from the toes to below the knee, rewrapping every eight hours. We find this aggressive approach to the control of edema not only increases the patient's comfort but leads to fewer long-term problems with edema, particularly in patients with more severe forms of deep venous thrombosis. When swelling is reduced and the legs have returned to normal size, the patients are measured for form-fitting elastic stockings. Our patients are instructed to wear the stockings for at least one year. If, at one year, they still have edema, the stockings should be worn for the remainder of the patient's life. We have not found diuretics useful in this setting.

RESULTS

The randomized trial of Arnesen, Hoiseth, and Ly comparing heparin therapy with streptokinase in the treatment of DVT[23] found that 71.4% of patients treated with streptokinase versus 23.8% of patients treated with heparin achieved a significant improvement on follow-up phlebograph.[28] Tsapogas and coworkers found comparable results with greater than 75% improvement in 10 of 19 streptokinase patients versus 1 of 14 heparin patients.[29] Kakkar and coworkers had a smaller group of patients but streptokinase was again superior to heparin.[30] In a patient with deep venous thrombosis less than five days old the expected success rate is approximately 70% with streptokinase versus 10–15% with heparin. We treated 23 patients with acute DVT using burst therapy. Fourteen of the patients had excellent results—defined as a normal noninvasive examination—at the completion of the treatment and maintained this result for at least six months. Five patients had good results, i.e., the test improved, and four showed no improvement.

Very few long-term follow-up studies exist that report the initial success achieved with streptokinase. However, Arnesen, Hoiseth, and Ly followed their original group of patients for approximately 6.5 years. They found 44% of the streptokinase-treated patients had normal veins by phlebograph versus 0% in the heparin group. Clinically 13 of 17 streptokinase patients were asymptomatic versus 3 of 18 heparin patients.[23]

SUMMARY

Acute deep venous thrombosis is a very common and serious problem faced by all physicians. A firm diagnosis and plan of therapy are crucial to the treatment of such patients. We feel that fibrinolytic therapy is the treatment of choice. Aggressive treatment of edema and the use of oral anticoagulants after the acute phase of treatment are equally important.

REFERENCES

1. Persson AV, Ekdahl K: The treatment of acute DVT with fibrinolytic agents. J Med, 1985 (in press)
2. Schafer AI: The hypercoagulable states. Ann Int Med 102:814–828, 1985
3. Griffin JH, Evatt B, Zimmerman TS, Kleiss AJ: Deficiency of protein C in congenital thrombotic disease. J Clin Investig 68:1370–1373, 1981
4. Stead RB: The hypercoagulable state, in Goldhaber SZ (ed): Pulmonary Embolism and Deep Venous Thrombosis. Philadelphia, WB Saunders, 1985, pp 161–178
5. Coon WW: Epidemiology of venous thromboembolism. Ann Surg 186(2):149–164, 1977
6. Haller JA Jr: Massive deep thrombophlebitis (Phlegmasia cerulea dolens), in Haller JA Jr (ed): Deep Thrombophlebitis. Pathophysiology and Treatment. Philadelphia, 1967, pp 18–21
7. Salzman EW: Heparin therapy in venous thromboembolism, in Bergan JJ, Yao JST (eds): Venous Problems. Chicago, Year Book Medical Publishers, 1978, pp 297–303
8. Coon WW, et al: Assessment of anticoagulant treatment of venous thromboembolism. Ann Surg 170(4):559–568, 1969
9. Verstrate M, Bory M, Collen D, et al: Randomised trial of intravenous recombinant

tissue-type plasminogen activator versus intravenous streptokinase in acute myocardial infarction. Report from the European cooperative study group for recombinant tissue-type plasminogen activator. Lancet, April 13, 1985, pp 842–847

10. Mueller HS, Dyer A, Greenberg MA, et al: The thrombolysis in myocardial infarction (TIMI) trial. New Engl J Med 312(14):932–936, 1985

11. Graor RA, Risius B, Young JR, et al: Peripheral artery and bypass graft thrombolysis with recombinant human tissue-type plasminogen activator. Presented at the 33rd Scientific Meeting of the International Society for Cardiovascular Surgery, June 7, 1985, Baltimore, Maryland (in press)

12. Collen D, et al: Coronary thrombolysis with recombinant human tissue-type plasminogen activator: A prospective, randomized, placebo-controlled trial. Circulation 70(6):1012–1017, 1984

13. Relman AS: Intravenous thrombolysis in acute myocardial infarction. New Engl J Med 312(14):915–916, 1985

14. Collen D, Topol EJ, Tiefenbrunn AJ, et al: Coronary thrombolysis with recombinant human tissue-type plasminogen activator: A prospective, randomized, placebo-controlled trial. Circulation 70(6):1012–1017, 1984

15. Sobel BE, Gross RW, Ronison AK: Thrombolysis, clot selectivity, and kinetics. Circulation 70(2):160–164, 1984

16. Bounameaux H, Vermylen J, Collen D: Thrombolytic treatment with recombinant tissue-type plasminogen activator in a patient with massive pulmonary embolism. Ann Int Med 103(1):64–65, 1985

17. Belkin M, Belkin B, Buckman CA, et al: Intra-arterial fibrinolytic therapy: Efficacy of streptokinase versus urokinase (in press)

18. Comerota A, Rubin R, Tyson R, et al: Intra-arterial thrombolytic therapy in peripheral vascular disease. New horizons for old problems. Am J Surg, 1985. Presented at the Society for Clinic Vascular Surgery, Rancho Mirage, California, April 13, 1985

19. Goldberg L, Ricci MT, Sauvage LR, et al: Thrombolytic therapy for delayed occlusion of knitted Dacron bypass grafts in the axillofemoral, femoropopliteal and femorotibial positions. Surg Gynecol Obstet 160:491–498, 1985

20. Urokinase Pulmonary Embolism Trial: Phase 1 Results. JAMA 214:2163–2172, 1970

21. Urokinase–Streptokinase Pulmonary Embolism Trial: Phase 2 Results. A cooperative study. JAMA 229:1606–1612, 1974

22. Physicians Desk Reference, Medical Economics Company, 1986, Oradell, New Jersey, Barnhart ER (publisher)

23. Arnesen H, Hoiseth A, Ly B: Streptokinase or heparin in the treatment of deep vein thrombosis. Acta Med Scand 211:65–68, 1982

24. Persson AV, Persson CA: Thrombolytic therapy for deep vein thrombosis. Am J Surg 150(4A):50–53, 1985

25. Persson AV: Treatment of acute deep venous thrombosis with emphasis on fibrinolytic therapy, in Bergan JJ, Yao JST (eds): Surgery of the Veins. Orlando, Grune and Stratton, 1985, pp 145–151

26. Persson AV, Robichaux WT, Jaxheimer EC, DiPronio E: Burst therapy: A method of administering fibrinolytic agents. Am J Surg 147:531–535, 1984

27. Wintrobe MM, Lee GR, Boggs DR, et al: Clinical Hematology, 8 ed. Philadelphia, Lea and Febiger, 1981, p 407

28. Arnesen H, Heilo A, Jakobsen E, Ly B, Skaga E: A prospective study of streptokinase and heparin in the treatment of deep vein thrombosis. Acta Med Scand 203:457–463, 1978

29. Tsapogas MJ, Peabody RA, Wu KT, et al: Controlled study of thrombolytic therapy in deep vein thrombosis. Surgery 74:973–984, 1973

30. Kakkar VV, Flanc C, Howe CT, et al: Treatment of deep vein thrombosis. A trial of heparin, streptokinase and arvin. Br Med J 1:806–810, 1969

Index

Page numbers in *italics* indicate illustrations. Page numbers followed by *t* indicate tables.